Health and Nutrition Secrets
that can save your life

RUSSELL L. BLAYLOCK, MD

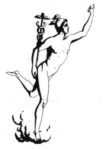

Health Press
Albuquerque, New Mexico

Published by Health Press
P.O. Drawer 37470
Albuquerque, NM 87176

Library of Congress Cataloging in Publication Data

Blaylock, Russell L., 1945-
Health and nutrition secrets that can save your life / Russell L. Blaylock.
p. cm.
Includes bibliographical references and index.
ISBN-10: 0-929173-48-1
ISBN-13: 978-0-929173-48-1

1. Self-care, Health. 2. Nutrition. 3. Hygiene. I. Title.
RA776.95.B535 2006
613--dc22
2006015920

Illustrations by Russell L. Blaylock, MD
Author Photo by Ron Blaylock

Disclaimer: The information presented in this book has been obtained from authentic and reliable sources. Although great care has been taken to ensure the accuracy of the information presented, the author and the publisher cannot assume responsibility for the validity of all materials or the consequences for their use. Before starting any regimen of vitamins or supplements, you should consult with your physician.

The editors have made every effort to identify trademarked products accurately within the text of the book; however, it is impossible to check each instance.

Dedication

I dedicate this book to my mother, Mrs. Jonnie Blaylock, and to my father, Mr. C.D. Blaylock, who laid the foundations for my life, gave me the gift of love and an untiring thirst for wisdom. I also dedicate this book to my dear brother Charles (Chuck), whom I will always love. His life was taken from him by a medical care system that encourages arrogance, narrow thinking, and cold-hearted treatment of patients. May all be protected from the types of doctors who were assigned to his care. I pray that he is now with our dear Lord. And to my beautiful wife, Diane, who has made the last thirty-one years of my life the most wonderful a man could ever ask for, and who remains forever my best friend and love of my life. To my two sons, Damien and Ron Blaylock, who have made my life meaningful and left me with a sense of pride I shall never outlive. To my daughter-in-law, Lindsay Blaylock, and especially to our two grandsons, Gabriel (Gabe) and Declan. And to Ronald Kempff, my wife's brother, a brave man who gave his life in service to his country during the Vietnam War.

Finally, a special dedication to Richard Wurmbrand, who, despite fourteen years of torture in one of the worst communist prisons of the world, not only survived, but unwaveringly held to his faith in Jesus Christ throughout it all. And to the organization he founded, Voice of the Martyrs, also dedicated to those who give their lives for our savior.

Acknowledgements

I would like to thank my lovely wife, Diane, for reading the manuscript and offering many helpful suggestions, and for her help in researching many of the topics in the medical center library. In addition, I thank her for her never-ending encouragement and support. I would also like to thank my grandson, Gabriel, for keeping me laughing and in a good mood throughout the difficult time during the preparation of the book.

I also thank Dr. William Daggett for critically reviewing the manuscript and making many helpful suggestions along the way.

Contents

Foreword

The environmental left would have us believe the world is a swirling mass of pollution, and that the earth's problems are all the result of capitalism, while American conservatives would have us believe that DDT is so safe you can drink it without harm. So what is the truth? Unfortunately, the truth has become a victim of political haggling. Most people would agree that debates about the best ways to make our world's food supply and environment safe should not be left to those who would return humanity to the age of Neanderthals versus those who are convinced that the megacorporation can do no harm. Reasonable solutions to real problems should be left to those still in possession of clear minds unsullied by the dogma of either politics or profit—certainly not the people who are currently responsible for social and environmental policies in this country.

Environmentalists are correct when they point out that something is very wrong with the way we evaluate the dangers of industrial chemicals, food additives and other modern creations. The Food and Drug Administration (FDA), Environmental Protection Agency (EPA), and other governmental regulatory agencies have become nothing more than the handmaidens of international corporations and worldwide financial conglomerates. A revolving-door policy exists that is designed to grease the palms of bureaucrats in charge of regulatory agencies, which then pass rules and regulations that favor profit-mongering conglomerates. In exchange, our bureaucratic heads are offered lucrative jobs or consulting fees.

This unfortunate cycle happens over and over again, the drug and vaccine approval processes being prime examples of lax regulation. For instance, the anthrax vaccine was not only approved, but our government (through the Pentagon) funded the company that was making the vaccine—*despite* the fact that this company had been cited numerous times for dangerous manufacturing violations. These breaches were simply overlooked and our fighting men and women have been forced to take a vaccine that is extremely dangerous, and possibly contaminated with mycoplasma.

Conservatives should take note that while they defend the soldiers of our armed forces against enemies, they choose to support a manufacturer that could single-handedly cripple our military and leave this nation vulnerable to its real enemies, to say nothing of destroying the lives of millions of innocent men and women.

It is also unfortunate that conservative politicians and pundits have been led to believe it is their mission in life as philosophical champions of capitalism to defend the corporate world, even international corporate conglomerates run by those who eschew the very foundations of conservatism. Conservatives will cry that I must be a liberal or environmentalist fanatic. In fact, I am a conservative and have been all my life.

Capitalism is very different from the opportunistic system modern corporations have invented for themselves. For a magnificent defense of true capitalism, see Ludwig von Mises' magnificent 1949 work, *Human Action*. Von Mises' student F.A. Hayek, eventually won the Nobel Prize for economics. Both of these great men recognized that the corporation, especially the international corporation, is in fact alien to the principles of capitalist economics, and they saw corporate collusion with the government as the greatest danger to a true free market—using the power of the government to prevent competition and to protect themselves from citizens who recognize the dangers that corporate activity poses to public health and safety.

Modern-day corporations act more like small governments, complete with massive bureaucracies, dictatorial heads and board rooms filled with corruption, intrigue and collusion with those in political power. These behemoths are not free market entities, but rather exist as a merger between capitalism and socialism, something that once was known by its true name: fascism or corporatism. Corporations are impersonal, bureaucratic, slow to change, resistant to criticism, and rely on incestuous relationships with governmental power structures for their continued existence. Further, I find it ironic that conservatives have chosen to support and defend international corporations when the vast majority of these corporations financially support our nation's political and military enemies.

Von Mises first pointed out that corporations use the power of government to prevent competition. Let's face it, corporations are responsible for most of the regulations in which our society is drowning. They themselves have literally choked off the free enterprise system they so loudly defend: they detest competition, yet are wrongly defended by conservatives who rightly extol the virtues of free enterprise.

As for environmentalists, the leaders (though not their followers) have a secret agenda that they rarely make public. They want to see a socialist world, one controlled by bureaucrats and politicians—*their* bureaucrats and politicians. Instead of a free market, a giant collectivist machine controlling all that we do would be forced on us.

I find it telling that the left in the West supported the Soviet Union throughout the Cold War as an example to follow. They extolled the virtues of the Soviet system in protecting the environment and preventing the rape of the world's resources. The irony is that socialism, not the capitalist West, produced the world's first nuclear reactor disaster. With the collapse of the Soviet political structure, suddenly we learned that the most massive pollution in the history of the world occurred in the socialist countries of the world—the Soviet Union and Eastern Block nations. Entire lakes were so polluted that not a single living organism could be found.

Millions of children were deformed by chemical pollution from factories and mining operations. In Romania, thousand of mentally deficient children are left to languish in filthy, poorly staffed, living hells run by the government: all the result of mass pollution and rape of the environment. Even when all of this was known to the West, these loud, often-obnoxious defenders of the environment, remained silent to this disaster. Most of the destruction and environmental contamination by socialist countries will take hundreds of years to correct, if it can be corrected at all.

My point is that there is plenty of blame to go around. The environmental problems we face should be de-politicized, not used as a forum to promote socialism or conservatism. God created the earth and gave it to us to care for as good stewards. We should fulfill that goal as his children.

Introduction

One of the most frequent questions I hear when I lecture on nutrition is: "If our nutrition is so bad, why are we living longer than ever before?" This is a good question, and a little examination will provide us with a bit of insight. Yes, we are living longer in terms of median survival, but we are not living healthier. Our nursing homes are filled with an alarming number of decrepit, sick, disoriented, demented, and crippled elderly. Most health experts have lamented that all of the degenerative diseases have been increasing in incidence, but even more alarming, they are occurring at a younger age. This is especially so with neurodegenerative diseases, such as Alzheimer's dementia, Parkinson's disease and amyotrophic lateral sclerosis (also known as ALS and Lou Gehrig's disease).

In my practice over the past twenty-six years, I have been amazed at people's poor health, usually beginning during early middle age. For example, I am seeing more forty- and fifty-year-olds suffering from significant difficulties with memory. They are wracked with arthritis, cataracts, macular degeneration, detached retinas, bursitis, tendonitis, hypertension, diabetes, asthma, chronic lung disease, kidney failure, heart disease, poor circulation, vertigo, digestive problems, poor hearing, aching muscles, fatigue, and poor immunity. In essence, they are in terrible shape, with many just barely hanging on.

The reason they are living longer, statistically, is that the medical profession is keeping people alive by using powerful medications, electronic gadgets, and surgery; that is, we won't let them die. Before the age of antibiotics, not so long ago, most deaths were due to infectious diseases, especially pneumonia. With the advent of powerful antibiotics that can kill virtually any bacterial organism, people have begun to live longer in larger numbers, and today we have a significant population of people living into their eighties and nineties. At the same time we now are seeing a virtual explosion of new, more resistant bacteria that continues to climb unabated.

Over the last thirty years, with the widespread intervention of cardiovascular surgery, we have also favorably impacted this country's number one killer, heart disease; which is not to say that we have reduced the problem of cardiovascular disease—far from it—but we have increased the number of people surviving heart attacks and strokes.

In fact, a recent cardiology conference reported that over the past ten years congestive heart disease has increased almost 600 percent. But, we can keep patients alive, often just barely, by using powerful drugs that force the diseased heart muscle to keep pumping.

Insulin, especially the newer recombinant human form, is keeping diabetic patients alive, but it has not reduced the number of diabetes sufferers or the complications associated with diabetes. In fact, the incidence of non-insulin dependent diabetes has increased 600 percent over the last decade and is now occurring even in teenagers in alarming numbers. In the not-too-distant past, this was a disease of middle age and beyond. Now we have drugs that can keep diabetics struggling through life.

This is not to disparage the tremendous advances we have made in medical science, yet we must face the fact that modern medicine has done little or nothing to prevent disease and lessen its traumatic impact on individuals. Likewise, it has done virtually nothing to improve our overall quality of life in terms of incidence and severity of degenerative diseases. I say "overall" because modern medical science has definitely improved the lives of diabetics, hypertensives, and cardiac patients, in terms of relieving some of their more disabling symptoms. Surgery is safer and less traumatic than ever before. Despite this, over our prolonged lifetime, we are sicker than ever. This simply doesn't have to be.

It is a crime that modern medicine has all but ignored one of the greatest weapons we have against disease—nutrition. Every medical journal, no matter the specialty, contains at least one article on the subject of nutrition. Annually, the peer-reviewed journals contain tens of thousands of articles on nutrition. Incredibly, most of this groundbreaking information is never read and is rarely implemented by the doctors who treat patients on a day-to-day basis. Yet, professors of medicine continue to wax eloquent about how they practice "evidence-based medicine," as if it were separate from nutritional science.

I remember as a neurosurgery resident seeing the neurosurgical intensive care ward filled with unconscious patients receiving only sugar water for nourishment: no vitamins, minerals, or trace elements were ever included in intravenous feedings. If these unfortunate patients didn't recover for several weeks or a month, sugar mixtures remained their only source of nourishment as they wasted away to almost nothing.

This tragic situation started me on a quest to learn more about nutrition, surgery, and the trauma patient. I learned that trauma to the body—even to the head alone—greatly increases the body's metabolic rate. In fact, the metabolic rates of many trauma patients resemble those of long-distance runners. Further study revealed that such stresses to the body cause a very rapid depletion of water-soluble vitamins and many minerals.

So we have patients with enormously high metabolic demands experiencing rapid depletion of nutrients, and we are supplying them only with sugar, water, and sodium chloride (salt)! Here I was in a medical center mecca, in a neurosurgical training program with some of the most famous neurosurgeons in the country, and we were providing medical care bordering on the medieval. That was the beginning of my studies into nutrition and disease.

While this book is about the vital role proper nutrition plays in preventing and treating diseases affecting all parts of the body, one of my main interests is protecting the brain. As a result, much of the book will deal with various ways of protecting the brain from injury and disease. Likewise, as will become obvious, the book will cover more than just nutrition. But first, let us take a quick look at the brain.

God's Greatest Miracle

Without question, the human brain is the most complex system in the entire known universe. All too often it is compared to a computer, but in reality, the human brain only vaguely resembles a computer, as with some of its more basic reflex activities and simple logical functions. In fact, a mouse's brain is more sophisticated, in terms of its ability to analyze data, than the most high-tech computer known—even the much-lauded Cray supercomputer. This is because even small brains have the ability to change their circuits and connections almost on demand, adapting constantly to changing external and internal conditions. In addition, they have the ability to fine tune the brain cells (neurons) by utilizing a wide array of neurohormones, neurotransmitters, and other information molecules. Unlike a computer, the brain has overlapping circuits that can, on demand, take over the function of damaged circuits. This is why some children can have literally half their brain (cerebrum) removed and still function almost normally.

Most of us who have used computers know that if you make even a small mistake in typing a URL or a file name nothing works. The computer is very demanding in terms of addresses and procedural operations. The brain, on the other hand, often needs only rudimentary information, a mere hint of what is needed, to deliver the needed information to consciousness.

The brain's ability to perform such incredible feats has been given the name "association functions." These association patterns in the brain change from day to day. For example, today we may recall the sound of a particular song being played on a radio that reminds us of the time we met someone special. Sometime later, it may also be associated with a tragic event that occurred in connection with the music. The computer, on the other hand, gives us the same information every time, based on set key words and functions. The construction of the brain allows us to reach into the memory files and extract information we thought was long-forgotten by using mechanisms that go far beyond even the most sophisticated computer. It also allows us to arrange these associated memories in any way we choose.

In addition, the brain gives us uniquely human qualities such as insight, empathy, love, compassion, hatred, anger, poetic and literary creativity, artistic expression, a sense of awe, and ecstasy. We can develop a love of virtue, patriotism, and honor or, at times, the opposite of these good qualities. Most of us have a strong sense of our creator and a need to think about Him and to pray to Him, things beyond the capacity of the computer to duplicate.

One of the most enchanting events in our life experience is the creation and birth of a baby. The very idea that a single cell can come together genetically to form a fully developed organism, with thousands of specialized tissues and organs, is not only intriguing, but has challenged our ability to understand even the most basic aspects of the process. While we know that genes are capable of being turned on and off, and that this plays a part in cell and tissue specialization, we still have no idea what initiates this process and how it is regulated.

Further, we know little about how the tissues that make up the arms, for instance, know to develop in the way they do. What signals the arms to stop growing so as to make the body symmetrical? What is it that controls the growth of the blood vessels and nerves, and how do they make the exact connections within the limbs? How does the median nerve, for example, know to travel down the arm, dipping and sliding beneath certain muscles and ligaments, until it finally spreads its fine nerve connections out into the skin and muscles of the thumb and index finger? The answer is that we simply do not know!

Compared to the development of the human nervous system, the development of the rest of the body is comparatively simple. The brain must not only develop dozens of specialized cell types, but most of these brain cells possess unique processes (dendrites and axons) that connect these components to each other in a three-dimensional way. There are approximately ten billion neurons in the human brain and ten times that many neuroglia cells. But there are trillions of connections among the nerve processes. A single neuron may connect to hundreds of other neurons, while still others can make over ten thousand connections.

These connections are not haphazard, but specific and exacting, yet are also capable of change on demand, especially as we learn and grow intellectually. On the tips of the connecting fibers there are hundreds of specialized microscopic connections, called synapses. Throughout our existence, these synapses are changing and developing, even into our eighties and nineties. This process is called brain plasticity: it allows us to develop new memories and adapt to our changing environment, both internal and external. The synapses secrete minute quantities of chemicals called neurotransmitters that relay messages to neurons down the line, creating a mystical symphony of instructions that appear on an EEG as wild squiggles and waves.

It is the increasing complexity of the growing brain that gives us an expanded capacity to learn and understand. It has been said that with aging the brain becomes much more complex, even though its speed of function slows down. So while a younger person may be able to compute faster, his father may possess a deeper understanding, something that we often call wisdom.

In the developing baby's brain, specialized processes called growth cones exist on the tips of the newly-created and always-probing nerve fibers. These growth cones act as beacons, guiding the nerve fibers to their final destinations. How they do that is also unknown. These growth cones are very sensitive to the mother's nutrition during the baby's intrauterine life and to the child's nutrition after birth. As we shall see, an excess of certain food additives can severely affect the growth cone function.

What We Have Learned

Research over the past twenty years has clearly shown that our early nutrition significantly influences our genes, affecting our health as adults. Poor nutrition can lead to programming for an early onset of cardiovascular disease, degenerative brain diseases, or even cancer.

Based on this research, it is reasonable to assume that good nutrition during our developmental years can program genes for good health later in life as well, allowing us to avoid serious diseases. To utilize to the best advantage what nutritional science has discovered, we must begin to use this knowledge even before the birth of our children. The results of good nutrition are enhanced through each generation, because our nutrition improves the genetic health of our reproductive cells, the sperm, and the ova.

In this book I intend to share with the reader some of the newer research, especially concerning your child's brain health as well as the continuing importance of good nutrition, that has been shown to affect us throughout life. In addition, there are older studies that have withstood the test of time and can offer tremendous insights in our quest to give our children and ourselves the brightest future possible. More and more we are learning that good nutrition can help prevent some of the terrible diseases that have afflicted mankind, especially during the twentieth century.

The first book I wrote, *Excitotoxins: The Taste That Kills*, told of a group of food additives, such as MSG and aspartame, that in my opinion, and based on numerous scientific studies, pose a serious danger to our neurological health. One of the driving forces that compelled me to write the book was my anger at what the food-processing industry had done to, and continues to do to all of us—but especially to our children. At the time I had two young children of my own. Fortunately, I discovered the serious danger imposed by such food additives in time to save my children from a life of misery. I felt I owed the same to other parents and their children. Christ told us to protect the children from evil. This was one form of that evil.

In this book I will cover more topics in more depth than I did in my first book. I will address hazards posed by environmental toxins, food toxins, and certain medical treatments and procedures, and discuss ways to enhance, through good nutrition, both general health and brain health. I will also discuss ways to make sure your children are protected from dangerous foods in schools and other places away from home.

While not all authorities will agree with this book in whole or in part, it is the result of my examination of a large number of scientific studies and my experience in the clinical setting. The opinions are purely mine. When writing any book one must necessarily limit the information to some degree. Some readers will complain that a topic important to them may have been left out or only briefly mentioned: unfortunately, this is a hazard of writing. I have tried to include all of the major factors affecting our health, especially those factors of which the general public is unaware but needs to know.

Growing up in the deep South, I was raised on fried foods: fried catfish, fried okra, fried shrimp and French fried potatoes. Even vegetables in the South are either fried or cooked in a bit of ham (fatback) to make them tastier. (Rarely did we eat raw vegetables, and salads consisted mostly of iceberg lettuce and tomatoes.) In the early days, frying was done in lard, a saturated fat product. In the early 1950s, lard was supplanted by vegetable oil for its ease of use and the claims that it was also healthy for your heart.

Desserts were expected after each meal except breakfast. Of course, breakfast usually included fried eggs, bacon or sausage, and occasionally pancakes drowned in butter or margarine with a heavy application of syrup or molasses. As if all of this nutritional junk was not bad enough, we usually added several slices of white bread, enriched of course, with each meal. My dad always enjoyed cornbread dipped in buttermilk with his breakfast. Having grown up in the country, he loved vegetables and insisted that they be served with each meal. Still, they were usually canned vegetables cooked in ham or fatback. Dad did have a garden and often we enjoyed freshly picked spinach, collard greens, okra, tomatoes, and radishes during the growing season.

My wife, Diane, grew up in a similar household in New Orleans, Louisiana. Fortunately, as most girls will, she avoided a lot of fried foods and ate more sensibly to maintain her shapely figure. Unfortunately, her family lived in the big city and a garden was out of the question. Most of their vegetables came from a can, again with added fatback.

When we both moved away from home to attend the university, our diets got even worse. Diane attended the University of Southwestern Louisiana (USL) and I attended Louisiana State University (LSU) in Baton Rouge, Louisiana. While still watching her diet, she ate more in the way of fast foods and occasionally some of the good Cajun foods. It is impossible to live in south Louisiana and not eat these wonderful recipes, at least on special occasions. As for me, I lived on pizza, hamburgers, and French fries. Rarely did I eat a vegetable unless I went home for a visit. My dad often kidded that all I ate was "meat, beans, and potatoes."

After we met and married, while I was still in medical school, our diets continued along the same destructive paths. In fact, I introduced my wife to the wonderful world of French fries. The only saving grace was that my dad was interested in nutrition and always encouraged me to take nutritional supplements, which I did throughout this period of nutritional darkness. Diane also took the supplements.

During her pregnancy, she was meticulous about her diet and avoided things obviously bad for both her and the baby. But at the time, I was not aware of the things that were known concerning nutrition and the development of a newborn. I had no knowledge about excitotoxins, fluoride, mercury, or the special fatty acids necessary for normal brain growth. After all, I was attending a modern medical university, where nutrition was virtually unknown. During my four years in medical school, we did not have a single class on nutrition. The same was true during my internship and residency. In fact, to provide your patients with nutritional supplements opened you up to ridicule from your colleagues.

Since these early years, I have come to realize that there are numerous nutritional discoveries that can help people avoid the heartache of bad health and greatly improve their energy, extend healthy life, and enhance their sense of well-being. This book is dedicated to sharing these discoveries with you.

Each chapter will treat a different topic. In the first chapter, the book will deal with the early years of child development and growth, because these years are so vital to a healthy adulthood. In addition, I will share newer information concerning excitotoxins and their effects, not just on the developing child, but throughout our lives. The reader should realize that nutrition is the fastest growing area of health science, with new discoveries being made every day. What has impressed me is that much recent scientific evidence is now validating what was suspected hundreds, even thousands, of years ago. For example, there is now excellent evidence that vitamins C and E in combination can dramatically reduce the incidence and severity of numerous degenerative diseases including Alzheimer's disease, Parkinson's disease, heart attacks, strokes, arthritis, and even cancer. A newer class of plant-derived chemicals, called phytochemicals, is being shown to have even greater disease-preventing and -reversing effects than vitamins.

What is especially exciting about nutrition is not just the possibility of prevention, but the *reversal* of diseases. The body has a tremendous ability to heal itself—including repair of the damage to our DNA. Certain vitamins, minerals, and special phytonutrients can promote this healing and strengthen our cells so that they are better able to protect themselves against future injury. In fact, recent evidence has shown that a common herb can rescue injured brain cells even when taken hours after the injury occurs!

Now let us begin our voyage into the wondrous land.

Health and Nutrition Secrets That Can Save Your Life
Section I

1
Do All Degenerative Diseases Have A Common Cause?

Most of us are certain that we cannot change what has happened in the past, and many nutritionists in the past would tell their patients that all that they could do was to change their diets and hope for the best. When I lecture on the subject of nutrition I am always asked, usually by someone in their seventies: is it too late for me to start these nutritional changes? This is a good question and one that has intrigued many nutritional scientists. My response is unequivocal: it is *never* too late. Your body's response to nutritional changes will not be as dramatic if you have spent seventy years practicing poor nutrition and as a result are presently suffering from one or more degenerative diseases; yet it is never too late to enjoy the fruits of good nutrition, particularly when the alternative is to continue down a path of assured destruction.

We now know that aging, as well as degenerative diseases, are the result of a lifetime of assaults on our cells. Medical science has realized that all disease occurs on a cellular, and even molecular, level. The process that results in what we call aging is slowly being understood. For example, we now know that from the time we are first formed in our mother's womb, our cells are producing destructive particles called free radicals, and that over a lifetime these free radicals chip away at our cells, like water wearing away a stone, until the cells are so weakened they begin to malfunction. We call this process aging, and in extreme cases, degenerative disease.

What the Heck Is a Free Radical?

You have probably heard the ads on TV about the importance of antioxidants, but have only vaguely understood what they do or what oxidation is. Oxidation is a common, everyday process—from rusting of metal left out in the weather to our need for oxygen to breathe. At the same time, oxygen is a powerful destroyer of life. All of us are aware that without oxygen we would quickly die; however, few of us are aware that this same life-giving oxygen is slowly killing us and making us sick.

All living organisms must produce energy to carry out the many functions of the body, from the beating of our hearts to thinking. This energy is derived from the food we eat, and the process that brings this about is a very complicated series of biochemical reactions called metabolism. During this breakdown process, electrons flow down through a series of step-like reactions, eventually producing the universal energy molecule, ATP (adenosine triphosphate).

During this carefully regulated chemical process, some of the electrons escape and act as very reactive particles we call free radicals. (About 95 percent of the oxygen that enters our cells goes to mitochondria, the powerhouse of the cell, but 3-5 percent of this oxygen escapes in the form of free radicals.) These particles can damage any part of the cell with which they come into contact. You can visualize them as red-hot particles bouncing in all directions within the cell, burning the DNA, the cell membranes and the proteins within the cytoplasm. When these particles burn proteins, they produce oxidized proteins called protein carbonyl products. This is important because many cellular proteins are, in fact, enzymes that allow the thousands of chemical reactions of metabolism to take place: when these enzymes are damaged, they can no longer function properly, and as a result, the cell becomes weaker.

When free radicals interact with the cell's membranes, they set up a chain reaction of destruction that spreads through the wall of the membrane in all directions like a wildfire. If you have ever touched a red-hot wire to a tissue paper, you will have an idea of how the fire spreads out from the point of contact, burning up the tissue. A cell has many membranes that enclose not only the cell itself, but also all of the little components inside, such as the mitochondria, nucleus, endoplasmic reticulum, and golgi apparatus. These cell membranes are composed of rows of fatty molecules arranged side by side in two layers, separated by the tails of the fat molecules. When the free-radical reaction begins, it is these fatty acids that are damaged.

Cell membranes are more than just a covering for the cell and its components. These membranes also contain numerous complex structures such as special pores, transfer enzymes, information molecules, and many receptors. So free-radical damage to these membranes severely affects cellular function. This process of oxidation of the fatty membranes is called lipid peroxidation. As we shall see, lipid peroxidation occurs in almost every disease we know of, especially chronic inflammatory diseases such as cancer, degenerative brain diseases, arthritis, lupus, diabetes, and rheumatoid arthritis.

Lipid peroxidation greatly affects organs with a high fat composition. Because the brain is 60 percent fat, it is especially vulnerable to the ill effects of the lipid-peroxidation process, and to toxic insults from lipid-soluble substances, such as mercury and pesticides.

After many years of oxidative injury, our cells' membranes begin to change, losing much of the soft, fluid-like quality we see in young cells. Gradually, over many years, they begin to stiffen, something we call a loss of fluidity. Stiff membranes have difficulty transferring nutrients in and out of the cell and in carrying on the numerous other functions of the membrane. As a result, our cells become sick.

Oxidation of a cell's DNA is even more perilous because DNA provides the instructions for the rest of the cell's function. In the case of the reproductive cells, the sperm, and the ova, DNA damage can even be transmitted to the cells of our children. Every cell has a system of enzymes whose function it is to repair this damage. Unfortunately, these DNA-repair

MICROGLIAL ACTIVATION ──────► GLUTAMATE RELEASE

PGE₂ (LEUKOTRIENES)

NO+O₂ (superoxide)

NOS ── Ca⁺⁺

PEROXYNITRITE

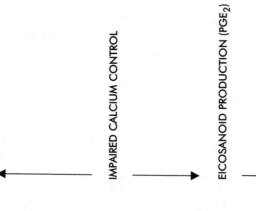
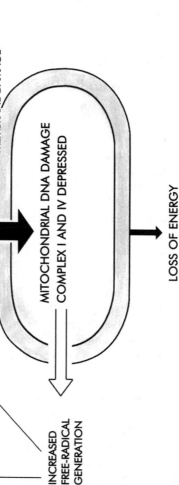

LIPID PEROXIDATION

MEMBRANE DAMAGE

FREE-RADICAL GENERATION

IMPAIRED CALCIUM CONTROL

EICOSANOID PRODUCTION (PGE₂)

INFLAMMATION

MITOCHONDRIAL DNA DAMAGE
COMPLEX I AND IV DEPRESSED

LOSS OF ENERGY

EICOSANOID GENERATION

INCREASED
FREE-RADICAL
GENERATION

FIGURE 1.1   This diagram illustrates the cellular processes that result in damage to mitochondria. Free-radical generation and lipid peroxidation products can severely damage mitochondria's ability to produce energy, thereby
initiating the production of even more free radicals. In addition, this cycle triggers the eicosanoid inflammatory pathway, and in the brain activates the excitotoxic processes linked to degenerative brain disorders and
aging.

enzymes are also made of proteins and, like all other protein enzymes, can become oxidized by free radicals. Indeed, as we age, our ability to repair DNA damage is impaired. Several studies have shown that this increases our risk of getting cancer as well as other degenerative diseases of aging. Oxidative DNA damage is found in most neurodegenerative diseases—including Alzheimer's dementia, Parkinson's disease, and ALS (Lou Gehrig's disease)—as well as in cancer.

A diet high in sugar causes proteins and DNA to become sugar-coated, a process called glycation. (Actually, these cellular components are not sugar-coated, but rather react chemically with very reactive sugar molecules, producing unstable molecules that generate free radicals.) In the nervous system we see a similar interaction of proteins in neurons, resulting in advanced glycation end products (or AGEs). These sugar-coated proteins are also seen in diabetes because of elevated levels of sugar in the tissues. What makes these glycolated proteins so dangerous is that they are more easily oxidized than normal proteins, which then increases the risk of protein and DNA oxidation in the cell, even beyond levels we would normally expect. This is one reason why diabetics have such a high incidence of complications and associated degenerative disease.

What Causes Free Radicals?

Metabolism

Thus far we have seen that free radicals are commonly produced during the normal energy-producing reactions within our cells; that is, it is part of life. What is less appreciated is the fact that if we increase our metabolism, we also increase free-radical production. So how do we increase our metabolism? One of the most common ways is by exercising. It is now known that intense exercise dramatically increases free-radical production and lipid peroxidation. This has been demonstrated in carefully conducted experiments in marathon runners and extreme athletes. There is also some evidence that extreme athletes have a higher incidence of free-radical diseases such as cancer, immune suppression, and cardiovascular disease.

Another way our metabolism is increased is by overactivity of the thyroid. Normally, the thyroid gland hormones regulate our metabolism. Overproduction increases metabolism (hyperthyroidism) and underproduction (hypothyroidism) slows metabolism. Persons suffering from hyperthyroidism require a greater supply of antioxidants to protect themselves against this increase in free-radical production. Medical practitioners rarely take this into consideration.

It was observed many years ago that underfeeding lengthens the life spans of several species of lower animals. This finding has been reproduced in scientific studies several times since then. At least two highly respected scientists maintain a very low food intake in an effort to increase their longevity. While no one has specifically connected free-radical generation to the phenomenon of aging, it is obvious that one of the effects of underfeeding is a reduction in the production of thyroid hormones and a slowing of metabolism. It is also well known that overfeeding, especially of high-energy foods like sugars and carbohydrates, dramatically increases metabolism and hence free-radical generation. So the whole effect of low-calorie diets may be related to decreasing metabolism and, therefore, a better way to increase longevity is to improve the body's antioxidant defenses rather than dramatically and dangerously lowering nutrient intake.

Along this same line, but less well-known, is the observation that low-protein diets also increase longevity and high-protein diets are linked to shortened life spans. If confirmed, this finding could diminish the popularity of the high-protein diets being advocated by some popular authors. We already know that high-protein diets increase the incidence of osteoporosis, heart disease, and kidney disease, and high-protein diets in certain diseases, such as Lou Gehrig's disease (ALS), have been shown to significantly elevate blood levels of several destructive amino acids, including glutamate and aspartate.

Inflammation

Infections, traumatic injuries, burns, and even stress all increase metabolism. In fact, with burns, severe infections, and extensive traumatic injuries, the metabolic rate can become very high, producing a dramatic increase in free radicals flooding the body. This explains, at least in part, the deadly nature of these disorders. Unfortunately, modern medical treatment rarely addresses the free-radical problem in the clinical setting. Rarely are such patients treated with increased antioxidants or any antioxidants at all, even though the medical literature clearly shows that rapid depletion of antioxidants is universal in all of these conditions—another example of the fallacy of so-called "evidence-based medicine."

As a neurosurgery resident in training, one of my responsibilities was to care for patients suffering from serious brain injuries. Having been interested in surgical nutrition, even as an intern, it amazed me to see these patients literally subsist on an intravenous infusion of water, salt, and glucose for weeks, with no other form of nutritional supplementation. These patients would come to us robust and healthy, and within three weeks to a month they would look like POWs in a communist gulag. It never dawned on anyone that the patients were literally starving, often to the point of death.

I knew from my own investigations into the metabolism of trauma that seriously injured patients have much higher metabolic rates than do persons at rest. In fact, their metabolisms are higher than those of persons running the Boston marathon! If these patients develop infections, which is likely in a starving person, their metabolic rates go up even higher. At the time we didn't know that much about free radicals, but it was obvious that unconscious people with very high metabolic rates needed more nutrition than sedentary people. Unfortunately, common sense does not always prevail in modern medicine.

After teaching myself how to administer high concentrations of nutrition intravenously or by a feeding tube inserted into the stomach, I started giving these patients an accelerated program of nutritional supplementation which included vitamins, minerals, trace elements and adequate amounts of proteins and carbohydrates. The results were dramatic in the salvageable patients: they regained lost weight, had fewer infections, and their neurological improvement exceeded anything I had seen before. Incredibly, it changed nothing as far as the protocol used by the chief of the service to treat trauma patients. They just kept right on starving patients. Unfortunately, little has changed twenty-five years later. I still see seriously ill patients lying in the hospital with IV bags containing only water, salt, and sugar.

Chronic smoldering infections and inflammations are also known to result in very intense generation of free radicals, a condition that has been demonstrated in such diseases as Lyme disease, viral hepatitis, encephalitis, lupus, rheumatoid arthritis, multiple sclerosis (MS), Alzheimer's disease, and Lou Gehrig's disease (ALS). All of these diseases improve with a judicious use of selected antioxidants. The reason for this is twofold.

First, inflammations and infections increase the metabolic rate, which as we have seen, increases free-radical generation. Second, the immune system attacks and destroys foreign invaders by releasing an intense barrage of free radicals from the white blood cells that have thronged to the site of the infection. For example, when bacteria invade your skin, your immune system sends a swarm of white blood cells and other immune cells to the site of invasion. As they approach the bacteria, the white blood cells dramatically increase their metabolism, producing a blast of free radicals which they release around the bacteria. It is the free radicals that kill the bacteria. So, you ask, why aren't the white blood cells also killed? It's because white blood cells have a very high concentration of antioxidants, about six times higher than normal cells.

When we have a smoldering infection that the immune system cannot kill outright, the free-radical attack by the body's immune system continues for years, leading to damage not only at the site of the attack, but to all tissues of the body. Increasingly, this is thought to be the basis of many so-called autoimmune diseases, such as rheumatoid arthritis and lupus. It may even explain many cases of arteriosclerosis. Ironically, even specialists treating these well-known free-radical diseases do not put their patients on increased doses of selected antiox-

Origin of Free Radicals

- metabolism
- inflammation
- stress
- environmental toxins
- ultraviolet radiation (sun and tanning beds)
- x-ray radiation
- low magnesium
- immune activation
- excitotoxins

TABLE 1.1

idants. When the body is severely deficient in antioxidants, white blood cells can no longer protect themselves from their own free radicals and, as a result, die in large numbers. This results in an impaired immune system, leading to a worsening of the infection.

Stress: Worrying Up Free Radicals

Most of us think of stress in terms of psychological stress: being overworked or worried about bills and our future. In fact, stress is defined as anything that upsets our normal state of well-being, and can include extreme physical exhaustion, trauma, and even infections. Yet, medical science has gradually come to realize that psychological stress can actually do *physical* harm. Recent experiments using stressed animals have demonstrated that unrelieved stress results in a dramatic increase in free-radical generation within virtually every area of the brain—cortex, striatum, and hippocampus. In such cases, free-radical overproduction is the result of oxidation of neurochemicals (epinephrine, norepinephrine, and dopamine) within the brain that are released during stress, producing significant injury to vital brain structures.

It has been shown in both experimental animals and in humans that chronic, unrelieved stress can produce permanent damage to the brain. Humans placed under the extreme stress of captivity, such as POWs and those subjected to torture and prolonged sleep deprivation, may never fully recover. Ironically, brief periods of stress interspersed with periods of rest actually strengthens the brain. The bottom line is that during periods of intense stress we need to increase our antioxidant defenses.

Environmental Toxins

The toxicity caused by many poisons found in nature, as well as man-made toxins, are known to do their damage, in large part, by generating free radicals within tissues. For example, aluminum has been shown to trigger an enormous number of free radicals in tissues, especially in brain tissue. The same is true for iron, lead, mercury, and cadmium.

Fluoride, even in the small amounts added to drinking water, is also a powerful generator of free radicals. When combined with aluminum, as in most public drinking water, toxicity to the brain is increased significantly. While the amount of fluoride in drinking water is in the range of 1-3 ppm, in toothpaste it can be as much as 1,500 ppm. Brushing your teeth with fluoridated toothpaste exposes you to very high levels of this extremely toxic compound.

As for pesticides and herbicides, many kill insects and unwanted plants by causing them to generate extremely high levels of free radicals in their tissues. The herbicide paraquat, for example, is known to produce incredibly high concentrations of free radicals in humans, so much so that it can completely destroy the lungs.

Another source of free-radical generation is the use of illegal drugs. Amphetamines, such as methamphetamine (meth) and dexadrine, can generate high concentrations of these destructive particles within the brain, leading to an increased risk of degenerative brain disorders, such as Parkinson's disease and Alzheimer's dementia, later in life. One designer drug, called MPTP, can cause severe, almost instant, onset of Parkinson's disease, after even a single dose. One of its modes of action is to produce free radicals within the part of the brain responsible for this disease. The effects are irreversible.

Processed foods are filled with numerous additives, most of which have never been tested to see if they increase free radicals within the body. But there is one, called carrageenan, that we know increases free radicals. A polysaccharide made from a seaweed, the substance is known to produce intense inflammatory reactions when injected into tissues. In fact, the intense reaction is so reproducible it is used when researchers want to study inflammation. As we learned above, inflammation is strongly associated with intense free-radical production within tissues.

Another food additive that has been shown to increase free-radical production is monosodium glutamate or MSG. This additive, used in the majority of processed foods, often in disguised names, has been shown to significantly increase free-radical production, not just in the brain but in many other tissues as well. What makes it particularly dangerous is that this increase in free-radical production persists for prolonged periods of time following even a single dose of MSG, an especially dangerous condition for a baby's developing brain, and in the elderly brain as well.

Finally, the artificial sweetener, aspartame (found in NutraSweet®, Equal®, Spoonful®, and others) contains multiple breakdown products and primary components (phenylalanine, aspartic acid and methanol) that have been shown to increase free-radical production. For example, formaldehyde and formic acid formed from the breakdown of methanol, have been shown to severely damage DNA, most likely by such a mechanism. Another component, aspartic acid, is an excitotoxin that increases free-radical generation within the brain, especially the parts related to memory and fine coordinated movements.

Radiation: The Sun

We have known for some time that radiation damages tissues by increasing production of free radicals throughout cells and extracellular tissues. One of the best examples of this effect is exposure to the sun: the sun's rays contain damaging radiation in the form of UVA and UVB wavelength light. These rays penetrate deep into the layers of the skin where they interact with skin cells and produce large amounts of free radicals, leading to damaged DNA, cell proteins, and membranes. When free radicals interact with the skin's collagen and elastic tissues, these fibers are weakened, causing sagging and wrinkling of the skin. This is why sun worshippers develop early and extensive wrinkling and sagging of exposed skin.

Fair-skinned people who sit in the sun for thirty minutes or more develop a deep reddening of the skin we call a sunburn—and it does burn. This is a good example of the destructive power of free radicals. With exposure under these conditions, so many free radicals are produced that the skin's antioxidant defenses are quickly depleted, leaving the skin totally unprotected against further free-radical injury. This is why the skin suddenly turns red. Repeated burning of the skin dramatically increases the risk of skin cancer, especially a highly fatal form called malignant melanoma. If you fall asleep in the sun for several hours, the destructive effect of free radicals can be so extensive as to cause your skin to break down, with the appearance of blistering and even ulceration of the skin. Extreme exposure to the sun can result in severe systemic effects we call sun poisoning: this will land you in the intensive care unit.

A good example of the vital importance of antioxidants in the skin is found in cases of a rare genetic disease called xeroderma pigmentosum, in which a person is born with virtually no antioxidant defenses, especially in the skin. Even mild exposure to the sun can cause extensive destruction and promote the development of multiple skin cancers. Even more frightening is that the risk of developing internal cancers also increases substantially. Antioxidant supplementation can significantly reduce the risk of developing these sun-related cancers.

Topical as well as oral antioxidants provide significant protection against free-radical damage to the skin and delay skin aging.

X-rays: Diagnostic and Therapeutic

Most of us at some time or other have had x-rays taken. In the 1960s and 1970s it was considered wise to have a yearly chest x-ray to catch disease early, a preventive measure especially for cancer. Today, for the same reason, the medical establishment encourages all women to have an annual x-ray series for early detection of breast cancer, but each time x-rays pass

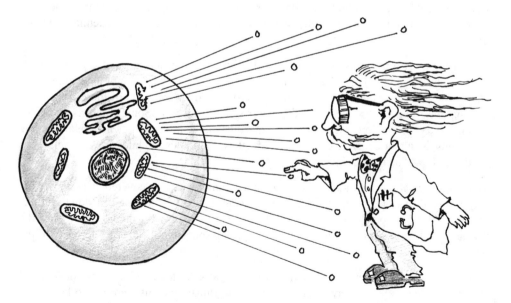

FIGURE 1.2   Demonstration of the intense bombardment by free radicals within a cell. These free radicals damage cell membranes, DNA, and protein enzymes.

through the body free radicals are produced. In the case of a chest x-ray or even a breast exam, this produces only minor elevation of free radicals and limited damage to the DNA with each dose—but the effect is accumulative.

More extensive radiological examinations, such as a lower and upper GI series or an arteriogram, can expose you to a significant amount of damaging x-rays. One estimate is that annual radiological breast exams increase the risk of breast cancer by 2 percent a year: over ten years you will have increased your risk 20 percent. This is not necessarily a call to avoid all mammograms, but you should increase your antioxidant defenses before you undergo such an exam. And there are other ways to screen for breast cancer that do not involve radiation, such as careful digital examinations, MRI scan, thermograms and ultrasound exams.

In the past, x-rays were used to treat benign conditions, such as scalp ringworm, scoliosis, tonsillitis, and to shrink the thymus gland. Being a new and untested tool, doctors thought it was harmless. It wasn't until a clever observer began to look at the high incidence of cancer and jawbone destruction seen in workers who painted radium watch dials that caution began to creep into this area. Madam Curie also died of cancer as a result of her extensive exposure to x-rays during her studies of the mysterious invisible ray.

Young girls exposed to gamma radiation to treat scoliosis were found later in life to demonstrate a very high incidence of breast cancer compared to those who had not been exposed. Likewise, children treated with radiation to rid them of ringworm infestations of the scalp were later found to have significantly increased rates of thyroid cancer, leukemia, and brain cancers.

One of the most tragic episodes in medical history occurred during the 1930s and 1940s when doctors using the new x-ray machine discovered a mysterious tumor appearing in the chest x-rays of small children. Suddenly, there occurred an epidemic of these dangerous-looking chest tumors discovered by the new roentgen machine. Some enterprising doctor decided to try the new roentgen-generating machine on the tumor. Sure enough, after a few treatments the tumor began to disappear. Ultimately, thousands of children were radiated to rid them of this "dangerous" tumor.

Thankfully, other doctors studied this so-called tumor—and discovered that it was the thymus gland! It seems the thymus gland is large during early childhood and slowly shrinks in size until it disappears from view later in life. Unfortunately for the young victims, the thymus gland is one of the major lymphatic organs responsible for the development of the immune system.

At one time, enlarged tonsils and adenoids were treated by the revolutionary non-surgical technique using the new x-ray machine. Those unfortunate victims were left to lead a life fraught with cancers of the esophagus, permanent immune suppression, and oral and facial cancers. I have seen one of these unfortunate people in my practice: the poor man now suffers a living hell every day of his life.

Now let us suppose that you are sixty-five years old and have poorly controlled diabetes. Your doctor decides you need to have a gallbladder x-ray series and an upper and lower GI series to find the cause of an unrelenting abdominal pain. By the time you have finished the x-ray series you will have a folder full of x-ray film that you can barely lift, and in the process will have received a significant dose of radiation to major areas of your body, including your bone marrow.

We now know that at the onset of diabetes, the body begins to produce an inordinate amount of free radicals and that the number of these free radicals increases dramatically as diabetic complications develop. Diabetes is even more treacherous for older people since free-radical production increases, the body's antioxidant supply is severely depleted, and tissues are much more vulnerable to the damaging effects of x-ray radiation. What to do?

If you know ahead of time that you will have an extensive radiological study, you should prepare yourself by increasing your antioxidant intake. Doing so will significantly lower your risk of cell, and especially DNA, damage. This has been shown in multiple studies. The antioxidants, alpha-lipoic acid, N-acetyl L-cysteine (NAC), and the carotenoids, are recommended in such cases. More about this in chapter nine.

Sometimes you face a situation in which you will be unable to plan ahead for an x-ray study. For instance, you may be in an automobile accident or develop an acute disease, such as a heart attack or stroke. It is for this reason that you should always keep your antioxidant defenses strong. In such cases, an ounce of prevention is certainly worth a pound of cure.

You may also face the unpleasant prospect of receiving very high doses of radiation when undergoing treatment for a cancerous disease. By concentrating the x-rays or gamma rays on the tumor, radiation oncologists are able to harness the destructive power of radiation against the cancer cells. The sensitivity of cancers varies: some tumors virtually melt away and others show next to no improvement under radiation therapy.

In the past, therapists were unable to direct radiation to the tumor alone and inadvertently radiated extensive volumes of normal tissues, resulting in hair loss, skin burns, and a breakdown of deep tissues. As a neurosurgery resident, some of my all-too-frequent cases were patients who had become paraplegic suddenly—even years later—following radiation treatment for chest tumors. The scatter radiation from the x-ray beam damaged the spinal cord resulting in prolonged radiation-induced free-radical damage. No one thought to increase the antioxidant defenses of these patients, even though the medical knowledge was available at the time—more evidence-based medicine.

Today, radiation oncology is much more sophisticated, using radiation types that spare the skin and concentrate the destructive beams mostly on the tumor. Still, some radiation does scatter into the surrounding normal tissues, and in patients with extensive tumors the health effects of this scatter effect can be significant. For twenty-six years I gave cancer patients powerful antioxidants before, during, and after their radiation treatments, with a significant reduction in complications and an improved effectiveness of the radiation against the tumor.

Radiation oncologists worry that using antioxidants during therapy will not only protect the surrounding normal tissue, but could also protect the tumor against the radiation as well. For this reason, many radiation oncologists will discourage their cancer patients from taking antioxidants. Several recent experiments have shown that specialized antioxidants not only do *not* protect the tumor from radiation injury, but actually enhance the x-rays' destructive power against the tumor, at the same time protecting normal tissues. This is because cancer cells are different, biochemically and structurally, from normal cells.

Because the body's immune defenses are concentrated in the bone marrow and lymph tissue, these sites are exceedingly sensitive to radiation injury. In addition, cells in these areas divide so rapidly they are much more sensitive to radiation injury. One thing you do not want to do during cancer treatment is to suppress the immune system, which is the most important destroyer of cancer cells. Even after your cancer is cured, your immune system runs a constant body-wide check (called immune surveillance) to make sure no new cancer cells appear. Antioxidants very effectively protect the immune system during radiation treatments, and are important even after treatment has stopped.

Low Magnesium and Free Radicals

Magnesium is one of the body's most incredible minerals. It plays a vital role in over three hundred biochemical reactions, protects the nervous system from strokes, excitotoxins, and other injuries, and acts as an antioxidant. A recent survey of a large number of healthy individuals found that over three-fourths were consuming less-than-recommended amounts of magnesium and two-thirds of that number had severe deficiencies. Further, certain medical conditions, such as cardiovascular disease, hypertension, diabetes, and renal disease, increase one's risk of low magnesium. Likewise, low magnesium levels increase complications associated with these diseases.

Magnesium is a mineral found mainly within the tissues and not the blood stream. Many doctors make the mistake of testing for blood levels of magnesium and conclude that normal findings indicate an adequate magnesium supply. This is just not true. You can have a normal blood value and very low tissue levels, which would put you at a very high risk for hardening of the arteries (atherosclerosis) and associated complications such as coronary heart disease, strokes, and peripheral vascular disease (poor blood supply to the extremities).

In addition, tissue magnesium deficiency puts you at a very high risk of developing a major neurological disease such as Parkinson's disease, Alzheimer's dementia, or ALS. One reason is that low magnesium levels in tissues double the number of free radicals in the body, and increase their killing ability over twofold. Adequate tissue magnesium levels are very protective against free-radical injury. In addition, magnesium dilates blood vessels, thereby improving blood flow to the brain, heart, and kidneys and, in addition, acts at the neuron membrane to prevent excitotoxic damage in the nervous system.

How Does the Body Protect Itself Against These Nasty Free Radicals?

In His divine wisdom, God equipped our bodies with a very efficient system to protect us against destructive free radicals. This system, or network, is composed of many parts that work more efficiently together than alone. In fact, most antioxidants when used alone can actually become free radicals themselves.

First, let us see how antioxidants work to neutralize these damaging particles. Chemically, a free radical is a particle possessing an unpaired electron in its outer orbital. To the non-scientist this means nothing. In nature, electrons always prefer to come in pairs. If they don't, they will steal an electron from whatever is close by. This process of stealing electrons is called oxidation. When free radicals are loosed in a cell, the unpaired electron begins to steal electrons from surrounding DNA molecules, proteins, and lipids within the membranes, as I discussed earlier.

Antioxidants work by supplying electrons to free radicals, thus sparing the cell's vital components. In the process, an antioxidant becomes a free radical itself, not as powerful as the free radical it neutralized, but still a mildly destructive chemical. This means that the antioxidant needs to be regenerated; it does this by borrowing an electron from another antioxidant. For example, vitamin C will regenerate vitamin E and vice versa. This is why our diets should supply fresh antioxidants, so that the renewal process can continue. There are special antioxidants, such as alpha-lipoic acid, that can constantly renew the antioxidant status of other antioxidants without being renewed itself. Special chemicals in fruits, vegetables, and herbs called flavonoids, have been found to be very powerful and versatile free-radical antioxidants, and can also renew the antioxidant status of several of the vitamins.

The Network

Neutralizing destructive free radicals is so important that God designed a unique and somewhat complicated system to protect us. This antioxidant network involves at least three tiers of protective molecules: (1) the vitamin, mineral and flavonoid network, (2) the antioxidant enzymes, and (3) special antioxidant molecules.

1) Vitamins, Minerals and Flavonoids

From extensive television advertising, most of us are familiar with vitamin antioxidants such as vitamin A, beta-carotene, vitamin C, and vitamin E. All are powerful antioxidants that neutralize a significant number of free radicals. Less well-known antioxidants are vitamins D and K, magnesium, zinc, and manganese. Also, there are over forty carotenoids and five thousand flavonoids from plants in the human diet that act as antioxidants.

Each antioxidant acts in a different place in the cells and tissues. For example, vitamin C is concentrated in the blood plasma, connective tissues, and within the cytoplasm of the cell. Vitamin E components are dissolved in the fatty parts of the cell such as the membranes and are not usually concentrated within the watery parts of the cell. Vitamin E is also an important part of the LDL cholesterol molecule. Carotenoids, such as beta-carotene, alpha-carotene, lutein, and lycopene generally are found in the fatty parts of the cell as well, but can enter the watery cytosol of the cell. Minerals like zinc and magnesium are found principally within the cell.

So we see that this vitamin/mineral antioxidant network is highly compartmentalized so that each has its own zone of defense, much like football or basketball. This is another reason that all of the vitamins and minerals are needed in balance to adequately defend cells. Vitamin E's major role is to defend the membranes while magnesium, zinc, and other antioxidants primarily protect the DNA and cellular proteins. Vitamin C plays a major role in protecting the watery spaces both inside and outside the cell. Alpha-lipoic acid can go anywhere.

It should also be appreciated that this portion of the antioxidant system is highly dependent on our nutritional intake of preformed vitamins and minerals, even though some of the vitamins can be manufactured from other precursors, as in the case of vitamin A from beta-carotene.

When an antioxidant encounters a free radical it is oxidized and becomes a free radical itself, milder than the one it neutralized, but still capable of causing problems. This is why we have numerous types of antioxidants in our bodies, each one regenerates the other. For example, vitamin C regenerates vitamin E and visa versa. This is why it is a bad idea to take just one type vitamin, soon it will fill your body with an oxidized vitamin, causing more harm than good.

The rate at which our antioxidants are used up depends on how many free radicals we are producing. A person with lupus or diabetes will require considerably more antioxidants than a person who is perfectly healthy. An extreme athlete, likewise, will require more antioxidants than will a person who exercises moderately. From this you can see that a diabetic who takes no supplemental antioxidants and develops an infected toe is more likely to die from this event than is a diabetic who maintains an adequate store of antioxidants. Antioxidants must be constantly replenished, and a good diet and careful supplementation accomplish this goal.

Phytochemicals: the Flavonoids

Plants contain thousands of antioxidants, mostly in the form of specialized complex chemicals called flavonoids, each of which is a unique molecule that plays a major role in nutrition. Plants also contain numerous vitamins and minerals that act as antioxidants: one group of vitamins is called the carotenoids, which includes about forty different varieties that humans consume. Most of us have heard of beta-carotene, but there are others such as alpha carotene, lutein, lycopene, canthoxanthin, zeaxanthin, and cryptoxanthin. Diets poor in fruit and vegetable intakes deprive us of these vital antioxidants.

In 1936, a Nobel Prize-winning biochemist by the name of Szent-Gyorgi isolated a factor from plants that had some rather unusual properties. He knew that seriously depriving an animal of ascorbic acid would engender bleeding gums and internal bleeding, and that the animal would finally die as a result of extreme sensitivity to stress—a condition we know as scurvy. Yet when he fed the animals his newly discovered plant extract they appeared perfectly healthy, with no signs of scurvy, no matter how long they were denied vitamin C.

At the time, he felt his new factor met the criteria for a vitamin, and based on the idea that the new bioflavonoid inhibited the increased capillary permeability seen with vitamin C deficiency, he named it vitamin "P" for permeability factor. Later, biochemists concluded it was not a vitamin, and the compound was given the name bioflavonoid. Since this early discovery, thousands of flavonoid compounds have been discovered, many possessing quite unique biological properties.

Recent studies have demonstrated that all of these compounds are powerful and extremely versatile antioxidants, acting against a whole host of dangerous free radicals. In fact, some of the flavonoids can neutralize special free radicals that cannot be neutralized by most of the antioxidant vitamins and network enzymes. It should be noted that there are other dangerous radicals besides oxygen radicals. For example, there are reactive nitrogen species that can be equally, if not more, destructive than oxygen radicals. Vitamins are poor at neutralizing these special types of radicals, while flavonoids are very efficient.

In addition, several of the flavonoids can remove (chelate) dangerous, free-radical-generating metals, such as iron, copper, aluminum, and some of the heavy metals including mercury, arsenic, and lead. This becomes especially important as we age, since iron and aluminum accumulation is common with aging, and is also very common in neurodegenerative disorders such as Alzheimer's disease and Parkinson's disease.

The antioxidant protection afforded by plant flavonoids makes sense when we realize that it is flavonoids and carotenoids that allow plants to survive in the glaring sun all day long. Normally, the sun's harsh rays would quickly destroy the leaves, but flavonoids block the damage, both by absorbing the harmful rays and by neutralizing the free radicals they generate. The same phenomenon occurs in humans.

Research into the medicinal properties of flavonoids has expanded almost exponentially in recent years. We are now finding that beyond their usefulness as antioxidants they may hold the key to controlling cancer, both as a preventative and as a treatment of established cancers.

2) Antioxidant Enzymes

The human body has several enzymes whose function it is to neutralize free radicals and other destructive oxidants. The first of these is superoxide dismutase or SOD. Actually there are three types of SOD: one associated with manganese, one with copper, and another with zinc, each of which has distinct locations and functions within the body. All function in converting the superoxide radical to hydrogen peroxide. Superoxide is a very destructive free radical and is found throughout the body. It has been estimated that over a lifetime we produce about three tons of superoxide radicals.

Deficiencies in zinc, copper, or manganese can result in malfunctions of these critical enzymes and can lead to serious disorders. For example, a deficiency in SOD in the spinal cord can result in a rare form of inherited amyotrophic lateral sclerosis. Stress is associated with an increased supply of SOD enzymes in the brain, as a reflexive protective mechanism.

When superoxide is converted into hydrogen peroxide, usually in the presence of free iron, all is still not well. If left alone the hydrogen peroxide can break down into the very destructive hydroxyl radical that can damage the cell's membranes and DNA, as well as other structures. It must be quickly neutralized to prevent irreversible damage. Two enzymes have the function of accomplishing this task: catalase and glutathione peroxidase, both of which convert hydrogen peroxide into harmless water. The brain contains very little catalase enzyme and is more dependent on the glutathione peroxidase enzyme. Deficiencies in either of these enzymes can lead to catastrophic diseases, as is seen with Parkinson's disease and possibly Alzheimer's dementia. Glutathione peroxidase enzyme is dependent on selenium.

Another important antioxidant enzyme is glutathione reductase, whose job it is to return the powerful antioxidant glutathione from its oxidized form to its reduced and functional form. Sometimes you will find that a chemical is in reduced form—but that doesn't mean it is in

---

The Antioxidant Network

I. Vitamin, Mineral, Flavonoid Network
- ascorbate
- alpha-tocopherol (vitamin E)
- carotenoids
- vitamins D and K
- magnesium
- zinc
- manganese
- plant flavonoids

2. Antioxidant Enzyme Network
- superoxide dismutase
- glutathione reductase
- glutathione peroxidase
- catalase

3. Thiol Antioxidants
- albumin
- alpha-lipoic acid
- glutathione

TABLE 1.2

lower concentrations. A reduced chemical is simply one that has fully paired electrons. Virtually all antioxidants must be in the reduced form to be effective. Glutathione, like the vitamins, becomes oxidized when it comes into contact with a free radical and must be restored. Lowering the level of this enzyme can lead to heightened sensitivity to free-radical damage. Glutathione is a powerful antioxidant found in every cell of the body. Prolonged free-radical production severely reduces glutathione levels and has been associated with virtually all degenerative diseases, including cancer.

While these antioxidant enzymes cannot be derived directly from food, they are dependent on the foods you eat for the building blocks needed to construct them. When the vitamin and mineral network is deficient, greater strain is placed on other parts of the antioxidant enzyme network to protect your cells and tissues. This can lead to early disease.

3) Special Antioxidant Network: the Thiols

The thiols portion of the network consists of a special group of antioxidant compounds containing an important sulfur-hydrogen linkage called a sulfhydral group. It includes alpha-lipoic acid, glutathione, and albumin. Two members of this group deserve special attention: alpha-lipoic acid and glutathione.

Alpha-lipoic acid is one of the most powerful antioxidants in the body, carrying out its antioxidant function throughout the extracellular tissues and within the blood and cells. This unique antioxidant is able to neutralize a wide variety of free radicals and, more importantly, restore other oxidized antioxidants to their functional reduced antioxidant state. For instance, it can convert oxidized vitamin C, called dehydroascorbate, to its reduced and functional form, ascorbic acid (ascorbate).

In the process of doing this, alpha-lipoic acid is converted to dihydrolipoic acid or DHLA. Unlike the vitamins, when oxidized, alpha-lipoic acid still acts as an antioxidant. Feeding alpha-lipoic acid to animals or humans does some remarkable things. It enhances cellular energy production; regenerates all of the other antioxidant molecules, including glutathione; acts as a metal chelating agent (removes dangerous metals); and increases cellular levels of coenzyme Q10 (CoQ10), a primary energy molecule. A coenzyme is an organic, nonprotein molecule that binds with a protein molecule (called an apoenzyme) to form an active enzyme, called a holoenzyme. Alpha-lipoic acid is a remarkable antioxidant that can be found in virtually every area of the body, including cell membranes. Severe stress, chronic inflammation and poor nutrition can all deplete alpha-lipoic acid levels.

Another powerful and universal antioxidant is glutathione. This antioxidant is especially important in protecting cells from an extremely wide variety of reactive oxygen species, many of which are resistant to other antioxidants such as vitamins C and E and the carotenoids. Glutathione is present in all cells, including brain cells. Several studies have shown that the lower a person's glutathione levels are, the greater their risk of cancer. We also know that one of the early events associated with Parkinson's disease is a fall in glutathione levels in the neurons associated with the disease (substantia nigra). Alzheimer's patients also have glutathione deficiencies. There are ways to increase the glutathione level in cells, even brain cells. Three of the best methods are supplementing your diet with ascorbate, N-acetyl L-cysteine (NAC), or alpha-lipoic acid. More about this later.

Oxidation and Disease: an Overview

Many years ago, it was proposed that a common event could explain many of the findings we associate with diseases of various sorts, such as diabetes, heart attacks, strokes, arthritis, lupus, Alzheimer's disease, and other degenerative diseases of aging. That common event appears to be the destructive oxidation of tissues by free radicals, a process I have already described.

Some have tried to separate disease from normal aging, while others have insisted that aging is a disease and that it is not normal for tissues to deteriorate with aging. This latter group of thinkers has grown in the last several decades to form a whole discipline dedicated to anti-aging medicine. Whether aging is a disease or a natural event, we know that both share a common factor: damage to cells and tissues by a constant barrage of free radicals, and other reactive molecules, over a lifetime.

Aging begins even before birth; in fact, free radicals are formed from the very moment of conception. They produce some damage, but because of the tremendous growth and reproduction of cells and tissues, it is inconsequential. Of course, some free radicals are necessary for normal development, since they act as signals for development and normal functioning of cells. As long as the production of free radicals is controlled, they do not present serious health consequences. We know that the antioxidant network is poorly formed in the early stages of development, and, as a consequence, the child depends on its mother for protection. This is why the mother's diet is so important. As the baby begins to develop its body features these antioxidant enzymes increase in concentration and continue to do so after birth, well into adolescence.

As these antioxidant-network enzymes increase in activity and concentration, so, too, must the other components of the antioxidant network such as the vitamins, minerals, thiols, and flavonoids; again, all heavily dependent on the child's and mother's diet. It should be remembered that not only is the child dependent on the mother for nourishment during gestation, but also soon after birth. This means that mom must maintain a healthy diet of fruits, vegetables, high-quality proteins, complex carbohydrates, and special fats to assure that the newborn baby's brain and body will continue to grow and develop to its maximum potential: this, of course, includes a highly functioning antioxidant network.

Now let us take a hypothetical case, one that is repeated millions of times in this country. Before a mother-to-be even realizes she is pregnant, her diet is that of the typical American and includes carbonated drinks, coffee or tea made with tap water, highly processed foods, regular consumption of red meats (usually seared over a hot flame), and plenty of french fries and snack foods cooked in either hydrogenated or polyunsaturated vegetable oil. Throughout this time, the baby's cells are struggling to form by dividing and moving in a dance of life that very quickly begins to resemble the shape of a baby in the making.

At this stage, the new baby is totally dependent on its mother for nutrition, which is delivered through a highly complex blood exchange system within the placenta. What the mother eats eventually ends up in the baby's blood stream, but, as we shall see later, not in the same concentrations. So all of this junk food, filled with numerous additives, bad fats, toxic amino acids, pesticides and toxic metals, flows into the tissues of the baby, not only depriving the baby of needed nutrients, but actually poisoning the developing cells.

As for the rest of us, free radicals appear to play a central role in virtually every disease you can name, either directly or secondarily. Of the diseases known to be related to free-radical injury, the best evidence exists for: lupus, multiple sclerosis, all of the degenerative brain diseases (Alzheimer's dementia, Parkinson's disease, Huntington's disease, olivopontocerebellar degeneration, and ALS), strokes, heart disease, arteriosclerosis, all infectious diseases (viral, fungal, mycoplasmal, and bacterial), rheumatoid arthritis, cancer, smoking-related diseases, diabetes, and all other inflammatory diseases.

Even when other primary mechanisms appear to be involved, such as autoimmunity in rheumatoid arthritis and lupus, it is the unrelenting generation of free radicals that causes the damage we associate with these diseases. Which disease will develop depends on the site of the free-radical attack. For example, in rheumatoid arthritis free-radical injury occurs within the joints. You must also appreciate that, even though the primary attack is within the joints, free radicals spill out into the blood stream causing damage to other far-removed tissues, including the brain, muscles, nerves, heart, and kidneys.

In lupus, injury is concentrated primarily in the connective tissues of the body. The reason the symptoms associated with lupus are so widespread and varied is that connective tissue exists throughout the body, and in all the organs. The brain and peripheral nerves are commonly affected in lupus for this same reason. This universal free-radical attack makes lupus an especially damaging and serious disorder, and antioxidants should play a major role in every autoimmune disease patient's care.

Even in cases that would seem far removed from the mechanism of free-radical injury, such as a stroke or a traumatic brain injury, these damaging particles do play a major role in the event's outcome. Experimental evidence clearly indicates that powerful antioxidants significantly improve the neurological outcome of both stroke and brain trauma, making the difference between a full and useful life or one of repeated hospitalizations, suffering, and disability.

Free radicals play such an important role in strokes and head trauma because the injured brain reacts by releasing enormous amounts of glutamate, which in these concentrations behaves as a powerful toxin (called an excitotoxin). Excitotoxins in turn generate enormous numbers of free radicals that injure the surrounding damaged, but still living, brain. If this free-radical attack is not stopped, this brain tissue will die as well. If it is protected, then the surrounding brain tissue can recover its normal function. With large strokes and injuries, even the surrounding normal brain will come under free-radical attack, since the excitotoxin accumulation extends far out into the brain. Excitotoxic destruction following a brain injury can persist for more than a week after the initial injury.

Several recent studies using animal models have shown that the use of antioxidant therapy can reduce the volume of destroyed brain in cases of strokes by more than 50 percent. Animals without antioxidant treatment had a very high mortality rate, and those which survived still had serious neurological deficits. The animals receiving antioxidants not only survived in greater numbers, but many appeared to be entirely neurologically normal. Unfortunately, most doctors treating strokes and head injuries do not use antioxidants in their patients' treatments. Actually, it is worse than that, because not only do they make no attempt to increase their patients' antioxidant defenses, they make no effort to even replace the antioxidants that might be lost due to the stress of injury or to pre-existing nutritional deficiencies.

Atherosclerosis, or hardening of the arteries, is a condition that has become epidemic in the industrialized world, especially in the United States. For many years conventional wisdom held that this fatty destruction of the arteries was due to excess cholesterol in the diet. This led to a national obsession with eating only foods that did not contain cholesterol or that boasted very low cholesterol content, thus creating a whole new industry for food manufacturers. More than fifteen years ago it was discovered that cholesterol is not dangerous unless it is oxidized, and the reason high cholesterol levels are associated with elevated rates of heart attacks, strokes, and peripheral vascular disease is that the more cholesterol you have in your blood stream, the more likely some of it will become oxidized.

Later it was determined that certain types of cholesterol were good and others bad, in terms of risk. Low-density lipoprotein or LDL cholesterol has been dubbed the bad cholesterol. On the other side of the coin, high-density cholesterol or HDL cholesterol is now considered to be a good cholesterol. The reason LDL cholesterol is bad is that it is much easier to oxidize than HDL cholesterol. But oxidized HDL cholesterol is just as dangerous as oxidized LDL cholesterol.

Recent research has challenged the cholesterol theory of atherosclerosis, however. Newer studies have shown that many people afflicted with heart disease and advanced atherosclerosis also have certain types of bacteria—including chlamydia, helicobacteria, and mycoplasmal organisms—growing within the fatty crud lining their arteries. It is thought that this chronic infection and the resulting attempt by an impaired immune system to clear the organism results in a focused, intense generation of free radicals within the wall of the vessel. The resulting damage leads to failed attempts by the body to heal the damage, a condition doctors call arterial plaque. This plaque build-up slowly occludes the vessels.

There is growing evidence that high antioxidant intake, especially from fruits and vegetables, dramatically reduces the incidence of cardiovascular disease and strokes. Even more exciting is the confirmed finding that eating large quantities of nutrient-dense fruits and vegetables can dramatically reduce damage *following* a heart attack or stroke; that is, antioxidants are effective even if taken after a heart attack. More about this in chapter ten.

Detoxification and Food Additives

If you have ever looked at the labels on processed foods, drinks, or soups you will see a long list of additives that resemble names seen only in a chemistry textbook, such things as allyl anthranilate and benzyl dimethyl carbinyl butrate. Remember, most of these compounds are foreign to the human body and must be detoxified or metabolized in some way. According to Ruth Winters' book, *A Consumer's Dictionary of Food Additives,* there is no toxicity information available on 46 percent of the chemicals added to foods and only 5 percent have had complete toxicity evaluation. Some food labels look more like labels from organic chemistry laboratories than what you would expect to find attached to foods. Yet we consume these processed foods as if safety has been assured.

It is also important to remember that the detoxification process depends on enzymes, mostly in the liver, but also within every cell, and that these enzymes must develop before birth. While much remains to be learned about the development of these detoxification enzymes, we do know that they are not fully developed in the unborn baby and for some of the enzymes, the levels are extremely low or non-existent. This puts an unborn child at extreme risk: the effects of a high toxic load can vary from catastrophic to mild and subtle. For adults, these same detoxification enzymes may be deficient, a condition not uncommon with aging and disease. As individuals, our detoxification capacity varies considerably.

One toxin that is especially dangerous to the developing fetus is the artificial sweetener, aspartame. This artificial sweetener is composed of a complex blend of two amino acids, phenylalanine and aspartic acid, joined by methyl alcohol. Methyl alcohol is a powerful toxin that is carefully regulated by the EPA. Recent studies have found that even low doses can be quite harmful to cells, especially to DNA. When methyl alcohol is consumed, it is converted in the cells to formaldehyde and formic acid, both potent toxins. Formic acid is the poison used by the fire ant that causes such intense pain. Formaldehyde is used as a preservative, and in the past, as an embalming fluid. It is also a known carcinogen.

Both phenylalanine and aspartic acid are normally found in the nervous system, but at higher concentrations both are neurotoxic. Phenylalanine is the toxic component seen in the child-hood disorder called phenylketonuria or PKU. In this disorder, phenylalanine accumulates in the blood and hence brain, in very high concentrations. Carriers for the gene develop blood levels of phenylalanine twice as high as those of normal people, when consuming an equal amount of aspartame. Aspartic acid is one of the excitotoxic amino acids, and has been shown to produce significant damage to the brain in higher concentrations. In addition, the metabolic breakdown of aspartame yields about a dozen toxic compounds, some of which have been associated with cancer induction and alteration of brain function. The fewer of these toxins and foreign chemicals you expose your unborn child to, the better. This applies to newborns, toddlers, adolescents and adults as well. All of the toxins produced by ingesting aspartame must be detoxified and this puts a strain on the body's ability to cope.

Conclusion

Free-radical production begins the very moment life begins and continues until we die. A small number of these free radicals are necessary for normal functioning of the body, for example, in the production of cellular signals and for the proper functioning of the immune system; yet any excess of these free radicals can slowly damage important components of the cells and surrounding tissues, leading to changes we call aging and/or degenerative disease.

With time, this accumulated damage becomes so extensive that cells begin to fail and many of the body's functions begin to go awry. Of particular importance is the damage done to the cell's energy-producing capacity. Energy within all cells is produced primarily by small islands of bacteria-looking particles called mitochondria. Ninety-five percent of all the oxygen entering our cells passes through the mitochondria's energy-producing system. About 3-5 percent of this oxygen is diverted into making free radicals.

These free radicals first damage the many energy-producing enzymes within the mitochondria itself, its DNA, and the membrane of the tiny structure. It is important to remember that mitochondria have their own DNA, which is ten times more sensitive to free-radical damage than DNA in the cell's nucleus. Because mitochondria have their own DNA system they can reproduce independent of the cell itself. If mitochondrial DNA is damaged by free-radical attack, the new mitochondria formed during its reproduction have a reduced ability to produce energy. As these divisions continue, more and more of the mitochondria are damaged. Soon, the cell contains mostly damaged mitochondria.

This means that the cell has less energy to carry out its many functions and, as a result, will produce even more free radicals. Soon cells begin to die and obvious illness develops. In Parkinson's disease, we know that this process begins very early and is localized mainly to special neurons in the brain responsible for motor movement. As we shall see later, neurons with deficient energy supplies are up to one hundred times more susceptible to excitotoxic injury and death, ultimately caused by free radicals.

We know that some diseases associated with severe muscle weakness and brain malfunction (encephalopathy), and a large number of strokes are caused by inherited mitochondrial malfunction. This inheritance is unusual in that it passes only from the mother, since sperm contribute no mitochondria to conception. Parkinson's disease is also suspected to have a maternal, mitochondrial lineage, so that if your mother had Parkinson's disease your chances for developing the disease are significantly increased.

Mitochondrial malfunction is not always inherited, as we have seen. More often, it is the result of chronic, decade-by-decade exposure to small injuries by free radicals that have accumulated during life. Three things can speed up and magnify this damage: a poor antioxidant defense network, increased free-radical production, and a combination of both. In all three cases, poor nutrition is the culprit. Now let us look at some specific conditions and what you can do to prevent them. If you have a pre-existing condition, you can still do much good by improving your nutrition.

2
The Remarkable Effect of Practicing Good Nutrition From the Very Beginning

Nutrition and the Gene

Research of the past twenty years has taught us that early nutrition may have a profound effect on development of, or protection from, later diseases, a phenomenon that goes beyond the direct effect on the disease itself. A growing body of evidence based on this research indicates that nutrition can actually control the genes for diseases. For instance, it is known that poor nutrition during infancy and adolescence seems to program the genes for early onset of major degenerative diseases such as cardiovascular disease, strokes, diabetes, and degenerative brain diseases. Further, good nutrition has the opposite effect, programming genes for a life free of major diseases.

Most lay people are of the opinion that genes are set at birth, thereby programming our cells to function in a certain way. For example, if we inherit a bad gene for an early heart attack, there is nothing that we can do to change our fate—it is locked in our system. To say otherwise would be to imply that through lifestyle changes we could, for instance, change the color of our eyes. This argument has been given a boost following the excitement generated by completion of the Human Genome Project. Recently, geneticists have announced that there appear to be more gene-controlled diseases than we ever thought in the past. Upon hearing this, many may conclude that we should eat, drink and be merry for tomorrow we die; our fate is locked into our inheritance.

Fortunately, not all genes behave in such a predetermined fashion. We now know that genes have switches that allow them to be turned on or off, and that numerous genes in our cells are continuously turned off and unused. For example, we know that a cartilage cell in the knee joint has all the genes necessary to be a brain neuron or a heart cell, but it remains a cartilage cell because the genes that would make it otherwise are turned off. Recent experiments have shown that brain cells can indeed be transformed into heart cells merely by turning on the heart-cell genes.

It is true that some of us carry genes that make us more prone to early heart attack, stroke, diabetes, autoimmune diseases, or cancer, yet for these genes to cause these diseases, they must be turned on. As long as they are off, we are safe. So what regulates these "on" and "off" switches? Several factors contribute, including stress, physical trauma, and environmental agents, but the most important element of all is nutrition. In fact, nutrition can override many of the chemical and environmental triggers for bad genes. We know that in juvenile diabetes (type I), genetic susceptibility is a major catalyst in those who develop the disease, but diabetes only occurs following early childhood exposure to particular environmental or infectious triggers. Exposure to a virus, cow's milk, or MSG all act to turn on the diabetes gene switch, allowing the disease to fully manifest itself. Without these triggering exposures, the disease may never manifest.

We also know that certain chemicals, viruses, physical irritations, and nutritional deficiencies can all result in the development of cancer. Yet the process may take years, even decades, to develop. The reason for this delay is that the switching on of cancer genes (oncogenes) has to occur in a certain sequence and involves numerous genes. This polygenetic basis of disease occurs in many diseases including hypertension, diabetes, lipid disorders, gout, arthritis, osteoporosis, and polycystic ovaries. Each gene contributes a small part of the puzzle that eventually results in the disease. If a piece is missing, the disease may not fully develop.

Certain vitamins and plant chemicals, called phytochemicals, can inhibit the activation of these cancer genes, and prevent a gene's instruction from reaching its destination in the cell's mechanism. This is how genes influence the function of cells, by ordering the secretion of special signaling molecules that instruct enzymes, for instance, to build a special protein that will promote the growth and spread of the cancer. Or in another instance, it will turn off a gene's instructions, preventing the information transcription.

Early Nutrition and Antioxidant Defenses

Another way that nutrition protects all of us from disease is by fortifying the body's antioxidant defenses. We have already seen the immense destructive power of free radicals: it is important to remember that under normal circumstances the cell is undergoing a barrage of attacks by free radicals resulting in the oxidation of the major components of the cell—the membrane lipids, the DNA, carbohydrates, and the proteins. These destructive effects are slow and accumulate over many years.

Dr. Bruce Ames, a leader in the field of free-radical biology, has estimated that each cell in our body undergoes about ten thousand free-radical attacks a day. In truth, even this startling figure underestimates the immensity of this attack. When we are ill with a virus or following an injury, the number of attacks may reach one hundred thousand per cell. Even extreme exercise and aerobics can drastically increase the number of free-radical attacks within a cell. So, throughout life we are exposed to conditions that increase our free-radical generation, and as a result, we suffer accumulative damage that eventually can result in a major disease.

Certain types of cells are more susceptible to free-radical injury than others. For example, cells that divide very rapidly, such as bone marrow or liver cells, can suffer devastating effects from high free-radical generation, as is seen with radiation exposure. Conversely, cells that do not divide at all are less vulnerable to DNA damage but in other ways are even more susceptible since the same cells must endure an ongoing attack throughout the life of the organism. For example, neurons generally do not divide after maturation of the brain is complete, sometime after birth. As a result, a lifetime of free-radical attacks can lead to severe degenerative diseases of the nervous system such as Alzheimer's disease and Parkinson's disease. There is overwhelming evidence that ALS (a spinal motor neuron disorder) is caused by free-radical destruction of spinal and brain stem motor neurons.

For these reasons, it is vital for us to build strong antioxidant defenses early in life, even before birth. For mothers, especially, this means that you must be sure you are adequately supplied with antioxidants and the nutrition necessary to complete the building of the other components of the antioxidant network (antioxidant enzymes and thiols) for both you and your child.

An additional advantage of practicing good nutrition is that it will help prevent viral infections and environmental injury to the genetic structures that can lead to premature onset of other disorders. Throughout childhood, infants and toddlers are exposed to hundreds of

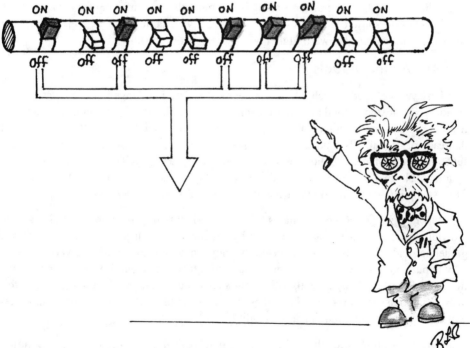

FIGURE 2.1 Genetic switches can either turn on or off instructions for cell processes. In many cases, these switches control harmful signals, but nutrition has been shown to be a major factor in controlling them.

viruses and bacteria, especially if they stay in day care facilities. With each viral invasion the body is subjected to a wave of free-radical generation that will continue as long as the virus persists: as long as the virus is active in your child, his or her immune system will be launching an attack to destroy it, and, as we have seen, the immune system kills foreign organisms by releasing a burst of intensely concentrated free radicals. Less free radical damage will occur if the immune attack ends quickly, again, emphasizing the importance of having a strong immune system in conjunction with a powerful antioxidant system.

There is compelling evidence that the immune system plays a vital role in brain development and that a weak immune system can severely impair later brain function, especially cognition—the ability to think. The connection appears to be between immune chemicals, called cytokines, and brain neurotransmitters, chemicals that allow brain cells to communicate with each other.

There is also evidence that antioxidant vitamins and minerals play a vital role in brain function. While much of this antioxidant research has focused on the elderly, there is also abundant evidence that brain function is affected during childhood as well. It may be that antioxidants protect the delicate brain-cell processes from destruction during life's ongoing free radical attack. One interesting finding is that most children suffering from ADD/ADHD and autism also show deficiencies in brain zinc, a vital antioxidant as well as immune-supporting nutrient. Again we find that both systems work together.

We Are All Individuals

In all my years of medical school, one of the most interesting things I learned was in gross anatomy. Our textbook for that course contained drawings illustrating the numerous anatomical differences among individuals. It was confirmation of something that I have always felt, that each of us is totally unique, not just in our minds, but in our anatomy as well as body functions. Physiologically, biochemically, anatomically, and psychically, we all are unique creations. No two brains are designed the same way or function exactly in the same way. This is why no two people think or feel the same way when faced with similar events.

The biochemist, Dr. Roger Williams, first pointed out the importance of biochemical individuality, and that we cannot use the hypothetical "normal person" to set nutritional guidelines and norms. In his many years of study, he demonstrated that we vary considerably in our ability to detoxify environmental toxins, metabolize our foods, and in our nutritional requirements. Only recently is it being appreciated that normal values for laboratory tests do not fit a specific person. Instead, we must rely on physiological or functional values, which take into account individual variability.

With the tremendous growth in the field of biochemical genetics, we have had further confirmation of this fundamental idea of individuality. The study of human genetics has demonstrated that there is a considerable biochemical variation within and between human populations, even between identical twins. Artemis P. Simopoulos, MD, a molecular geneticist, stated that DNA sequencing has demonstrated "how unique each one of us is, and the extent to which genetic variation occurs in human beings."

This genetic uniqueness is so prevalent that we cannot really extrapolate nutritional recommendations from one population to another, because they may have significantly differing methods of metabolism of the same food chemicals; that is, a person from Alaska metabolizes food differently than a person from Mississippi. Our metabolic individuality is also determined by constitutional factors, such as age, sex, developmental size, and parental factors, as well as environmental factors, such as time, geography, climate, occupation, education, and diet. All of these factors coalesce to influence our individual chances of surviving in a hostile world.

Another important finding has been that DNA-repair enzymes can vary as much as 180-300 times among individuals. This is critically important when we consider that our ability to repair free-radical-damaged DNA can mean the difference between developing cancer, degenerative brain diseases, or other devastating disorders and enjoying good health. Recent studies have shown that people who develop certain types of cancer have an impaired ability to repair damaged DNA. Similar defects in DNA-repair enzymes have also been seen in cases of Alzheimer's dementia. Free radicals also damage DNA-repair enzymes, as do several of the toxic metals.

This genetic and biochemical individuality can either place us at a high risk of certain diseases or a very low risk. For example, persons lacking a detoxification enzyme called glutathione transferase M1 show an increased risk of developing lung and bladder cancer, especially if they smoke. People with low liver-detoxification capacity due to other enzyme defects also show a high rate of carcinogen-induced cancers because of an inability to detoxify specific cancer-causing chemicals.

Another genetic toss of the coin can play a major role in your risk of developing two particularly devastating diseases. It has been shown that persons carrying the apolipoprotein E4 gene (apoE4) are at a very high risk of developing Alzheimer's disease and heart disease. Even having one copy of the gene increases your risk. One autopsy study found that 85 percent of those diagnosed with Alzheimer's disease were positive for the apoE4 gene. People with the apoE4 gene that suffered head injury were also found to have more long–term residual neurological damage, and were more likely to become demented than those not possessing the gene. This is especially true for boxers. Even mad cow disease (Creutzfeldt-Jakob disease) is more common in individuals possessing this gene.

So, how could one gene produce such a high incidence of such diverse diseases? It appears that people with this gene have an exaggerated inflammatory response, and both diseases— Alzheimer's and heart disease—are the result of prolonged inflammation, as we shall see. In addition, individuals possessing the apoE4 gene also have lower levels of antioxidant enzymes and therefore less protection. Those lucky enough to have the apoE2 gene have a significantly lower risk of developing these inflammatory diseases.

Again, we see that although individual variation in genetic inheritance can drastically influ-ence our risk of disease, neither is our genetic code a "Last Will and Testament." Nutrition can alter the course of high-risk genes, not only by turning these genes off but also by inhibiting the resulting bad effects produced by them, in this case increased inflammation. In such cases, it is important to start your defense as soon as possible, before irreversible injuries can occur.

A recent review of genetic influence on disease found that 50 percent of the variation in plasma cholesterol concentration, 30-60 percent of the variation in hypertension, and 75 percent of the variance in bone density is genetically determined. In the latter case, it has been found that the vitamin D receptor gene type is of particular importance for bone density in premenopausal women, since this gene controls calcium absorption.

Postmenopausal woman with the BB genotype (homozygous dominant) were found to have difficulty absorbing calcium when dietary supply was low, whereas those with the recessive bb genotype (homozygous recessive) had better calcium absorption. When the poor absorbers (BB type) were given high doses of calcium in their diets, they were able to maintain normal calcium levels. At RDA levels of 800 milligrams (mg) of calcium, women with the BB genotype will not be able to maintain normal blood calcium levels: they will require at least 1,200 mg of calcium a day.

A recent study of seventy-two elderly women with normal vitamin D levels found that those with the bb genotype had normal spinal bone densities no matter their calcium intake. This means they would not need to take calcium supplements. Those with the BB genotype lost mineral density and required higher calcium intakes to maintain their bone density. Those having one of each of the genes, noted as Bb, had bone densities that varied with calcium intake, that is, the higher the intake, the better the bone density. So, this means that some women might need additional dietary calcium intake after menopause but that a lucky few will not. Yet, it should be understood that control of bone mineralization (strength) is deter-mined by more than calcium intake.

Many doctors, who should know better, have their patients taking 1,500 mg of calcium a day to prevent osteoporosis. They do this out of a mistaken impression that, unless supplemented with additional calcium, all women will develop osteoporosis. Ironically, these are the same doctors who think it is ridiculous to supplement the elderly with additional vitamins and other minerals.

The problem with taking a lot of excess calcium is that calcium is also associated with many destructive reactions in the cell, and these injuries can be accelerated by increasing tissue calcium levels. This is true of Alzheimer's disease, Parkinson's disease, and all other neurodegenerative diseases. It is also true with degenerative diseases of every kind. We know that as we age we lose some of our ability to regulate cellular calcium levels. This means more calcium will leak into the cell, triggering free-radical generation, release of inflammatory chemicals called cytokines, and can lead to increased cell death. We also know that elevating calcium intake can increase the excitotoxic reaction in the brain as well. Later, I will discuss the best ways to improve bone mineral density and protect you from osteoporosis.

Have you ever wondered why some people develop Parkinson's disease and others do not? There is growing evidence that those destined to develop the disease have a defect in iron metabolism within a specialized area of the brain called the striatum. One of the earliest changes in the disease is an accumulation of iron in the part of the brain called the substantia nigra, located deep within the center of the brain. Most likely, the defect is based on a defective gene. There is also evidence that Parkinson's patients have an inherited defect in mitochondrial function, which is responsible for cellular energy production. Both of these defects can lead to destruction of the neurons controlling our motor movement. It is also critical to note that the destruction is carried out by an intense generation of free radicals caused by a combination of excess iron and low energy supply. Again, all of this damage can be mitigated by the judicious use of nutraceuticals and changing one's diet.

Your Nutrition and Your Child's Future

Most books and articles about prenatal nutrition and child development focus on health after conception, that is, after a woman realizes she is pregnant. In reality, nutrition—both the mother's *and* father's—impacts a child long before conception: both the sperm and ova are derived from tissues that are also subject to free-radical attack. This fact is especially important for the mother, because she carries the same ova cells throughout her reproductive life.

Many things we do, and to which we are exposed, have an affect on these delicate reproductive cells. For example, the huge number of free radicals produced by exposure to pesticides and heavy metals, extreme exercise, and prolonged poor nutrition will produce the same cellular damage to the sperm and ova as it does to other cells in the body. In fact, because of the rapid turnover of sperm cells, their nutritional needs may be even greater than cells that divide less often.

In both cases, sperm and ova cells must be protected from the many environmental and internal assaults to which they will be exposed over a lifetime. Sometimes, protecting these cells requires a little imagination and forethought. For example, the young girl who lies on the beach for hours each summer, and then makes regular winter visits to her favorite tanning booth, risks severely damaging her ovaries. The sun's gamma rays are especially destructive—even to internal organs—and without antioxidant protection, this damage can be significant.

Nutrition and the Sperm

Several nutrients significantly improve sperm function and survival. For example, zinc supplementation has been shown to improve sperm counts and motility, which increases the likelihood of successful conception. L-carnitine is another supplement found to improve sperm function and survival.

We know that sperm, like all other cells, depend on the B vitamins for energy production and cell maintenance. These include thiamine, riboflavin, niacinamide, pyridoxine (B_6), panthothenic acid (B_5), folic acid, and methylcobalamin (vitamin B_{12}). The best source of these nutrients is a good wholesome diet consisting daily of five to ten servings of fruits and vegetables, adequate high-quality proteins, and complex carbohydrates low on the glycemic index. Minerals, including magnesium, zinc, chromium, and other trace elements also play a vital role in sperm health.

Unfortunately, most of us do not eat such a healthy hypothetical diet. A recent study of children below age four found that fewer than 25 percent were eating the recommended five servings of fruits and vegetables daily. Adults fared even worse, with fewer than 4 percent even knowing they should be eating ten servings of fruits and vegetables a day. Interestingly, these studies counted french fries as vegetables. As a result, most of us require dietary supplementation—which is not limited to vitamins and minerals but also includes phyto-chemicals.

Sperm, like all cells, must be protected from free-radical injury. Increased testicular heat from taking hot baths or wearing tight underwear can increase free-radical production in the testes, thereby injuring the DNA within the sperm. Such detrimental practices are also associated with increases in testicular cancer in young men as well. Free-radical injury to the sperm, due to extreme exercise, exposure to environmental toxins, poor nutrition, and radiation exposure, can damage the genetic material that contributes to future life. Adequate free-radical protection demands good nutrition in terms of antioxidant minerals, vitamins, and plant flavonoids.

One of the most harmful things a young man can do to his future children is to expose his sperm to the damaging effects of illicit drugs. Proponents of legalizing marijuana rarely address the well-demonstrated fact that tetrahyrocannibol in the marijuana leaf is very genotoxic; that is, it causes the DNA to break in multiple areas.

This means that because you have chosen to smoke marijuana, your children's DNA may be permanently damaged. Other such drugs may also endanger the sperm's genetic integrity. Even smoking is genotoxic because of the large number of free radicals generated by chemicals in cigarette smoke. Studies have shown that the children of smoking males have a higher incidence of all cancers, with an incidence three to four times higher of brain tumors. Over twenty million children and young adults smoke and take illicit drugs on a regular basis: we are creating a society doomed to poor health, populated by citizens whose intellectual capacity will be severely limited.

Nutrition and the Ova

The same factors listed above can also damage the genes within the ovum. More teenage girls are smoking today than ever before, and many will become addicted to cigarettes. Free-radical production associated with smoking causes accelerated aging of all of the body's tissues, including the reproductive cells in the ovaries. A significant number of these same young women are also engaging in drug use, which is very damaging to reproductive cells.

Another common practice among young women is starvation dieting to maintain their image of a supermodel. Often these diets are quite extreme, and young women will skip meals and maintain diets devoid of important nutrients, especially antioxidants. Unfortunately, these diets also include aspartame- and MSG-containing products that can have a deleterious effect on the DNA within the reproductive cells of the ovaries. I will discuss this in more detail later.

Recently, we have become aware that certain types of fats play a vital role in the formation of a baby's brain, and that when these fats are missing from the mother's diet, the baby may later suffer learning difficulties and behavioral problems. One of the most important of these fats is called docosahexaenoic acid or DHA. This fat plays an important role in the formation of the synaptic connections within the brain. These connections allow the various parts of the brain to communicate with each other and communicate with the body as well.

Several recent studies, conducted in both animals and humans, have shown that babies who receive adequate amounts of this vital fat have better functioning brains and higher IQs. Those with low amounts of DHA demonstrate learning difficulties and visual problems. For the unborn baby, the source of this important fat is from the mother's blood, transferred by the placenta. After birth, it must be supplied from the mother's breast milk. Only recently have commercial formulas added DHA. Not surprisingly, several studies have shown that breast fed babies have better brain function and visual acuity than formula-fed babies.

Many teenage girls and boys are also on junk-food diets high in "bad fats." These fats include corn oil, sunflower oil, safflower oil, peanut oil, and, to a lesser degree, canola oil. These oils share several unwelcome characteristics. They increase inflammation, depress the immune system, and impair enzymes necessary to convert other oils (linolenic fats) into DHA oils. This results in a severe depletion of "good fats," which include fish oils and flaxseed oil. Fish oils are composed of two types of fats, EPA and DHA, both of which play a role in protecting the baby's brain from injury.

The brain uses large amounts of DHA for construction of synapses and dendritic connections. EPA is found only in small amounts in the brain, but does seem to play an important role in its function. Consuming flaxseed can enhance the body's store of DHA, but it must be first converted by an enzyme, delta-desaturase. Some people have a poor supply of this enzyme, or what they do have has been damaged by chronic disease, high intake of partially hydrogenated oils, viral infections, or by a high insulin level. In the course of my nutritional practice, I have seen several people who have been unable to convert flaxseed oil to DHA and EPA. This condition can be measured by a metabolic profile test.

In both men and women, extreme exercise can also damage reproductive cells by generating enormous amounts of free radicals. Although aerobics is popular among young women, and such exercise is a good way to keep a trim figure and to feel better, less depressed, and more energetic, the problem with this kind of exercise is that most people do not correspondingly increase their antioxidant intake. This imbalance can lead to severe free-radical injury to all tissues, leading to rapid aging and an early onset of several degenerative diseases. More importantly for those who intend to become parents is the increased risk of genetic damage to their children, including early onset of cardiovascular disease, diabetes, strokes, hypertension, or other degenerative diseases.

As much as possible, everyone should avoid exposure to pesticides, fluoride, toxic metals, and food-additive excitotoxins.

One of the breakdown products of aspartame, an excitotoxin, is formaldehyde. Using a radioactive tracer method, it has been clearly demonstrated that the formaldehyde formed from aspartame accumulates near the DNA in cells, resulting in numerous deletions and strand breaks in the nuclear material. Even more frightening is the finding that the damage is accumulative, so that even drinking one diet cola a day can produce significant genetic damage. There are also several reports of severe aspartame addiction, characterized by the daily consumption of a gallon or more of aspartame-sweetened beverages.

Fluoride—in the forms of fluoridated public water, dental treatments, and fluoride toothpaste—is another oft-ignored but very real danger. Risk to the unborn has been virtually ignored, but we have evidence that it is real and substantial. I encourage everyone to avoid exposure to fluoride. I will discuss fluoride in more depth in chapter four.

Other toxic metals, in particular lead, mercury, and cadmium, are especially dangerous to the developing brain. As we shall see, all of these metals can significantly damage neuron development, and result in impaired brain function.

Finally, food-additive excitotoxins have been shown to have a deleterious effect on the formation of the brain during its critical growth period during the last trimester and the first two years of life, the so-called brain growth spurt. We already know that the ovaries contain numerous glutamate receptors exactly like those found in the brain. And study after study has demonstrated that excitotoxins cause brain damage; if it turns out that glutamate receptors in the ovaries are affected in the same way as are those in the brain, then future generations may be endangered by our eating foods high in certain food additives.

Feeding the Brain During the Growth Spurt

Because of the brain's rapid growth and differentiation early in life, it requires significant amounts of special nutrients. Nutrient deficiencies at this critical period can cause varying degrees of disruption in the development process. Each nutrient plays a special role in brain development. Water-soluble vitamins, such as folate, vitamin B_{12}, thiamine, riboflavin, pantothenic acid, biotin, and ascorbate are critical for normal neuron metabolism, neurotransmitter synthesis, and energy production. They also play a major role in gene function and protein synthesis. Fat-soluble vitamins, especially vitamin A, the carotenoids, and vitamins D, E, and K also play a major role in brain formation and specialization. In addition, vitamins, minerals, and flavonoids play a vital role in protecting the brain from free radicals, which can destroy the delicate projections formed during development.

Free-radical generation during this critical period is also influenced by heavy metals (lead, mercury, arsenic), MSG, aspartame, infections, high fevers, hypoglycemia, and pesticides. During such exposure, a developing baby will need additional protection, and this is why good nutrition is so important. All of the antioxidant defenses, even antioxidant enzymes such as SOD and glutathione peroxidase, depend on our nutrient intake. Flavonoids from fruits and vegetables are especially powerful and versatile antioxidants.

Folate, or folic acid, has gotten a lot of well-deserved attention lately for the role it plays in preventing birth defects. The most common birth defects involve the nervous system, and both folate and vitamin B_{12} are essential for the formation of the nervous system's intricate patterns. Recent studies have found that babies with neural birth defects, such as meningomyelocele (an open spine), hydrocephalus, or anencephaly, frequently have elevated homocysteine levels. Homocysteine is a unique amino acid utilized in the metabolic pathway for DNA maintenance and for the formation of a special substance called S-adenosyl methionine (SAMe) used in many cellular reactions. The conversion of homocysteine for these reactions requires three vitamins: pyridoxine (B_6), folate, and vitamin B_{12}. Even minor deficiencies can result in dangerous elevations in homocysteine.

We have known for some time that supplementing diets with folate can significantly reduce the incidence of neural tube birth defects, as well as other birth defects. What is less well-appreciated is that homocysteine and its breakdown products are also excitotoxins, similar to monosodium glutamate. While it is possible that some of the damaging effect is related to its excitotoxicity, most likely it is the interference with DNA synthesis and maintenance of metabolism that causes problems. Homocysteine levels are also elevated in Alzheimer's disease, and in some individuals who suffer heart attacks and strokes.

Despite what many doctors think, vitamins and minerals are not something invented by the health food industry; they are part of our biological system. Without them all life stops and you die. Vitamin and mineral deficiencies can often lead to disease, and you do not have to be embarrassed about taking vitamin and mineral supplements. The medical and scientific literature supporting nutritional supplements is extensive and goes back over a hundred years. I know many doctors who religiously take supplements themselves but will not recommend them to their patients because of fear of being ridiculed by their colleagues. This is intellectually and morally dishonest.

Because our food has become adulterated by processing methods and certain growing practices, supplementation is more important than ever. Stress has become an integral part of human existence, and stress rapidly depletes our nutrients, especially our antioxidants. In addition, numerous pesticides, herbicides, foreign organic chemicals, fluoride, mercury, aluminum, and other toxic substances, are assaulting our bodies. All of these compounds must be detoxified, putting a heavy demand on our detoxification systems—all of which are dependent on nutrition.

Are the Effects of Nutrient Deficiencies During This Period Reversible?

There is, indeed, some evidence that at least some of these effects are reversible. First, let us look at the developing brain of the infant.

Conventional wisdom has always held that severe nutritional deficiencies during the period of rapid brain growth produces permanent changes in the infant's brain that lead to lower IQ and impaired mental functioning for life. Recent evidence, based on two long-term studies, has cast some doubt on these long-held beliefs. Over a period of several years, researchers studied impoverished children exposed to various diets and social conditions in rural Guatemala and in Cali, Colombia.

In the Guatemala study, researchers followed the progress of children in four impoverished villages in 1969-77 and during a follow-up period in 1988-89. Two thousand children up to age seven, and their mothers, were included in the first study. Two villages were chosen randomly to receive a high-protein, high-calorie drink called Atole containing 11.5 grams of protein and 163 Kcal of energy per cup. The other two villages received a drink without protein and only 59 Kcal of energy, called Fresco. Both drinks contained vitamins and minerals. The drinks were given to the children twice a day, seven days a week throughout the study period.

The follow-up study involved 70 percent of the original participants, at which time they were from twelve to twenty-six years of age. Extensive examinations were done, which included tests of participants' growth, cognitive function, educational achievements, ability to process information, reaction time, literacy, numeracy, general knowledge, tests of reading comprehension, and short-term memory. Motor and mental tests were performed during the first two years of life and the preschool period, and repeated during adolescence using an extensive battery of tests.

Researchers found that children with a low intrauterine growth rate (IUGR-1), when examined from infancy to age twenty-four months, lagged behind normal children in mental development. The preschoolers showed statistically lower verbal scores at thirty-six months but not at forty-eight months of age when compared to normal children. In the IUGR-1 children, performance on memory tests depended on growth after birth, with the taller babies showing better memory than the shorter ones. The taller babies had better nutrition.

The study's real surprise came when children reached adolescence: by this time, there was no difference between the small babies at birth and the normal children, in terms of the school programs. Also, extensive psycho-educational testing at eighteen years of age found no statistically significant difference between the IUGR-1 babies and normal-growth-rate babies. Researchers concluded that intrauterine growth deficiency had only a modest effect on the eventual intellectual outcome of these children; that is, the deleterious effects of poor nutrition during the developmental years reversed itself during adolescence or middle school years.

The test indicated that adequate supplementation allowed this reversal to take place. In fact, the children who were given the nutritional supplement Atole (the high-protein, high-calorie supplement with vitamins and minerals) during intrauterine life through age twenty-four months significantly enhanced their cognitive performance by eighteen years of life on a wide range of cognitive tests. Supplementation also enhanced their information-processing as well. These benefits were less obvious in children who were older than two when the test first began. Also, the Fresco supplement was significantly less effective than the Atole.

The weakness of the study is that babies with very low birth weights were excluded. This means that severe nutritional deficiency could, and most likely does, severely impact brain development and may produce permanent changes in the brain. Whether nutritional supplementation could reverse such defects is possible but was not tested in this study.

The second study in Cali, Colombia studied the effects of providing health services and educational stimulation in the intellectual function of children born to impoverished mothers. These children were also given nutritional supplementation, but treatment did not begin until the children were older—at 42, 56, 60, and 72 months of life. Despite the late onset of treatment and educational stimulation, the cognitive test scores of these children were nearly the same as those of middle- and high-income children. When tested two years later, the beneficial effects persisted. The earlier the stimulation began, and the longer it persisted, the greater the benefit.

When we consider both of these studies together, we see that they conform to common sense: everyone needs to practice good nutrition before conception, and women should practice good nutrition throughout pregnancy and during breast-feeding. We should provide our children with educational stimulation, love, and warmth. In this way, they will develop not only intellectually, but psychologically and spiritually as well. The importance of these studies is that they emphasize that application of good nutrition is never too late.

What About Adults?

One of the great concerns of those who have reached middle age is, have I deteriorated so much that things are hopeless? As a result of this way of thinking, most people will just eat what they enjoy and live out what life they have left. What many of these people do not consider is that they won't just die after they've finished enjoying themselves: the lucky ones may suddenly die of a heart attack or get hit by a car. Yet for most of us, that will not happen.

I remember walking through a hospital with a doctor friend of mine, a fellow in his middle years, when he suddenly stopped and peered thoughtfully into a ward full of sickly looking elderly people. I stared with him at the elderly patients scattered about the room, with their emaciated legs wrapped in tangles of stained sheets, mouths open in perfect ovals, sunken eyes staring off into some netherworld, unaware of little but their pain and humiliation. IV bags could be seen dangling from metal poles and catheters coursed from under the stained sheets, attached to bags of cloudy urine, filling the room with a heavy smell of death. The doctor slowly shook his head back and forth, looked up at me with doleful sadness and said, "These are the golden years."

You see, most of us will not be spared the pain and suffering of age. Rather than dying that death we all dream about—going peacefully in our sleep—we will instead undergo a series of health crises, such as multiple heart attacks with years of medication and limitations on our activity, maybe even a loss of employment. Or, we may suffer from a stroke that leaves us paralyzed and unable to speak, dependent on others for the simplest things, such as eating or going to the bathroom.

Frequently, we may suffer from slowly progressing arthritis, undefined aches and pains, unexplained weakness, headaches, deteriorating vision, difficulty concentrating, and a memory that fails us more often than not. Still others will be crippled by diabetes or a neurodegenerative disease such as Parkinson's disease or Alzheimer's dementia. Unfortunately, all of these so-called diseases of aging are now occurring in younger people, not just the elderly. We are seeing Parkinson's disease in forty-year-olds and type II diabetes in teenagers.

My experience with treating many such patients has been sobering, especially when you consider that for most of us life doesn't have to end this way. Extensive scientific studies on nutrition and nutritional supplementation have demonstrated that many disorders associated with aging can be avoided, or at least significantly reduced, by following simple nutritional guidelines and avoiding behaviors that increase our risk. The earlier such programs are begun, the more effective they are. A program of good health will reduce disease and complications of disease at any age.

Nutrition can alter the course of even a major disease, such as heart attack. It has been shown experimentally that tying off one of a dog's coronary arteries will induce a heart attack, and the amount of destruction to the heart muscle can be extensive. If that same animal is fed powerful antioxidants before the heart attack, the amount of heart tissue destroyed can be reduced by half. Incredibly, feeding antioxidants soon after the vessel has been tied off protects the heart muscle.

In the past it was thought that the damaging effects of a heart attack or stroke were due to death of the tissue fed by the artery, that is, a direct loss of the oxygen and glucose supply. Now we know that much of the damage is caused by the build-up of toxic free radicals and lipid-peroxidation products. In strokes, damage results from brain cells releasing glutamate, triggered by a loss of oxygen and glucose.

Free radicals are also generated during a heart attack. These radicals destroy not only the tissue fed directly by the artery but also seep into surrounding normal heart tissue, causing extensive damage to a much wider area. Free-radical accumulation following bodily trauma has been measured in numerous animal and human studies, and is no longer theoretical. Because free radicals can kill in such a wide zone, it is vital to protect as much of the tissue as possible.

So we see that good nutrition and antioxidant supplementation can significantly protect us from disease, but if a disease does occur, its seriousness can also be greatly reduced. This is true not only in heart attacks and strokes, but also in diabetes, hypertension, lupus, rheumatoid arthritis, chemical toxicity, cancer, and a host of other diseases. Now let us look at some specific examples of diseases caused by environmental toxins.

3
Mercury: The Silent Killer

Mercury is considered by toxicologists to be one of the most poisonous naturally occurring substances on the earth. Because of its tremendous toxicity, it is carefully regulated by the EPA, the Occupational Safety and Health Administration (OSHA) and other regulatory bodies. The amount allowed in the atmosphere is fewer than 50 ug/M³, fifty-millionths of a gram per cubic meter of air. In the summer of 1990 the EPA banned the use of mercury-containing interior latex paint after discovering that levels of mercury in the urine of occupants living in recently painted houses could reach 118 micrograms (ug) per gram of creatine, a level associated with human toxicity. Such levels could produce subtle neurological damage such as memory loss, irritability, difficulty concentrating, and tremors.

Previous experience with mercury has already demonstrated that high mercury levels in the environment could produce widespread injury to humans, as well as to wildlife. For example, between the years 1932 and 1968 in Minamata Bay, Japan, the world witnessed one of the two largest outbreaks of mercury poisoning in history. During this extended period the Chisso Factory of Minamata produced and dumped one hundred tons of mercury into the Minamata Bay in the process of manufacturing acetic acid, used in making vinyl chloride for floor tiles and artificial leather. By 1982 over 1,773 residents of the area were suffering from severe mercury toxicity, and 456 of these people eventually died. A follow-up study found that in truth over five thousand people were suffering from mercury-related neurological diseases. Most of the survivors continue to suffer severe neurological effects of the exposure.

In 1971 Iraqi officials reported that 6,530 people were severely damaged by, and 459 people died from, ingesting corn treated with a mercurial fungicide. Later, more accurate figures indicated that 50,000 people were poisoned and over 5,000 died.[1] The problem began following a major drought, during which the government decided to switch to a more resistant variety of wheat ordered from Mexico. Because of a single typographical error in labeling, a fungicide containing the infinitely more toxic methylmercury had been used on the wheat. The illiterate peasants of Iraq used the wheat to make their pita breads and other cereals. Similar but smaller scale disasters occurred in Sweden, Canada, Pakistan, the United States and Guatemala.

In one tragic case of self-inflicted mercury poisoning, an ingenious fellow managed to kill himself and three family members when he attempted to smelt silver from dental amalgams in a frying pan, not knowing the "silver" was in fact mostly mercury.[2] An autopsy study demonstrated severe destruction of large areas of his brain. A second similar incident resulted in the deaths of four people: mercury levels in that case were so high that the house had to be demolished.[3]

The reason I cite these cases is not to compare high-level mercury exposure to low-level but first, to emphasize the destructive nature of mercury on the nervous system, and second, to point out the danger caused by the American Dental Association's (ADA) refusal to publicly state that dental amalgam fillings contain a high level of mercury, and that the mercury escaping from them can cause serious harm to humans.

High-dose acute or chronic exposures were responsible for casualties in all of the cases cited above. More recently, increased scrutiny has focused on effects of chronic exposure to low levels of mercury in its various forms. You may recall that for many years scientists insisted that lead, another hazardous metal, was only dangerous following high-dose exposure: it took twenty years for medical and toxicological science to acknowledge that exposure to even minute amounts of lead could be devastating, especially to the nervous system of the developing neonate and small child. It is also important to remember that before science officially recognized the destructive effects of lead, people who tried to raise early warnings about low-level lead toxicity were ignored or labeled "alarmists" by elitists in the fields of toxicology and medical science. The same thing is now happening with mercury and those who promote the use of products containing mercury: warnings are being ignored.

Many of us are being exposed to levels of mercury that have been demonstrated to significantly affect the nervous and immune systems and other biological structures. For instance, children and adults are being exposed to mercury in a multitude of ways: through vaccines, medications, broken thermometers, antiseptics, industrial usage, contaminated fish, and dental amalgams. Mercury use is so widespread in certain industries that many workers are occupationally exposed every day to this toxic metal (see Figure 3.1). Most of us will also recall that when we were sick as children and running a fever, our parents would frighten us with stories of a horrible death if we bit into the mercury thermometer in our mouths. It was true: entire households have been poisoned when mercury from a broken thermometer was vacuumed up.

In the 1940s children began appearing in pediatricians' offices with flushed faces, pink hands that constantly shed skin, and signs of various neurological illnesses. Because of the light pink coloration of their faces and hands the condition was named "pink disease." In 1950 fifty-seven children died of the mysterious disorder. Doctors and scientists were baffled as to its cause and suggested everything from an infectious disease to food allergies. Some noted that many of its features resembled mercury poisoning, but they were ignored until it finally came to light that a teething powder used by the children contained high concentrations of mercury: when the teething powder was withdrawn from the market "pink disease" disappeared.

There now exists an enormous body of medical literature documenting the deleterious effects of chronic low-level mercury exposure. Effects of such exposure can vary significantly depending on the predominant tissue and/or organs involved, as well as other factors.

```
+----------------------------------------------------------+
|            Symptoms of Mercury Poisoning                 |
|  • personality changes      • insomnia                   |
|  • unusual irritability      • apathy                    |
|  • timidity or shyness       • impaired concentration    |
|  • weakness                  • suicidal disposition      |
|                                                          |
|  TABLE 3.1                                               |
+----------------------------------------------------------+
```

Although mercury exposure can damage many bodily systems, the nervous, immune, and cardiovascular systems suffer the most adverse effects of such chronic exposure, and there is growing evidence that mercury toxicity plays a vital role in a significant number of cases of Alzheimer's disease as well as other neurodegenerative diseases. First let us explore the history of mercury toxicity.

Where Does Mercury Come From?

Mercury occurs naturally across the earth due to degassing of the earth's crust. This constant release of the earth's supply of mercury into lakes, streams, and oceans releases anywhere from 25,000-150,000 tons per year; however, most human contact with this deadly toxin comes from man-made sources such as dental amalgam, beauty creams, mirrors, medications, vaccinations, coal-burning, and other industrial uses. Fossil fuels such as coal may contain as much as 1 ppm of mercury. It has been estimated that as much as 5,000 tons of mercury are released into the atmosphere every year from burning coal and natural gas and refining petroleum products.

A very dense element with many unusual physical properties, mercury is the only common metal that exists as a liquid at ordinary temperatures. Due to its high surface tension, it beads easily when spilled and its high density led to its use in barometers. Its high rate of thermal expansion is fairly constant over a wide range of temperatures which makes it an obvious, though far from safe, choice for use in thermometers.

Mercury can occur in three forms: in its elemental form as a pure metal, or combined with other elements to form organic and inorganic compounds. Rarely found uncombined in nature, mercury is usually encountered as cinnabar, mercuric sulfide ore. For commercial use, the metal is easily separated by roasting the ore in air. It is then purified by repeated vacuum distillation, and combined with other metals to form compounds and organic salts that are applied in a wide range of industrial uses. Mercury, when it combines with other metals, also forms a special kind of alloy called an amalgam; one such amalgam—of mercury, silver, and tin—is used in dentistry for filling teeth. Organic mercury, compounds of mercury that contain carbon, can be found as methyl-, ethyl- and phenylmercury in nature.

Two forms of mercury, mercury vapor from metal mercury and the organic compounds, methylmercury and ethylmercury, should be of particular concern to readers. Metallic mercury (such as that found in dental amalgam) constantly releases a vapor that is similar to the clouds of smoke emitted from dry ice, except that mercury vapor is not only invisible but dangerous.

Human methylmercury exposure comes mainly from eating contaminated fish; unlike metal mercury, the methylmercury compound is highly absorbable from the gastrointestinal tract. Elemental mercury and mercury salts, although fairly inert when deposited on the bottom of waterways, are converted to organic mercury by microorganisms—a similar process occurs in our mouths when bacteria comes into contact with the mercury in our fillings. In nature, methylmercury enters the food chain where it is biomagnified up to 100,000 times in predacious fish. Consumption of toxic fish and of game birds and mammals that feed on fish is the main risk to humans.

Large sea animals, such as sharks, swordfish, and large tuna have some of the highest mercury levels of any edible seafood—and the highest levels of all are found in whales. Canned tuna is taken from smaller species and has considerably less mercury than larger tuna. Periodically, high mercury levels are also found in various fresh water species. This is especially a problem where hydroelectric plants have stagnated the waters, and where mercurial fungicides drain into lakes and streams near farmland.

Seafood is periodically checked for methylmercury levels and warnings are released to the public when concentrations exceed safe levels. The problem lies in the fact that we do not know the full effect of chronic absorption of even small concentrations of methylmercury.

Mad as a Hatter

Most of us have heard this expression, but few people are aware of its tragic source. The phrase originated in Britain where felt hat-makers used quicksilver (mercury nitrate) in making hats. The ingredient was a trade secret in the industry from the 1600s to the 1800s. Unfortunately, as a result of exposure to the toxic metal, a significant number of workers were afflicted with poor memory, inappropriate behavior, shyness, and a tremor that resulted in the labels "mad hatter" and "hatter's shakes."

Similar problems afflicted cinnabar miners. Cinnabar, ground into the pigment vermilion, is valued chiefly as the source of metal mercury. After years of working in mines, workers would often suffer from crippling neurological and mental disorders. Many powerful men were reduced to frail, trembling weaklings wracked with multiple neurological problems. The same conditions also existed in mirror-manufacturing plants where mercury was used in combination with tin to make the mirrored surface. But perhaps the most widespread use of mercury was in medications, especially those used to treat syphilis.

These medications were combined in creative ways and used in both children and adults. Mercury was combined with chalk and honey of rose and made into plasters, ointments, and even suppositories. Intravenous injections of mercury, as well as specially designed inhalations of mercury vapor were given for syphilis. Inunction, the use of mercurial ointments, was common. Another interesting compound called unquentum hydrargyri dilutum (USP or blue ointment) was rubbed along the inner thighs, chest, back, or abdomen as a daily treatment for syphilis.

One ingenious delivery method, described as an "improved technique," involved direct inhalation of mercury vapor produced by heating amorphous mercury over an alcohol lamp. A tube, which was held in place by a headband, ran from the generating apparatus to the patient's nose. The medical textbook in which this treatment appeared stated that the patient could thus read and be comfortable for hours. Another method of delivery involved a bib soaked with 90 percent mercurial ointment. The mercolint bib was fitted over the chest and back and worn until the blue fabric turned white, a sign that all of the mercury had been absorbed into the patient's body. The author stated that it was the best method to use with children. It is interesting to note that this 1927 textbook of medicine, one of the most presti-

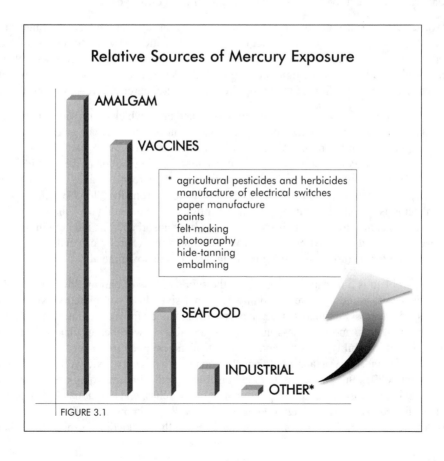

Relative Sources of Mercury Exposure

AMALGAM

VACCINES

* agricultural pesticides and herbicides
  manufacture of electrical switches
  paper manufacture
  paints
  felt-making
  photography
  hide-tanning
  embalming

SEAFOOD

INDUSTRIAL

OTHER*

FIGURE 3.1

gious of its time, had no restrictions for use by pregnant women before their sixth month of pregnancy.

The use of mercurial medications to treat syphilis became so common throughout the industrialized world that millions of people already tormented by the debilitating effects of syphilis were also forced to endure acute mercury poisoning. It is interesting to note that one of the most common diagnoses for admission to mental hospitals during this period was neurosyphilis (called "general paresis of the insane"). One can only speculate as to how many of these unfortunate individuals were in truth suffering from neurological mercury toxicity, rather than syphilitic damage to the brain. The use of mercury to treat syphilis was one of the greatest medical disasters of all times, since it had little effect on syphilis itself.

While mercolint bibs may be a thing of the past, dentists have been using a special mixture or amalgam, consisting of mercury, tin, zinc, and other metals for filling teeth for over 150 years. This so-called "silver filling," composed of approximately 50 percent mercury, constantly releases vapor that is highly absorbed by the tissues of the mouth and nose. Today, Americans get over 180 million amalgam fillings every year.

So we see that mercury poisoning has been a problem throughout the history of industrialized nations. Unfortunately, the problem is not getting better, only worse. Our knowledge about the effects of long-term exposure is somewhat limited, but a significant number of recent studies have shed some light on the potentially serious effects of such exposure. One problem we have is our limited ability to directly measure mercury levels in living tissues.

Most studies involve measurements of hair, blood, and urine which do provide a reasonable measure of acute and subacute mercury exposure, but tell little about actual soft tissue accumulation (i.e., in the brain). We have autopsy studies that provide enough information to make reasonable conclusions concerning organ levels during the life of the individual, but we still do not know about the dynamic movement of mercury in a living system. For example, when mercury is absorbed, how does it move from the blood plasma into the central nervous system? Does it move from other tissues into the brain over time? How long does it take mercury to leave the body once it has been absorbed? The half-life in the brain has been calculated to be extremely long. We also know that exercise can cause mercury to move throughout the body, increasing the brain load of this toxic metal.

Another problem is our inability to measure the subtle effects of chronic low-level toxicity of virulent compounds. Acute poisoning with massive doses of mercury is clinically obvious, with such symptoms as abdominal cramping, kidney failure, tremor, hallucinations, muscular weakness, and numbness in the hands and feet. Lower mercury levels frequently cause unusual irritability, timidity, and suicidal tendencies. Even lower levels may produce symptoms that most physicians would not even connect to mercury toxicity. Symptoms such as frequent colds, joint pains, autoimmune disorders, and subtle neurological dysfunction, such as an inability to think clearly, poor memory, headaches, and emotional disorders, may never be linked to real but undiagnosed metal toxicity. We do know, as I will show, that even very low levels of mercury can interrupt numerous cellular functions, especially in brain cells (neurons). There is growing evidence that low-level chronic mercury exposure is associated with numerous disorders, including multiple sclerosis, Alzheimer's dementia, Parkinson's disease, and ALS.

How the ADA Is Covering Up a Medical Disaster

Dentists began using mercury amalgams to fill cavities over 150 years ago. Amalgams are, in fact, mixtures of various substances used to fill cavities, and include 45-52 percent mercury, 30 percent silver, and small amounts of zinc, tin, and copper. Mercury amalgams began to be used because they were so much cheaper than gold and true silver fillings. Use of amalgams eventually became so widespread that the American Society of Dental Surgeons, the first dental society in the United States, attempted to put a stop to its use by requiring its members to sign a pledge that stated: "It is my opinion and firm conviction that any amalgam whatever is unfit for the plugging (filling) of teeth."

So many dentists were removed from the society because of amalgam violations that the society itself finally collapsed by 1850. Profits from using the new amalgams were just too great to resist. As a result, the ousted members formed their own society in 1859 called the American Dental Association. Today, the ADA is one of the best-funded dental organizations in the world, with over $27 million in annual dues and $10 million more from grants and support from dental product manufacturers and advertisers. Not surprisingly, it uses its money and political clout to further its often-nefarious aims. The ADA is ranked as one of the thirty largest PACs in the nation.

As Dr. David Kennedy, a dentist opposed to the use of dental amalgams, states in his book, *How to Save Your Teeth*, the ADA makes the official claim that "Amalgam restorations continue to be shown safe for the vast majority of dental patients … indeed for the vast majority of patients the benefits of using amalgam restorations far outweigh any risk." As we shall see, there is considerable evidence that mercury from dental amalgams is extremely hazardous to human health.

Mercury was already known to be a danger to human health when amalgams were first introduced in the United States over 150 years ago. So how can the ADA justify their stand on safety? They simply tell the unwary public, as well as their own members, that "Mercury is made virtually harmless when it combines with other metals used to produce amalgam." Dr. Kennedy states unequivocally, "This is an out-and-out lie." As we shall see, Dr. Kennedy is right on target.

Another distortion of the truth is that mercury in human tissues comes primarily from the diet, especially from seafood. In truth, we get almost seven times more mercury from dental amalgams as from fish and other seafood. In an attempt to stem the rising tide of dentists publicly expressing concerns about using amalgam, the ADA then tried to make it unethical for dentists to remove the toxic substance from their patients. They added in their code of ethics the following language: "The removal of amalgam restorations from the non-allergic patient for the alleged purpose of removing toxic substances from the body, when such treatment is performed solely at the recommendation or suggestion of the dentist, is improper and unethical."

Now you might conclude from the wording that the ADA has a legitimate point, since an unscrupulous dentist could frighten his patients into paying for a very expensive procedure, whether or not it was based on good science. The real problem is that the ADA leadership knew that medical doctors were generally unaware of the issue of amalgam toxicity, and so would not be inclined to send their patients to a dentist for removal of amalgam fillings. This keeps the issue "in house."

As a further safeguard against dental rogues breaking ranks, many local and state dental boards will revoke dentists' licenses for removing dental amalgams. Many dentists have already had their licenses revoked for even *refusing* to use dental amalgams in their practices. In other words, the ADA forces dentists to harm patients so the organization can continue the charade that amalgam fillings are safe.

Is Mercury Absorbed From Dental Amalgam Fillings?

This is the pivotal question—and the one most often denied by the ADA. That mercury does indeed leak from dental amalgam was first discovered in 1926 by the German scientist, Dr. Alfred Stock.[4] His findings were confirmed in 1979 by Dr. Gay and co-workers[5], and again in 1981 by Dr. Carl Svare.[6] Dr. Svare conducted experiments in volunteers among his dental students to see if the amalgams in their mouths released mercury. One student, growing hungry, left during the long wait to be tested and returned eating a slice of pizza. When she was tested, the doctor was shocked to see that she had enormously high mercury levels in her readings. Thinking it might be the pizza that contained the mercury, he had it tested. When the levels came back negative, he had her repeat the breath test, but this time had her chew on a piece of rubber tubing. Once again her mercury vapor levels were sky high.

Based on this "chewing gum study" other researchers repeated the experiment under better controlled conditions and found similar results[7]: chewing dramatically increases release of mercury from dental amalgams. The EPA sets the maximum acceptable dose of mercury, other than from air, at 10 ug. The average dental amalgam filling contains 750,000 ug of mercury, so the store of mercury in fillings is considerable.

One researcher found that chewing gum for five minutes led to a threefold increase in the release of mercury vapor from amalgam fillings, while chewing in controls without fillings had no effect on mercury levels. When test subjects rinsed with hot water he saw a further increase in mercury vapor release. His conclusion was that the amalgam alloy is unstable and constitutes a source of long-term mercury exposure that is toxicologically unsuitable as a dental filling material.[8] A large number of people chew gum, not just for five minutes but for hours at a time. In addition, nearly everyone consumes hot food and liquids on a daily basis. People who do both have the highest mercury vapor levels and hence the highest blood and tissue levels.

In another study, Zander and colleagues found, in examining ninety-three males and females aged eighteen to sixty-three years of age, that those with dental amalgams had significantly higher urine mercury levels than subjects without amalgams.[9] In addition, urinary mercury levels were highly correlated with the number of amalgam surfaces. (Dentists count amalgam fillings according to the number of sides of the tooth containing amalgam, called surfaces.) They concluded that mercury exposure from dental amalgams is greater than from food or other sources.

Several studies have shown that mercury vapor from dental amalgams can reach levels of from 6 to 150 ug/M^3.[10] The EPA banned mercury-containing latex paint for producing mercury vapor levels of 2-3 ug/M^3. While you might spend an inordinate amount of time in your house, your teeth follow you everywhere.

One study involving thirty-five subjects found that chewing markedly elevated oral mercury levels which then slowly declined over ninety minutes when chewing was stopped. Those with twelve or more mercury amalgam surfaces had levels reaching 29 ug a day, whereas those with four or fewer had 8 ug of mercury released daily. These levels alone exceed by a factor of eighteen those set as allowable mercury exposure from all sources.

Another consideration is manipulation of your fillings by a dentist. A high-speed dental drill can release mercury levels as high as 4,000 ug/M^3 eighteen inches from the drill. (Remember, 50 ug/M^3 is the limit set by the EPA for safe occupational exposure.) This high concentration of mercury is absorbed by the tissues of your mouth and distributed throughout your body. The dentist and his assistant share in this mercury cloud. In fact, even unwary patients sitting in the waiting room are exposed to high mercury vapor levels.

It is also important to realize that approximately 80 percent of the mercury released by your fillings is being constantly absorbed and stored in your body. For example, if your fillings release 12 ug of mercury a day, in a week you will have absorbed 67.2 ug, and in a month 288 ug. A small portion of that dose will be excreted, but most of it will be stored in your body. We already know that absorbed mercury accumulates in the nervous system. In fact, studies have shown that brain levels of mercury increase about three- to fourfold in those with dental amalgams compared to those without. Mercury from amalgams was found to saturate gum tissues as well as the jawbone itself.

It should be appreciated that not all people release mercury from their amalgams at the same rate. One Swedish study found that some people release as much as 23-63 ug/g of creatinine of mercury daily, indicating a daily uptake of 100 ug a day, well within the toxic range.[11] This number is five to ten times higher than the average found in the general population of Sweden.

Every day, we do many things that increase the release of mercury vapor from amalgam fillings: chew gum, brush our teeth, use a water pick, have dental work done or our teeth cleaned, and consume hot foods and drinks. Even undergoing general anesthesia poses a risk due to oral manipulation by the anesthesiologist during intubation and mechanical stimulation to the teeth by the endotrachial tube.

Removing amalgams without taking special precautions dramatically increases mercury blood levels for over a month. One study found that immediately following removal of amalgam fillings, plasma mercury levels rose three- to fourfold and tissue levels rose by 50 percent. Also, such a concentrated release of mercury vapor can severely exacerbate pre-existing neurological conditions.

Once amalgam fillings are removed, mercury levels will slowly decline. One study, in which seventeen people had their amalgams removed, found that mercury levels actually increased 30 percent during the first week, slowly declining over the next twelve months.[12] In this study the mean half-life of blood mercury was ninety-five days. Unfortunately, removal from the nervous system is incomplete and occurs at a much slower rate.

A final study clearly refutes the ADA's lie that mercury is not released from amalgam fillings. In this study, subjects of all ages were examined for the concentration of mercury in their saliva prior to and after chewing.[13] The data were obtained following ten minutes of chewing sugar-free gum. In the study group, children had an average of three fillings, thirty- to thirty-four-year-olds had the greatest number of fillings, and older individuals had an average of five fillings. (In older people, the lower average was due to the fact that many had lost teeth.)

Researchers found a direct correlation between the number of amalgam fillings and mercury levels in the subjects' saliva, although values varied considerably. People at the low end of the curve tested for less than 5 ug/l of mercury in their saliva and those at the high-end had values over 1,000 ug/l. Approximately 1.7 percent of the subjects had mercury values greater than 400 ug/l. In all, 30 percent of the people examined had mercury values above those suggested by the World Health Organization (WHO) as being acceptable. It is important to note that WHO admits there is actually no truly safe level of mercury exposure.

Extrapolating from this study, we see that when we are dealing with very large numbers of people, for example 200 million in the United States alone, this puts over sixty million people at a very high risk of mercury toxicity. Within this number are a significant percentage of people with low levels of antioxidant defenses and other metabolic derangements that place them at even higher risk.

It is critical to note that two age groups were found to be in the highest risk categories for mercury absorption from dental amalgams: women of child-bearing age (twenty to thirty-nine years) and children between the ages of six and nine. As we shall see, it is the developing child's brain that is most at risk.

A word of caution concerning animal studies. Often we assume that the effects of toxin exposure in animals correspond to those in humans, but this is not always so. For example, compared to humans, cats have a tenfold higher resistance to the uptake of methylmercury across the blood-brain barrier. To produce chemical imbalance (ataxia) using mercury in cats requires a minimum dose of 46 ug/kg/day and blood levels of 6-8 ppm. In humans, ataxia occurs after a dose of only 4 ug/kg/day or 0.6 ppm of mercury. This means that humans may be much more sensitive than animals to mercury. We find a similar phenomenon with amphetamine. Many animals have physiological and biochemical systems quite different than humans, yet as far as we can tell, humans, rats, and mice appear to react similarly to mercury exposure.

What About Dentists?

I know that as you read this material your first reaction will be anger at your dentist, but remember that your dentist has been lied to, just as we have. Their union, the ADA, has done all they can to cover up information—not only about mercury toxicity but also about the dangers of fluoride (which I will discuss in much more detail in the next section)—and to give false assurances to their members that rumors of toxicity are nothing more than baseless scare tactics by health fanatics.

Dentists should be out in the forefront fighting this battle: this is an opportunity not only to redeem themselves, but also to help in the battle to prevent others from being harmed by the dangerous practice of using amalgam fillings. In all actuality, the dentist and his or her assistants are at the highest risk for mercury toxicity.

The first lie perpetuated by the ADA leadership, as well as professors in dental schools, and among practicing dentists was that mercury vapor does not escape from amalgams because it is bound to other metals in the amalgam that render it inert. As you have seen, this is not true—and they knew it. Knowing they had no defense scientifically, they then resorted to making removal of dental amalgams a violation of ethical standards, and finally they influenced licensing boards to pull the licenses of recalcitrant dentists who refused to maintain the lie. Recently, the ADA has even gone to far as to distribute brochures to dentists' offices assuring patients that amalgam fillings present no danger. This is unconscionable.

Mercury levels in 15-20 percent of dentists' offices have been shown to exceed OSHA limits for ambient mercury exposure.[14] A recent study is even more alarming, for the dentists, their assistants, and patients. In this study, measurements were taken from the dental aspirator vent (the little tube the dentists hangs in your mouth) to see if the vapor contained high levels of mercury.[15] The study demonstrated that, after twenty minutes of operation, at the dentist's level (which is also the patient's level) mercury vapor concentration was ten times higher than the current safety limit set by OSHA.

Mercury vapor build-up occurred within the tubing, and researchers noted that as the vacuum motor heated up, the mercury vapor level increased. They then tested the air being released beyond the bacterial filter and found that because particulate amalgam was trapped in the filter, even greater mercury vapor contamination occurred. In this study, the mercury vapor by the end of the day filled the work area and ventilation systems pumped this vapor out into the patient waiting area. Unsuspecting patients had no idea that they were receiving a significant dose of mercury even as they waited to be seen.

While a patient will be exposed to dangerously high levels of mercury vapor only while undergoing treatment, the dentist will suffer the effects of prolonged and cumulative exposure. One study conducted in Singapore compared dentists who use amalgams with those who did not, and found that dentists exposed to dental mercury restoratives had higher aggressive mood scores when tested with a battery of psychological tests.[16] They also did poorly on a wide variety of other neuropsychological tests, including immediate and delayed recall. Similar results were found among American dentists who use dental amalgams in their practices.[17] This study found that older dentists in particular, when compared to controls matched for age and other variables, were found to be significantly impaired for memory retrieval and other neurobehavioral functions.

A more recent test of the effects of occupational dental exposure to mercury found a mean urinary mercury level among nineteen exposed dentists of 36 ug/l.[18] This is seven times higher than the estimated national average for dentists. These dentists were examined with a battery of tests including a Profile of Mood Scale, a medical questionnaire, and six behavioral tests. The results were analyzed by multivariate regression technique to evaluate the dose effect while controlling for age, race, gender and exposure to alcohol. They found a strong correlation between urinary mercury levels and poor mental concentration, emotional liability, sensory irritability and mood scores. In conclusion, they stated that the results provided evidence for subtle preclinical changes in behavior associated with chronic low-dose exposure to mercury.

It is interesting to note that in several European countries—Germany, Austria, Denmark, and Sweden—the use of dental amalgams has either been banned or is in the process of a scheduled phase-out. The largest producer of dental amalgams in Germany announced that it would no longer provide the substance to dentists because of pending and future lawsuits.

California's 1992 Watson law (written by then State Senator Diane Watson, now a congresswoman) required the state's Dental Board to list the risks associated with amalgam so that consumers would be able to make informed choices knowing that "silver" fillings are mostly mercury, and that such content poses health risks. The law also requires dentists to get permission from patients before placing hazardous substances in their mouths. Unfortunately, most dentists have simply ignored this law and refuse to post the warning.

Furthermore, many insurance providers—including Medicaid and Medicare—will pay for amalgam fillings but not for safer non-mercury composites, but the additional expense of composite fillings would pay for itself in the improved health of recipients, and recipients would be far less susceptible to onset of neurological diseases in later life.

How Does Mercury Harm You?

Mercury harms biological systems in many ways. Like its cousins, cadmium and lead, mercury greatly increases free-radical production within the cell and lipid peroxidation in the cell membrane. In fact, much of the damage done by mercury results from free-radical injury, which involves all of a cell's components.

Once absorbed, mercury is distributed to all parts of a cell with a set distribution: 48 percent resides in the mitochondria, 38 percent in the nucleus, 8 percent in the cytoplasm, and 7 percent in the microsomes.[19] In the cell's nucleus, mercury binds tightly to all of the nucleic bases of DNA and as a result is mutagenic, causing the cell to mutate.[20] Mercury has also been shown to damage the membrane lining the mitochondria, thereby impairing its ability to regulate calcium levels in the cell, which can trigger cell death. Once mercury triggers lipid peroxidation within the cell membrane, additional destructive chemicals—with interesting names like peroxyl ions and 4-hydroxynonenal—are produced, greatly magnifying the original damage. Recent studies have also shown that mercury, even in low concentrations, can impair a cell's protective antioxidant systems. One of the ways this occurs is by binding with the cell's principal protection molecule, glutathione. One molecule of mercury has been shown to bind with two molecules of glutathione, leading to its inactivation and removal.

Mercury inhibits the function of several antioxidant enzymes, which puts cells at great risk and, as we have already seen, many diseases are associated with impaired antioxidant protection, including diabetes, hypertension, cardiovascular disease, strokes, and neurodegenerative diseases.

Mercury inhibits two other enzymes, called glutathione reductase and glutathione synthease, which are responsible for free-radical protection. Another antioxidant system impaired by mercury is called superoxide dismutase (SOD). Its job is to convert the dangerous superoxide free radical into peroxide. The peroxide is then converted to water by another enzyme called glutathione peroxidase. This enzyme is also inhibited by mercury. Several experiments have demonstrated the poisoning power of mercury on all of these protective antioxidant enzymes. When these enzymes and antioxidants are crippled by mercury, the nervous system, as well as the rest of the body, is completely vulnerable and defenseless against the free radicals generated both by the mercury itself and by other processes.

One study of forty-two workers in a chloralkali plant that uses mercury found that workers exposed to mercury vapor experienced significant decreases in their antioxidant enzyme levels, as well as increased lipid-peroxidation levels.[21] So this effect of mercury is not unique to experimental animals, but occurs in humans as well.

It has also been shown that sensitivity to mercury toxicity is directly related to the existing antioxidant protection in a person's cells prior to the exposure. For example, if you practice poor nutrition and as a result have poor antioxidant defenses before being exposed to mercury, you are more likely to suffer greater toxicity than someone with adequate antioxidant protection and good general nutrition. Certain nutrients, such as vitamins C and E, magnesium, zinc, alpha-lipoic acid, and selenium, are especially important: they not only act as powerful antioxidants, but some can actually remove mercury from tissues. It is interesting to note that the idea of a variable sensitivity to mercury toxicity was known as far back as 1888. Dr. W.R. Gowers, one of the great men of neurology, noted in his textbook in 1900 on diseases of the nervous system, *A Manual of Diseases of the Nervous System*, under the chapter on mercury poisoning: "The weakly suffer more readily than the strong, and individual differences in susceptibility vary greatly."

Another way mercury can damage cells is by interfering with protein synthesis, the building of proteins for the cell. Rats exposed to inorganic mercury experience dramatic reductions in protein synthesis, primarily because of mercury binding to RNA and DNA.[22] During the period of rapid brain growth, interference with DNA or RNA function, and hence protein synthesis, retards brain development.

In addition, mercury also binds very tightly to special chemical bonds called sulfhydral groups (-SH), which are found throughout living systems. This is very important because many of the hundreds of enzymes within the body depend on these sulfhydral groups for their activity. These enzymes are concerned with everything from energy production, DNA repair, cell signaling, membrane structure, digestion of proteins, and antioxidant protection.

Mercury also poses special risks to the brain. In the nervous system, a loss of energy production—which accompanies mercury toxicity—increases the brain's release of glutamate, leading to even further damage. Brain cells deprived of energy are up to one hundred times more sensitive to glutamate excitotoxic injury and death than cells with normal energy supplies. This damage by glutamate further increases free-radical production, leading to a vicious cycle that ends in the death of the surrounding brain cells in large numbers, a mechanism that may be responsible for many neurodegenerative diseases.

In its metallic form mercury is poorly absorbed from the GI tract but constantly releases highly absorbable mercury vapor, especially through the mucous membranes lining the mouth, nasal passages and lungs. Once absorbed it can exist as the mercury ion, Hg^{+2}, which has difficulty entering most of the brain due to poor penetration through the protective blood-brain barrier, but can enter certain parts of the brain, such as the hypothalamus, that do not have a barrier system.

The organic form of mercury, called methylmercury, on the other hand, easily penetrates the brain, yet at a slower rate than other tissues of the body. Dental amalgam releases mercury that can exist in all three forms: as a vapor, as the ion, and as methylmercury (the major source of methylmercury, though, is from seafood).

We know that certain forms of mercury, such as methylmercury and phenylmercury, are highly lipid soluble, which makes the brain especially susceptible to mercury accumulation. These forms of mercury are found in vaccines as the preservative thimerosal. Once in the brain, it tends to attach itself to protein structures, especially to the cell membrane, where it can disrupt membrane functions.[23] By binding to the cell membrane, mercury changes the membrane's fluid-like quality, making it stiffer and causing the cell to age faster.[24]

The brain is unique in that neurons depend on special microscopic, tube-like structures within the cell, appropriately called neurotubules, for their function. These neurotubules are manufactured by the cell from a substance called tubulin. We know that mercury interacts with tubulin causing it to unravel. Studies in rats have shown that doses of mercury corresponding to those seen in humans can cause a 75 percent increase in tubulin inhibition. As

I will discuss later in this chapter, defects in tubulin construction appear to play a major role in Alzheimer's disease.[25]

Mercury can also affect neurotransmitters in the brain. For example, mercury has been shown to inhibit the uptake of the neurotransmitters dopamine, serotonin, and norepinephrine into their synaptic storage depots.[26] When a neuron secretes a neurotransmitter to convey a message to its neighboring neurons, the chemical messenger must be quickly removed or the message will become scrambled, and in some cases, the neurotransmitter itself acts like a toxin. If levels get too high, as we have seen with glutamate, neuron death can occur very quickly. This is especially important in newborns and people with neurological diseases, since they are much more vulnerable than mature or healthier individuals.

What causes the brain to be especially vulnerable to mercury toxicity is its total dependence on critical energy supplies, and its high content of polyunsaturated fatty acids that are known to be susceptible to oxidation injury (lipid peroxidation). The brain utilizes energy at an enormously high rate, consuming 25 percent of all of the blood's glucose and 20 percent of all the oxygen, even though it comprises only 2 percent of the body's weight. Even in the deepest of comas, the brain's metabolic rate is slowed by only 50 percent.

Also important is the fact that the brain tends to retain more mercury than other organs, such as the kidney.[27] One estimate of mercury's half-life in the brain is ten years, meaning it would take ten years for half of the mercury accumulated in the brain to be eliminated under normal conditions. Longer half-lives have been proposed.

Compounding the problem is the fact that the brain accumulates mercury in concentrations ten times higher than the plasma.[28] This means that the nervous system is especially vulnerable to even very low concentrations of mercury. Minute exposures occurring over long periods of time can accumulate in the nervous system, and because the brain is so energy-dependent, this small amount of mercury can produce significant neurological problems.

A frequent finding in mercury toxicity is its accumulation in the cerebellum of the brain.[29] One study found the distribution of mercury in the cerebellum indicated high levels in certain of its cells.[30] Overall, the highest concentrations of mercury were found in the cerebellar nuclei. This distribution was the same in both adults and infants. So why is it important that mercury accumulates in the cerebellum and in its nuclei? Because modern neuroscience indicates that the cerebellum acts as a central control for much of what we consider higher brain functions, such as the initiation and planning of motor movements, as well as storing new information and planning new types of movements. There is even evidence that it plays a major role in memory and learning. In the past we thought that the cerebellum's only function was coordination.

Another recent finding is extremely important for children who suffer from seizures. One study found that seizures were easier to induce in the offspring of rats exposed to mercury during their pregnancy than in control animals not exposed to mercury during development.[31] Researchers concluded that mercury exposure during development damaged the brain system that normally suppresses the spread of seizures, in addition to causing widespread neuron loss.

This could help to explain why some children develop difficult-to-control seizures early in life. If the mother has multiple dental amalgams, consumes large amounts of mercury-containing seafood, is occupationally exposed to mercury, or is exposed to any combination of these conditions during pregnancy, her baby's brain could be damaged in such a way as to encourage intractable seizures. Any dental work, including professional cleanings, she may have had during pregnancy would also greatly increase risk to the developing baby: vigorous cleaning of the amalgam surfaces generates a large amount of mercury vapor that quickly enters the baby's system.

A recurring finding in mercury poisoning is muscle weakness and fatigue, and some have proposed that chronic exposure to mercury may explain chronic fatigue syndrome. While I do not agree with this hypothesis, I do think that it contributes to the problem. A recent study documents the effects of mercury on muscle. In this study of five dental technicians and one dentist, age thirty-five to fifty-five, who presented with findings compatible with chronic mercury toxicity, needle biopsies of the subjects' leg muscles were examined using both light microscopy and transmission electron microscopy.[32] Researchers found damage to the muscle fibers, as well as to the capillaries supplying blood to the muscle. Chronic fatigue and weakness would certainly be compatible with mercury selectively damaging muscle cells' energy enzymes.

It may be that a combination of viral invasion, secondary to immune suppression (either due to mercury toxicity or other causes) leads to the chronic release of inflammatory chemicals called cytokines. These cytokines cause the fatigue we associate with flu or other viral illnesses. Mercury further complicates the problem by damaging the immune system and interfering with muscle energy production.

While some will insist that methylmercury is the culprit in most cases of neurological toxicity, there is good evidence that this is not true. In fact, the inorganic mercury found in dental amalgams was shown to be a more powerful neurotoxin than methylmercury by an order of magnitude.[33] As I stated before, there is experimental evidence that methylmercury breaks down in the brain into the ionic form (Hg^{+2}).

In summary, we have seen that mercury, even in concentrations too low to cause cell death, can affect multiple neuron cell functions, such as membrane transport, calcium regulation, energy production, neurotransmitter control, free-radical production, excitotoxicity, enzyme function, DNA stability and repair, and antioxidant defenses. We have also seen that by improving our nutritional defenses we can significantly reduce the toxic impact of mercury toxicity. Nutrition can protect the nervous system on many levels by strengthening cell membranes, protecting DNA, chelating mercury, enhancing mercury removal, improving cellular energy production, reducing inflammation and protecting the detoxifying enzyme systems in the cells and liver.

We have also seen that federal and state standards for safe levels of mercury exposure are far too high and should be lowered tenfold or more. We should also keep in mind that there is, in fact, no safe level of mercury exposure. It is critical that pregnant women and their babies be protected from mercury exposure at all costs. Injecting babies with numerous mercury-containing vaccines and using amalgam dental fillings is both ludicrous and unconscionable!

Now let's take an in-depth look at the specific kinds of damage for which mercury is responsible in each stage of human life.

Mercury's Effects on Babies and Children

The development of the brain is a marvelous event that has, as yet, defied our ability to completely understand this God-given phenomenon. But we do know many intriguing things about this process. Basically, the brain must be constructed from a mere three layers of cells that differentiate into numerous types of specialized cells which in turn sprout out into trillions of spiny processes, each molded into a three-dimensional architecture of incredible exactness. During this intricate process, the brain makes far too many connections and must remove a large number of them by a process called pruning, just as you would prune a fruit tree. This pruning process is extremely precise and requires a critically timed release of higher concentrations of glutamate. Too much glutamate for too long a time and the brain will be overpruned; too little, and the connections will form a mass of confusing signals.

As this delicate molding process takes place, special enzymes make their appearance in the brain, again in a specifically timed sequence. Mercury, as an enzyme poison, interferes with this meticulous process, causing the brain to be "miswired." The process of miswiring can result in anything from mild behavioral and learning problems to major disorders such as autism and other forms of cerebral malfunction. Another way mercury seems to interfere with this process is by altering the careful balance of calcium within the cell. We know that calcium passing into the cell, and within compartments of the cell, plays a major role in the transmission of signals that direct the development process as well as neuron function.

In part, special bulbs, called growth cones, located at the end of the neural fibers direct this process of neural pathway development in the brain. These specialized cones direct the nerve fiber to its correct location in the three-dimensional maze that makes up the immature brain. How the growth cone does this depends to a large degree on calcium, and heavy metals like mercury and cadmium interfere with this calcium-directed process. As a result, the nerve fiber gets lost and the brain is miswired. The final effect of this miswiring process depends on the severity of the miswiring. Mercury has been shown to affect this growth process at concentrations in the micromolar or even sub-micromolar range.[34] In other words, it happens with exposures that are extremely small.

In simple terms, the reason for this disorganization of brain development is that mercury poisons the chemicals used to induce these cells to migrate to their assigned locations. Brain cells normally align themselves in functional columns, which on stained slides have beautifully layered patterns of light and dark. In the past, neuroscientists classified these patterns in elaborate maps (cytoarchitectonic maps). The process of brain development is very complex and beyond the scope of this book, but basically we know that toxins, like heavy metals, can disrupt many of the intricate steps in brain formation.[35]

As you know by now, one of the central processes in brain injuries and degeneration is the formation of free radicals. For example, in Down's syndrome there is a fourfold increase in these destructive particles.[36] A recent study found that exposure of brain neurons (caudate, hippocampus, cerebellum, and frontal cortex) to as little as 1-5 uM of methylmercury significantly increased free-radical generation in all of the cells.[37] A micromole is one-millionth of a mole weight, an infinitesimally small amount of mercury.

One of the ways mercury induces free-radical formation is by damaging a cell's mitochondria.[38] Because of this loss of energy-producing capacity, the neuron becomes infinitely more susceptible to excitotoxic injury and death even in the presence of normal levels of the neurotransmitter, glutamate. The cycle continues until the cells begin to die or the dendritic fibers shrink. It is these dendritic fibers that make the trillions of connections in the brain.

Destruction of the spiny dendrites can occur independent of the death of the neuron. This is especially important when considering chronic exposure to very low concentrations of mercury. By removing the mercury and supplying nutrients to the neuron, we may be able to regrow these dendritic spines that are so critical to brain function. Synapses are also very sensitive to free-radical injury and lipid peroxidation.

Neurotransmitters, like most other things in the brain, appear in a set pattern, a sequence which is carefully controlled during brain development but can be disrupted by environmental toxins such as mercury. For example, mercury has been shown to cause a sudden release of acetylcholine in the brain, which can not only interrupt developmental signals but can be directly neurotoxic.[39]

It has been well-demonstrated that even minor changes in the structure or function of these cells, or their processes, can have profound consequences on behavioral, neurological and learning functions, as well as other body functions. It must be remembered that the nervous system connects to all parts of the body and exerts either a direct or an indirect influence on body function. For example, the brain has intimate bi-directional connections with the immune system, endocrine system, and gastrointestinal tract. We know that MSG-induced injuries in a newborn's hypothalamus can result in profound depression of the immune system that may last a lifetime. The same is true for endocrine malfunction; that is, we see a loss of the normal flow of growth hormone, reproductive hormones, and adrenal hormones with MSG-type hypothalamic injuries.

When we consider the effects of small concentrations of mercury on the developing brain, we must appreciate the subtle effects that can result. Medical science generally assumes a substance is safe if it does not cause an obvious abnormality on neurological function or behavior. For example, if a substance does not cause a seizure, loss of movement, or obviously impaired learning, it is considered generally safe. Unfortunately, this is very naïve and dangerous thinking. The human brain is a very complex structure that can withstand significant injuries with only subtle changes in function, yet even these subtle effects can have a devastating impact on our children's ability to function normally throughout life.

But of special concern is mercury's ability to do two things in the brain. One is to activate the brain's immune system (microglia), and another is to poison the glutamate re-uptake system.

The amino acid, glutamate, is used by the brain as a neurotransmitter, mainly to cause excitation of special brain cells, used for communication between neurons. But, *overex-citing* the brain can also be very dangerous: it can lead to seizures, and destruction of brain cells by a process called excitotoxicity. For this reason, the amount of free glutamate allowed to move around in the brain's extracellular spaces is carefully controlled by the brain under normal circumstances.

This control system involves a family of protein-carrier molecules whose job it is to bind with the free glutamate and carry it to a nearby cell called an astrocyte, where the glutamate is safely stored. Even microscopic increases in free glutamate can trigger a destructive process that causes neurons to commit suicide. Under certain conditions, even normal levels of glutamate can kill brain cells.

Mercury is unique among metals in that it can selectively block the glutamate re-uptake system, even when present in incredibly small concentrations. When the system is blocked, free glutamate accumulates in the brain's extracellular spaces, triggering excitotoxicity. The glutamate transporter continues to be impaired since mercury stays in the brain for such long periods of time.

We know that the infant brain is four times more sensitive than the adult brain to excitotox-icity. This is because many of the infant brain's protective systems are immature and poorly developed. Not surprisingly, glutamate plays a critical role in brain circuitry formation, including the operation of the growth cones that guide neural fibers in the developing brain.

Introduction of mercury during this delicate process can cause glutamate levels to rise too soon or accumulate in high concentrations, resulting in miswiring of the brain. The effects of this miswiring can be subtle or devastating, depending on many conditions: the dose of the mercury, when it was given, and the nutritional status of the baby.

Subtle changes may result in minor behavioral problems, such as some difficulty with memory and cognition, or a loss of anger control. As a child, these conditions may be classed as attention deficit disorder (ADD), attention deficit hyperactivity disorder (ADHD), or one of autism spectrum disorders. In more severe cases, the damage may result in full-blown autism or Asperger's syndrome. As we shall see in chapter seven, early changes in glutamate levels can also disrupt the endocrine system, resulting in reproductive problems, hypothyroidism, and adrenal gland malfunction later in life.

Localization of Mercury in the Immature Brain

Acute, high-dose, mercury poisoning in adults is characterized by a localization of the toxin in the occipital lobes of the brain, especially in an area called the calcarine cortex, which is the part of the brain controlling vision. This may explain the loss of color vision and tunnel vision seen in mercury miners. Remember that the cerebellum is a primary site of localization of mercury in both adults and children. Chronic exposure in children has a somewhat different brain deposition, with localization more commonly found in the amygdala, neocortex, and temporal lobes.[40]

Significant but lower accumulations of mercury also occur in other parts of the brain. In children exposed to high-dose mercury, we see widespread destruction of neurons in the brain accompanied by scarring (called gliosis), but more importantly we see grossly abnormal development of brain-cell layers (referred to as the cytoarchitecture of the brain) with isolated clumps of malformed brain cells and disorganization of the cells in the cortex of the brain.[41] This was the sort of damage seen in the Iraq and Minamata poisonings.

Most studies of mercury's effect on brain development have concentrated on methylmercury rather than inorganic mercury, but, as we have seen, dental amalgam releases both methylmercury and inorganic mercury, and within the brain methylmercury can undergo

---

How Mercury Damages Cells

- Inhibits enzyme function.
    Na+/K+ ATPase
    mitochondrial enzymes
    glutathione reductase
    glutathione synthease
    superoxide dismutase
- Binds to nucleic acids.
- Induces astrocyte swelling.
- Inhibits protein synthease.
- Inhibits neurotubules.
- Inhibits dopamine, serotonin, norepinephrine.
- Inhibits cytokine production.
- Inhibits glutamate transport proteins.
- Increases free-radical production.
- Encourages lipid peroxidation.
- Binds to cell membranes.

TABLE 3.2

demethylation to form inorganic mercury. We have also seen that inorganic mercury can be more toxic to the brain than the organic form (methylmercury).

The concentration necessary to produce abnormal development of the brain has not yet been accurately determined; nevertheless, we know from the Iraq incident that mercury levels as low as 10 ppm can adversely affect neural development. The problem with trying to determine toxicity levels during development is a problem of measurement and of time. The time span between exposure and the appearance of a neurological problem can be quite long. As I pointed out before, toxic injuries that affect higher cognitive functions, such as performing complex mathematical computations or logical thinking would not appear until the teenage years. So until a child reaches that age he or she may appear to be perfectly normal, both intellectually and behaviorally.

We are also limited by our ability to test for more subtle mental and behavioral functions; that is, our inability to test for a problem doesn't necessarily mean a problem doesn't exist. Rather, it may mean that our instruments or methods are not sensitive enough to identify a specific problem. As I mentioned earlier, studies have found a close correlation between the number of dental amalgams in a mother's mouth and mercury tissue levels, including brain levels, in her baby. This finding has been reproduced in both humans and experimentally in sheep using radioactive tracers to track the mercury. Toxicity to the baby while in the mother's uterus can occur without the mother showing any signs of mercury toxicity.[42]

One obvious question is: if mercury is so toxic to the developing baby, why are any babies born normal? The answer is the same as for adults. Sensitivity to toxicity depends on a number of variables, such as the condition of the antioxidant network, state of general nutrition, presence of natural metal chelators, differences in DNA-repair enzymes, biochemical differences, and genetic differences. We know that mercury uses a cysteine transport system in the placenta and that neutral amino acids can block mercury transfer to the baby. A mother who consumes these amino acids during pregnancy would naturally transfer less mercury to the baby.

One important study demonstrated that the state of selenium nurture plays a major role in protection against mercury toxicity, especially in the unborn. Experiments have shown that animals fed diets with low amounts of selenium were most affected in terms of neurobehavioral function when exposed to mercury.[43] Those with the highest selenium diets had the greatest protection. This would mean that babies born in the Midwest, which has a high soil selenium level would be less vulnerable than babies born in New Jersey, which has a low selenium soil. The problem is that most people do not eat foods grown locally, which means it is almost impossible to know the selenium content of produce purchased at a grocery store.

In the study cited above, selenium did not reduce the amount of mercury in the baby's brain, but stimulated the production of the protective antioxidant selenium-containing enzyme, glutathione peroxidase, and bound the mercury so as to make it non-toxic.

At least one other study indicates that selenium supplementation in those with pre-existing low selenium levels may reduce mercury hair levels,[44] which give a crude indication of brain levels. Twenty-three people in the study were supplemented with 100 ug of selenomethionine for four months and experienced a 34 percent reduction in mercury levels.

In another experimental animal study using 344 pregnant Fisher rats given methylmercury in high concentrations, experimenters found that feeding the mothers garlic juice reduced fetal mortality rates by 37 percent and could significantly inhibit developmental damage to the fetus caused by the mercury.[45] Mercury levels in the dams were decreased in the liver by 67 percent, 47 percent in the kidney, and 58 percent in the brain. In the fetus, mercury levels were lowered 56 percent in the liver, 47 percent in the kidney and 37 percent in the brain. It is not known what the active factor in the garlic juice is, but numerous possibilities exist, including the presence of selenium, methionine, and cysteine.

In one experiment, researchers using sheep as a study animal implanted twelve amalgam fillings containing radioactive mercury (203Hg) for a tracer, in the teeth of the pregnant ewes.[46] At intervals of one to three days for 140 days they collected blood, feces, urine, and amniotic fluid. The radio-labeled implants were inserted after 112 days of gestation, and the labeled mercury began to appear in the amniotic fluid as well as in the maternal and fetal blood by day two. Mercury was found in all of the tissues examined, with the highest levels in the kidneys and liver of each adult animal and in the liver and pituitary gland of each fetus. The placenta was shown to accumulate mercury progressively, so that the mercury tended to concentrate in higher levels in the baby than in the mother.

How long mercury stays in the body depends on a particular tissue's or organ's ability to flush the metal. The half-life for the kidney is sixty-four days.[47] This means that for every sixty-four-day period, half of the mercury in the kidney will be excreted in the urine. For the body as a whole, the half-life is fifty-four days, and for the brain it is one year. Other studies have shown a much longer half-life in the brain, as long as ten to eighteen years.

Studies on mercury miners, and those exposed during industrial accidents, indicate that mercury can remain in the brain as long as ten years after a single exposure, but the damage produced by the mercury can last over thirty years.[48] The victims of the Minamata exposure, when examined twenty years later, were still severely neurologically impaired. The same is true for victims of the Iraq fungicide catastrophe.

The form mercury takes in the body can also influence its half-life, due to the ways in which the different forms are distributed to bodily systems. One study, using mice injected with radioactively labeled mercury, found that inorganic mercury entered most areas of the body but methylmercury entered the brain in concentrations fourteen times higher.[49] The mercury from dental amalgam is inorganic mercury, but is partially converted to methylmercury by bacteria in the mouth. As a result, mercury vapor from dental amalgams is especially toxic to the brain; once in the brain in its converted state, the mercury's half-life is suddenly increased. Other studies have shown that inorganic mercury is also distributed to the brain in similar distribution patterns as methylmercury.

Can Mercury Enter Breast Milk?

This question should be of paramount importance to those readers contemplating parenthood or for those who already have a baby on the way. One study, in which mercury levels were examined in Swedish women on a diet high in seafood known to have a high mercury content, found that breast milk mercury levels were 20-30 percent higher than the mother's blood mercury levels.[50] A second part of the study found that inorganic mercury from dental fillings existed in the milk in concentrations 40-80 percent higher than in the mother's blood. This means that mercury amalgam fillings pose a greater danger than mercury from seafood to the developing child. Total mercury levels correlated with the number of amalgam fillings in the Swedish women; that is, the greater the number of fillings, the higher the mercury level—both in the mother and in her breast milk.

Another review of all published studies on mercury and breast milk concluded that significant elevations of mercury occur in some women's breast milk and can exceed the highest tolerable daily intake of 0.5 ug/kg proposed by the World Health Organization (WHO).[51]

From the available literature, it is obvious that the major source of mercury in breast milk is from dental amalgams in the mother. Based on this research, it is recommended that young women should avoid having dental amalgam fillings placed before and during pregnancy, and they should avoid having them removed during pregnancy, which as you will recall can cause a sudden elevation (up to a fourfold increase) in blood and tissue mercury.

In fact, a recent study documented that any dental procedure during pregnancy that involves manipulation of amalgam fillings increased the mercury levels in the mother.[52] Even more frightening, mercury levels in the newborn babies were significantly higher when their mothers had had dental treatments. Babies are significantly more sensitive to mercury toxicity than their mothers. Because the placenta concentrates mercury as it passes into the baby's blood stream, exposure during pregnancy causes significantly higher levels in the baby's blood than in the mother's[53].

From what we have learned so far, no one should have dental amalgam fillings. One writer noted that under present FDA standards, dental mercury amalgams would never get approval. In most states, if you were to throw one of your fillings on the ground you would face a stiff fine by the EPA for polluting the environment. Furthermore, dentists must follow strict guidelines in handling mercury amalgams in their offices, yet 15-20 percent of dentists' offices were in violation of OSHA rules on safe mercury vapor levels.

Behavioral and Neurological Effects of Mercury Exposure During Childhood

According to the National Academy of Sciences, 12 percent of America's sixty-three million children under age eighteen are suffering from one or more mental illnesses. There is growing evidence that many of these developmental disorders are related to environmental toxicities and that of all the environmental factors, heavy metal exposure during critical periods of brain development plays the most important role. Likewise, good nutrition plays the most critical role in normal brain development and in protecting the brain against toxic effects. There is abundant evidence that poor nutrition during the period of brain development can lead to a loss of DNA, reduction in supportive brain cells (astroglia), poor myelination of the brain, and impaired dendrite formation.[54]

The developing brain is more vulnerable than the mature brain to a multitude of toxic insults, including exposure to heavy metals such as arsenic, lead, cadmium, and mercury. Remember, the brain undergoes its most rapid growth during the third trimester of intrauterine development and this continues until two years after birth. By four years of age the brain has reached only 80 percent of its full growth. Many complex processes occur during this critical period: trillions of synaptic junctions are interconnecting, neural pathways are probing their way to their final destinations, and the brain is progressively coating its neural fibers with a protective carapace of fatty myelin.

Over seventy years ago medical doctors recognized an unusual syndrome in those exposed chronically to low levels of mercury, something they named erethism. This syndrome is characterized by unusual irritability, timidity or shyness, weakness, and at times delirium. More recently, we have had added to the list insomnia, apathy, impaired concentration and memory, abnormal motor coordination, suicidal tendencies, and personality changes. Children exposed to higher levels of mercury have had these symptoms persist for as long as eighteen to thirty years following exposure.[55]

As with lead toxicity, many of the effects of mercury poisoning have been ignored because of their subtle nature and the difficulty in specifically connecting symptoms to mercury exposure. This is a problem that plagues all toxicologists, chiefly because of the long delay between exposure to the toxin and the manifestation of symptoms. For example, damage to the parts of the brain concerned with higher mental functions will not become evident until a child begins to utilize such functions, usually during adolescence. Likewise, effects on reproduction will not become evident until after puberty.

As our sophistication in measuring the subtle effects of toxins improves, we will be better able to connect exposure to effects. For example, when children were tested for the effects of exposure to methylmercury from seafood, no obvious neurological effects were seen using standard behavioral tests. Yet, when the same children were tested with sensitive instruments that can measure subtle changes in brain function, such as visual and auditory evoked potentials, significant changes were noted.[56]

One report of two adolescents, aged thirteen and fifteen, who were unintentionally exposed to high levels of mercury vapor for three months, found that both suffered from a diffuse encephalopathy (brain dysfunction).[57] When examined a year later, they had improved on psychiatric testing but continued to have defects in visual perception, construction skills, nonverbal memory, and conceptual abstractions. These symptoms persisted despite the removal of the mercury from the blood by chelation, demonstrating that actual destruction of widespread parts of the brain can occur, and that even during adolescence, the brain is more sensitive than an adult's.

In one unusual case, mercury poisoning was caused by a child's obsession with making silver bullets.[58] It seems the child had a sudden brainstorm, as children will, of making silver bullets by heating a combination of lead shot and mercury from a thermometer. Air samples from the child's home demonstrated mercury levels four times higher than maximal industrial limits. As a result, the child and several family members suffered severe neurological poisoning.

The presence of inorganic mercury and methylmercury in the body together has been shown to intensify the toxic effects of either alone.[59] Remember, dental amalgams produce both inorganic mercury and methylmercury. It has been shown that the common bacteria in the mouth (*Streptococcus sanguis*, *S. mutans*, and *S. mitiors*) can all convert inorganic mercury from mercury amalgam fillings into methylmercury,[60] which easily enters the nervous system.

One of the arguments given by those who defend the safety of dental amalgams is that there is no clear-cut evidence of mercury poisoning from dental amalgams. Certainly, other than the fellows trying to extract silver from amalgam in a frying pan, that is true, yet we also have abundant evidence that the mercury vapor arising from dental amalgams produces in utero levels in babies which can cause abnormal brain development. We also have considerable data relating the number of dental amalgams to toxic levels of mercury in the tissues, levels known to produce organ and cellular malfunction. Such correlations have been demonstrated in people with Alzheimer's dementia as well.

Clear correlations were seen between adult maternal and infant-cord blood mercury levels and deficits in language, attention, and memory among 917 children living on the Faroe islands when examined at birth, one year, and at seven years of age.[61] These children were chosen because they have a diet high in whale meat, which has very high mercury levels. Fine motor function deficits were particularly associated with maternal hair mercury levels at the time of birth. The children's hair mercury levels were significantly predictive of their performance on memory tests for visual information. The greatest risk appeared to be during later gestation, during the brain growth spurt.

Multiple vaccinations, especially in newborns, are another major source of childhood mercury exposure because of the mercury-containing thimerosal preservative. Over twenty-two vaccinations are now recommended for children before the age of two! I will discuss vaccinations in more detail in chapter six.

Effects of exposure can vary from subtle to major malformations but even minor degrees of maldevelopment can have unacceptable consequences. Say, for instance, a low concentration of mercury has resulted in minor miswiring of your child's brain. Outwardly, the child may seem perfectly normal. Even a battery of psychological and learning tests may show little, yet he may have difficulty handling subtle abstract concepts, enough difficulty to cause problems in higher math or complex thinking in later years. This impairment will limit his ability to advance in a very competitive world.

Maybe he just has trouble thinking clearly or remembering blocks of facts. With a different set of injured neurons or misdirected brain pathways, he may have difficulty with anger and impulse control, or develop a phobia that otherwise may never have appeared. It is also possible that he could suffer from an endocrine disorder such as thyroiditis, reproductive problems, or growth impairment, all of which have been associated with chronic low-dose mercury exposure. The number of possible problems is almost limitless.

Mercury Exposure in Adulthood

While young women of child-bearing age have been warned not to have dental amalgam fillings because of the deleterious effects on the developing baby, there is some evidence that exposure to mercury can reduce fertility itself. In one study conducted in the mid-1990s, 418 registered dental assistants in California who had become pregnant during the four years preceding the study were interviewed by phone. Detailed information was taken regarding the handling of amalgam, and the number of menstrual cycles without contraception it had taken them to get pregnant. Dental assistants not working with dental amalgam served as controls. Dental assistants that prepared thirty or more amalgams a week were only 63 percent as likely to get pregnant as were unexposed women after controlling for variables. An unexplained observation was the finding that dental assistants exposed to lower levels of mercury were actually more fertile than non-exposed controls.

In a German study of women who had repeated miscarriages, a direct correlation was found between the load of mercury in the tissues and the number of miscarriages.[62] In this study 111 women with repeated miscarriages were examined for heavy metal toxicity as well as detailed hormone (progesterone, estrogen, prolactin, and thyroid stimulating hormone) and immunological studies (natural killer cells and T-cell subpopulations). It was proposed from the findings that mercury alters the mother's immunity to such an extent that it interferes with normal immunological tolerance seen during a normal pregnancy. When a woman becomes pregnant the baby exists within her as if it were part of her own tissues. The mother's immune system is thus altered to prevent her body from automatically rejecting this new entity. This condition is known as immunological tolerance: mercury appears to significantly alter this process.

Mercury's effects on the endocrine system can be significant, especially in cases of chronic exposure. The above study also found that women experiencing primary miscarriages (the first of a series of miscarriages) had lower progesterone levels, and higher mercury levels, following provocative chelation tests for mercury. Other studies have shown that mercury directly inhibits progesterone production in the ovary's granulosa cells, and has a profound effect on estradiol as well. Women with both primary and secondary miscarriages had higher mercury levels than did women who had never had miscarriages. Another study found that the incidence of luteal insufficiency (low progesterone) was significantly increased in women with ten or more amalgam fillings.[63]

Based on the scientific studies linking excess mercury with multiple miscarriages and infertility, it is obvious that the effect of mercury on fertility needs to be explored in more depth.

Pregnant women with numerous dental amalgam fillings should protect themselves and their babies by taking supplemental antioxidants, especially selenium and alpha-lipoic acid. They should also avoid taking megadoses of vitamins to avoid possible toxic effects to the baby. I would suggest 100 ug of selenium a day, double RDA levels of the B vitamins, 25 mg alpha-lipoic acid a day, 400 IU natural form vitamin E (mixed tocopherols), and 400 mg of magnesium a day.

Effects of Mercury on the Immune System

The internal damage caused by mercury exposure is not limited to the nervous system. The immune system can also suffer severe injury.[64] Like the nervous system, the immune system is highly complex and involves many elements, including cellular components, cytokines, special hormones, and antibodies. It is also important to remember that the immune and nervous systems are intimately connected, both directly and indirectly, a connection that is especially important during development.

Low levels of mercury have several significant effects on the immune system. For example, one study involving eighty-one males occupationally exposed to mercury vapor, as compared to thirty-six controls, found that mercury stimulated T-lymphocytes including T-helper and T-suppressor cells in the exposed workers.[65] In another study of forty-four workers exposed to mercury vapor, the majority with levels below the accepted toxicity limit of 50 ug/gram of creatinine, demonstrated increased levels of several humoral immune parameters, such as IgG, IgA, and IgM.[66] This study found that mercury levels considered to be safe could stimulate humoral immunity, that is, antibodies.

So why is humoral immunity important? Because elevated humoral immunity coupled with T-cell malfunction leads to autoimmunity, a condition where the immune system inadvertently attacks various tissues in the body. There are numerous autoimmune disorders, including thyroiditis, rheumatoid arthritis, primary adrenal insufficiency, and lupus. In fact, we have good evidence that at least part of the damage caused by many neurodegenerative diseases is related to autoimmune reactions to cells in the nervous system.

In one study that used mice bred for autoimmunity, test animals were exposed to mercury vapor several hours a day for ten weeks. All mice receiving concentrations of mercury (480 ug/week/per kilogram body weight) developed auto-antibodies to their own DNA (antinuclear antibodies).[67] The lowest dose of mercury capable of producing antinuclear antibodies was 170 ug/week/per kilogram. Researchers found immune complexes within the kidneys, as well as deposited in the blood vessel walls. What this means is that anyone unlucky enough to have an increased genetic risk for any of the autoimmune diseases is at even greater risk of precipitating the disease after exposure to even low doses of mercury.

Further confirmation of the possible link between autoimmunity and mercury exposure comes from another experiment using autoimmunity-bred mice implanted with dental amalgam.[68] The amalgam triggered an autoimmune reaction with elevations in IgG auto-antibodies toward nuclear protein, and deposits of immune complexes, indicating a strong connection to the length of exposure and the dose of mercury used. This research confirms numerous other studies: exposure to mercury from amalgam fillings can chronically stimulate the immune system leading to autoimmunity.

There is growing evidence that many autoimmune diseases do not develop until some environmental trigger activates the process. In juvenile diabetes we know that cow's milk, certain viruses, and even MSG can trigger the onset of the disease. Mycoplasmal infections may trigger rheumatoid arthritis. Now we can add another trigger for several autoimmune disorders: exposure to low levels of mercury. The amount of mercury released as a vapor from dental amalgam fillings and dissolved into the saliva may be sufficient to trigger a disorder.

One recent observation may indicate a particularly dangerous complication associated with mercury exposure. In a Swedish study conducted on people before and after dental amalgam removal, researchers demonstrated that the number of resistant microorganisms found in the colon (but not in the mouth) increased significantly, by almost fivefold.[69] The colon is a major site for microorganisms responsible for postoperative wound infections, and as we shall see later, may play a critical role in autism. Bacterial resistance has become a major public health problem, and has been recently blamed on the overuse of antibiotics. Now we have evidence that dental amalgams may be to blame, at least in part. Unfortunately, neither the Centers for Disease Control and Prevention (CDC) or the ADA are doing anything to correct this situation.

A particular type of white blood cell, the macrophage, plays a critical role in ridding the body of viruses, especially the herpes simplex type II virus. A recent study demonstrated that mice injected with low doses of mercury chloride before being infected with the virus had viral titers one hundred times higher than the control mercury-free mice.[70] It appeared that the effect was caused by mercury inhibiting the release of important immune-related chemicals, called cytokines (interferon-alpha/beta and TNF-alpha), by the macrophage. These cytokines are essential for the macrophage's antiviral activity. In a human study, mercury was shown to inhibit the ability of neutrophils to kill the *Candida albicans fungus*, again an especially important factor in autism.[71]

The interaction between the immune system and the brain is especially significant during early development. For example, several special chemicals secreted by macrophages can adversely affect the brain, especially the immature brain. These powerful chemicals are released in rather high concentrations following prolonged immune stimulation (infections, vaccinations, or exposure to inflammatory chemicals). In a fairly recent study, researchers found that mice exposed to mercury responded by secreting large amounts of a special, very damaging, cytokine called interleukin-1 (IL-1).[72] The increase in IL-1 production started six hours after the mercury dose was administered and reached a maximum concentration at forty-eight hours. The higher the dose of mercury, the greater the immune response.

This is important because IL-1 has been shown to inhibit a special carrier protein that clears dangerous levels of glutamate away from neurons. Excess glutamate, especially during brain formation, can cause variable disruptions of the brain's development. In the elderly, it can result in damage to special groups of neurons, a condition that may lead to neurodegenerative disease. We also have evidence that mercury can initiate an intense inflammatory response in tissues, followed by persistent inflammation.[73] Again, this is critical to our understanding of the relationship to many brain disorders and mercury exposure.

Mercury and Multiple Sclerosis

Based on compelling evidence, the consensus in the medical community is that MS is an autoimmune disease. The big question is: what triggers this autoimmunity? There is growing evidence that a chronic viral infection (Herpes virus 7) plays a major role in this disorder, yet we also know that environmental and nutritional conditions can alter the course of the disease. High-fat diets, low in omega-3 fatty acids (from seafood) and high in omega-6 fatty acids (from vegetable oils), promote the disease and increase the severity of complications. Likewise, high antioxidant intake combined with a low-fat diet and increased DHA intake can reduce the severity of MS.

We also know that certain metals, such as mercury, iron, and aluminum, make symptoms worse. Aluminum accumulates in the fatty covering of nerve pathways (myelin) and may interact with iron to promote dramatic increases in free-radical production, greatly aggravating symptoms. Mercury, by interacting with iron, may produce the same effect, and may also interfere with normal nerve function.

One interesting study of forty-seven MS patients with mercury amalgams compared to fifty patients who had had their amalgams removed found that those with amalgams had more mental problems.[74] The study used a questionnaire of eighteen mental health symptoms and found that those with amalgams had 43 percent more symptoms than those who had their amalgams removed. The symptoms associated with mercury exposure included more frequent occurrences of depression, hostility, psychotic episodes, obsessive-compulsion, and significantly more incidents of anger.

Common sense would seem to dictate that you would not want a known neurotoxin implanted in your mouth when you have a major neurological disease. The same is true of receiving mercury-containing immunizations for the flu every year and consuming seafood that contains mercury.

Does Mercury Cause Cancer?

It has been established that mercury damages chromosomes,[75] and we have known for quite some time that gene mutations are closely correlated to the development of cancer. For example, methylmercury and mercury chloride have been shown to cause kidney tumors in male mice. Studies of those exposed occupationally, such as chloralkali and nuclear weapons workers, dentists, and dental technicians, indicate that exposure to low levels of mercury may increase the risk of lung, kidney, and brain tumors.[76] Better studies on these groups of high-risk individuals need to be done. No one has specifically examined the relationship between dental amalgams and brain tumors, but there is suggestive evidence that they are related.[77]

The effect of mercury on the immune system should be of major concern to both cancer patients and their doctors. We know that survival rates in cancer patients are directly related to the competence of the immune system. When it is operating inefficiently, cancer rates are high and survival is low. It has been proposed that a special immune cell, called a macrophage, plays a major role in fighting cancer, and as we have seen, mercury impairs macrophage and neutrophil function. It also impairs immune cytokine generation, and can significantly impair immune resistance to cancer and cancer growth. I personally feel that cancer patients should be asked about dental amalgam fillings, seafood consumption, and other heavy metal exposures. If any of these are present, provocative mercury testing should be done.

Effect of Mercury on the Elderly

In my practice, I see a considerable number of elderly people suffering from either age-related memory loss or a major neurological disease, and over the years one thought has haunted me: How many of these poor people are suffering needlessly because of some environmental hazard? What a tragedy it would be to know that some common treatment— a dental filling or flu vaccination—could produce or contribute to older people being struck down by horrible diseases.

Flu vaccines contain 25 ug of organic mercury! These vaccinations, which offer little protection against yearly flu virus strains, are heavily promoted by the CDC, Public Health Department and most physicians. Many hospitals have made flu vaccinations of the elderly a part of routine admission orders. This, in my view, is criminal.

Some forms of mercury, such as methylmercury, phenylmercury, and ethylmercury, are very fat-soluble. This means that an obese person can sequester a considerable amount of mercury in his or her body fat, as well as in his or her nervous system. What happens when we suddenly lose a lot of body fat, when we diet or lose weight as we age? It would make sense that it would be released into the bloodstream, to be redistributed mainly into the brain and kidney. This could cause abrupt increases in mercury levels without additional outside exposure. Unfortunately, no one has done such studies to see if this is happening. Once again, there is suggestive evidence, and at least one study did find a redistribution of mercury in the body.[78]

What about the elderly person who goes to the dentist for bridgework, to have a filling replaced or for other dental procedures? We know that any manipulation of teeth containing amalgam significantly increases the burden of mercury in the body and brain. Even having your teeth cleaned significantly augments your risk. It has been proposed that having two types of metal in close contact—a gold cap overlaying an amalgam filling, for instance— greatly increases the mercury release.

When I explain the dangers of mercury amalgams to patients, many are relieved to tell me that they have had all of their teeth removed. Unfortunately, this does not protect them against mercury poisoning: the very process of pulling teeth that have amalgam fillings significantly increases mercury levels, often as much as fourfold. This mercury is locked into tissues for a prolonged period of time, especially in the brain and spinal cord and, unless this heavy metal is removed, it will continue to do great harm. The process of removal involves a special procedure that I will describe in detail later.

In the brain, mercury quickly attaches itself to proteins, mostly enzymes. One particularly important molecule affected by mercury is glutathione, which is found in every cell in the body, and is especially important in the central nervous system (the brain and spinal cord). Because glutathione contains sulfhydral groups, mercury attaches to it very tightly and can remove glutathione from the cell. As we have seen, one molecule of mercury can inactivate two molecules of glutathione. So why is glutathione so important? Because of its ability to neutralize such a wide variety of very destructive free radicals and lipid-peroxidation products. We know that one of the earliest precursors of Parkinson's disease, one that occurs decades before the first clinical signs appear, is a loss of glutathione in the affected area of the brain (the substantia nigra). Similar losses of neuronal glutathione occur in Alzheimer's dementia and ALS.

Mercury damages virtually every enzyme and information molecule in the brain, including DNA. Many of these enzymes are involved in energy production for the brain, and a loss of the ability to produce adequate amounts of energy is a precursor to all neurodegenerative diseases. In both Alzheimer's disease and Parkinson's disease, such brain-cell energy losses can occur over a decade before the first symptoms develop. We also see a loss of the antioxidant enzymes, especially superoxide dismutase and catalase. Because mercury, as well as other metals, can produce such an enormous number of free radicals in the brain, a loss of antioxidant defenses becomes even more critical.

Immune alterations by mercury exposure are also important as we age. We know that as we age we tend to become immune to ourselves. Numerous reports on normal aging have noted antibodies against various tissues, especially against the brain. Mercury has been shown to induce immune complexes against brain structures, and as we have seen, can induce prolonged inflammatory effects. Because mercury also impairs white blood cell function, we may become more susceptible to infections and infectious illnesses.

Mercury and Neurodegenerative Diseases

The connection between exposure to mercury in its various forms and degenerative diseases of the nervous system is fairly strong. Many of the symptoms of chronic low-level mercury exposure closely resemble the neurobehavioral symptoms seen in many neurodegenerative diseases. For example, the asthetic-vegetative syndrome (micromercurilism) caused by exposure to low levels of mercury, is characterized by decreased productivity, loss of memory, loss of self-confidence, depression, fatigue, and irritability, many of which symptoms are also present in the dementias. Also, the studies done on dentists exposed to mercury vapor demonstrated impaired memory recall. It is also interesting to note that one of the complications listed in the 1927 edition of Sajous's *Analytic Cyclopedia of Practical Medicine* under mercury poisoning is paralysis agitans, also known as Parkinson's disease.

A more recent study of nine exposed workers from a thermometer plant found symptoms of Parkinson's disease in four, which eventually cleared in all but one. They also experienced loss of muscle power, tremors, and atrophy of muscle mass, all symptoms associated with motor neuron injury, as in ALS. We know that there is a tremendous overlap in these diseases, with about 30 percent of Parkinson's patients showing signs of dementia and a smaller number having features of ALS; this is consistent with the effects of an environmental toxin.

Connection to Amyotrophic Lateral Sclerosis

In ALS the motor neuron cells in the spinal cord and motor neuron cells of the brain stem are primarily affected. The mystery has always been why these cells are singled out in this disease and why the disease suddenly appears later in life after so many years of normal function. The answer may be an environmental toxin, or even a combination of toxins. Several studies have shown, for instance, that mercury is selectively taken up by motor neurons in the spinal cord.

In one study, Wister rats were exposed to mercury vapor at a concentration of 50 ug/M3 for six hours a day, five days a week, extending from one to eight weeks.[79] A special autometallographical technique was used to identify the mercury in tissue sections taken from the animals and was quantified using cold atomic absorption spectroscopy. At the end of the selected time periods, sections were made of the spinal nerve ganglion (dorsal root ganglion) and the spinal cord. Representative sections were made from the cervical, thoracic, and lumbar spinal cord. After two weeks of mercury vapor exposure, mercury granules had accumulated heavily in all motor neurons in each of the areas of the spinal cord. Electron microscope analysis showed that the mercury was localized primarily in the large motor nerve cells.[80]

Human studies of mercury's relation to ALS have not made the same strong connection. For example, in a fairly recent examination of fifty-three ALS patients using provocative testing with the mercury chelator DMSA, researchers found no difference between ALS patients and controls in either lead or mercury excretion.[81] In truth, this still leaves us short of an answer, since some have suggested that those who are unable to excrete mercury on provocative testing may be at a greater risk of neurological disease than those who secrete greater amounts. We have already seen that the nervous system holds onto mercury much tighter than other tissues and organs, and there is some question as to the ability of even chelation drugs, such as DMSA, to remove mercury from the nervous system.

Confirmation of a potential link to ALS comes from several other studies. In one study of persons suffering from ALS, researchers found several metal-related problems when other internal organs were examined.[82] The ALS patients had significantly elevated levels of iron in their kidneys and liver as compared to controls. They also had mercury levels two times higher in their kidneys and 17 percent higher in their liver than did controls. Despite this, the differences were not statistically different than the controls because of the wide variations in mercury levels among people.

This might mean that the mercury was tightly bound in these patients, preventing its removal by such chelators as DMPS and DMSA. Despite the fact that some ALS patients possess the same mercury levels as those free of the disease, it may be that ALS patients have several contributing factors that make them much more sensitive to mercury. For example, they may have a weakened antioxidant defense network in their motor neurons, genetic differences in metabolism, impaired detoxification mechanisms, nutritionally impaired cellular energy production, lower selenium levels, an altered blood-spinal cord barrier, associated toxins (such as other toxic metals, pesticides and herbicides), low magnesium levels, or different levels of metallothionein in the affected neurons. Metallothioneins, found throughout the body, are low-molecular-weight proteins and polypeptides of extremely high metal and sulfur content; they are thought to be necessary for intracellular fixation of the essential trace elements zinc and copper, in controlling concentrations of the free ions of these elements, in regulating their flow to their cellular destinations, in neutralizing the harmful influences of exposure to toxic elements such as cadmium and mercury, and in the protection from a variety of stress conditions. There are numerous reasons for a differential effect with similar exposures to toxins, all of which have been well documented in the scientific literature.

A final study deserves examination. In this study, mercury chloride was injected into the abdominal cavities of test mice to see if mercury accumulated in the motor neurons of the spinal cord.[83] Researchers used an extremely low dose of mercury (.05-.2 ug/g of body weight). When examined five days later mercury granules were detected in the cell bodies of the spinal and brain stem motor neurons. The mercury still persisted in the motor neurons eleven months later, indicating that this type of neuron in the spinal cord and brain stem acts as a sink for mercury and then holds onto the mercury tenaciously. This would also explain why it would be so difficult to chelate the mercury out of the nervous system of ALS patients.

It may also explain why the disease does not manifest until later in life. First, the mercury accumulates slowly, over many years. This would include all sources of mercury from seafood and dental amalgams, as well as any other environmental exposure. In the case of dental amalgams, we have seen that accumulation can occur at a rate of 2-17 ug per day. At this rate, it would take many years for the body to accumulate enough mercury to actually kill neurons, but during this time the cells are being damaged by the mercury, impairing their ability to produce energy and dramatically increasing free-radical generation while at the same time depleting neurons of their antioxidants. There is overwhelming evidence that free-radical generation by excitotoxins is a central process in this disease.

Mercury also damages cellular DNA and RNA, two factors founds in ALS. Progressive disruption of the cell's homeostatic mechanisms would necessarily lead to eventual cell death (by apoptosis and necrosis). A final piece of the puzzle has recently been supplied, and that is the connection between mercury poisoning and excitotoxicity. There is growing evidence that excitotoxicity plays a major role as the final destructive event in all neurode-generative diseases; when the neurotransmitter glutamate cannot be removed from the body safely, the nervous system is eventually damaged.

Recent studies have shown that deactivating the transport proteins necessary to safely elimi-nate glutamate from the body causes the substance to accumulate. Soon afterwards neurons begin to die off. ALS can actually be induced in experimental animals by this process. Mercury, even in extremely low concentrations, acts as a powerful inhibitor of these gluta-mate transport proteins. In fact, levels that do not affect other cellular functions can inhibit the glutamate transport protein.[84] Once the excitotoxic process begins, enormous numbers of free radicals are produced, further injuring the cells.

It should be noted that mercury is not the only substance that can deactivate the glutamate transporter molecule, inflammatory cytokines and infectious agents may do so as well. For example, we know that certain viruses can also hinder these glutamate transport proteins.

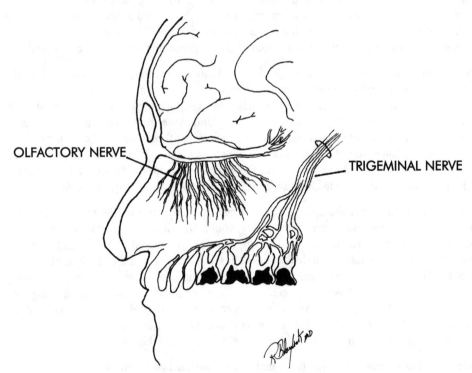

OLFACTORY NERVE

TRIGEMINAL NERVE

FIGURE 3.2 Midsection view of the head demonstrating how mercury can saturate and pass up the olfactory nerve filaments in the nose and the trigem-inal nerve filaments in the mouth to reach the brain.

Further research should be done on this possible connection, especially in light of the occasional case of ALS that resolves with amalgam removal.

We have good experimental and human pathological evidence that prolonged free-radical injury to neurons and astrocytes precedes most neurodegenerative diseases by decades. We also have overwhelming evidence that neural energy impairment plays a pivotal role in these diseases. Autopsy studies of large numbers of Alzheimer's victims have consistently shown elevations of mercury, as well as other toxic metals, within the parts of the brain characteristically damaged by the disease. So, I think those who dismiss these concerns out of hand are themselves not using good science and certainly are not using common sense.

Mercury and Alzheimer's Disease

Autopsy studies of Alzheimer's patients have consistently demonstrated elevated mercury levels in the affected areas of the brain.[85] Likewise, there is a direct correlation between brain levels of mercury and the number of amalgam fillings.[86] To better understand the relationship between mercury toxicity and degenerative diseases of the brain, it is necessary to examine the cellular events that occur with these disorders and relate them to the mechanism of toxicity of mercury.

Hippocrates described dementias over twenty-four hundred years ago in an historical text, but, it wasn't until 1907 that the pathologist Alois Alzheimer described the changes in the brain associated with dementia occurring before age sixty-five, often referred to as presenile dementia. At the time it was thought to be a different disorder than senile dementia of old age, but since Alzheimer's first studies we have come to realize that these are actually the same disease. These changes include atrophy of several localized areas of the brain, including, but not limited to the prefrontal, temporal, and inferior parietal lobes.

It was also noticed that some of the earliest changes occurred in the olfactory (entorhinal) part of the brain, and included a special, small but very critical collection of neurons, called the nucleus basalis of Meynert. This tiny nucleus sends fiber connections over a wide expanse of the cerebral hemispheres of the brain. In experimental animals, lesions of this nucleus can lead to pathological and chemical changes in the brain very similar to those seen with Alzheimer's disease in humans.

When radiolabeled mercury within dental amalgam was implanted in the teeth of sheep so that its movement could be traced by scanners, it traveled up the olfactory nerve filaments in the nose, into the olfactory bulb within the cranial cavity, and then into the hippocampus and septal area where this vital nucleus is located. What makes this observation so important is that these are the areas of the brain where the earliest changes of Alzheimer's disease occur.

When neuropathologists examine the brains of those dying of Alzheimer's disease they see numerous darkly staining microscopic bodies referred to as plaques (senile or neuritic plaques) scattered throughout the affected parts of the brain, but the severity of the disease does not correlate with the number of these plaques. In fact, numerous plaques may also be seen in persons with normal memory functions, although the plaques are somewhat different in structure.

Another microscopic particle, called a neurofibrillary tangle, is of more interest, because its presence *does* correlate with the severity of the disease. Inside this inclusion body we find what are referred to as paired helical filaments. Although sort of twisted around one another like DNA, these bodies are actually failed attempts to make neurotubules, unique structures that make up a vital part of neurons and are concerned with cellular communication and neurochemical transfer.

The process whereby neurotubules are constructed involves some rather complicated brain chemistry. For our purposes it is sufficient to know that the proper assembly of these structures depends on the addition of just the right amount of phosphate units, a process called phosphorylation. In Alzheimer's disease we see excessive phosphorylation of the tau protein, an essential building block of neurotubules. We also know that several factors can interfere with the healthy construction of neurotubules, including certain free radicals and lipid-peroxidation products, immune complexes, cytokines, excitotoxins, and certain toxic metals, such as mercury and aluminum.[87]

With this background, let us look at some of the studies linking mercury exposure and Alzheimer's disease. An article by Dr. Wenstrup and his co-workers in the journal, *Brain Research*, reported the results of a study of thirteen trace elements in Alzheimer's patients versus control patients matched for age and gender.[88] They looked at the level of these elements in the subcellular fractions (mitochondria, nuclei, and microsomes) in the whole brain and temporal lobes of the brain. They found markedly elevated levels of mercury in the microsomes as well as significant losses of selenium in the same areas. Zinc was decreased in the nucleus of the cells and rubidium was deficient in both the nuclei and the microsomes. This is particularly important since both zinc and selenium play a major role in detoxifying mercury. In addition, low rubidium levels indicate impaired membrane function.

A separate study, which also examined metal accumulation in Alzheimer's disease, demonstrated that mercury accumulation in the nucleus basalis of Meynert was the largest metal imbalance found in the Alzheimer brain to date.[89] Remember, it is this nucleus that connects widely to all areas of the brain damaged in Alzheimer's disease, and is the site most often damaged in the disease. When it degenerates, we see associated degeneration of the acetylcholine-using (cholinergic) neurons concerned with orientation and memory.

A more recent study examined blood levels of mercury in Alzheimer's disease patients compared to patients with major depression and to normal people who were used as controls.[90] Blood mercury was found to be two times higher in the Alzheimer patients than in both sets of controls. Mercury levels were three times higher in those with early-onset Alzheimer's dementia than in controls. Furthermore, a significant correlation was found between the high mercury levels and the presence of increased amounts of beta-amyloid in the spinal fluid. Interestingly, beta-amyloid is the principal component found in neuritic plaques.

I have already mentioned the role that neurotubules play in cellular communication within the brain; abnormal production of neurotubules produces the microscopic neurofibrillary tangles seen scattered throughout the affected brain areas associated with Alzheimer's disease.[91] Experimental studies, in which rats were exposed to low-dose mercury vapor, showed that tubulin assembly was reduced 41-75 percent—a truly drastic amount![92] By interfering with the ability of the brain to create one of its chief components, mercury can inflict devastating effects upon brain function that may take years to manifest.

In addition, there is good evidence that mercury also alters the cell membrane, significantly interfering with its function. Not only must the membrane regulate fuel and oxygen entry, it also controls numerous neurohormones, information molecules, peptides, neurotransmitters, ion traffic regulation, and bio-electric functions. The form of mercury appears to make a lot of difference in terms of the effect on the cell. For example, phenylmercury, the form used in vaccines, is more lipid soluble than either methylmercury or inorganic mercury, making its entry into the brain easier.[93]

Also, phenylmercury is more likely to be stored in subcutaneous and abdominal fat stores, which can be suddenly released with drastic weight loss, thereby redistributing the mercury to the nervous system. This may be especially important in the long-term health of people who yo-yo diet.

The bottom line is that all forms of mercury can significantly disrupt the excitability of the neuron membrane and synaptic information transmission in the hippocampus of the brain, which not only controls the memory process but also integrates other higher cerebral functions such as fear, love, empathy, logic, and sensory comprehension into meaningful forms.

Because mercury interacts with so many enzymes, it can also disrupt the ability of the mitochondria to produce energy. When a neuron loses its ability to generate adequate energy, it becomes significantly more sensitive to excitotoxic injury and death. Another mitochondrial effect is also gaining attention: the ability of mercury to disrupt the normal regulation of calcium in the neuron. One of the central features of the excitotoxic mechanism is the elevation of cellular calcium, which in turn triggers a whole series of destructive processes.

Mitochondria are normally quite efficient in removing excess calcium, but this protective system fails when mercury is present. Keep in mind that because of mercury's almost universal toxicity, several destructive processes occur simultaneously. (1) Glutamate accumulates outside the neuron as its normal carrier is poisoned. (2) This causes more calcium to enter the cell. (3) Mercury interferes with the intracellular calcium regulation system, thereby magnifying the excitotoxic effect. (4) Cellular energy is reduced, leading to increased free-radical formation and increased sensitivity to excitotoxicity. (5) Mercury alters the cell membrane, affecting neuron excitability. (6) Destructive processes are then triggered, resulting in the death of numerous neurons (both by apoptosis and necrosis).

One possibility that has not been adequately explored is the effect of mercury on autoimmunity toward the brain. Antibodies to brain proteins have been described in several studies, but are usually present only in low levels; however, the process seems to be intensified in people with neurodegenerative diseases, including ALS, Parkinson's disease, and Alzheimer's disease. Numerous studies have shown that mercury precipitates enhanced autoimmunity to body tissues other than the brain,[94] and more research might yield some interesting results.

We now know that inflammation of the brain plays a major role in the development of Alzheimer's, but what causes the inflammation? Several possibilities exist: chronic viral infections, genetically controlled autoimmunity triggered by environmental agents, and elevated free-radical generation. We already know that chronic viral diseases trigger excitotoxicity, which can indeed produce many of the changes we see in Alzheimer's disease. Mercury can also trigger antibodies to neural proteins, resulting in a state of chronic inflammation, just as in all other autoimmune diseases such as lupus and rheumatoid arthritis. No matter the etiology, excitotoxicity is the common element that eventually induces the disease.

Once inflammation occurs, special immune cells, called microglia, are activated and dispersed throughout the brain. (Because it is somewhat isolated from the body's other organs, the brain actually possesses its own immune system.) A fairly recent study found that mercury tends to accumulate in high concentrations in microglia for long periods of time, even after a single exposure.[95] Defenders of the safety of dental amalgam will counter that this study was done with methylmercury, and the consumption of fish is the major source of this form of mercury. But, as we have seen, methylmercury is also produced from the mercury vapor released from dental amalgams. In addition, this same study found that methylmercury tends to break down into mercury ions (Hg^{+2}) within the brain, so that it may be that even in the brain, inorganic mercury is the most toxic form.

Once microglia are activated, especially chronically, they begin to pour out special chemicals called cytokines, which regulate the immune process. In addition, they invoke a powerful inflammatory process that triggers excitotoxicity and its associated generation of large numbers of free radicals. Because the inflammatory process is prolonged, we begin to see all the changes characteristic of Alzheimer's disease. This is why anti-inflammatory drugs so successfully reduce the incidence and severity of this dementing disorder.

Another recent finding emphasizes a connection to neurodegenerative disorders. Once activated, microglia begin to secrete large amounts of two excitotoxins, glutamate and quinolinic acid, significantly worsening the excitotoxic attack already underway. This process also damages the energy-production system and increases free-radical production. All of these events can be triggered by low levels of mercury, as well as other toxic metals, such as iron and aluminum.

The obvious question is: If all this is true, then why doesn't everyone eventually develop a degenerative brain disease? In fact, the incidence of all of these diseases is increasing significantly, and they are appearing at an earlier average age. But we must still consider many factors when examining the effects of a toxin on individuals in a population. We have known for a long time that sensitivity to a toxin depends on the host's resistance to the substance; some people will be very sensitive and others quite resistant to the same quantities of a toxin.

Anything that increases free-radical generation will reduce the antioxidant network's efficiency and greatly magnify the toxic effect of mercury or any other toxin. Most diseases—including diabetes, hypertension, strokes, head injuries, infections, and even aging itself—do just that. There are many other conditions in everyday life that contribute to hypersensitivity, including lupus, rheumatoid arthritis, all other autoimmune diseases, chronic viral infections, fever, metabolic diseases, tumors of the nervous system, other metal toxicities (lead, cadmium, aluminum, and iron), Lyme disease, MSG and aspartame ingestion, and multiple immunizations. Vigorous exercise, such as Iron Man contests and marathons, also greatly increases free-radical damage to all tissues of the body and increases the likelihood of heavy metal toxicity.

People with longstanding poor nutrition are at much greater risk than the well-nourished for developing a neurodegenerative disease following mercury exposure.[96] As we have seen, nutrition plays a major role in protecting the brain from injury, including mercury toxicity. Selenium, alpha-lipoic acid, magnesium, zinc, the antioxidant flavonoids, and vitamins all help protect us from mercury toxicity. Earlier I said that one of the central events in all degenerative diseases is a loss of the cell's ability to produce sufficient energy: nutrition plays a major role in preventing energy loss by the neurons, a condition that can be alleviated by nutrients such as acetyl-L-carnitine, CoQ10, and the B vitamins.

Genetic susceptibility also plays a role, since people who carry both copies of the apoE4 gene have a much higher risk of getting Alzheimer's disease than those with the apoE3 gene. Recent studies using cell cultures have shown that this is due to the fact that those with apoE4 genes also have lower levels of antioxidant defense enzymes than those with apoE3 genes. Exposure to conditions that increased free-radical generation and lower antioxidant defenses markedly increased a neuron's sensitivity to mercury toxicity.[97]

Dr. Boyd Haley found that the apoE4 molecule contains no sulfhydral chemical groups, whereas the more protective apoE3 and apoE2 forms contain several such sulfur-containing chemical groups. The sulfhydral chemical group binds with mercury, thereby preventing toxicity, so those who inherit two apoE3 genes have significant protection against cellular mercury poisoning, whereas those with only apoE4 genes have none.

We must also consider levels of lifelong mercury exposure. For example, a person who has had numerous dental amalgams and repeated dental procedures that disturbed these fillings are expected to have a higher likelihood of developing the disease, a correlation demonstrated in human studies. Increased risk may also be expected in people with diets high in methylmercury-containing seafood, and in those who are occupationally exposed to mercury—from working in a printing shop or at an insect extermination service, for example. Finally, alcohol consumption must be taken into account when computing a person's risk factors for developing Alzheimer's: we know that ethyl alcohol blocks the glutamate receptor in the brain, which in small quantities would actually decrease excito-toxicity, but in binge-drinking the alcohol itself is neurotoxic, creating a hypersensitivity to glutamate excitotoxicity. (The glutamate receptor seems to play a major role in memory; the fact that alcohol blocks this receptor is thought to be the explanation for the amnesia that occurs with alcoholism.) Glutamate hypersensitivity explains, in part, why the brain atrophies with chronic alcohol abuse. Furthermore, the same amount of mercury exposure would be more toxic to an alcoholic than to a non-drinker.

Mercury Exposure and Parkinson's Disease

All of the comments I have made concerning Alzheimer's disease also apply to Parkinson's disease. Like Alzheimer's and ALS, Parkinson's disease is associated with free-radical and lipid-peroxidation damage to a very restricted part of the brain called the substantia nigra and its connections. Like the others, excitotoxicity appears to play a central role in the disease process itself. There is strong evidence that iron toxicity is also critical in this disease. Some feel that the free-radical generation caused by mercury is related to the fact that it causes free iron to be released from its binding protein, ferritin.

On top of all this, those destined to get Parkinson's disease seem to possess an inherited weakness in their ability to detoxify toxins, both those formed within the body during metabolism and those ingested or inhaled. A recent study, in which one hundred Parkinson's patients were compared to two hundred matched controls, found that Parkinson's patients had a genetic defect that altered their ability to form conjugating enzymes, a vital method of cellular detoxification,[98] and a condition that would make them more susceptible to oxidative stress in the part of the brain causing the disease. Mercury, by increasing free-radical generation (oxidative stress) and poisoning the antioxidant network, would greatly magnify the effects of this inherited weakness.

In one case report, a female dentist, age forty-seven, developed Parkinson's disease within eighteen months of the onset of her first symptoms.[99] Her baseline urinary mercury was 46 ug. With chelation using penicillamine, it increased to 79 ug and then continued to fall during the week of treatment. During the period of the treatment, she improved clinically and then stabilized. It was noted that this represented a new possible cause of Parkinson's disease in the absence of other signs of mercury poisoning. Penicillamine is not the best choice for chelating agents, especially for removal from the brain. In addition, the treatment period was too short and should have included a more complete program for mercury toxicity reduction.

In another study, researchers looked at environmental factors such as pesticide exposure, well-water drinking, and heavy metal, solvent, and animal exposures possibly related to Parkinson's disease.[100] They discovered a very strong correlation with pesticide exposure, a finding that has been confirmed repeatedly in other studies. Interestingly, they also found that patients with Parkinson's disease had a significantly higher number of dental amalgam fillings than did controls. The study also found that having a relative with the disease compounded all of these factors indicating a genetic sensitivity to these toxins.

I again emphasize, all of the neurodegenerative diseases I have discussed can—and frequently do—overlap, which would indicate a common cause. Why one person would develop Parkinson's disease and another ALS may depend on a multitude of factors such as associated toxins, nutritional factors, associated viral injuries, genetic sensitivities, biochemical differences, and timing of exposure to the toxin. In my previous book, *Excitotoxins: The Taste That Kills*, I demonstrated how simply altering the dose of a toxin could make the difference between an animal developing ALS or dementia. The same may hold true for mercury.

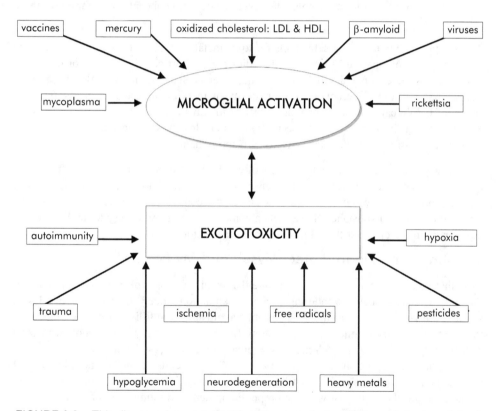

FIGURE 3.3   This diagram demonstrates the numerous factors that can induce excitotoxicity, leading to degeneration of various parts of the nervous system. Notice the intimate connection between microglial activation (brain immune activation) and excitotoxicity. Also note the connection between excitotoxicity and free-radical generation. In the real world, many of these factors operate simultaneously.

Mercury is extremely toxic to numerous organs, tissues, and cells, but especially to the brain. Like lead, the medically acceptable definition for mercury toxicity is constantly being revised by health authorities. Levels that we considered safe ten years ago are now known to be quite toxic. The reason for these ongoing revisions is that scientific instrumentation for measuring the toxic effects of these metals has become much more sophisticated. Also, we now know a lot more about the biological systems being affected by the metals. Finally, our ability to test for subtle changes in neurological function has also improved.

In the past, toxicity determinations were based on evaluations of obvious effects. Mercury levels high enough to cause obvious confusion, dementia, or a loss of sensation in the limbs were used to determine safe levels—any level below that needed to cause these effects was considered safe. With our ability to measure biochemical functions in cells and tissues, we can now measure toxicities on a molecular level that occur at concentrations far below these early estimates of safety.

Another problem with setting safe levels for toxic metals is that we have no idea what they do over a very long period of time. Most studies are of short duration, weeks or months at most. Also, we rarely consider the effects of these metals on certain individuals whose sensitivities may be quite different from the majority of individuals tested. There is always a subset of individuals whose biochemistry differs in ways that can produce profound toxic effects not seen in others; often these individuals are lost in statistical analysis involving large numbers of people. No one seems to care about them.

Finally, we simply do not know the effects of combining various toxic metals. While there is some evidence that their toxicities are synergistic, we do not know for sure in many cases. For example, substance A may have no toxicity at low concentrations when used alone. The same may be true of substance B. Yet, when combined they may be very toxic. We are just now beginning to discover the effects of such combinations.

So What Can I Do to Protect Myself and My Family?

Now that you have seen the terrible damage that even low doses of mercury can create in the body, you are probably wondering what you can do to reduce your risk. First of all, you should limit your exposure as much as possible: avoid amalgam fillings, refuse vaccinations that contain mercury (thimerosal), stop eating fish high in mercury, and do not live near a coal-burning facility. If you already have amalgam fillings, and you are not presently pregnant or nursing, you should have them removed by a dentist trained in the safe removal of amalgam. The fillings cannot just be removed by any dentist; rather a special protocol must be followed by a dentist with the proper equipment and training, and by a nutritionist or physician trained in proper mercury removal techniques.

The dental protocol has been worked out by the International Academy for Oral Medicine and Toxicology (IAOMT) and tested to make sure the method prevents elevation of mercury blood levels following removal of amalgams. Studies in people having amalgams removed and utilizing the protocol have demonstrated there is no rise in blood levels of mercury with amalgam removal. These patients were followed for sixty days to be sure there was no delayed release. Removing dental amalgam fillings without following the IAOMT's precautions has been shown to cause a three- to fourfold elevation of blood mercury that can persist for as long as sixty to ninety days.

As for vaccinations, parents should insist that their children receive only vaccines without thimerosal. Manufacturers are slow in producing mercury-free vaccines, but as a parent you should insist they be free of this toxic metal. (See chapter six for a more detailed discussion of childhood vaccinations.) The practice of inoculating the elderly every year against the latest flu viruses is ludicrous. Recently the CDC recommended lowering the age for yearly flu shots from age sixty-five to fifty-five and some pediatricians are now recommending flu shots for small children. *All of these vaccines contain the mercury-containing thimerosal preservative, and small children and elderly people are the two most vulnerable age groups to mercury toxicity!*

It is not a good idea to keep mercury thermometers around the house, as accidental breakage can wreak havoc. It may be hard to believe that such a small volume of mercury can cause a major catastrophe, but it absolutely can.

Increased risk of mercury poisoning is associated with several occupations and hobbies. Dentists and people involved in the manufacture of dental amalgam, barometers, and thermometers are at increased risk. Certain disinfectants contain mercury. Embalmers, pesticide workers, those who work with wood preservatives, fireworks and explosives, photographers, electroplaters, jewelers, chlorine workers, bronzers, fur processors, taxidermists, farmers, and tannery workers are all at risk. It is interesting to note that in Goldfrank's *Textbook of Toxicology* one method of exposure is listed as "home amalgam extraction."[101]

If you have already been exposed to mercury and have elevated tissue levels, special steps must be taken to reduce your toxicity. Even before removal you must begin taking supplements known to reduce toxicity and improve tissue removal.

Selenium

Selenium is a sulfur-containing molecule that binds tightly to mercury, and has been shown to neutralize some of its toxic effects. An essential metal in the body, it is required for normal health and plays a vital role in immune function and cancer prevention, and is also a vital component of the selenomethionine-containing antioxidant enzyme, glutathione peroxidase.

There is also evidence that selenium may increase removal of mercury from tissues. It is particularly effective within the brain, normally a difficult place to reach during mercury detoxification. Selenium supplementation should be started as soon as mercury toxicity is suspected. In high doses—greater than 1,500 ug—selenium can have some toxic effects of its own. Recommended doses are based on kilogram weight, so divide your weight, or the weight of your family member, in pounds by 2.2 to get kilograms.

The dose is 1-4 ug/kg/day. For adults the dose is 200ug a day of selenomethionine.

Alpha-Lipoic Acid

This is a truly a remarkable substance that provides many protective functions. Most important for mercury toxicity is that alpha-lipoic acid is a very powerful antioxidant and, in addition, binds tightly to mercury even in the nervous system, neutralizing its toxicity. Alpha-lipoic acid easily penetrates the blood-brain barrier, so that it can reach into the brain to remove the damaging metal.

Alpha-lipoic acid also increases cellular levels of glutathione, a major neutralizing molecule for mercury; it enhances cellular energy production, is a powerful and versatile antioxidant (as dehydrolipoic acid or DHLA), and chelates iron.

In general, in adults the doses needed to remove mercury from the brain are very high, 600-800 mg a day. Intravenous doses have been attempted, but it is very difficult to dissolve alpha-lipoic acid in water. Significant hypoglycemia can be a problem with large intravenous doses and can occur with R-lipoic acid taken on an empty stomach. I usually suggest taking three to four small doses daily, rather than a single large dose. Suggested dose based on weight in kilograms is 10 mg/kg/day.

Vitamin E

In vitro (in artificial-environment tests), vitamin E can completely block mercury toxicity in neurons; but while it can significantly reduce damage in the body, it cannot afford complete protection against toxicity.

Vitamin E actually exists as eight subtypes, four tocopherols and four tocotrienols. Most of us are familiar with the d-alpha tocopherol form. The ability of the various forms to inhibit mercury toxicity, or for that matter any heavy metal toxicity, varies considerably. The least potent as antioxidants are the dl- and the d-alpha tocopherol acetate forms. Guess which forms are most commonly sold in pharmacies and even health food stores. You guessed it, the dl- and d-alpha tocopherol acetate forms. This form of vitamin E is the least absorbed from the GI tract, has the least penetration into the brain, and has the lowest antioxidant power. The best forms are the natural or mixed tocopherols; in particular, a form called d-alpha tocopherol succinate has been shown to have the greatest antioxidant power. These are more expensive, but money spent on an ineffective antioxidant that cannot reach the problem is a total waste of money and creates a false sense of security.

The dose based on weight in kilograms is as follows: 10 IU/kg/day

N-acetyl L-cysteine (NAC)

Mercury causes a loss of glutathione, a vital antioxidant molecule caused by mercury binding to the sulfhydral chemical groups in the glutathione molecule. Remember, glutathione is lost in most neurodegenerative diseases long before clinical symptoms begin to appear. N-acetyl L-cysteine, commonly called NAC for short, can effectively chelate mercury. It is also a very effective and safe way to improve cellular glutathione levels.

Unfortunately, recent evidence indicates that NAC may actually worsen the neurological effects of mercury by increasing brain levels of the toxic metal.[102] It does this by binding to the mercury in the blood and tissues and re-distributing it back into the nervous system, acting as a carrier for mercury. Since no one has shown that mercury, when bound to NAC, is harmful, I would recommend a limit of 500 mg a day for an adult.

Fortunately, mercury is carried into the brain by using one of the amino acid carrier sites (large neutral amino acid transport system (LNAA). Normally, the various amino acids compete with each other for use of these carrier sites, and the branch chain amino acids (leucine, isoleucine and valine) share the same carrier used by mercury when it is bound to NAC. It has been proposed that, to prevent NAC-chelated mercury from entering the brain, one might increase the intake of branched-chained amino acids in the diet, which include L-leucine, L-valine, and L-isoleucine. Other amino acids, such as L-tyrosine, L-phenylalanine and L-tryptophan, can also inhibit uptake of mercury into the brain, but some may have significant side effects of their own. I prefer the branched-chained amino acids. L-methionine also competes with mercury for absorption, but is less effective.

Because cellular glutathione is so vital to cell function and protection, and NAC is one of the more efficient ways to increase cellular glutathione levels, it should be used, but in lower doses, and in conjunction with the branched-chained amino acids. Alpha-lipoic acid also increases glutathione levels, so that the two work together.

I would recommend taking limited amounts of NAC during therapy, until this controversy is settled.

> 100 mg twice a day from eight to thirteen years of age.
> 250 mg daily for age fourteen to eighteen.
> 500 mg daily after age eighteen.

The branched-chained amino acids can be purchased as a combination of leucine, valine, and isoleucine or you can use L-leucine alone. L-leucine can cause hypoglycemia at any age. Should you develop the symptoms of hypoglycemia, such as nervousness, trembling, and anxiety, stop taking it. Take only during the course of treatment. *Also, do not give l-leucine to infants and small children because of the danger of hypoglycemia.* Otherwise, the dose should be:

> From ages four to ten: add 250 mg to food at dinner.
> Ages eleven to sixteen: add 500 mg to each meal.
> Adults: 1,000 mg with each meal.

Nutraceuticals: Vitamins, Minerals, and Flavonoids

Vitamins and Minerals

The ability of neurons to resist mercury toxicity is dependent on the overall health of the cell and there is abundant evidence that vitamins and minerals play a vital role in keeping our cells healthy. You should always remember that these nutrients serve as essential cofactors in normal metabolism. For instance, most of us know that a severe deficiency of vitamin C will lead to scurvy, which left untreated can lead to death. Likewise, most people understand that a severe thiamine (vitamin B_1) deficiency can lead to beriberi, a potentially fatal condition if left to run its course.

For some unknown reason, though, many people do not consider that less severe nutritional deficiencies, which may not cause outright cell death, can still result in less-than-optimal overall cellular and physical health. Cells that function at minimized capacity make us more susceptible to injury and disease, which has been shown numerous times in the scientific and medical literature.

Modern research and human studies clearly demonstrate that even minor deficiencies in one or more nutrients can lead to disease. We know, for instance, that even a single deficiency in one of the B vitamins can cause profound impairment of the immune system. A recent study among juvenile inmates in a correctional facility and young people in public schools demonstrated significant improvements in behavior simply by correcting even a single subclinical nutrient deficiency. The stronger and healthier our cells, the better they will be able to resist injury, disease, and heavy metal toxicity; and if injured, the more likely our cells will recover.

Vitamins C and E may be the best-known of the antioxidant vitamins, but many others play a vital role in suppressing and controlling free radicals. All of the carotenoids, such as alpha and beta-carotene, lycopene, phytofluene, phytoene, canthoxanthin, lutein, and zeaxanthin, possess powerful antioxidant properties. Zinc, magnesium, and manganese can all neutralize free radicals. Zinc and manganese make up part of the antioxidant enzyme superoxide dismutase (SOD) which neutralizes the powerful superoxide free radical. The special fatty acid component called DHA, derived from omega-3-oils, has been shown to stimulate the production of SOD as well. Magnesium plays a part in the function of over three hundred enzymes, many of which produce energy, and can also protect the brain against excitotoxicity.

In one study, in which various compounds were tested for protective activity against mercury toxicity, researchers found alpha-tocopherol, selenium, trolox, and probucal all offered powerful protection against lower doses of mercury.[103] These compounds' protective abilities proved far less effective in cases of high-level mercury poisoning (such as the tragic Iraqi and Japanese incidents). The protective effects of vitamin E occurred even when given two days after the mercury exposure.

Some have recommended high doses of vitamin C as an antidote for mercury poisoning, but a recent study using large amounts of intravenous vitamin C found no evidence of increased mercury removal from the body. Such doses of vitamin C may protect the body in other ways, perhaps as an antioxidant, and there is also evidence that ascorbic acid can protect the brain against excitotoxicity.

Zinc has also been shown to protect the nervous system from mercury toxicity. This could be secondary to its antioxidant effects, or possibly because zinc plays a major role in metallothionein metabolism. This large molecule is unusual in that it contains numerous cysteine amino acid units. You will recall that cysteine binds very tightly with mercury and other heavy metals, such as lead and cadmium. One metallothionein molecule can hold up to a dozen molecules of mercury, making it a very efficient scavenger of mercury. Cells, especially in the liver, react to mercury poisoning by producing large amounts of metallothionein. Three forms of this unique molecule have been discovered. Types I and II are found in most cells, including in astrocytes in the brain. Type III is found only in neurons.

In special animal models of mice with no type I or II metallothionein (MT-knockout mice), Aschner and his co-workers at the Department of Physiology and Pharmacology at Wake Forest Medical University have shown that by selectively inserting genes that overproduce type I metallothionein in brain cells, the animals were dramatically protected against methylmercury toxicity.[104] This may offer a novel way to treat mercury poisoning in the future, if a way to stimulate metallothionein production can be found. In states of deficiency, we know that zinc supplementation will enhance metallothionein production.

A word of caution: while normal zinc levels are protective, high levels have been found to increase damage in the presence of mercury or in cases of excitotoxicity. The hippocampus normally contains naturally high concentrations of zinc.

Flavonoids

Flavonoids are a group of highly complex molecules found in all plants; over five thousand have been described thus far, and these God-created chemicals have been shown to possess many miraculous properties. They are very powerful and versatile antioxidants, reduce inflammation, improve blood flow to the brain, chelate several dangerous metals, improve cell-membrane quality, protect the blood-brain barrier, strengthen blood vessels, inhibit viral replication, and increase glutathione levels. Recent studies have shown that blueberries, strawberries, and spinach are excellent sources of flavonoids that protect the brain from metal toxicity.

As metal chelators, flavonoids show powerful effects against iron and copper, two of the most powerful generators of destructive free radicals, especially in the brain. In fact, it has been hypothesized that the free radicals generated by aluminum, mercury, and lead may be secondary to the fact that they trigger the release of iron from its storage molecule. If true, then flavonoids would play a dual role in protecting the nervous system from free-radical injury: directly as antioxidants, and indirectly by chelating iron and copper. Direct chelation of mercury by flavonoids has not been examined.

Recommendations

Quercetin plus vitamin C 500 mg
This common flavonoid possesses powerful cancer-inhibiting properties, and is a versatile antioxidant, iron chelator and anti-inflammatory. Adults take one or two three times a day.

Curcumin 500 mg

This is also a powerful flavonoid with many of the properties of quercetin. Take one to two, three times a day.

Hesperidin 500 mg

Hesperidin has been shown to powerfully chelate iron in the nervous system. Take one twice a day.

Zinc 15 mg daily

Higher does may be used only for a short duration, and only under competent medical supervision.

Eat lots of fresh fruits and vegetables.

Eat between seven and ten servings of nutrient-rich fruits and vegetables every day. You may want to use a Vita-Mix blender for better results. Drink twelve ounces twice a day.

Other Mercury-chelating Compounds

Mercury combines with malate and citrate to produce harmless compounds that can be removed from the body. An additional advantage is that it should remove the mercury from the nervous system as well, since the organic compounds and magnesium all enter the brain fairly easily. Citrate and malate are both normal byproducts of metabolism. By combining magnesium with the malate and citrate you can get double your protection, since magnesium protects neurons from excitotoxicity, and in addition, protects tubulin from mercury toxicity and promotes its formation. Malate and pyruvate have also been shown to protect against excitotoxicity.

The Thorne Research company makes a product called magnesium citramate that offers both malate and citrate. I would recommend two capsules twice a day. The magnesium will also help prevent heart attacks and strokes, as well as offer considerable brain protection against a number of neurological diseases.

Other Things to Remember

Until getting your amalgams removed, you should avoid chewing gum, tobacco, or pencil-ends. You should also avoid eating hot foods and drinking hot liquids. If you do consume hot foods or beverages, immediately afterwards either drink a very cold glass of water or eat frozen blueberries. The frozen blueberries not only will cool the amalgam but also will enhance your antioxidant defenses, especially in the brain. Cooling amalgam fillings has been shown to reduce the escape of mercury vapor significantly.

Brushing your teeth has also been shown to increase mercury vapor release. Either brush around the fillings or use a mouthwash instead, until you can get the fillings removed. Avoid toothpaste containing fluoride. Fluoride is a highly reactive metal and will complex with the mercury, which could increase its release. You should also avoid having your teeth cleaned, since the cleaning process can greatly increase mercury release from the fillings. Once your fillings have been removed, you can resume your regular cleaning program.

The removal of dental amalgam fillings should only be done by a dentist trained in its safe removal. The International Academy of Oral Medicine and Toxicology has a very specific protocol that must be followed to prevent dramatic rises in mercury levels that can follow attempts to remove mercury amalgams by conventional means. I would suggest that you call the IAOMT office for a list of names of dentists in your area using this approved method of filling removal. It is interesting to note that the vapors released during removal of fillings is so toxic that dentists are urged to wear a special mercury filter gas mask during the procedure. The EPA has determined that air levels of mercury above 50ug/M^3 are definitely toxic. High-speed drilling of the tooth during filling removal has been shown to release mercury concentrations as high as 4,000 ug/M^3.

Two days before you have your fillings removed, I advise that you take DMSA to lower your tissue and blood levels as low as possible. This chelating medication powerfully binds mercury in your tissues and promotes its elimination in your urine. This should be supervised by a physician trained in the use of the drug. If this chelator is used, you will have to have a test to see that your kidney function is normal (usually a BUN and a creatinine). I emphasize once again: *all chelation should be supervised by a physician expert in the procedure.*

Following removal of your fillings, you will have to undergo a prolonged period of chelation using DMSA. I would also recommend continuing all of the supplements I mentioned above throughout your treatment. Because of the difficulty in removing mercury from the nervous system, intermittent treatment over a prolonged period of time will be required. I suggest four days of oral chelation followed by two weeks off. This can be repeated until urine provocative testing indicates no further mercury is being released. How long this will take is dependent on your own body. For some, it may take only a few months. Others may require years of treatment.

Some have advocated using intravenous calcium or disodium EDTA intravenously or orally during treatment. Of some concern is the observation by Duhr and colleagues that when mercury complexes with EDTA it forms a compound that, in the brain, can powerfully inhibit a process (tubulin polymerization) that closely resembles a pathological event seen in Alzheimer's brains.[105] The experiment was done in isolated human neurons and not in live animals. In humans, EDTA does not pass through the blood-brain barrier very easily and only low concentrations would be expected to enter the brain. In this study, it was found that the presence of EDTA could increase the toxicity of mercury to tubulin tenfold. But, they were using EDTA concentration fifty to five hundred times higher than the mercury. They also found that magnesium offered significant protection against this toxicity. Magnesium has been shown to promote normal microtubule formation in the brain, again emphasizing the importance of magnesium in our diet.

Oral chelation with EDTA would make more sense, since a significant amount of the body's circulating mercury is excreted into the hepatic circulation (liver) and enters the gastrointestinal tract, primarily the large bowel. One study found that in humans, mercury excretion into the bowel is twenty times higher than into the urine.[106] If this is not removed, it will be reabsorbed. Oral EDTA would bind the mercury and prevent its absorption. Only about 5 percent of oral EDTA is absorbed.

One commercial product holds promise as a comprehensive oral chelation agent for many heavy metals, including mercury. This product, called Garlic Plus, not only contains EDTA but also garlic, which has been shown to prevent mercury toxicity to developing embryos and may protect adults as well. Garlic extract has also been shown to efficiently remove mercury from the brain.

Because garlic can effectively remove mercury from the nervous system, I recommend taking aged garlic extract daily. The dose is 300-600 mg three times a day. This method is the safest way to chelate brain mercury over a long period of time—without the danger of toxicity. If you eat mercury-containing fish, season it with garlic or take garlic extract with the meal to prevent absorption of the mercury.

The product also contains MSM (methylsulfonylmethane), dl-methionine and other components that reduce heavy metal loads, primarily in the bowel, and prevent their absorption. My only problem with the supplement is that it contains carrageenan, which has been shown to powerfully promote inflammation in tissues and may promote accelerated bowel cancer growth. For this reason, I would not use the product over prolonged periods of time. The evidence indicates that removal of the recirculated mercury from the intestines and bowel is critical to effective removal from the tissues. This should be done at the same time as DMSA chelation is being used.

Along this same line, to further remove mercury from the bowel, I would recommend daily enemas for one week during the removal process, and then at least weekly for the next month. This is especially important for those suffering from chronic constipation and those with especially high mercury burdens. A complete colon cleansing is vital.

Over twenty years ago it was noted that the consumption of alcohol could alter absorption of mercury. A study done in 1978 using mice found that intoxicated mice exposed to ethanol exhaled eight times more mercury vapor over a twenty-four hour period than did control mice.[107] While this caused excitement among those who wanted to drink their alcohol, caution was being advised. A follow-up study done eight years later, using rats given a dose of methylmercury once a day for ten days, demonstrated a significant increase in neurological injuries and mortality when they were exposed to alcohol at the same time.[108]

This seemed to settle the question, but unfortunately the waters were muddied by a third study, this time done in humans as well as animals, that indicated ethanol was protective.[109] In this study, three human subjects were exposed to 65ml of ethanol over thirty minutes before being exposed to mercury vapor. Only two controls were used. Researchers found: (1) reduced retention of mercury in the body, (2) an observed increase in the rapid phase of vapor loss by expiration, (3) increased storage of mercury in the liver, and (4) a marked reduction in mercury uptake by red blood cells. The experiment, when repeated in animals, produced the same results.

It may have been that the response to alcohol combined with methylmercury differs from exposure to metallic mercury vapor. We know the distribution in the body is different, as well as its elimination. There may be biochemical differences in the two forms of mercury on cellular components as well. The human study was also done with a single exposure to mercury vapor, whereas in the other experiments, mercury was allowed to accumulate in the body over ten days. This could have an impact on the eventual outcome of these two experiments.

Two things need to be said about ethanol. First, it is a neurotoxin in its own right, so the negative effect found in mice may have been an additive toxic phenomenon. Second, alcohol inhibits the catalase enzyme, which normally converts metallic mercury to the ionized form (Hg^{+2}). This will increase blood levels of metallic mercury by allowing the mercury to leave the organs and tissues, where it can more easily be eliminated. But, you must remember, elimination of metallic mercury depends on chelation being used, even though some increase in mercury elimination by the kidneys and GI tract will naturally occur. The only way I can see for alcohol to play a role in the elimination of mercury from a practical standpoint is by combining the chelation treatments with the alcohol consumption or by taking garlic extract. This way the gradient is away from the tissues and into the urine. But, this still doesn't overcome the problem of redistribution to the brain once mobilized, as well as the direct toxicity of the alcohol on the brain.

A recent study in which animals were either exposed to mercury alone, alcohol alone, or mercury and alcohol in combination clearly demonstrated a significant enhancement of mercury toxicity by alcohol on the nervous system when compared to mercury alone.[110] In this study, there were no outward symptoms of mercury toxicity or alcohol intoxication in the animals, but objective testing of nervous system functioning by EEG, cortical evoked potentials and conduction velocity of nerves, clearly showed a toxic effect that was dose dependent. In essence, this combination could possibly keep the flow of mercury always moving out of the body, but at the same time would markedly increase the toxicity of the mercury on the nervous system. I would not advise using this combination of alcohol and chelation until its success has been properly evaluated.

Finally, here is a word about a treatment that was considered the standard in treating cinnabar miners at the turn of the nineteenth century. This treatment involved sweating the mercury out of the body, and was done in a steam bath or similar arrangement. In my home state of Mississippi, you could easily accomplish the same thing by doing any form of work outdoors during the hot summer. A recent review of sweating as a treatment for mercury removal found it to be very effective.[111] The only drawback for this treatment, especially if you use a steam bath, is the negative effect of heat on neurological disorders, such as MS, Alzheimer's disease, Parkinson's disease, and ALS. This has been well-documented for multiple sclerosis. In fact, one of the tests for MS is the "hot bath test." Patients experience a sudden, and at times, dramatic worsening of their symptoms when placed in hot bath water. The effect is usually temporary, but can leave permanent worsening in a few patients.

The search for more effective methods of removing mercury from the brain is in progress. Until then I recommend the following method.

Testing

Have a twenty-four-hour urine test for mercury excretion or a stool mercury test. This is done without chelation to see how much mercury is being released on a daily basis. Also, if the mercury levels are extremely high, provocative testing may go beyond the measuring capability of the test.

Take DMSA, under a doctor's supervision, at a dose of 10 mg/Kg in two divided doses, daily for two days prior to the test. Two weeks before the test you should also start on the following supplements. (Doses given are for adults. Consult discussion above for other doses.)

Selenium 200 ug
Take once a day.

Alpha-lipoic acid 200 mg
Take three times a day with meals.

Vitamin E succinate (alpha-tocopherol succinate) 600 IU
Take twice a day.

Buffered vitamin C 500 mg
Take three times a day.

Multivitamin/mineral supplement.

Garlic Plus™

All of your urine is to be collected for twenty-four straight hours as instructed in the testing kit information. Keep the urine in the refrigerator and tell your children it is not a new drink. They will think it is gross, but they will survive. If it is not cooled, the test will be invalid. Follow the instructions exactly.

Once the test results come back, your doctor will proceed with your treatment. Continue with your supplements as before. If your mercury levels indicate that you are at a significant risk of mercury toxicity, you will have to determine the source of the mercury.

Treating Mercury Toxicity

Start DMSA at a dose of 10 mg/kg/day on an empty stomach. Divide this into two equal doses. Do not eat for at least one hour after taking the DMSA and drink only distilled water during that time. Take the DMSA for four days and then stop. After two weeks, start again for four more days and then stop. At that point you should be re-tested. You can start the urine collection on the last day you take the DMSA. Use the Great Smokies Diagnostic Laboratory Toxic Urine Screen test to follow your progress.

If your mercury is still elevated, repeat two more cycles, followed by a repeat in the toxic screen test. Continue this until your mercury levels are undetectable. Some suggest that chelation must be continued for several months or even a year in cases of obvious neuro-logical problems. Instead, I recommend taking garlic extract at a dose of 600 mg three times a day for at least one year. You can take it permanently without experiencing any side effects. Garlic is also excellent for reducing atherosclerosis.

You should take 50 mg of zinc with each dose of DMSA. This is because DMSA also binds to zinc and can cause significant zinc loss as well. Because DMSA binds more actively to mercury than zinc, the DMSA will deposit the zinc in the tissues where it is needed, and remove the mercury. Likewise, because of its affinity for mercury, even small amounts of DMSA can be effective.

Side effects of DMSA

On rare occasions serous allergic reactions can occur. Most reactions are mild and subside when the DMSA is discontinued. On very rare occasions bone marrow suppression can occur, leading to a drop in neutrophils and platelets, an effect that subsides when you stop taking the drug.

Persons with impaired kidney function should take DMSA cautiously and only under the supervision of a physician experienced in its use. Usually, much smaller doses are used in such cases.

I have found that using the higher dose of DMSA, 30 mg/kg/day can make some people feel poorly. For that reason, and the fact that DMSA works well at 10 mg/kg/day, I recommend the smaller dose which usually prevents side effects and is well tolerated.

Monitoring During Therapy

The need for evaluation of kidney function before instituting DMSA therapy is not absolute. Elderly persons, especially those with obvious health problems, should have a renal-function evaluation done. This can be done by ordering a BUN and creatinine study (blood test) before beginning chelation. Persons with known kidney disease should have DMSA administered only by a medical practitioner knowledgeable in the use of DMSA or other chelating drugs.

One problem I see frequently among those who administer chelation therapy, even among well-known practitioners, is a failure to do follow-up studies on heavy metal levels, as well as levels of trace minerals. This is especially important when using EDTA, since it can chelate numerous necessary metals, in addition to the harmful ones.

In general, a toxic metal screen (which includes a survey of metals found naturally in the body) should be done after the first two rounds of DMSA therapy and repeated at two months and then every six months until therapy is completed. Remember, DMSA will also bond with other metals, including zinc. Lost minerals must be replaced.

Conclusion

There is some good news on the mercury front. Many readers may have noticed that mercury thermometers have quietly disappeared from store shelves. Also, Vermont won a major battle at the end of 2001 when a federal appeals court upheld a 1998 law that requires labeling on all consumer products in that state that contain mercury (including fluorescent light bulbs, batteries, and others). With the support of many other states, the state was able to successfully battle a well-funded lawsuit by the National Electrical Manufacturers' Association that sought to void the label requirements based on the notion that such wording would violate the member companies' Constitutional rights by interfering with interstate commerce and infringe their First Amendment rights by compelling speech.

In other heartening developments, California Congresswoman Diane Watson has proposed a law that would phase out mercury amalgam fillings within five years. Also, the same California Dental Board that fought her original 1992 law for nearly a decade was finally dissolved by the state Legislature in 2001—an unprecedented act—due to its ongoing refusal to abide by state regulations. A new Board was appointed in the first part of 2002.

The Rhode Island legislature has passed a law requiring that insurance companies provide alternatives to dental amalgam. And in Maine, children on Medicaid-funded programs are no longer required to get amalgam fillings simply because they are on a low-income insurance plan.

4
Fluoride: What Have They Done to Us Now?

"Fluoridation is the greatest case of scientific fraud of this century."
Robert Carton, Ph.D., former EPA scientist, 1992

"Regarding fluoridation, the EPA should act immediately to protect the public. Not just on the cancer data, but on the evidence of bone fractures, arthritis, mutagenicity and other effects."
William Marcus, Ph.D., Senior EPA toxicologist, 1992

If the last chapter didn't scare you, this one should. Not that it is my intent to scare you; rather, I am trying to inform you of the real dangers you and your family face every day. Unfortunately, this world is inhabited by some people who seek a profit at any cost and have no concern for public welfare and safety. The fluoride story will powerfully demonstrate that we are indeed correct to be suspicious of megacorporations. We will see how these institutions have done everything in their power to avoid civic responsibility and to manipulate the government, scientific institutions, and the medical and dental professions, all in the name of empty profit.

Most of us have been led to believe by a powerful propaganda network that fluoridation of drinking water, regular brushing with fluoride toothpaste, and regular fluoride treatments are not only a good way to prevent cavities, but that the practice of fluoridation itself is very safe. Nothing could be further from the truth. Those who promote this viewpoint have an ulterior motive and, as we shall see, it is *not* your health.

What Is Fluoride?

A fluoride is a compound composed of the highly reactive element fluorine plus another element (or elements). For example, when fluorine combines with hydrogen the compound, hydrogen fluoride, is formed. Fluorine also combines readily with elemental metals, such as calcium and sodium, and the new compound then exhibits metallic properties; it is these compounds and their potential to accumulate in human tissues with which we will be most concerned.

The halogen fluorine is a yellowish, poisonous, highly corrosive gas. Halogens are a class of nonmetallic chemical elements which also include chlorine, bromine, and iodine, and are used industrially to kill pathogenic organisms—and can kill human cells as well. One halogen, chlorine, can kill all life forms including viruses and even prions (short for "proteinaceous infectious particle," a nucleic-acid-free protein which can transmit infectious disease, and is responsible for such infamous conditions as mad cow disease and Creutzfeldt-Jakob disease).

Fluorine is the least dense and most active member of this chemical class: it can even displace oxygen from water. And, because it is *so* reactive, it never occurs uncombined in nature. Fluoride is also a byproduct of the aluminum, steel, and fertilizer industries. It is essential to remember that fluoride is so reactive it can eat through steel, glass, iron, aluminum, and most other substances: it joins mercury as being one of the most poisonous substances on earth.

The compounds of the element are widely used in many industrial processes. For example, hydrofluoric acid (a water solution of hydrogen fluoride) is used in glass etching, and sodium fluoride in high concentrations is used in rat poisons and pesticides—in smaller concentrations, you will find it in your toothpaste. A common ingredient of many pesticides, sodium hexafluorosilicate (also known as sodium silicofluoride), is added to drinking water. In concentrations smaller than those used to destroy plant pests, the experts tell us the substance is not only safe, it also prevents cavities and encourages good dental health.

History of Fluoride in Cavity Prevention

Officials who loudly promote fluoridation of public water claim as their motivation the prevention of dental cavities. They frequently cite studies comparing tooth decay rates in fluoridated areas to unfluoridated areas, which purport to show dramatic reductions in tooth decay in children—as much as a 60 percent difference. If this were true, and fluoride were indeed safe, it would be a truly miraculous substance, but this still would not justify putting it in the water supply because we are being medicated and have not even been given a *choice* in the matter, as you will see. As it stands, there is in fact no credible evidence that fluoride added to the water supply reduces cavity rates at all, and several studies have convincingly demonstrated that the incidence of cavities is actually higher in fluoridated areas.

Shortly after the turn of the century it was noticed that children in certain areas of the country had a high incidence of damaged teeth. Further investigation disclosed that this mottling of their tooth enamel, now known as "dental fluorosis," was caused by elevated contents of naturally occurring fluoride in certain water systems. This finding motivated the American Dental Association and the U.S. Public Health Service to call for the removal of fluoride in the water from these areas. H. Trendley Dean of the U.S. Public Health Service in 1930 conducted the original work on this problem.

At this juncture, Dr. Gerald Cox took up the banner and suggested that using a smaller dose of fluoride could not only prevent dental fluorosis, but could even prevent cavities. He suggested adding 1 ppm of fluoride to the public drinking water. He made these proclamations without any studies, human or otherwise, to suggest that it would be effective or safe. What makes this so interesting is that Dr. Cox was on the staff of the Mellon Institute, and the Mellon family owned the Aluminum Company of America (Alcoa). One of the major waste products produced in the aluminum industry is fluoride. Because of its intense corrosive ability and extreme toxicity, disposal of fluoride had, up until that time, been a very expensive and controversial proposition. So what could the aluminum industry do with all of this toxic fluoride? After all, safe disposal cost the company millions of dollars every year. Ironically, the answer was to come from government.

Fortunately for Alcoa, Andrew Mellon, its founder, was also the Treasury Secretary. Interestingly, the U.S. Public Health Service at that time was under the direct control of the Treasury Secretary. Dr. Dean, who eventually came to support adding 1 ppm fluoride to public water supplies as a safe and effective way to reduce dental caries, became known as "Mr. Fluoridation," and was chosen by the USPHS to head up the fluoridation studies.

As Dr. John Yiamouyiannis noted in his excellent book, *Fluoride. The Aging Factor*, the American Medical Association (AMA), on September 18, 1943, (as fluoridation was first being proposed) cautioned that fluoride was a powerful protoplasmic poison, and because of its widespread presence in nature, toxic accumulation could be a major problem if water was fluoridated. On October 1, 1944, the *Journal of the American Dental Association* also noted that "the potential for harm outweighed those for good." It would behoove the Association's present membership to remember that in this same article, the ADA recognized that as little as 1.2-3.0 ppm of fluoride in drinking water was associated with "developmental disturbances in bones as osteosclerosis, spondylosis, and osteoporosis, as well as goiter."

Despite these cautionary warnings, Dr. Cox convinced Dr. J.J. Frisch, a Wisconsin dentist, to actively promote fluoridation of the water supply. According to historians of the era, Frisch led the charge with the frenzy of a religious zealot and turned it into a political crusade.

These developments were, of course, just what Alcoa's owners wanted. In 1944, according to Hearings before the Committee on Interstate and Foreign Commerce held on May 25-27, 1954, Alcoa hired a powerful attorney, Oscar Ewing, and paid him an annual salary of $750,000, even though Alcoa wasn't facing any major litigation. A few months after being hired, he left the company to accept a job as Federal Security Administrator, a position that put him in charge of the USPHS and under the direct control of—you guessed it—Treasury Secretary Mellon. It should also be noted that he made a great deal of fanfare about leaving such a well-paid job to serve his country. Not surprisingly, Ewing launched a vigorous nationwide campaign to promote fluoridation of public water supplies.

The fluoridation effort was no small project, and certainly not one that Ewing intended to lose. He hired the best public relations master money could buy: Edward L. Bernays, labeled by *The Washington Post* as "the original spin doctor." In addition to his other credentials, Bernays was also the nephew of Sigmund Freud. Bernays knew the best route to take was to get the endorsement of the dental and medical professionals, since the public depended on their wisdom in these matters, and generally trusted them.

By using all of the powers at their command Mellon's fluoridation team convinced the city council of Grand Rapids, Michigan, to allow its water supply to be fluoridated, with the city of Muskegon serving as an unfluoridated control in the experiment. The project was to begin on January 25, 1945, and would be the first U.S. city to add fluoride to its drinking water. Two things need to be understood at this point. First, the recommendation was accepted just three months after the dire warnings expressed by both the AMA and the ADA. Second, even at that time there was significant evidence that fluoride was toxic to cells in small concentrations, yet these devious men proceeded despite the fact that no human studies had been published on the safety of adding fluoride to Grand Rapids' water supply. The people of Grand Rapids were to be unwilling test subjects.

Opponents of the fluoridation project were quickly labeled by the masterminds of Alcoa's PR group as loonies and right-wing extremists who saw fluoridation as a communist plot. I remember these charges very well in the 1950s, having grown up during that period. Suddenly making a complete reversal of their previous stance, the USPHS and the ADA began to endorse widespread fluoridation, even before a single study of the Michigan experiment had been completed that could show fluoridation was safe, much less that it reduced cavities. But there was a compelling reason they didn't want to wait on the results of a study, namely because initial results were showing that tooth decay rates in unfluoridated Muskegon had decreased as much as fluoridated Grand Rapids. In fact, tooth decay rates were falling in all industrialized nations well *before* fluoridation. Why? Because of better hygiene and nutrition.

The fluoridationists' shenanigans were recognized as early as 1952 by Dr. A.L. Miller, a U.S. representative from Nebraska who was also Chairman of the Special Committee on Chemicals in Foods. He noted how strange it was that high officials of the USPHS would do a complete about-face on the acceptability of fluoridation—and within only three months of advocating extreme caution. Dr. Miller also noted that he could find no original studies by the AMA or the ADA, or any other evidence for fluoridation's usefulness. All those associations did was refer to each other for confirmation. Representative Miller also noted the convenient connection between Oscar Ewing in his position as Federal Security Administrator and his representation of Alcoa, which was anxious to get rid of its toxic fluoride waste.

In his book on this subject, Dr. Yiamouyiannis also points out that dissenting dentists were either censured or lost their ADA membership. Dental scientists themselves were controlled by the power of USPHS grant money: those who criticized fluoridation simply saw their grant monies dry up, a very effective tactic still used in many other areas of politicized science.

The list of people involved in the fluoridation conspiracy reads like a rogues' gallery. For example, there is John Small, the USPHS' fluoridation expert since the 1960s. His sole job is to stem any criticism of fluoridation from any quarter, and he does his job very well. One of his major tasks is to harass, intimidate, and virtually destroy anyone who dares to publicly speak or write about the dangers of fluoridation. As an example of his viciousness, I will share the story of Dr. Yiamouyiannis, who was once the biochemical editor of the Chemical Abstracts Service, the world's largest chemical information center. When John Small learned that Dr. Yiamouyiannis was writing critical reviews of fluoridation, he contacted the problem doctor's immediate superior and expressed his displeasure. In ensuing conversations with this superior, Dr. Yiamouyiannis was told that $1.1 million in federal funding was in jeopardy if he did not cease and desist his criticisms of fluoridation. The good doctor was warned several more times and finally—unwilling to suppress the truth about fluoridation dangers—he was forced to resign. So much for the independence of science.

The ADA Fights Back: the Grand White Paper on Fluoridation

After his forced resignation, Dr. Yiamouyiannis was appointed director of the National Health Federation, where he continued his battle against fluoridation. In 1978 his pivotal testimony before a Pennsylvania court convinced the presiding judge to ban fluoridation of all public water supplies in the region.

Terrified their pet project was in jeopardy, the ADA hurriedly put together a "White Paper on Fluoridation," which set the tone for future dealings with its enemies. Opponents of fluoridation were henceforth to be labeled as "self-serving" and "self-styled experts" unqualified to speak on the issue. The leaders of the ADA suggested that dental associates convince their politician patients of the virtues and safety of fluoridation while they had them in the chair. The paper also suggested that the EPA, CDC, National Centers for Health Statistics, National Institute of Dental Research, and state dental societies all work together to move on communities considered ripe for the implementation of fluoridation.

Incredibly, this seminal paper even included a suggestion for behavioral profiling of opponents so that they could be better dealt with. It said that public debates about safety

Fluoride...

- causes dental fluorosis.
- damages DNA repair enzymes.
- increases risk for osteoporosis.
- increases risk for cancer (bone, oral, bladder, lung).
- causes genetic damage.
- causes skeletal fluorosis.
- causes abnormal brain development.
- causes hypothyroidism.
- reduces fertility in males.

TABLE 4.1

would be deferred to the USPHS and state health departments, who would assure a trusting public that no studies existed indicating a problem with small concentrations of fluoride being added to water. Of course, this was—and continues to be—a bold-faced lie. Even by the 1960s there was significant scientific evidence indicating that, even at the low levels proposed by fluoridationists, the substance is toxic to humans.

The War Council Meets to Plan Strategy

Individual choice is utterly repugnant to such single-minded collectivists, who always resort to compulsion when citizens reject their grandiose plans. So it comes as no surprise that the powerful proponents of fluoridation decided to cull their immense resources, and scheduled a meeting to deal with growing public dissension. Fluoridation was all-out war in the minds of these crusaders, and it would be fought as such.

On August 9 and 10, 1983, members of a planning committee met at the University of Michigan to organize their troops and plan their strategy. The powerful forces of government and industry had joined hands in this battle to the finish. This "war council" was sponsored by the Department of Health and Human Services, the Public Health Service, Centers for Disease Control, Center for Prevention Services, Dental Disease Prevention Activity, Dental Health Plan of Michigan, Blue Cross/Blue Shield of Michigan, and Medical Products Laboratories.

The ostensible purpose of the meeting was to discuss the status of the antifluoridation opposition, to analyze their opponents' motivations, to assess a need for a national fluoridation policy, and to evaluate legal challenges.

It is interesting to note that one of the speakers, Dr. William T. Jarvis, warned that when he allowed fluoridation debates in his dental classes, "Invariably, each class became more antifluoridationist as a result of the debate." Dr. Sheldon Rovin also warned that participants should avoid local referendums on fluoridation. Why? Because fluoridation opponents would convince the public to reject fluoridation by presenting the scientific facts concerning the danger. And incredibly, Dr. D. Scott Navarro of Blue Cross/Blue Shield, as chairman of his workshop, suggested that taxpayers themselves should bear the cost of litigation when proponents had to defend fluoridation before the courts!

The ADA Struggles to Cover Up Fluoride Dangers

The passage of the Safe Drinking Water Act in 1974 presented a terrible dilemma for the ADA. The EPA set the maximum allowable concentration of fluoride at 1.4 ppm for warmer climates and 2.4 ppm for cooler climates. The reason for this disparity is related to the issue of *total body accumulations* of toxic substances in body tissues, which—as I showed with mercury—remain in the body for a very long time after exposure. With fluoride, the concern is with potentially dangerous accumulations in bone. The EPA's assumption was that people in warmer climates drink more water than those who live in cooler climates, and would thus store a greater total amount of fluoride over the same period of time.

The reason for the ADA's concern was that fluoride levels being added to drinking water were very close to those the EPA recognized as toxic levels. As we shall see, toxicity actually occurs at concentrations below those being added to water. The ADA asked EPA officials to raise the recognized toxicity levels to 8 ppm to lessen public fears of the fluoridation program. As a result, the EPA held hearings, inviting ADA representatives to attend. Lisa Watson, the ADA's delegate at these hearings, was shown a slide of a child's horribly eroded and crumbling teeth due to dental fluorosis. She was told that this had resulted from exposure to 4 ppm of fluoride occurring naturally. When asked if she considered this to be a significant health problem, her response was "no," that it was a cosmetic problem. She didn't stand alone in that conclusion.

A bogus report prepared by the government and sent to the EPA scientists concluded that dental fluorosis did not occur below 2 ppm. This was clearly a lie, since other studies clearly demonstrated its occurrence at 0.8 ppm. The report also concluded that "teeth with fluorosis are desirable." How desirable are teeth that are crumbling, pitted, and mottled with dark brown spots? Repair of fluorosis is very expensive, even more so than cavities.

EPA scientists were not convinced by the dog-and-pony act and refused to raise the toxic limits to 8 ppm. The vote was ten to two in favor of leaving the toxic limits at 1.4 and 2.4 ppm for children up to age nine. Unsurprisingly, given the government, industry, and forces embroiled in the debate, the report was later altered, officially raising toxic levels to 4 ppm—completely without the committee's knowledge or consent.

Now let us backtrack for a bit to a very interesting part of the fluoridation story, one which illustrates well how the dovetailing interests of industry profit and government protectionism collude to suppress truth and destroy public trust.

The Atomic Bomb and Fluoridation of Water

This astounding report is the result of the intrepid efforts of two medical journalists, Joel Griffiths and Chris Bryson, who have labored against all the forces of government secrecy to provide us with this critically important investigation. Consult their 1997 article, "Toxic Secrets: Fluoride And The Manhattan Project," for a complete account of the sordid politics behind fluoridation of our water supplies.

The story begins during World War II in 1943 with the Manhattan Project and the creation of the atomic bomb, one of the most secret projects in our nations' history. The manufacture of high-grade uranium for nuclear bombs required huge amounts of fluoride—millions of tons of it in fact—and many parts of the project were farmed out to America's manufacturing firms, such as the industry giant DuPont. Handling such enormous quantities of fluoride proved to be a monumental task, chiefly because of the escape of the fluoride into the atmosphere.

In the early 1940s, the E.I. DuPont de Nemours Company chemical factory in Deepwater, New Jersey, was one of the largest fluoride producers on the Manhattan Project. The manufacturing process continually released clouds of toxic fluorine gas into the atmosphere, covering nearby farms and orchards. At the time, these farms produced some of the highest quality produce in the area: their peaches went directly to the Waldorf Astoria Hotel in New York and the Campbell's Soup Company bought up tomatoes from the region. But by the summer of 1944, farmers began reporting blighted and "burned" crops. Peaches would no longer grow, and whole orchards were abandoned. Animals were also affected. Horses began to walk stiff-legged and some cows became so sick they could graze only by crawling on their bellies. Farm workers who ate the crops became sick as well, and many vomited continually for up to two days after eating the produce.

Not unlike most disasters involving the government, a massive cover-up ensued. Eventually, the Pentagon intervened directly and engineered a whitewash of the disaster that included token pay-offs to the injured farmers who had filed suit against the government in 1946 once the war ended. These lawsuits sent ripples of fear throughout the government (as recently released secret memos from the period indicate), and raised concerns that future suits would raise public awareness of the dangers of fluoride in manufacturing and defense, thus impeding the government's ability to continue its atomic research—the cornerstone of this country's international superiority following World War II. At the center of it all sat two major players from the Atomic Energy Commission: Dr. Harold Hodge and his immediate superior, Colonel Stafford L. Warren, Chief of the Medical Division.

It is important to note that plans for testing of animal and human subjects began even before the Deepwater incident. A declassified Manhattan Project memo marked SECRET and dated April 29, 1944, addressed to Colonel Stafford Warren reads: "Clinical evidence suggests that uranium hexafluoride may have a rather marked central nervous system effect...It seems most likely that the F [code for fluoride] component rather than the T [uranium] is the causative factor." The memo-writer then seeks approval from Warren for a program of animal research on CNS effects, suggesting that worker confusion may result from fluoride poisoning. Strangely, the proposal attached to the request—which Warren approved the very same day—and the study itself *have disappeared from the National Archives*. Harold Hodge is named in the memo as the author of the missing proposal.

Planning also began in 1943 for human studies. It was obvious that researchers would need a large-scale human experiment to justify what they were proposing; that is, using fluorida-tion of the public water supply to prevent cavities. The first experiment would involve two matched cities in New York State, one to have its water fluoridated and one to serve as a control. The town of Newburgh was to have 1 ppm of fluoride added to its water supply and Kingston was to serve as a control, since its natural fluoride content was less than 0.15 ppm.

The central research facility for fluoride testing was to be the University of Rochester, under the direction of our old friends Hodge and Warren. It is important to emphasize that these studies were not really about reducing cavities so much as deflecting bomb-related law suits. Another declassified memo, this one dated May 2, 1946, and addressed to General Leslie R. Groves, states that agencies "are making scientific investigations to obtain evidence which may be used to protect the interest of the Government at the trial of the suits brought by owners of peach orchards in...New Jersey."

Furthermore, it is crucial to know that the University of Rochester had already been used as a testing facility for toxic effects on humans of radioactivity. In a Pulitzer Prize-winning article in the early 1990s, Eileen Welsome revealed the cruel and unethical tests that had been performed in Rochester without the knowledge or consent of the unfortunate victims who were injected with lethal doses of radioactive plutonium. It is now obvious that the University of Rochester enjoyed a very cozy relationship with the federal government and funding of highly questionable secret research during this whole period.

The fluoride deal was worked out by a special committee of the New York Health Department. Not surprisingly, none other than Dr. Harold Hodge—chairman of the special committee—was appointed director of the fluoride study program, tasked with establishing the safety of fluoride to combat cavities. He would eventually become the nation's leading proponent of water fluoridation.

Other committee members included Henry L Bennett, a captain in the Manhattan Project's medical section, and John W. Fertig, who was a member of the Pentagon's super secret research and development office. These men's military affiliations were kept secret and special care was taken to conceal their secret mandate. Dr. David B. Ast, Chief Dental officer with the State Health Department was appointed officer in charge of the Newburgh project.

Dr. Ast stringently denied, even until his death, knowledge of the Atomic Energy Commission's involvement in the study, but a recently released secret memo indicates otherwise. Ast not only attended a secret wartime Manhattan Project conference in January 1944, he also accompanied Dr. Hodge on a government-sponsored trip to investigate the DuPont spill that decimated crops and injured people and livestock.

Only a few months after the ADA's Michigan experiment began, Newburgh's water was fluoridated in May 1945 and Dr. Hodge and his committee worked out in detail what kinds of studies would be done over the following decade on the exposed population. Not surprisingly, these scientists conducted secret studies (called Project F) on Newburgh's population separate from those that had been formally announced. These studies included tests of tissue and blood levels of fluoride and possible toxic effects of chronic exposure. The New York State Health Department cooperated fully by shipping blood, tissue, and placental samples directly to Dr. Hodge's laboratory at the University of Rochester.

In the course of the study, Dr. Hodge hit upon a grand idea. He knew that atomic bomb workers had experienced a dramatic decrease in cavity incidence—because exposure to high levels of fluoride had caused their teeth to fall out. Fewer teeth, fewer cavities! This handy statistical method would be used again and again, when later studies "demonstrated" that fluoride reduced cavities in children less than six years old. They too had fewer teeth, but this fact is never mentioned in published study results.

The final conclusions of the Newburgh study were published in the *Journal of the American Dental Association* in 1956. It essentially stated that small concentrations of fluoride placed in the drinking water were found to be safe. The study itself is still classified, so that we may never know what was really discovered concerning the toxicity of chronic exposure to low doses of fluoride in large populations. In fact, the report is missing from the files of the University of Rochester, the Atomic Energy Commission, and the U.S. National Archives. Very convenient!

As a comparison, it is interesting to note that Bryson and Griffiths did find one study in the National Archives that formed the basis of an obviously censored article that appeared in a 1948 issue of the *Journal of the American Dental Association*. These journalists compared the actual study with the journal results, irrefutably showing that the government suppressed information about the very real health risks posed by fluoride exposure. For example, the secret government study stated that many of the men in the study exposed to fluoride had no teeth—yet the published version made no mention of this vital fact. It simply stated that the men exposed to fluoride had fewer cavities. While we have only one study, and many were completed which have disappeared, it is this missing research upon which is based the alleged safety of water fluoridation.

Problems with the Newburgh Experiment

This famous massive population experiment, which began in 1945, was loudly proclaimed seven or eight years later to have shown that indeed fluoride did reduce cavities in Newburgh. A figure of 60 percent reduction in cavities was reported. In fact, the results were tainted just like the original, but still secret, Atomic Energy Commission report that also showed a 60 percent reduction in cavities. As you will recall, the "reduction" in tooth decay was because the subjects had 60 percent fewer teeth. The children of Newburgh were found to have fewer teeth and a delay in the appearance of new teeth.

In 1995 another comparison was made between the cavity incidence of still-unfluoridated Kingston with fluoridated Newburgh. Researchers found little difference in cavity incidence in seven- to fourteen-year-olds. Statistically, the children in Kingston had slightly fewer cavities than those in Newburgh. But, there was one major difference: children in the fluoridated community of Newburgh had twice the incidence of dental fluorosis. So now let us address the essential question: Does fluoridation of drinking water reduce cavities in children?

Does Fluoridation of Drinking Water Actually Reduce Cavities?

This, obviously, is the most important question, since it is the sole justification for adding fluoride to the public water system. According to conventional academic wisdom, the basis for fluoridating water to prevent cavities hinges on a study conducted in 1933-1934 by the United States Health Service, led by Dr. H. Trendley Dean, in which communities with naturally fluoridated water were compared to communities having low levels of fluoride in their water. Bauxite, Arkansas, was chosen as the study city, since it had a natural level of fluoride of 14 ppm. Researchers claimed that Bauxite had a dental caries (tooth decay) rate of 39 percent compared to unfluoridated communities of 65 percent. This sounds very impressive.

Numerous studies have now shown that cities with fluoridated water, when compared to unfluoridated cities, either have no reduction in cavities or the unfluoridated cities have an even lower incidence of caries. If fluoridating the water could reduce the incidence of cavities, then fluoridated San Francisco should have a drastically lower incidence of cavities than unfluoridated Los Angeles. In truth, Los Angeles has a lower incidence of tooth decay than San Francisco.

The USPHS used thirty-nine thousand school children to carry out one of the largest U.S. studies ever done on fluoridation and tooth decay. The results of this important study were not made available to the public until Dr. John Yiamouyiannis forced the release of the report under the Freedom of Information Act. Once he reviewed the data, he realized why they wanted it kept secret: it clearly demonstrated that the incidence of tooth decay in fluoridated and unfluoridated areas was no different. When confronted with this damaging information, the defenders of fluoridation stated that there was a difference in children below age six. Once again it was shown that in the fluoridated group tooth eruption was delayed or prevented, resulting in fewer teeth. It was the old idea: fewer teeth, fewer cavities.

In 1981 Ziegelbecker reviewed all published studies and found no evidence of cavity reduction by fluoridating water supplies.[112] In another study of eight developed countries, Mark Diesendorf looked at the data on decayed, missing and filled (DMFT) teeth over a thirty-year period and found no difference between fluoridated and unfluoridated cities.[113]

In reviewing the literature on fluoridation and tooth decay, nothing I found convinced me more of the dreadful error of fluoridation of public water supplies than the testimony of Dr. John Colquhoun, a man of incredible integrity and courage. All of us are vulnerable to error and being led astray, either by the deception of others or by our own desire to believe. But, it takes a man of enormous courage and conviction to admit publicly that he has been in error, and to endure the scorn of his colleagues in an effort to correct his error. Dr. Colquhoun is such a man.

As a dentist of high repute, he was chosen to promote the new program of fluoridation in his home city of Auckland, New Zealand's largest city. From his position as the Principal Dental Officer, he led the battle to fluoridate not only Auckland but the rest of New Zealand as well, whose population had been resisting government efforts. Because New Zealand's dental care system was socialized, Colquhoun was able to collect large amounts of data on tooth decay rates, especially in poor areas. He wrote widely quoted papers on the dramatic fall in tooth decay rates in the fluoridated city. Like others today, he attacked his colleagues who dared to disagree, sometimes viciously. His success in promoting fluoridation was so phenomenal that he was elected president of the Fluoridation Society.

In 1980 he was chosen to make a world tour to further study fluoridation efforts by colleagues in other countries. Before he left, his superiors confided in him that new evidence had arisen indicating that tooth decay was already declining in unfluoridated school districts at a rate equal to that of the fluoridated areas. He was told that the elite members of the fluoride "team" would soon discover the cause of this problem and correct it.

Colquhoun's world tour took him to North America, Britain, Europe, and Australia, where he met all of the experts promoting fluoridation in their respective countries. Much to his surprise, he discovered that these experts were having the same problem as his colleagues in New Zealand. They were finding dramatic declines in tooth decay of equal magnitude in both fluoridated and unfluoridated communities. Again, they had no explanation.

On his return, Dr. Colquhoun reviewed the dental statistics collected on all children living in Auckland, and to his surprise he found that children living in unfluoridated areas had fewer fillings and better overall dental health than those in fluoridated areas. It is important to remember that New Zealand's dental program is completely socialized, so that all children receive essentially the same care.

At this juncture, Dr. Colquhoun requested dental statistics from the rest of New Zealand, and was told that they were not to be made public. Review of the information made clear why: it clearly demonstrated that the number of children with perfect teeth was greater in the unfluoridated areas. Such a revelation would have endangered the fluoridation program, since its sole stated goal was to reduce dental caries in youth. The data were eventually published.

Meanwhile, in the United States, fluoridation promotion experts refused for many years to release their own data comparing fluoridated and unfluoridated areas, surveys that clearly demonstrate no difference in tooth decay rates between fluoridated and unfluoridated areas. Other large population studies in Missouri and Arizona have shown similar results.

In fact, some studies have shown a direct connection between cavity incidence and fluoridation levels. For instance, when Dr. Steelink reviewed dental records of all school children in Tucson, Arizona, some twenty-six thousand children, he found higher cavity occurrence in fluoridated areas. In fact, the higher the fluoride intake, the greater the number of cavities. Similar results were seen in Australia, Britain, Canada, Sri Lanka, Greece, Malta, Spain, Hungary, and India.

India is an interesting anomaly in this story, in that it has been leading the fight *against* fluoridation for a long time. Why? Because naturally high fluoride water levels in that country have created ongoing health problems in many Indian communities. In a thirty-year study of over 400,000 children, Dr. Teito and his team found that as fluoride levels in the water increased, tooth decay also increased.

So what can account for the steep drop in tooth decay in *this* country? A review of dental statistics clearly indicates that tooth decay began to decline sometime in the 1930s. Fluoride wasn't added to toothpaste by Proctor & Gamble until early 1960, so brushing with fluoride toothpaste could not have had anything to do with this decrease. One of the most important factors in improved dental health was better overall nutrition and greater consumption of fruits and vegetables (greatly assisted by the introduction of refrigerators about this time). Others have pointed to the eightfold increase of cheese consumption, which has been shown to inhibit tooth decay, most likely due to its high calcium content.

Not to be outdone, fluoridation proponents began to rig their studies to purposefully show that fluoridation reduces cavities. A good case in point is the famous Hastings Fluoridation Experiment. Dr. Cloquhoun obtained the data on this often-cited study by using his country's version of our Freedom of Information Act. He found that, to begin with, dentists were ordered to change the way they diagnosed tooth decay, toughening the criteria of what could be called a cavity, so that fluoridationists in his country could report a dramatic fall in cavities with the introduction of fluoridation.

Even more devious, New Zealand fluoridationists originally included the city of Napier as an unfluoridated control. Then suddenly, without explanation, they dropped Napier from the study. Why? Because tooth decay rates in unfluoridated Napier actually declined even more than the fluoridated city, and researchers couldn't let the public know that, so they just eliminated the "problem" from the study. Similar deceptions were used in the Grand Rapids, Newburgh, Evanston and Brantford studies in the United States. This is not only bad science but criminal behavior, since by then studies had demonstrated that fluoride was associated with dental fluorosis, skeletal fluorosis, osteoporosis, increased cancer rates, lower fertility, weakened bones, genetic damage, and even damage to the brain. There was, and is, absolutely no justification for adding fluoride to drinking water!

The Cancer Connection

Most regulatory agencies responsible for public safety cite preventing cancer and lowering risk as the major criteria in limiting exposure to potentially toxic substances. In general, wide margins of safety are adopted for safe doses and toxic or cancer-causing doses. The differential recognizes wide variances in human sensitivity to various cancer-causing agents, and also takes into consideration the problem of accumulation and long-term exposure to known toxins. We know that each of us possesses unique metabolic and biochemical differences, and our individual responses to a toxin can vary widely. For example, if you give one hundred people a large dose of arsenic, most will become violently ill and many will die. But some will be able to consume the very same dose with very little toxic effect. In fact, it may take massive doses of arsenic to kill such a person. The same is true for all toxins.

There are many reasons for our variable tolerance to poisonous substances, including: our ability to detoxify poisons, our antioxidant defenses, strength of our DNA-repair enzymes, degree of absorption of the toxins, differences in our cellular enzymes, age differences, presence of pre-existing diseases, genetic inheritance, exposure to other toxins at the same time, and the strength of our immune system. To complicate matters, there exist many as yet unknown or poorly understood factors.

In a paper published in the journal, *Cancer Research*, in 1984 Dr. Takeki Tsutsui and his co-workers demonstrated that fluoride could indeed induce cancer (fibrosarcoma) when injected under the skin of hamsters.[114] This original research was confirmed by other independent laboratories, including the Argonne National Laboratories. Of special importance, the Argonne Labs found that fluoride enhanced the cancer-causing ability of other chemicals as well.[115]

Clinical studies on humans also demonstrated precancerous transformation of cells in patients who had received fluoride as a failed treatment for osteoporosis.[116] These precancerous cells reverted to normal when fluoride treatments were stopped.

Alerted by these studies, other researchers examined the effects of exposing animals to a concentration of 1 ppm in drinking water, and observed a 25 percent increase in tumor growth in mice.[117] This 1965 study was available to all of the government agencies pushing fluoridation of city water systems at that time, as well as to the Proctor & Gamble company, who made the decision to start adding large amounts of fluoride to toothpaste. The importance of this study cannot be stressed too highly. Consider that there are hundreds of thousands of cancer patients in the United States alone, and cancer has become one of the two leading causes of death in this country since the end of WWII (along with heart disease). The idea that fluoride could increase the growth rate of cancers in the population by 25 percent is truly frightening.

The next step in connecting fluoridation of drinking water to cancer involved a careful look at the incidence of cancer in fluoridated cities versus unfluoridated cities. This important study was carried out in 1977 by Dr. Dean Burke, former chief chemist at the National Cancer Institute, and Dr. John Yiamouyiannis. They compared the cancer death rates in the ten largest fluoridated cities with rates in ten matched unfluoridated cities. The cities' cancer death rates were very similar during the period just prior to fluoridation, but once public water supplies were fluoridated, they found a strong association between cancer death rates and fluoridation. In fact, fluoridated cities demonstrated a 10 percent increase in cancer deaths following the first thirteen to seventeen years of fluoridation.

To appreciate the enormity of this number, that means that during this period, for a city the size of San Francisco with 6.6 million people, fluoridation could potentially be responsible for hundreds of new cancers. Who wants to volunteer to be the one to die? But there are no volunteers: fluoridation has been forced on you and millions of others.

That fluoridation of drinking water is a significant risk factor for cancer has even been proven in several court cases, one in Pennsylvania and one in Illinois. The judges in these cases not only cited fluoride added to water as a cancer risk but also as a risk to health in general.[118]

To confirm what they had discovered in the first cancer study, Drs. Burk and Yiamouyiannis conducted a second study of cancer deaths rates in all cities east of the Mississippi River with populations greater than ten thousand, and again found statistically significant elevated death rates in fluoridated cities as compared to unfluoridated cities.[119]

As a result of these studies, Congress became concerned with the effect of the fluoridation program and began hearings on the subject in 1977. The US Public Health Service tried to allay Congressmen's fears by presenting data that refuted Drs. Burke and Yiamouyiannis' studies. But the USPHS' study was seriously and flagrantly flawed, a fact addressed in the course of the hearings: it contained significant mathematical errors and left out 80-90 percent of the data pertinent to the issue.

Congress, not convinced by the USPHS' answers, ordered them to conduct a study that would definitively answer the question of whether fluoridation of drinking water causes substantial cancer risk. In an effort to carry out this mandate, the USPHS obtained the services of the Battelle Memorial Institute in Columbus, Ohio, to carry out the studies. On February 23, 1989, the Institute announced the results of its careful research.[120] Of particular importance, they had discovered that exposure to fluoride in drinking water caused a rare form of liver cancer in male and female mice called a hepatocholangiocarcinoma. The incidence of these cancers was, yet again, dose-dependent—the higher the dose of fluoride, the greater the incidence of the cancer.

This tumor is so rare that it was the first one of its kind the project leader of Battelle Labs had ever seen in his years of testing carcinogenic substances. The USPHS actually tried to deny that the observed growths were cancerous tumors at all, but when the slides were later examined by the scientist who had first described this rare cancer he confirmed that the growths were indeed hepatocholangiocarcinomas.

A second part of the study revealed that there was also a dose-dependent relationship between fluoride consumption in drinking water and cancer of the mouth. Exposure of the tissues had produced a precancerous lesion called oral squamous cell metaplasia. At 11 ppm there was a 2 percent incidence and at 45 ppm a 12 percent incidence. While this may seem far above the doses most people would be exposed to, consider that fluoride treatments at dentists' offices contain 15,000 ppm of fluoride, which soaks into the tissues of the mouth. Also the use of fluoride varnishes, plus fluoride mouthwashes and toothpaste all add up to very high levels of fluoride in direct contact with the tissues of the mouth.

It is not unreasonable, given the Battelle study's findings, to conclude that the cumulative effect of all this fluoride exposure would produce oral cancers in a small, but significant, percentage of people, especially if they engaged in other risky practices such as smoking and chewing tobacco. An examination of fluoridated communities compared to unfluoridated communities confirms our fears: oral cancers are more common in fluoridated communities. Once again, the incidence is related to the number of years the community has been fluoridated, the data indicating a 33-50 percent increase in oral cancers in fluoridated communities.

Cancer of the Bone

That fluoride is linked to bone cancers has been known for a long time. But, like so much of this unwelcome information, it has been kept from the public. In fact, Proctor & Gamble Company's scientists found a link between fluoride ingestion and cancer formation in bone at a time when they were adding fluoride to Crest toothpaste. This information was not voluntarily released but required the good old Freedom of Information Act to pry it loose. According to Dr. Yiamouyiannis, other studies by Proctor & Gamble confirmed that fluoride was linked to precancerous bone lesions.

Battelle Labs also found a link to bone cancers. In their carefully conducted studies they found a rare form of bone cancer called an osteosarcoma, significantly increased in male rats exposed to fluoridated drinking water. At 45 ppm the incidence was 2 percent and at 79 ppm, 5 percent. In humans this highly malignant cancer most often occurs in males younger than twenty years old. Remember that fluoride accumulates in the body, primarily in the bones, and several studies have found bone fluoride levels in fluoridated areas to be several thousand parts per million.

If there is a connection between bone cancer and fluoridation, we would expect bone cancer rates in young males should have gone up in fluoridated areas—and they have. A study by the National Cancer Institute found that the incidence of osteosarcoma was 50 percent higher in fluoridated communities in men up to age nineteen, when compared to unfluoridated areas.[121]

In 1992 the New Jersey Department of Health published a study showing osteosarcomas occurred at a rate three to seven times higher in males in fluoridated areas as compared to unfluoridated areas.[122] A review of three major studies found that overall, the incidence of osteosarcomas in young males increased 70 percent with fluoridation of drinking water.[123]

Other Cancers

Industrial exposure to airborne fluoride has been related to lung cancer in several studies. In one such study, cancer of the lung was 35 percent higher, larynx cancer 129 percent higher, and bladder cancer 84 percent higher in cryolite workers exposed to high levels of fluoride as compared to non-exposure rates.[124] Cryolite, or sodium aluminum fluoride, is a mineral that occurs naturally on the west coast of Greenland and only a few other places in the world. Due to its rarity, the compound has been synthesized for use as a flux in aluminum production. Cryolite contains about 50 percent fluoride.

With ever-increasing accumulations of fluoride in our water, foods, medicines and dental treatments, dangerous side effects of high levels of fluoride exposure are being seen. And unless stringent and drastic measures are taken now, future generations will be unable to escape high-level exposure and its destructive consequences.

Fluoride and Genetic Damage

Closely connected to the cancer issue is the risk of genetic damage with low-dose fluoride exposure. In fact, twenty-two separate animal studies have already linked genetic damage to fluoride exposure. We know that DNA damage occurs constantly and that our survival is dependent on a system of healthily functioning DNA-repair enzymes whose job it is to fix injuries induced by a daily barrage of free radicals. We also know that impaired DNA repair mechanisms are associated with increased cancer risk.

In 1976 Dr. Wolfgang Klein and co-workers demonstrated that cells exposed to 1 ppm fluoride exhibit a 50 percent reduction in DNA-repair-enzyme activity.[125] Not only does this increase cancer risk, it also encourages aggravation of degenerative diseases of the nervous system, such as Alzheimer's disease, Parkinson's disease, and Lou Gehrig's disease (ALS), as well as other degenerative diseases of aging. When unrepaired DNA damage occurs in reproductive cells, the damage is passed on to children as well.

Another study, by Dr. Aly Mohamed of the genetics department at the University of Missouri, demonstrated that as little as 1 ppm of fluoride could result in chromosomal damage in cells from the testes and bone marrow. Overall, the genetic damage increased with length of exposure and increasing dose. At 1 ppm, 25.7 percent of the bone marrow cells showed DNA damage at three weeks and 32.1 percent at six weeks. At 10 ppm, 35.5 percent of the marrow cells had DNA damage at three weeks and at six weeks, 46 percent were damaged. Remember that 1 ppm is the amount added to most municipal water systems. Because fluoride concentrations increase with time and by cooking, even 10 ppm can be attained in real life situations, especially in hot areas of the world.

Incredibly, even the studies done by Proctor & Gamble, makers of Crest toothpaste, found that 1 ppm of fluoride could cause genetic damage in Chinese hamsters' ovary cells.[126] The lowest dose of fluoride inducing genetic damage in human cells was found to be 0.6 ppm.

More recent evidence, presented in peer-reviewed scientific journals, clearly shows that fluoride causes chromosomal damage. For example, Dr. Anuradha and co-workers in the journal, *Archives of Toxicology*, July 2000, demonstrated that fluoride activates a destructive reaction in human cells (activation of caspase-3) that results in severe DNA damage.[127]

In another study, researchers looked for chromosomal aberrations in the white blood cells of workers in a phosphate fertilizer factory, and reported a significant elevation of such DNA damage that was both dose- and time-dependent,[128] meaning that the amount of damage depended on how long workers were exposed and how concentrated the fluoride was. Remember that fluoridating water means a *lifetime* of exposure, and the dose is accumulative, since 50 percent is retained in the tissues of the body with each dose. There is even evidence of a connection between total fluoride exposure—the sum from water, food, and other beverages, and airborne fluorides—and Down's syndrome.[129]

Skeletal Fluorosis: Making Us All Cripples

One of the most devastating effects of long-term, low-level fluoride exposure is skeletal damage, a condition referred to as skeletal fluorosis. In general, this condition is classified in stages, phase one presenting as arthritis-type pains and stage three as debilitating crippling. In countries with naturally high fluoride levels, skeletal fluorosis is quite common and considered a major medical disaster. Some villages have been described wherein every single resident has been afflicted with a twisted, bent spine leading to severe crippling. Death rates in such villages begin to skyrocket at about age fifty. In very advanced cases, the spine is so contorted and overgrown that the nerves and spinal cord are gradually crushed, leading to severe neurological injury.

While other countries are researching fluoride-induced problems such as skeletal fluorosis, very little is being done in the United States. In fact, cases of skeletal fluorosis are not recorded or tracked in this country, and most medical textbooks do not even mention the subject. Could it be because those who control our government, and thus our access to information, are afraid of the American public rejecting fluoridation of their drinking water because of the unavoidable dangers it poses?

In 1937 Dr. Kai Roholm of Denmark completed what is now considered a classic study of fluoride toxicity in cryolite workers. His study found that exposure to fluoride in concentrations between 0.2-0.35 mg/kg of body weight could result in skeletal fluorosis. The severity of bone damage depended on the length of the exposure, since fluoride accumulates in the bones.

Those exposed at these levels for two-and-a-half years showed early stages of fluorosis, mainly arthritic pains. Those exposed for four-and-a-half years advanced to phase two bone changes, with increased stiffness and reduced range of motion in the joints. If the exposure continued for eleven years, there was a high incidence of crippling of the spine and other bones.

At this point, let us rejoin the saga of Harold Hodge. In the early years of the fluoridation *putsch* in this country, Hodge relied on and quoted Dr. Roholm's figures in his own research, substituting pounds for Roholm's metric units—*without performing the proper mathematical conversions*. This allowed Dr. Hodge to eventually report that skeletal fluorosis was not a danger unless daily fluoride intake of 20-80 mg occurred for ten to twenty years. Dr. Hodge did not publicly correct this glaring and very critical error until 1979, long after his older figures had been cited repeatedly by fluoridation promoters to demonstrate the wide margin of safety for fluoride exposure.

The National Academy of Science and National Research Council also never volunteered to correct Dr. Hodge's error. It was only the insistence of U.S. Senator Bob Graham of Florida and Dr. Robert J. Carton, a senior official at the EPA, that finally forced the public correction of Hodge's scientific debacle many decades later. At long last, it was finally established that as little as 10-20 mg of fluoride per day for ten to twenty years will cripple an otherwise healthy individual. But even these figures understate the danger, since the appearance of crippling skeletal changes is dependent not just on daily dose of fluoride, but on the *total cumulative dose*. For example, if you ingested or inhaled 2.5-5 mg of fluoride a day for forty years, you would have an extremely high risk of developing crippling bone damage. Bear in mind that some cities have been fluoridating their water for over fifty years now.

Professor Hardy Limeback, a leading Canadian fluoride authority and previously a strong proponent of fluoridation, has been conducting studies on the effects of water fluoridation in Canada. He is also a Professor of Dentistry at the University of Toronto. One of his findings is that people growing up in fluoridated Toronto had bone fluoride levels twice as high as those living in unfluoridated Montreal.

In 1977 the National Academy of Sciences admitted that fluoride intake in fluoridated communities was as high as 3 mg per day, rather than a previously low figure they had given of 1.5 mg per day. The bone retains fluoride and may do so at concentrations as high as 2 mg a day. The average person growing up in a fluoridated community for forty years can accumulate 10,000 ppm of fluoride. In 1993 the National Academy of Science admitted that when bone ash accumulated fluoride at levels of 7,500 to 8,000 ppm, stage two and three skeletal fluorosis was likely to occur. It is at this latter stage that we see crippling of the skeleton.

One of the greatest problems in convincing the public of the danger of adding fluoride to water is that those pushing for fluoridation have ignored studies showing the dangers of cumulative doses. Furthermore, most of their calculations leave out other sources of fluoride, such as toothpaste, mouth rinses, fluoride tablets, fluoride dental treatments, fluoride in foods, industrial airborne exposure, pesticides, and medications. Many antibiotics, anesthetics, and other medications also contain fluoride. In fact, pesticide exposure alone can exceed the recommended optimum daily fluoride intake for both adolescents and children.

Over the past thirty years of my neurosurgical practice, I have been intrigued by the large number of spinal stenosis cases I have seen. In this condition, the bone and ligaments surrounding the spinal nerves become thickened and overgrown with numerous bone spurs. As the hole in the center of the spine narrows, it compresses the bundle of nerves contained within. These nerves supply sensation and movement to the legs, bladder, and bowels. Weakness and numbness of the legs accompanies worsening compression of the nerves, with eventual total loss of the ability to control bowels and bladder. If untreated, the person will become wheelchair-bound and depend on either a permanent catheter or an adult pad.

With the prolonged exposure of our elderly population to fluoridated drinking water, plus other sources of fluoride, it is no wonder that we are seeing this condition more and more. Incredibly, the medical community has expressed no interest in pursuing the possible connection to fluoride exposure.

Fluoride, Fractures and Fragile Bones

The second most frequently cited claim of fluoride's health benefits is that it strengthens bones. Many doctors have even suggested it as a treatment for osteoporosis. But carefully conducted studies have demonstrated conclusively that not only does it not strengthen the long bones, such as the femur and radius, it actually weakens them. To date we have over eight studies reported in peer-reviewed medical journals demonstrating increased hip fractures with fluoridation. Most studies have shown that fluoride treatments do increase the density of the axial skeleton (the spine) but clinical studies have not shown a significant reduction in spinal fractures in the elderly.

In one review of all articles reporting on the use of fluoride to treat postmenopausal osteoporosis, Dr. Louis Avioli, professor at the Washington University School of Medicine, concluded that the use of fluoride was accompanied by so many complications and side effects that it was not worth using in cases of postmenopausal osteoporosis, especially since it increased the risk of hip fractures and other stress fractures in the arms and legs.

One study examined Utah's Mormon community and demonstrated that fluoridation increased the incidence of hip fracture by 27 percent in women and 41 percent in men.[130]

Another interesting study by Dr. Mary Fran Sowers and co-workers examined 827 women aged twenty to eighty years in three rural Iowa communities over a five-year period for bone mineral density and incidence of fractures.[131] The study was unusual for several reasons. First, they looked at both young, premenopausal women as well as postmenopausal women. Second, they compared water systems not only containing varying amounts of fluoride but also concentrations of calcium.

What they found was that the communities with the highest fluoride water content also had the highest incidence of fractures and reductions in bone mineral density when compared to communities with higher calcium contents and no or low amounts of fluoride. Most shocking was that even the young women in fluoridated communities had significantly reduced bone mineral density than did women in the control community or in communities with high calcium levels in the drinking water. Bone mineral density measures the strength of the bone and estimates the likelihood of fracture.

The young women, as well as postmenopausal older women, had a significantly higher risk of having fractures of the wrist, hip, and spine than did those living in the control community or the community containing high calcium levels in the drinking water. The incidence of multiple fractures in all age groups of the study was 220 percent higher in the community with high drinking water fluoride content.

The importance of appropriate calcium intake cannot be overemphasized. Fluoride drastically lowers calcium levels by binding tightly with this essential mineral and removes substantial amounts of calcium from the blood, bones, and teeth, which become demineralized and weakened. One study using a CT scanner to measure bone density found that fluoride did increase the amount of cancellous bone (spongy, lattice-like bony tissue) but reduced the strength of the cortical bone (firm outer layer).[132] So, it may be that fluoride weakens the bone by diverting calcium from the cortex of the bone, which accounts for most of its strength, to the cancellous bone, which provides very little strength. Fluoride also is toxic to osteoblast type cells, which normally lay down calcium in the cortical layer of the bones.

In the past I have been a critic of our nation's obsession with calcium supplementation. Doctors have been leading the charge to convince women, especially postmenopausal women, to gulp down a daily allotment of calcium in every form imaginable, from Tums to crushed oyster shells. My objection has been based on the effect of excess calcium on the degenerative process, especially in the brain—a condition I discussed earlier—yet, supplemental calcium may actually afford some protection against some of the toxic effects of fluoride, especially dental and skeletal fluorosis. Unfortunately, one fairly recent study indicates that even calcium supplementation may not be protective against fluoride-induced calcium loss.[133] If this is so, the only solution is to remove fluoride from drinking water and teeth-cleaning products.

Taken together, these studies indicate that certain groups of individuals are at significantly increased risk of fractures when consuming fluoridated drinking water and using fluoride-containing products. This includes people with low calcium intake, renal disease, parathyroid disorders, genetic risk for osteoporosis, and diets low in magnesium and vitamin C intake.

Fluoride and the Brain

As we have seen, the brain is one of the most metabolically active organs in the body, highly dependent on its energy supply for proper functioning. As a consequence, anything that interferes with energy production will interfere with nervous system function. Fluoride poisons the enzymes used to make that energy.

Because many toxicology studies amply demonstrated fluoride's toxic effects on cells in experimental animals, one of the chief questions that kept popping up was: what effect does fluoride have on brain function? Available evidence indicated that the effects can be quite severe and cumulative. A summary of several reports on fluoride toxicity of occupationally exposed workers found that 25 percent of the workers exposed to cryolite who developed skeletal fluorosis also showed signs of nervous system effects such as difficulty thinking, fatigue, and memory problems.[134] Similar neurological effects were seen in other workers exposed to high levels of fluoride.

Other studies have described generalized progressive fatigue and a decline in mental acuity seen in persons living within three miles of a factory emitting hydrogen fluoride gas. Unlike cryolite workers, these individuals were exposed to much lower levels, emphasizing the extreme toxicity of fluoride. In another experiment, volunteers were asked to submit to a special psychomotor test in which they were to track a moving target before and after receiving a drop of water under their tongue, containing varying doses of fluoride (0.1, 1, 10 and 100 ppm).[135] The fluoride resulted in an increased rate of errors in attempting the test. One unusual finding was that the two highest doses of fluoride actually increased response time, a phenomenon that may be related to excitotoxicity.

The Developing Brain

It is accepted that a baby's developing nervous system is much more vulnerable to toxins than the mature adult brain. China, which has areas with naturally high fluoride levels in the water, has supplied us with much information on the toxic effects of fluoride. One study compared two villages matched for population, one with 4.12 ppm fluoride in the water system and the other with 0.91 ppm fluoride. It was found that children born in the high-fluoride village had a statistically significant lower median IQ as compared to its sister city. Dental fluorosis was present in 86 percent of children in the high-fluoride village and only 14 percent in the low fluoride village. You may recall that the ADA, as well as the U.S. regulatory agencies, insist that at 4 ppm, fluoride is safe for children and pregnant women.

Other studies have confirmed the findings of the Chinese research. In fact, one study found that there was a ten-point drop in IQ in the medium-severe fluorosis areas compared to low fluoride areas.[136] It is important to realize that these effects conform to a bell-shaped curve, with the number of children having IQs below seventy increasing as much as 21 percent, as well as a marked decrease in the number of children having IQs in the higher range. So you have more severely impaired children as well as fewer highly intelligent children. Fluoridation represents nothing less than the chemical dumbing-down of future generations.

Two Critical Studies

Two fairly recent studies have demonstrated the brain toxicity of fluoride in animals. In both studies, fluoride concentrations in the brains of test animals were equivalent to those achieved in humans through fluoridation programs, other environmental fluoride accumulations, use in toothpaste and mouthwashes, and dental treatments. It is important to remember that these studies were concerned with total body accumulations. With time, just as we saw with mercury, the retained fluoride reaches a level where it is extremely toxic.

In the first experiment, reported by Dr. Phyllis Mullenix and co-workers, 532 rats were exposed to different doses of fluoride in drinking water during three stages of life: prenatal, weaning, and as adults.[137] In the prenatal part of the experiment, researchers injected a fluoride solution under the mother rats' skins on the seventeenth through nineteenth days of pregnancy. When born, some of the baby rats demonstrated unusual hyperactivity. Strangely, only the males were affected.

The concentration of fluoride used in this phase of the experiment was comparable to that already seen in some parts of the country, and as the amount of fluoride increases in our environment due to widespread water fluoridation and contamination of foods, these levels will be increasingly more common. For example, humans ingesting drinking water containing 5-10 ppm fluoride will have similar blood fluoride levels as the animals used in these experiments. Plasma fluoride levels of 1.44 ppm, a level almost six times higher than the toxic levels seen in these experiments, have been found in children treated with fluoride gels in dentists' offices.[138]

In the Mullenix experiment, hyperactivity appeared to be caused by fluoride acting on the hippocampus of the temporal lobes of the brain, a part of the brain that plays a vital role in emotions, learning, and behavior. The reason only newborn males were affected can be attributed to gender-specific differences in brain development. We already know that many drugs act differently on males and females at this early stage of life.

Behavioral effects were different when animals were exposed to fluoride either soon after birth or as adults. The subjects in this case became sluggish, like human couch potatoes. Specific behavioral impacts depended on the timing of fluoride exposure during brain development. There was also a direct correlation between the level of fluoride accumulated in the brain (hippocampus) and behavioral effects in adult females, but not adult males.

Researchers also examined seven different regions of test animals' brains after fluoride exposure and found the substance in all seven areas. This study is particularly valuable because previous researchers had insisted that fluoride could not breach the blood-brain barrier.[139] It also proved that with long-term exposure, fluoride not only enters but accumulates widely in all areas of the brain.

The experiment is noteworthy not only for its scientific findings but also because the Forsyth Dental Research Institute, which commissioned it, attempted to destroy the research when it became obvious that the results would damage the fluoridation campaign. So who is Dr. Phyllis Mullenix? Her credentials are impeccable: she is considered one of the top toxicologists in the country, and at the time of her fluoride research held major research positions at Harvard University's Department of Neuropathology and Psychiatry and the Forsyth Dental Research Institute.

The design of Dr. Mullenix's research project was one of the most advanced and objectively based known. It used a computer pattern recognition system that removed usual human biases from interpretation of test results. For example, normal behavioral patterns of newborn and adult rodents were written into the computer program itself, producing a rigid standard for interpretation of results on all the test animals.

In one interview, she said the first portent that her findings had become unwelcome came when she was ordered to present her findings to the National Institute of Dental Research, a division of the National Institutes of Health (NIH). As she walked the Institute's corridors she began to realize that she was not dealing with objective, unbiased observers. The walls were plastered with posters extolling the "Miracle of Fluoride" and ridiculed those opposed to fluoridation. She was preparing to give a lecture on the dangers of fluoridation to fluoridation zealots!

She was quickly dismissed from her position at Forsyth after her presentation to the National Institute of Dental Research. Why? Because her research did not pertain to the dental field, they said. I ask: if fluoride toxicity *doesn't* pertain to the dental field, what does?

She was also pried for the name of the journal scheduled to publish her groundbreaking work. She refused, knowing inordinate pressure would be applied to the editorial staff of the journal to retract the article. Prior to the NIH's vicious attack on her character and the integrity of her science, she had submitted her research findings to one of the most prestigious journals in the field of neurotoxicology, the *Journal of Neurotoxicology and Teratology*. It had been immediately accepted for publication as a new and important finding in the field of toxicology.

Not long after her dismissal, the Forsyth Dental Research Institute received a quarter-million dollar grant from the Colgate Company, and before she could retrieve her specially designed equipment from their building it was destroyed by a mysteriously appearing water leak in the ceiling.

Following her dismissal from the Forsyth Institute, Dr. Mullenix received an unfunded appointment at Boston's Children's Hospital. In a moment of unguarded candor, officials there admitted they were frightened of the fluoride supporters' power to evaporate funding for "out of line" institutions.

Another vital piece of research involved a study of the brain effects of combined aluminum and fluoride exposure. This experiment is especially important because these two metals frequently occur together in foods and beverages. Aluminum occurs naturally to some extent in drinking water, but is also added as a clarifying agent. Given that fluorine and fluoride compounds are some of the most reactive substances known to man, this fact is of particular significance when we are talking about fluoridated drinking water and the aluminum containers in which so many drinks and food products are sold.

For this reason, any fluoride-containing product in an aluminum container, including fluoridated toothpaste in aluminum tubes, aluminum cans, aluminum cookware, and aluminum-containing foods mixed with fluoridated water, can potentially form the harmful aluminum fluoride compound AlF_3.

Entry of aluminum into the brain past the blood-brain barrier often involves special carrier molecules or combinations thereof. For example, albumin can carry aluminum into the brain, especially when magnesium deficiency is present. Recently, it has been shown that when aluminum combines with fluoride there is increased transport of both into the brain.

In an attempt to further examine this process, and study the resulting brain toxicity of the mixture, Varner and co-workers gave twenty-seven adult male Long-Evans rats distilled water containing fluoride as either aluminum fluoride at 0.5 ppm or sodium fluoride at 2.1 ppm.[140] Because relative fluorine concentrations in the two compounds differ, the doses were calculated so that both groups of animals received a comparable dose based on the form in which it was ingested.

While there were no differences in the body weights of the two groups, the animals who drank the aluminum fluoride water died in greater numbers. At the end of the experiment, researchers examined brain, kidney, liver, and spleen tissues, observing several important effects. First, the animals drinking the aluminum fluoride water demonstrated a progressive decline in appearance, with sparse hair growth, dry, flaky, copper-colored skin and a generalized unhealthy appearance. This was thought to be secondary to the damaging effect on the animals' kidneys, since aluminum levels in the animals drinking the aluminum-fluoride water were nearly double that of the control animals and animals drinking sodium fluoride treated water alone.

Additionally, animals who drank the aluminum fluoride water had brain levels of aluminum higher than animals drinking the sodium fluoride water, and levels over twice as high as those drinking plain distilled water. Control animals had both aluminum and fluoride in their brain tissue. This was because the Purina Rodent Lab Chow that all the animals ate contained from 150-8,300 ppm aluminum, and also contained fluoride.

This is important because there is a strong link between brain aluminum levels and neurodegenerative diseases such as Alzheimer's disease and Parkinson's disease. Histological examinations of test animals' brains indicated that damage was concentrated in the left hemisphere of the brain, with a significant reduction in neuron density. This loss of brain cells was greater in animals drinking aluminum fluoride water than in those given sodium fluoride or distilled water. The damaged neurons exhibited clumping, enhanced protein staining, and destructive chromosomal changes. Similar damage was seen in the blood vessels supplying this part of the brain as well, a consistent finding in Alzheimer's disease.

This type of damage to the brain's blood vessels could lead to the same changes in the blood-brain barrier we see in Alzheimer's disease. Animals exposed to both aluminum fluoride and sodium fluoride showed a buildup of vascular ß-amyloid in the lateral posterior thalamus. ß-amyloid is a commonly seen inclusion in the brains of those with Alzheimer's disease.

Especially frightening is that severe brain changes were observed following consumption of water containing only 0.5 ppm of the aluminum fluoride compound. You will recall that most communities are adding 1-1.5 ppm fluoride to drinking water. When combined with aluminum naturally found in drinking water, as well as numerous other sources of aluminum, an extremely brain toxic compound is formed. This brings into serious question the assurances being given by the ADA and the EPA that a fluoride level of 1 ppm in drinking water is safe. You must also take into consideration that the developing brain and the elderly brain are much more sensitive to such injuries.

Many conditions in the elderly make them much more susceptible. For example, they are more likely to be deficient in antioxidant nutrients, have long-term brain cell injury secondary to aging and disease, suffer from cerebrovascular disease, have other metal toxicities and low calcium levels. With aging, all of these conditions lead to severely weakened brain cells that are much more sensitive to injury by such toxins.

Other Effects on the Brain

An early change that has been observed in the brains of those developing Parkinson's disease is a significant reduction in the energy molecule, CoQ10. Animal experiments have indicated that chronic fluoride exposure at levels equal to accumulated concentrations high enough to produce fluorosis can significantly lower brain CoQ10 levels,[141] which may be the result of a dramatic increase in brain free-radical formation caused by the fluoride.

Fluoride, and especially aluminum fluoride, has been shown to interfere with brain cells' ability to form their normal skeletal structure (called a cytoskeleton).[142] This process is vital during fetal brain development, and it also plays a significant role in the ongoing health of brain cells.

We know that cell membranes play a vital role in all cell functions, and their exact composition must be carefully regulated to preserve normal functions. One recent study found that rats who were fed fluoride for seven months experienced a 10-20 percent reduction in brain phospholipid contents, depending on the concentration of fluoride used.[143] Fluoride when combined with aluminum was found to inhibit an important cell-membrane enzyme called phospholipase D. Interestingly, neither fluoride nor aluminum alone had any effect on the enzyme; it was inhibitory only when they were combined.

One of the most common sources of aluminum fluoride complexes is in liquids packaged in aluminum cans, a combination that is especially hazardous with acidic fruit juices and diet drinks. Acidic juices leach aluminum from the wall of the can and disperse it throughout the juice. Most canned fruit juices, especially grape juice, also contain added fluoride. Grape juice can contain as much as 6 ppm fluoride. Remember, the fluoride itself is highly reactive and will leach aluminum from the can as well. Soft drinks also present special hazards. While all soft drinks containing fluoride will leach aluminum from the can, diet sodas may be worse than regular sodas because the fluoride content, at least in one study, was higher in the diet drinks. Although most aluminum cans now have inner linings, the coating may be defective and can also be fractured during shipping.

To prevent local supplies from altering a soda's standardized taste, most water used in soft drinks is normally filtered of all impurities or is manufactured using distilled water. Ironically, the Coca-Cola Company bottles and sells water (under the name Dasani) purified by the reverse osmosis method, which removes fluoride from water, but their soda actually contains fluoride. Presumably, Dasani is the same water they use to make their soft drinks and it would make sense that Coke should actually be fluoride free. That it isn't would indicate that they are purposefully adding fluoride back in.

Furthermore, the longer a canned drink sits, especially at higher temperatures, the more aluminofluoride compound will be created in the drink. This would be a major consideration, for example, in the millions of diet soft drinks donated to soldiers in the Persian Gulf. These drinks sat in the blazing heat, over 105° F, for weeks. In addition, the drinks contained the toxic sweetener, aspartame, which in the heat breaks down very quickly into the carcinogenic compound, diketopiperizine, as well as formaldehyde and formic acid.

Another potential source of aluminofluoride is fluoridated toothpaste packaged in aluminum tubes. Toothpaste typically contains from 1,000-1,500 ppm fluoride, a very high concentration of fluoride. In fact, this much fluoride could easily kill a child or an elderly person with low calcium levels or a bad heart.

Other Effects of Fluoride

Because of its ability to poison enzymes and react with many biological components, fluoride can cause mischief in many parts of the body. Another important property of fluoride is its intense affinity for hydrogen. Hydrogen bonds are found throughout the biological system, but normally have considerably less binding strength than we see with fluoride. The reason this is important is that healthy biological molecules depend on a particular shape or conformation to work properly. Even minor alterations in this precise shape will cause the molecule to become ineffective. When fluoride binds to these molecules so intensely, the shape of the molecule is significantly altered, and as a result many critical reactions do not take place properly within cells.

Of particular importance are the reactions that occur between fluoride and proteins, many of which make up vital enzymes used by the cells for everything from energy production to DNA repair.

Fluoride and the Thyroid

Because of the problem of fluoride accumulation in our environment, serious multiple organ disorders are likely to begin occurring soon throughout the population. For instance, there is compelling evidence that the thyroid accumulates fluoride from the environment. In a study of fluoride concentrations in various human organs, Yiamouyiannis reported that the thyroid gland contained 4 ppm of fluoride after prolonged exposure.[144] Also, in a chart in which he compares thyroid fluoride concentrations of human body tissues before and after water fluoridation programs were instituted in the 1940s, he found that no organ contained more than 0.68 ppm fluoride before 1940. This change represents a drastic accumulation of this toxic substance in our population, caused purely by the fluoridation program. Further, only the kidney, at 2.3 ppm, came anywhere close to the thyroid gland in its ability to accumulate fluoride.

According to the USPHS, we are now approaching daily consumption of fluoride in the range of 8 mg/day—a huge amount. Fluoride tends to accumulate in most organs, and there is good evidence that this dose is now accumulating at an increasing rate. Even the notorious Dr. Harold Hodge admitted that chronic exposure to fluoride could alter thyroid structure and function.[145]

Another study using rats found that adding 1 ppm of fluoride to their drinking water could significantly lower thyroid levels of the hormones T4 and T3.[146] In truth, this study does not demonstrate effects of equivalent doses of fluoride to humans, since fluoride is absorbed poorly in both rats and mice. Dr. Mullenix found that rats and mice must receive a dose of fluoride fifteen times higher in their drinking water to reach equivalent human blood levels. What that means is that you would have to give a mouse 15 ppm fluoride to test the effects of 1 ppm fluoride in humans.

A more recent study using 288 mice found that the occurrence of goiter, combined with either a deficiency or excess of iodine, was dependent on fluoride exposure.[147] In this experiment, fluoride excess caused stimulation of the thyroid for one hundred days followed by 150 days of depressed function. Researchers also found that the rate and severity of dental and skeletal fluorosis was higher in the iodine deficient animals exposed to fluoride. Not only does fluoride affect thyroid function, low thyroid function also enhances fluoride-induced destruction of teeth and bones.

Numerous other studies have also linked thyroid problems with elevated fluoride exposure. If we examine the incidence of goiter (hypothyroidism) in different areas of the world based on water fluoride content, we see some remarkable parallels. For example, India has a very high incidence of goiter and a very high incidence of fluorosis (though, as I discussed above, fluoride occurs naturally in that country's water supplies). Belgium, on the other hand, has a moderately low incidence of both fluorosis and goiter. In China, we see the same pattern: very high fluoride levels accompanied by a very high incidence of goiter. This same pattern has held up in ten countries examined worldwide. When we combine the epidemiological evidence with the above-cited research we see strong evidence for a connection between hypothyroidism and fluoridation.

With the strong connection between early hypothyroidism and intelligence, it is obvious that the importance of this connection goes far beyond just not having energy to get through the day, or suffering from cold intolerance. The thyroid gland plays a major role in the formation of the brain during early development, and hypothyroidism during this stage can lead to severe mental retardation (cretinism). It has also been noted that the incidence of Down's syndrome is 30 percent higher in fluoridated communities than unfluoridated ones.[148] Down's syndrome is associated with thyroid dysfunction.

Sexual Maturity, Infertility, and Fluoride

A recent study compared males living in areas with high fluoride levels in drinking water to men matched in age who live in very low-fluoride areas, and found the first group had significantly lowered testosterone levels.[149] This study used two test groups of men drinking high-fluoride water, one group of which suffered from fluorosis and one group who drank the same water but did not have fluorosis. A separate set of controls consisted of men who drank only water containing very low fluoride levels. The lowest testosterone levels were observed in the men with fluorosis who drank high-fluoride water. Those without fluorosis who drank that same high-fluoride water also had low testosterone, but not as low as the men with fluorosis. The only men with normal testosterone levels were those who drank the water containing low fluoride concentrations.

Higher levels of fluoride have also been shown to reduce sperm motility and produce alterations in the area of the testes that produce sperm.[150] Other studies have demonstrated that even low levels of fluoride can render mice infertile.[151]

For the globalist seeking to control world population, water fluoridation could certainly offer an effective method of achieving an international reduction in births without having to announce an unpopular plan of enforced contraception. The world's population could be significantly reduced in the guise of preventing tooth decay in children, and the effect would increase with time as the contamination of foodstuffs and medications continued to grow. I am not saying that is the purpose of fluoridation, but it could be a reason for its continued support by high-ranking government officials, foundations, and those on the international scene.

Things They Never Told You

Over a hundred years ago, Frederic Bastiat, the brilliant nineteenth century French economist, wrote an essay titled, "What is Seen and What Is Not Seen," which attempted to show that economic activity does not exist in well-controlled isolation, and in fact often engenders a series of unintended, unfortunate, and uncontrollable effects. He says, "Of these effects, the first alone is immediate; it appears simultaneously with its cause; it is seen. The other effects emerge only subsequently; they are not seen; we are fortunate if we foresee them."[152]

Bastiat's analysis describes perfectly the sinister history of water fluoridation, an economic event masquerading as a public health campaign that involved, and still involves, enormous amounts of money and powerful political influence—and uncountable tragic side effects. No one in any position of real power has ever dared to clash with these powerful forces. I can only hope this book will begin to change that.

Fluoride Overflow: Accidents That Can Sicken and Kill

Most of us never give a second thought to the safety issues of how fluoride is added to our drinking water. As with so much, we just leave it up to the "experts." Few of us are even aware that numerous communities across the nation shut down their fluoridation equipment at the turn of the millennium because officials were afraid the equipment might fail, allowing dangerous fluoride overflows into drinking water. I ask: if it could happen during Y2K, why shouldn't we be concerned that it could happen at anytime? After all, this equipment must operate, usually by computer, all the time, adding just the right concentration of fluoride to the water. The truth is that exactly such a thing has happened. People became ill, and some have even died as a result. So, you're asking, why haven't we heard about this? The obvious answer is that the people who have so much invested in fluoridation have kept it quiet out of fear that it would make all too clear to the public the real dangers presented by water fluoridation.

In August 1993 residents of the little town of Popularville, Mississippi, became the unfortunate victims of a fluoride overspill. It came to light when patrons of a Pizza Inn suddenly began to get sick, complaining of stomach cramps, nausea, and burning in their mouths. The manager called city officials and learned that his customers had been poisoned by an overflow of fluoride at the water treatment plant. Fifteen people ended up in the hospital,

Aluminum-Fluoride Complex (AlF3)...

- is neurotoxic at 0.5 ppm.
- impairs brain-cell cytoskeleton.
- reduces brain phospholipids.
- inhibits phospholipase D in neuron membrane.
- lowers brain CoQ10 levels.
- produces widespread neuron loss in hippocampus.

TABLE 4.2

and over forty are known to have been poisoned. Given the scale of this disaster, many others must have been affected, but they never reported it to town officials. What those unfortunate people didn't know, and weren't told, is that the sudden elevation in fluoride would produce silent injury to their bones, thyroid glands, and brains that might not manifest itself for years or even decades. Pregnant women carrying developing babies, and small children exposed to these high levels of fluoride have a high risk of having permanent damage to their brain, as Dr. Mullenix's research has so cogently demonstrated.

A similar accident occurred in New Haven, Connecticut, in 1986. This time fluoride levels reached 51 ppm for over twelve hours: remember normal levels are 1 ppm. At least fifty-five people suffered full clinical effects of acute toxicity, with vomiting, diarrhea, fever, and skin rashes. Again, we can only guess at the extent of the chronic effects caused by the accumulated dose of this high fluoride level.

More recently the city of Middletown, Maryland, experienced a toxic spill of even more horrendous proportions. In this case fluoride overflowed to the tune of 70 ppm, much higher than the level set by the EPA as the limit for serious toxicity. City residents were warned by radio and television not to drink the water, but those without radios or TV sets, or who were not tuned in, suffered the consequences. Worse still, city officials did not even conduct a follow-up survey to determine the extent of human injury caused by this massive spill. Why? Because they didn't want a public record of the event, and certainly did not want the general public to be aware of the health dangers caused by the spill.

The highest recorded levels of fluoride occurred in Hooper Bay, Alaska, when the water tested at 150 ppm after a major spill! One death was attributed to the spill and 260 people were poisoned before the problem could be contained. The accident was explained away by officials who concluded that the spill had been caused by old equipment and an untrained operator. Another spill, this one in Chicago, caused the deaths of three dialysis patients and made five others extremely sick. Unlike the others, this overflow was actually investigated by the Centers for Disease Control, yet no public report has been forthcoming.

During the month of February 1992, Rice Lake, Wisconsin's fluoridation equipment failed and spewed extremely elevated concentrations of fluoride into the water system for two days before residents were notified. Fluoride levels reached 20 ppm during this time period and later measurements showed the water contained 92 ppm of fluoride. Approximately forty children suffered abdominal pains, vomiting, and diarrhea after attending an arts and crafts show at their school.

Don't assume that the city officials will necessarily tell you about an accidental spill. In the city of Annapolis, Maryland, in 1979, malfunctioning fluoridation equipment poured high levels of fluoride into the water system for nine days, during which time the city officials issued no warning to the public concerning the hazard. City council members were not informed of the tragic event for six more days. When asked why the city had kept this secret from the public and elected representatives, a public health official stated that he didn't want to endanger the fluoridation program. During this period of protectionist silence, one dialysis patient died and one other was left seriously brain injured. The damaged patient's wife sued the city for $480 million, and the case was eventually settled out of court for an undisclosed sum.

Most Americans have never heard of these accidents, and, as a result, no one seems to worry much about the safety of the water we are drinking. But, in addition to the cases I have cited above, numerous other incidences have occurred throughout the United States—and continue to occur. It would make sense that many smaller spills probably occur every day and are never reported. It seems a good time to start worrying!

Environmental Accumulation of Fluoride

One of the most obvious problems associated with fluoridation of the water supply, completely ignored by the fluoridation proponents, are the accumulative effects of adding this toxic chemical to drinking water. Unfortunately, those who have been entrusted to protect us from public harm have not yet officially recognized it as an obvious hazard. And that is actually part of the problem: we trust governmental organizations, such as the EPA, OSHA, and the CDC, to look after us. We believe that they will always tell the truth, and that they are above reproach. As you have now seen, nothing could be further from the truth. We must start thinking for ourselves and not accept the word of the chosen elite and "experts" in society who have a vested interest in continuing the dangerous practice of fluoridation.

When fluoride is added to something as ubiquitous as water, accumulation in the environment is inevitable. This means that fluoride levels will not only accumulate in food products and beverages, but the rate of that accumulation begins to increase exponentially. Fluoride already occurs in numerous medications, anesthetics, toothpaste, mouthwashes, dental treatments, fluid replacement for children, foods, fruit juices, teas, milk, meats, bottled water, industrial exposure, pesticides, animal feeds, and contaminated ground water. It has been estimated that we are now consuming 8 mg of fluoride daily in the United States. This is *eight times higher* than even the proponents of fluoridation recommended as necessary and safe for human consumption, an amount that has led to 30-60 percent of America's children suffering from dental fluorosis, and to a growing number of the elderly suffering from crippling skeletal fluorosis. Furthermore, nervous system injury inevitably accompanies these conditions.

Given the strong connection between bone cancer and fluoride exposure, how many young men are dying or being crippled due to this insane policy? Likewise, how many are suffering from hypothyroidism, cancer of the thyroid, ADD, autism, intellectual dysfunction, and an early onset of Parkinson's disease, Alzheimer's dementia, and other neurological disorders? All of these conditions can be expected to increase, and to occur at an earlier age, as the total fluoride content in our food and water supply increases. We should not forget that fluoride has been shown to significantly decrease fertility in men. As total daily exposure rises to 15-20 mg a day, what will happen to our population? These are serious questions that must be answered.

Once the majority of our food supplies and water supplies are contaminated, along with our soils, no one will be able to escape the hazards of fluoride toxicity. Just think of it. The apple you eat for a snack will contain fluoride, so will the chicken you eat for dinner, the orange or grape juice you have at breakfast, the potatoes you eat with your sandwich, the sugar you put in your coffee, butter for your toast, even your cereal! When foods are washed in water containing fluoride, they become contaminated. When you cook your vegetables in fluoridated water, the water evaporates, and the concentration of the fluoride increases. Soon, a single day's food consumption will also mean an unacceptably high level of fluoride exposure.

One of the greatest sources of food- and beverage-borne fluoride is tea. One study found concentrations of 50-125 ppm in fifteen varieties of tea, a dramatic rise in just the last two decades. A Polish study found levels up to 340 ppm in sixteen varieties of teas. Why tea? Because some plants tend to accumulate fluoride in greater concentrations than others.

This contamination of tea by fluoridation is a double tragedy because tea is an excellent source of some very important anticancer flavonoids and antioxidants. By contaminating teas with fluoride, one is denied safe access to these remarkable medicinal phytochemicals. Decaffeinated coffee is also contaminated by fluoride, because often the water used to decaffeinate the coffee contains fluoride.

Shrimp and canned sardines can have very high levels of fluoride (61 mg/kg). Infant cereals may contain anywhere from 0.9-2.1 ppm fluoride. Strained meats, also used in infant and toddler foods, can contain as much as 5.2 ppm fluoride. Deboned beef may contain 14-42 mg/kg of fluoride. Commercial grape juices contain as much as 6 ppm fluoride, as do most American wines. This is because the grapes in some vineyards are sprayed with fluoride solutions as a pesticide, which soaks readily into the grapes.

From these examples, we can see that already we have seriously contaminated our food and beverage supply. But, there is one instance where the danger is higher than in all of these examples, and that is drinks packaged in aluminum cans and bottles, including beers, fruit juices, sodas, and other popular drinks. As we shall see later, aluminum is also very toxic, especially to the nervous system. And, as we have seen, when aluminum is combined with fluoride, even in minute concentrations, it forms a very powerful brain toxin.

So in the case of diet drinks in aluminum cans, the very brain-toxic aluminum fluoride compound co-exists with multiple toxins found in aspartame, thus creating the most powerful government-approved toxic soup imaginable. With the strong association among aluminum, excitotoxins, aluminum fluoride complexes, and Alzheimer's disease, it would be completely irresponsible to encourage people to consume this toxic mixture. Yet, this is done literally billions of times every year in advertising. It is important to remember that the aluminum can has been around for only about three decades, and most toxin-related diseases take years of accumulation to produce the full clinical expression of the disorder.

A commonly used pesticide, Norflurazon, also contains a large amount of fluoride. It is used on numerous crops including apples, raisins, potatoes, lettuce, blueberries, strawberries ,and tomatoes. The fluoride not only clings tenaciously to the skin of the fruits and vegetables, but also can soak into the pulp of the plant as well. Once the "fresh vegetables" arrive at your supermarket, they are placed in display bins and intermittently sprayed with a fine mist of tap water that often is fluoridated, adding further to the fluoride burden of the plant.

My children loved the taste of one brand of orange juice from Florida, but because of my research in this area, I decided to call the headquarters of the orange juice company and ask if they used local drinking water. Their representative said, "Yes." I then asked if the local water was fluoridated and again she answered, "Yes." After a long pause she asked me if I was allergic to fluoride. I preceded to tell her of fluoride's toxicity.

Because orange juice contains so many phytochemicals, shown in numerous tests to have powerful health benefits including anticancer effects, I am hesitant to tell people to stop drinking orange juice or eating oranges. A safer course may be to squeeze your own from organically grown oranges. You must investigate the organic grower, though, because some use fluoride-containing pesticides.

If your schedule will not permit this, I would suggest reconstituting low-acid orange juice concentrate using distilled water. Unfortunately, the same safeguards do not apply to grape juice concentrate, since fluoride is mixed with the grape concentrate in rather high concentrations.

Dental Fluorosis, a Measure of Toxicity to the Brain

Unfortunately, there are no studies in which brain levels of fluoride have been measured in humans, particularly comparing fluoridated to unfluoridated areas. But, we do have one good general measure. We know that the presence of dental fluorosis indicates toxicity to other parts of the body including the brain. A study done by the National Institute of Dental Research in the mid-1980s found that 66 percent of children growing up in fluoridated communities showed signs of dental fluorosis.[153] The incidence is certainly higher today. Obviously, we are in a crisis situation.

Fluoridation defenders, and those who support the use of fluoride for alleged prevention of tooth decay, respond that dental fluorosis is not a major concern; it is merely a cosmetic problem. This is a very dangerous lie. Dental fluorosis provides a measure of fluoride accumulation within the bones, thyroid, brain and other organs. In India, where water fluoride levels are naturally high, dental fluorosis occurs in virtually the entire population. If we do not stop the fluoridation process, this could happen in our own country.

The Straw that Broke the Camel's Back

If all this isn't enough, dental and pediatric societies encourage their members to promote fluoridation treatments, as well as fluoridation of community water supplies. Numerous patients and friends have told me their pediatricians tell them to add fluoride pills to baby formula, and to start their children on fluoride treatments as soon as they are old enough. These experts have even encouraged adding fluoride to Pedialyte, an electrolyte fluid mixture primarily used for sick babies. This is unconscionable! These pediatricians are taking the word of the American Dental Association, which as we have seen, has a vested interest in promoting the use of a toxic product.

Dentists tell young parents that their children should use fluoridated toothpaste and are even promoting a fluoride varnish for these young children, a varnish which releases a continuous supply of fluoride into the mouth and is reapplied every six months or every year.

The ADA also suggests that only a pea-sized portion of toothpaste be used and that children below the age of six be supervised by their parents while brushing with fluoridated toothpaste. The Association began to issue this warning as a result of the growing public discussion of fluoride toxicity by opponents of fluoridation. As we all know, few parents in fact abide by this precaution, and many small children load their toothbrushes with a huge glob of toothpaste and brush unsupervised. I have spoken to many parents who say their small children walk around the house sucking on their toothpaste-soaked toothbrush. Toothpaste contains anywhere from 1,000-1,500 ppm fluoride, enough to kill any small child. With such a huge glob of toothpaste, the child may absorb 10-20 ppm fluoride. When they complain of a stomach ache or develop behavioral problems, parents rarely connect the fluoride consumption to the problem.

Worse still, our nation's marketing-obsessed culture encourages manufacturers to create toothpastes that appeal to children's love of sweets. Where is the sense in adding such copious amounts of sweetener to a product that's supposed to *prevent* cavities? One brand, called Barbie Sparkling Bubble Fruit Toothpaste, made by the Colgate Company, is both sweetened and fruit-flavored. Another, by Oral-B, is labeled Fruity Flavor Anticavity Fluoride Toothpaste. Both tubes carry the standard warning to keep the product out of the reach of children under six years of age, and to seek professional help or contact the local poison control center should the child swallow this product; yet both these products also bear the ADA's seal of approval.

So let's review. Fluoride is so toxic you should supervise children under age six while they are brushing, never let them use more than a pea-sized portion of toothpaste, and you should also be sure they do not swallow the toothpaste. But then, to encourage the children to brush, you put Barbie's name on it, plus you make the toothpaste sweet and fruity—which encourages them to swallow it. Finally, there are dental professors who say that children under six shouldn't brush with fluoridated toothpaste at all, but then the ADA endorses these products. A somewhat schizophrenic policy to say the least.

The Grand Deception

The form of fluoride being added to our water supply has never been tested in laboratory experiments. Virtually all laboratory experiments use either sodium fluoride or a close chemical relative. The only large, long-term study ever done using the type of fluoride—hexafluorosilicic acid or sodium hexafluorosilicate—being added to drinking water, is now being conducted on millions of unsuspecting individuals in the United States, Australia, New Zealand, Ireland, and Great Britain.

Remember that the fluoride being added to our water supplies is obtained from the smoke-stack scrubbers of fertilizer and metal factories. This toxic goo contains more than just fluoride. It also contains arsenic, cadmium, mercury, lead, and polonuim-210, a radioactive element that decays into lead. Polonium-210 emits five thousand times more alpha-radiation than an equal amount of radium. Despite numerous efforts by concerned scientists, even those working for the EPA, not one study has been commissioned by anyone—in either government or private industry—to study the toxicity of fluorosilicic acid on humans.

It is also known that fluoridating water supplies increases the amount of lead in the drinking water substantially. A Canadian study found that lead levels were twice as high in fluoridated water systems when compared to unfluoridated systems. A Dartmouth University study of 280,000 children also linked fluoridation with high lead levels in children. This is because fluoride is so reactive it leaches lead from pipes and lead-lined faucet fittings. According to Dr. Robert Carton, who spent twenty years as an EPA scientist, when the cities of Seattle, Washington, and Thermont, Maryland, stopped fluoridating their water, lead levels dropped by half.

With all the concern about lead toxicity in the young, especially its effects on neurological functions, should we just ignore this well-established fact? Lead, even in very small concentrations, can have a profound effect on the developing nervous system leading to significant impairment in learning and behavior. Elevated lead levels in children have also been well-correlated to hyperactivity, substance abuse, increased violent behavior, and crime. Combine this with the toxicity of mercury, arsenic, aluminum, and chlorine, as well as fluoride itself, and you have a very toxic mixture being consumed every day by individuals at substantially increased risk of any one of a number of diseases—from cancer to degenerative brain disorders to accelerated aging.

In 1993 the U.S. Department of Health and Human Services concluded that there exist a subset of individuals that are especially susceptible to fluoride toxicity. These include the elderly, those with calcium and/or magnesium deficiencies, and those with vitamin C deficiency, plus persons having cardiovascular disease or renal disease. Together this includes tens of millions of people. To be thorough, though, we must also include the very young (from the unborn to adolescents) and those with neurological diseases, those with thyroid disorders and individuals undergoing the stress of disease, surgery, and chronic unrelieved stress. This includes virtually everyone in the world.

One question I am frequently asked is: if fluoride is so toxic, and those promoting its use know it, aren't they afraid of the toxicity as well? They are in fact frightened of fluoridated water. When I asked a well-known opponent of fluoridation this question, he said that the mayor of Sacramento, California, Mayor Golding, stated as she voted for fluoridation of the city's water, that she didn't have to worry about fluoride toxicity because she had a reverse osmosis filter. He further stated that all you would have to do is walk the halls of the Capitol building and see all the purified water dispensers in the offices of those who have used their political power to force water fluoridation on millions of helpless and under-informed individuals.

These defenders of water fluoridation do not seem to care a whit that the poorest members of our society will be most harmed, since they will not be able to afford expensive reverse osmosis filters and distillation devices. They are also more likely to be deficient in antioxidant vitamins and minerals, and to suffer from medical conditions that will make them more vulnerable to the toxicity.

The Politics of Water Fluoridation

Those promoting fluoridation for profit have fine-tuned their methodology to an art. Technically, adding fluoride to drinking water is a violation of the Safe Drinking Water Act. Under the statutes of this act, it is illegal for the federal government to promote fluoridation of drinking water by endorsing, supporting, requiring, or funding such efforts. So how do fluoridationists get around this impediment? They use federal block grants. You see, they merely offer the block grants for unspecified use by the city being targeted, and then simultaneously have the state health departments and the American Dental Association move their well-funded forces into the area, screaming for fluoridation.

One may ask the question: If all this is true, why haven't EPA officials spoken out? In fact, some have. In 1990 Dr. William Marcus, senior toxicologist in the Office of Drinking Water at the EPA, was fired for daring to question the validity of a long-awaited government animal study on the safety of fluoride in drinking water. He found that the study was purposely designed to protect the fluoridation supporters' claim that fluoride in drinking water is safe.

The study in question, carried out by the National Toxicology Program for the EPA's Office of Drinking Water, purported to show that fluoride in drinking water was not connected to onset of cancer, but researchers purposely downgraded the definition of a tumor so it would appear that there was no connection between fluoride and a rare bone cancer called osteogenic sarcoma (also called osteosarcoma). Congress had mandated the study because of a real concern over the connection between increased cancer rates seen in epidemiology studies comparing fluoridated and unfluoridated communities. In truth, the study not only demonstrated a direct link to osteogenic sarcoma, but found that effects were dose related.

Dr. Marcus took his superiors to court and won not only his case and his job, but was also awarded $50,000 in damages. It was determined that the EPA also shredded important evidence during the trial, and had intimidated other EPA scientists who wished to support Dr. Marcus.

In November 1991 Dr. Bob Carton, vice-president of the union representing all twelve hundred scientists, engineers and lawyers at the EPA headquarters presented evidence of fraud in the preparation of the EPA's fluoride drinking water standard. This evidence was presented to the Drinking Water Subcommittee of the Science Advisory Board of the EPA. Carton received no response, but EPA headquarters now has fluoride-free water dispensed throughout their building.

Protective Measures

The stakes are so high, it is imperative that the public become involved in the battle to preserve clean water and food. Until that battle can be won, you must avoid fluoride as much as possible. This means no fluoride toothpaste, mouthwashes, or treatments by the dentist.

When you tell your dentist that you do not want fluoride treatments, he will jump up and down, turn red in the face, and while pointing toward his or her ADA certificate, tell you how all the scare stories are lies. You must understand that he or she is most likely mercury toxic and it makes him or her irritable. Just stick to your guns. Fluoride treatments are big business, and there are a lots of dentists in competition. The main problem is that most dentists do not realize that they have been lied to by the ADA.

This is especially important for the very young and for pregnant mothers. Drink only purified water, free of fluoride. This means you will have to purchase water that is either distilled or treated by reverse osmosis. For those who can afford it, a home distillation or reverse osmosis unit will save you the trouble of purchasing bottled water.

Fluoride is so caustic that it will damage the reverse osmosis filter within a few months, and it must be changed regularly to maintain the purity of your water. Foods cooked in water will also require fluoride-free water. As I stated previously, concentrations of fluoride increase as fluoridated water evaporates, and because it is so reactive, fluoride clings tenaciously to the vegetables or pasta being cooked. At that point, it becomes impossible to remove.

Some studies have indicated that calcium, magnesium, vitamins D and E, and certain amino acids can significantly reduce the toxicity of fluoride. The amino acids glycine and glutamine can both increase excitotoxicity, so I would not advise them as a protective measure. As for vitamin D, it has been shown experimentally to protect the embryos of pregnant animals exposed to fluoride.[154]

I recommend 500 mg magnesium a day in a highly absorbable form, such as magnesium lactate, malate, or gluconate. I do not recommend magnesium aspartate, since aspartate is an excitatory amino acid. Take 1000 to 2000 IU of vitamin D_3 a day. Vitamin E should be either in the alpha-tocopherol succinate form or the natural form, often called mixed tocopherols. The natural form contains four different types of tocopherols found naturally in biological systems. The dose is 400-800 IU a day.

Calcium supplementation is the present rage, although—as I discussed earlier—not everyone needs it to prevent osteoporosis. Further, cellular calcium leakage may play a significant role in aging and many diseases. But we also know that calcium is a very effective antidote for severe acute fluoride poisoning, and with people being exposed to such large acute doses of fluoride, blood calcium levels can fall to dangerously low levels, resulting in vascular collapse and cardiac arrest. Given this dilemma, I would recommend 1,000 mg of calcium citrate a day. Do not take calcium supplements made from a living organism, such as oyster shells or animal bone. These sources contain arsenic, lead, cadmium, and other contaminants.

It is especially important, in light of the extensive fluoridation of water supplies and foods, to avoid aluminum at all cost. This means aluminum cookware, aluminum cans and containers, aluminum in medications (both prescription and nonprescription), baked goods, and all other food sources. I am frequently asked about deodorants containing aluminum. I have no information on the absorption of aluminum through the skin, but it is certainly possible. If it can be avoided, it should be, until reliable data are available.

As you can see, to avoid toxic metals and other substances takes eternal diligence and tireless reading of labels. As with so many other modern-day hazards, eating fresh-grown foods and avoiding processed foods are the best ways to protect yourself.

Conclusion

In conclusion, I want to emphasize that I do not favor the government treating us as imbecilic children who must be constantly watched over and cared for by "benevolent" bureaucratic appointees. Fluoridation of water is a deliberate use of community drinking water to medicate millions of people. Remember that throughout modern history, there have been corrupt people who sought to use the public water system as a means of medicating the public, the most evil even going so far as to suggest adding tranquilizers to the water supply to keep the population docile. Fluoridation is an obvious abuse of public trust and a clear violation of the law.

What is so strange to me is that Americans have acquiesced to adding fluoride, a clearly recognized, very powerful toxin, to the water supply—not to prevent some deadly disease, but in hopes of preventing something as minor as tooth decay. The fact that these programs have been approved by the voting public does not make it any less criminal. It merely means that the proponents of this disaster have been able to convince—through coercion and outright lying—51 percent of the public to agree to this deadly policy.

No one told voters that the fluoride content of their foods, beverages, and water would continue to increase, so that even if they wished to avoid the poison, they would not be able to. No one cared about the indigent and those living on limited incomes who would not be able to afford filtered water or the expensive in-home filtration systems used by wealthy government bureaucrats, ADA elite, and state officials.

No one gave the choice to the pregnant woman who wanted to protect her unborn children from the devastating effects of high fluoride concentrations in her baby's body. The choice has been denied to the child whose teeth have been destroyed by dental fluorosis, especially to children of poor families that cannot afford the expensive dental work required to correct this devastating condition. And no one gave the choice to elderly persons who will spend their waning years crippled from skeletal fluorosis or devastated by a neurodegenerative disease. They have all been forgotten.

Again, this is not a problem of free enterprise, as has been suggested by some opponents of fluoridation. Rather, it is an example of corporatism, collusion between corporations, and the government operating totally outside the free market system. Corporations are an anomaly of the free market and were condemned as such as early as the 1940s by two leading philosophers of free enterprise, Ludwig von Mises and F.A. Hayek. They saw the corporation as an entity that used the power of government to stifle competition, the life-blood of free enterprise. They also saw that these institutions are similar to government itself in that they are inevitably heavily bureaucratized, and slow to respond to new and innovative ideas.

The collusion between the aluminum and superphosphate fertilizer industries and the government has resulted in the fluoridation of 75 percent of America's drinking water—at a profit, no less. Hayek, in his waning years, came to understand that free enterprise without the firm foundation of natural law and a moral order would degenerate into chaos and legal plunder of the nation. Only the light of truth can halt this process.

5
Other Toxic Metals to Avoid

While we know a great deal about heavy metal toxicity, many questions remain to be answered. For example, how do low levels of these toxic metals chemically interact when they occur together? Do they react synergistically? Does the treatment of heavy metal toxicity cause more problems than no treatment at all? All of these questions demand answers. Because of limited space, I will discuss other toxic metals together in one chapter. Unfortunately, this also means that I will be forced to omit discussions of some toxic metals that we encounter on a less-frequent basis in our daily lives.

In the past, a substance was considered toxic only if we could observe obvious symptoms following exposure, but with the advent of better methods of examining events on cellular and even subcellular levels, we now recognize that subtle toxicities can disrupt cellular function without producing obvious clinical toxicity—a condition known as subclinical toxicity. It may take years for such toxicity to produce obvious signs and symptoms. As you know by now, the ultimate effect a toxin will have on a particular individual depends on numerous variables, such as genetic susceptibility, the strength of the antioxidant system, age, associated toxicities such as alcohol abuse, smoking and exposure to other toxic chemicals, concomitant diseases, nutrition, and physical conditioning.

We must also consider the subtlety of some symptoms of toxicity. Rather than obvious signs such as nausea, vomiting and abdominal cramps, some people may experience no more than vague feelings of fatigue, cloudiness of thought, memory lapses, irritability, depression, or minor aches and pains that may be put off by a doctor, or attributed to stress, menopause, or old age. My experience has been that many doctors tend to shrug off patients' symptoms that do not fit the disorders and diseases with which they are familiar, and I have seen numerous patients whose doctors had attributed chronic symptoms to stress, and whose illnesses actually ended up being tied to very high lead and/or mercury levels. Had these patients' elevated metal levels not been discovered and treated, these hapless people would have spent the remainder of their lives miserable and sick.

Because so many physicians are totally unfamiliar with heavy metal toxicities, they never even consider them as a possibility when diagnosing sickness. Worse still, doctors sometimes classify difficult-to-diagnose patients as "crocks" or "depressed" and hand them off to someone else to deal with. Also, many doctors maintain very stringent definitions of toxicity, and often use criteria that are either outdated or based on poor medical evidence. Because they do not recognize subclinical toxicity, their patients continue to suffer. *More evidence-based medicine.*

Cadmium Toxicity

Cadmium is a soft, silvery-white metal grouped with zinc and mercury on the periodic table, and appears to be a potent neurotoxin to the developing nervous system of the fetus and newborn baby. Like mercury, it is very reactive in the presence of vital sulfhydral-containing enzymes and proteins in the body.

Cadmium is found naturally in the environment, though never in its elemental state, usually in association with zinc. Some of the most common sources of cadmium in our environment are as a byproduct of zinc smelting and burning of fossil fuels. It is also associated with mining operations, battery production, incineration of municipal waste, and with sludge-based and phosphate fertilizers. Approximately thirty-six hundred tons were used in 1985 alone for metal-plating processes, in paint pigments, plastic stabilizers, and in Ni-Cad (nickel cadmium) batteries. As a component of many disposable consumer goods, cadmium eventually ends up in landfills, much of which is burned, releasing this toxic substance into the atmosphere.

The primary source of exposure for most individuals who do not work in a cadmium-based industry is from food sources. The average daily uptake has risen to approximately 10-30 ug. Many leafy plants absorb cadmium from the soil, especially when sludge-type fertilizers are used. Organ meats, such as kidney and shellfish also contain significant amounts of cadmium.

Inhalation of cadmium released from factories, landfill incineration, and cigarettes is the second major source of exposure. Second-hand smoke is dangerous as well, and presents a particular danger to newborns and small children. Absorption of cadmium from the lungs varies from 30 percent to as high as 90 percent.

Once cadmium enters the body, only 1-5 percent is absorbed from the gastrointestinal tract in adults, but in newborns absorption is much higher, sometimes as much as 55 percent. Once absorbed, the metal quickly binds to the membranes of red blood cells, and to albumin, where it is quickly removed by the liver and especially the kidney. Not surprisingly then, the kidneys are the principal sites of cadmium toxicity. As with mercury toxicity, metallothioneins are considered to be the principal method of detoxification within the liver, kidneys, and cells.

Effect on the Unborn and Newborn

Cadmium toxicity in the developing brain has been studied extensively in experimental animals, and results clearly indicate that—as with most toxic substances—developing babies are at the highest risk for toxicity. Early studies concluded that the placenta acted as an efficient barrier against passage of cadmium from the mother to the baby, but we now know that higher elevations can pass through the placenta. Perhaps of more importance, though, is the observation that cadmium interferes with the passage of other important trace elements needed by the baby's developing brain.

In most studies, elevated cadmium levels have not been found in the unborn baby's brain, but in newborns, cadmium will pass into the brain in rather high levels. In fact, one day after birth, baby rats' brains will absorb ten to twenty times more cadmium than during adulthood. At this age the blood-brain barrier has not matured and therefore more cadmium can enter the brain than at any other stage of life. As the baby matures and grows, its brain becomes less vulnerable to the accumulation of cadmium—yet this does not mean that it is immune to cadmium toxicity. Toxicity in older animals seems to appear by way of a more indirect route.

Most studies have shown that exposing animals to cadmium during gestation produced behavioral changes in their offspring. One study found that such exposure did not increase cadmium levels in the baby's body, but it did produce a significant decrease in body iron levels. Iron is critical for growth, especially of the developing brain. Reduced zinc levels have also been seen following exposure of the mother to cadmium.

Pregnant animals given high levels of cadmium in their drinking water had babies of low birth weight. These newborns were also hyperactive, but later in life became hypoactive—couch potatoes. These animals also experienced significant problems with motor coordination and behavior.

After birth, most of the damage done by cadmium is to blood vessels supplying the brain. It has been observed that the most rapidly growing areas of the brain are also the areas most sensitive to damage. While it is the neonate that is most susceptible, even adults will show toxic damage to their brain following chronic exposure to cadmium in drinking water.

One interesting finding in animals exposed to cadmium early in life was that even though they showed no neurological effects at the time of exposure, they did develop behavioral

Cadmium...

- increases prostate cancer.
- causes hypertension.
- decreases testosterone production.
- blocks calcium receptors.
- decreases acetylcholine receptors.
- increases dopamine.
- impairs myelin formation.
- increases free-radical production.
- decreases reduced glutathione.
- decreases superoxide dismutase.

TABLE 5.1

changes later in life. This may be because of interference with critical brain pathway formation that is needed later in life, when behavior becomes more complex.

Human studies have also identified significant problems following early exposure to cadmium. One study, in which researchers looked at the levels of cadmium and thirteen other metals in normal and learning disabled children, found a good correlation between cadmium and lead levels in learning disabled children.[155] In another study, Marlow and co-workers also found that hair cadmium levels were consistently higher in mentally retarded children and children with borderline intelligence than in controls.[156]

The question remains: which of these two toxic metals, cadmium or lead, is responsible for the most destructive health effects? A possible answer was discovered in another study that found elevated cadmium more strongly affected verbal IQ, but elevated lead levels had more pronounced effects on performance IQ.[157]

One study, in which lead and cadmium levels were measured in both mothers and their newborn infants, found a significant relationship between exposure to these metals and the children's development. Lead was associated with problems with perceptual skills, whereas cadmium was associated with motor problems *and* perceptual skills. Exposure to these metals seemed to have no effect on memory or verbal skills.

The lesson here is that many toxic metals not only have specific brain localizing effects, but also overlap in terms of parts of the brain affected. This emphasizes the importance of looking at all of the heavy metals, not just one, when searching for causes of neurological toxicity.

Cadmium Toxicity in Adults

Overt toxicity in adults usually occurs in an industrial setting. For example, workers in electroplating, cadmium-battery, plastics-manufacturing, paint, textile, and phosphate fertilizer factories are at increased risk.

Exposure not related to occupation may come from many sources. As I mentioned, smokers inhale significant quantities of cadmium. A single pack of cigarettes can release up to 2 ug of cadmium: each cigarette emits between 0.1-0.2 ug of cadmium, depending on the number of puffs and depth of inhalation. Second-hand smoke is also a risk to those confined with smokers. I shudder when I see children closed up in a car while their parents eagerly puff away on cigarettes.

Non-smokers are also at risk. While food represents the major source of exposure, clear plastic wrap used to cover dishes also contains cadmium and should not be microwaved or in any way heated. It should be safe in the refrigerator. Drinking water can be a source of cadmium; in most instances levels are relatively low, but plumbing can increase cadmium water levels since both plastic (PVC) and metal pipes contain the metal.

Like most metals, cadmium tends to accumulate in the body over time. Once absorbed from the gut, it travels to the liver, where it combines with metallothionein molecules, which act to neutralize the metal. From there, the bound cadmium is excreted from the kidney, but if liver functions are impaired (due to disease, hepatitis, alcohol abuse, metabolic disorders, or drug toxicity), the neutralizing protein may be unable to do its job properly, in which case the cadmium is not excreted, but distributed to other organs, including the brain. By middle age, our body cadmium levels may be as high as 20-30 mg.

Chronic exposure to high doses of cadmium can also result in altered calcium metabolism, leading to a loss of calcium from the skeleton (osteomalacia). This disease was first discovered in Japan, where it was called *itai-itai* ('ouch-ouch') disease, an aptly named disorder that causes walking to become very painful due to brittle bones, skeletal deformities and numerous microfractures. Other common complaints include back and joint pains, rigid spinal movements, and thin, deformed bones that hurt when pressure is applied. I have seen one patient who tested for very high cadmium levels with early onset of joint pains, fatigue, and muscle tenderness and had been previously diagnosed with fibromyalgia and chronic fatigue syndrome.

In some studies, exposure to even low levels of cadmium has been associated with high blood pressure (hypertension). Experimentally, adding 5 ppm cadmium to drinking water produced elevated blood pressure. Adding zinc reversed this effect, and lowered blood pressure to normal. In other studies even concentrations as low as 0.1 ppm caused hypertension.

Subsequent studies have found an anomalous effect. When low doses of cadmium were given, test animals developed hypertension, but high doses induced low blood pressure. The cause of the hypertension appears to be related to the blocking of two enzymes needed to break down the hormone norepinephrine, which normally constricts blood vessels and raises blood pressure. If it cannot be cleared from the blood vessel walls, the vessels remain constricted and the blood pressure elevated. Why higher doses lowered blood pressure is still a mystery.

The natural question is: is cadmium responsible for hypertension? Unfortunately, the answer is not entirely clear. Several studies have found a direct correlation between elevated cadmium levels and hypertension in humans,[158] while others found no correlation at all.[159] It may be that some people are especially sensitive to the effects of cadmium. For example, we know that calcium and zinc deficiencies increase one's sensitivity to the toxic effects of cadmium, increasing absorption of the metal as well. Excess zinc is known to reduce cadmium toxicity, so that those with elevated tissue levels of zinc would likely be less affected. Low iron and vitamin C levels can also increase cadmium toxicity.

Effects on Reproduction

Studies of men exposed to industrial levels of cadmium have shown statistically higher incidences of prostate cancer. Experimentally, injection of cadmium into test animals resulted in damage to the testicles and eventually led to testicular tumors. Long term, low-level exposure in experimental animals also led to testicular and prostate tumors.[160]

In cases of heavy exposure, cadmium accumulated in the testes and reduced testosterone production. The mechanism of action is unknown, but cadmium is not thought to have a direct effect on the prostate and testes. It may be that cadmium has an indirect effect on zinc and androgen hormone production. There is no direct evidence that low-level cadmium exposure is a cause of prostate cancer in humans, but it also doesn't hurt to err on the side of safety.

In pregnant women, the placenta does appear to be an effective barrier against cadmium reaching the baby in the uterus, but large doses can breach this boundary. A study of 102 mothers and their newborns found that babies with elevated hair cadmium levels also had decreased birth weight.[161]

Effects on the Brain

Cadmium is known to have profound effects on calcium metabolism, not only in bone but also in the nervous system where calcium is used as a signaling device. Calcium stimulated by neurotransmitters enters special channels in the neuron membrane and once inside the cell, stimulates a whole series of reactions that cause the neuron to fire. Cadmium can block this calcium channel, thereby preventing the neuron from functioning properly.

As we have seen, one of the brain's most common neurotransmitters is glutamate, which interacts with several types of receptors on the neuron. Cadmium blocks one of these receptors (NMDA receptor) and stimulates two others (kainate and AMPA receptors).

Earlier, I said that excessive quantities of glutamate and other excitotoxins in the brain can result in neuron death that is associated with everything from Alzheimer's dementia, Parkinson's disease and Lou Gehrig's disease (ALS), to strokes and brain injury. This destructive process depends on calcium entry into the neuron triggered by the excitotoxins. Cadmium, in tissue culture, blocks this toxicity. At first, this might seem to be a good thing, but cadmium, even in low concentrations, has been shown to reduce cell survival. It appears that calcium blockage is so efficient that the cell cannot survive.

Next to developing babies, persons with neurological disorders would be at the most risk of cadmium toxicity. This is because neurological disease weakens neurons, reduces antioxidant levels and contributes to deficiencies of trace elements such as selenium, zinc, calcium, and magnesium.

Cadmium has been shown to decrease brain levels of 5-hydroxytryptophan, a metabolic precursor of the neurotransmitter serotonin, as well as to reduce the number of receptors to another neurotransmitter, acetylcholine (muscarinic site in the cortex and striatum). The levels of dopamine in the brain, on the other hand, were increased. This is especially important for newborns because these neurotransmitters play a critical role in how the brain eventually develops. Dopamine elevation has been associated with behavioral changes, such as confusion and an inability to relate with the real world.

The age during which exposure occurs also plays a major role in how neurotransmitters are affected. For example, exposure to cadmium at an early age results in a decrease in serotonin levels in the brain, while exposure later in life causes an increase. The effect on brain dopamine levels does not vary with age at time of exposure.

Cadmium affects the nervous system in many other ways, including inhibiting important enzymes.[162] It has also been shown to alter myelin formation and maintenance. And like so many heavy metals, cadmium not only increases free-radical production, it also interferes with the brain's ability to neutralize free radicals. Similarly, it increases lipid peroxidation in neurons.

One of the more important effects related to free-radical damage is cadmium's ability to lower levels of reduced glutathione in certain brain regions. Reduced glutathione's major role is protecting the nervous system from cadmium toxicity, as well as other oxidizing toxins. Cadmium also reduces the level of another antioxidant molecule, superoxide dismutase (SOD).

Increasing cellular glutathione levels can reduce cadmium toxicity. Glutathione binds cadmium and helps the body remove it before more damage can be done. Again, this emphasizes the importance of always keeping antioxidant levels high through good nutrition and supplementation. High doses of vitamins E and C, the carotenoids, flavonoids, and alpha-lipoic acid, can increase glutathione levels as well as assist in neutralizing free radicals.

Lead: Destroyer of Young Lives

Most of us are already familiar with lead toxicity, especially with the numerous lawsuits and media attention that have focused on the danger to children. In the not-too-distant past, leaded gasoline presented the greatest source of lead exposure. In 1968 alone, 500 million pounds of this metal were released into the atmosphere. Once federal guidelines were established in the 1970s, lead levels began to fall—by an astronomical 78 percent during the period from 1976 to 1991.

Other common sources of lead include soil, cans, paint, plaster, pipes, solder, newsprint, ceramic glaze, some herbal products, and even enclosed shooting ranges. Of particular concern today are herbal sources of lead contamination. Some herbs imported from China are not carefully checked before being placed on the market in this country, and some of these products may also contain mercury. American-made herbal products have not been implicated in this problem.

Strange as it may sound, indoor shooting ranges are a source of lead exposure. Lead bullets produce a vapor that can be absorbed through the lungs when discharged from a firearm. It is important to use only ranges that are well-ventilated. Jacketed ammunition will also further reduce your exposure to lead from bullets.

While most modern houses have PVC pipes, even modern faucets have lead-containing joints that can be a significant source of lead in drinking water. Remember, fluoridated water leaches even more lead from the pipes and faucets, greatly increasing your risk of lead poisoning from this source. Recall that one of the studies I mentioned in chapter four found that fluoridated cities have water lead levels twice as high as unfluoridated communities.

Our average lead intake ranges from 0.1 to greater than 2 mg a day. It is known that elevated levels of blood lead are associated with a high risk of stillbirth and miscarriage. When blood levels are greater than 30 ug/L/day, there is a greater risk to the health of the mother as well. Recently, levels as low as 10ug/g were found to impair cognitive function in children. Studies are now being conducted to see if levels as low as 2.5 ug/g are also harmful to brain function. Combined with zinc, calcium, and selenium deficiencies, even low lead levels can be quite toxic, especially to the brain.

Lead Toxicity and the Brain: the Child

As always, lead poses the greatest dangers to the unborn and the small child, but the danger continues to be significant throughout life. In children, even blood lead levels as low as 0.5 to 10 micromoles can adversely affect the development of the brain leading to mental retardation, impaired visual-motor coordination, and permanent cognitive problems.[163] It is also known that children absorb lead much easier than adults,[164] especially when they also suffer from an iron deficiency. Unlike cadmium, lead passes through the placenta without difficulty.

In 1991 the Centers for Disease Control set the maximum acceptable level of blood lead at 10 micrograms per deciliter (10 ug/dl). At least one study found that children with blood lead levels from 7-10 ug/dl developed behavioral and cognitive impairment.[165] Of particular concern is the estimate that 17 percent of children in the United States alone may have levels exceeding 15 ug/dl. According to studies done by the EPA, levels of 50-75 ug/dl can cause a five-point drop in IQ—even when controlled for other factors, such as socioeconomic status, age, and level of education.

Lead has several very toxic effects on brain cell function. For example, it is known to inhibit neurotransmitters, including acetylcholine, glutamate, and dopamine, and to inhibit the function of the GABAergic system. Acetylcholine plays a major role in memory as well as motor functions of the brain, dopamine plays a critical role in many of the automatic motor systems of the brain as well as the emotional parts of the brain, including the limbic system and striatal system, and the GABAergic system functions to reduce overstimulation of specific brain actions. All of these neurotransmitters are important for normal cognitive development, behavioral function, and motor functions of the nervous system; schizophrenia and Parkinson's disease have been linked to damaged neurotransmitter function.

The connection between lead exposure and parkinsonism was strengthened by the observation of a high incidence of the disorder in postal workers exposed to lead-sulfate batteries for up to thirty years.[166]

One of the most powerful effects of lead, which is of major concern during brain development, is its effect on the glutamate neurotransmitter system. Lead has been shown to powerfully inhibit part of the glutamate system (called the NMDA receptor). So why is this so important? As we have seen, glutamate is one of the most important stimulating molecules for normal brain development. Fluctuations in its level in the developing brain can significantly affect how the numerous brain pathways will eventually develop. This may explain why lead toxicity in newborns results in widespread behavioral and intellectual problems.

A second way lead alters brain function is by acting on the memory system. We know that one of the most important aspects of toxicity is related to long term potentiation, or LTP, a fancy phrase that describes an organism's ability to learn and *remember* solutions based on recurring experience with a particular stimulus. Studies have chemically linked LTP development to proper calcium transport and glutamate activity in brain cells; memory is severely affected when this system is affected by dramatic chemical changes. Exposure to lead throughout development acts as a powerful inhibitor of LTP because the system is highly dependent on normal glutamate function.[167] It has been shown that lead can easily permeate the blood-brain barrier, especially in newborns and small children.[168]

Lead also alters brain function by interfering with cellular calcium, which plays a very critical role in brain cell function. In fact, lead has a greater attraction for calcium's cellular receptors than calcium itself does. As we have seen before, excess cellular calcium triggers any number of destructive processes (eicosanoid cascade, free-radical generation, cytokine activation, etc). Lead, being more active than calcium, has been shown to trigger these destructive processes in the cell powerfully.[169]

Lead, like the other heavy metals I have discussed, markedly amplifies free-radical generation induced by excess glutamate, thereby magnifying glutamate's excitotoxicity.[170] This situation could be expected to worsen degenerative diseases, even if the metal is present only in small concentrations—doses many toxicologists would not expect to cause toxicity.

Studies consistently find that lead toxicity depends on duration and timing of exposure, concentration of lead, and the strength of cellular defense systems. You may recall that the body has many defenses against metal toxicity. For example, we know that calcium, zinc, and magnesium protect against lead toxicity. The presence of antioxidant enzymes are also extremely important: levels of SOD, reduced glutathione, and glutathione peroxidase, determine how sensitive we will be to lead toxicity. A well-functioning metallothionein system is also vital to good health.

```
┌─────────────────────────────────────────────────┐
│                                                   │
│                      Lead...                      │
│                                                   │
│  • inhibits acetylcholine production.             │
│  • lowers IQs in children.                        │
│  • is associated with neurodegenerative diseases. │
│  • increases free-radical production.             │
│  • promotes lipid peroxidation.                   │
│  • stimulates excitotoxicity.                     │
│  • inhibits proper memory functions.              │
│  • is associated with violent behavior.           │
│  • increases anxiety.                             │
│                                                   │
│ TABLE 5.2                                         │
└─────────────────────────────────────────────────┘
```

Breast Milk and Lead Exposure

From 1971-1972 the average concentration of lead in human breast milk in the United States was 0.07 ug/ml. Because of efforts to reduce lead in the environment, levels are now down to 0.001-0.02 ug/ml, a significant improvement. Based on this low figure, and the fact that about 47 percent of lead is absorbed by a baby's GI tract—combined with the breasts' efficient lead filtering system—total exposure will be 0.25 ug a day. So, in most instances, lead exposure from breast milk is not a major concern. (Umbilical cord blood was found to have lead levels two to five times higher than breast milk.)

The same level of certainty cannot be applied to baby formulas reconstituted with tap water, especially in fluoridated areas of the country. You may recall that fluoridated communities have almost twice the lead levels in their water as unfluoridated communities. I would, therefore, discourage all mothers from using any commercial baby formulas; if you must, at least do not use anything but distilled or properly filtered water to reconstitute the formula. You must also add DHA to the formula.

Lead, Violence, and Social Behavior

Several studies have shown that lead-intoxicated children experience intellectual difficulties, as well as problems with hyper-irritability and violent outbursts. A recent study of children exposed to high levels of environmental lead found that children with higher bone lead levels were more aggressive, exhibited delinquent behavior,[171] and demonstrated many other antisocial behaviors.

These findings may be explained by the fact that lead exposure early in life can affect brain serotonin levels. In a recent study, exposure to even low levels of lead early in life caused significant damage to this system in the brain,[172] which plays an important part in regulating violence. Furthermore, several studies of prison populations have linked low serotonin levels to violent behavior. The neurotransmitter, dopamine, also plays an important role in behavioral functions, and is similarly lowered by lead exposure during critical periods of brain growth.

The social cost of lead toxicity cannot be adequately assessed because of the subtle nature of some of its effects, but we do know that several studies have shown that lead-exposed children require more remedial education than do children free from lead exposure.[173]

The same is true of behavioral problems. A study of 1,782 eight-year-old children in Boston found that lead levels correlated with elevated scores on tests measuring anxiety and/or withdrawal, and scores measuring inattentiveness, nervousness, and aggressive behavior.[174] There was also some correlation to extreme behavior problems. In another study, children with high blood lead levels were three times more likely to have significant behavioral problems than children with lower lead levels.[175]

One recent study demonstrated that lead levels in children are higher during the summer than in colder months.[176] Researchers examined three sources of lead-containing dust—floor dust, windowsill dust, and carpet dust—and found that lead levels in children were higher during summer months because of the increased amounts of dust tracked into the house. This may help to explain some of the irritability of youngsters during the summer months. Although it may be a stretch, elevated lead levels in our nation's young people may also contribute to heightened acts of violence during hot weather.

Lead in Those With Pre-existing Neurological Diseases

One factor not often considered in cases of lead toxicity—both in children and adults—is the presence of an abnormal nervous system before the exposure. For people with autism, cerebral palsy or Down's syndrome, the brain is far more vulnerable to a number of common insults, such as aging, free-radical generation, and viral illnesses. And because their brain cells are already weakened, people with these diseases are less able to battle the adverse effects of lead and will suffer greater injury than those their age with normal nervous systems.

In adults, who have already endured years of free-radical damage, adding a little lead to the mix can push their systems beyond tolerance, leading to early aging and neurodegenerative diseases. As we shall see later, many neurodegenerative diseases are associated with increased levels of toxic metals in the parts of the brain associated with each of these diseases. A lifetime accumulation of one or more of these metals can result in severe damage to the nervous system at a time during adult life when it is most vulnerable, from middle age onward.

Why You Are at Special Risk After Middle Age

Lead, like aluminum and fluoride, preferentially accumulates in bones. In fact, 80 percent of ingested lead ends up in bones, where it is stored for a lifetime. Remember that lead has a very high affinity for calcium, and accumulation in the skeleton can begin even before birth. Lead exposure is especially dangerous during early childhood as bones undergo rapid growth and remodeling. Not surprisingly, lead also tends to accumulate in teeth during childhood.

In addition to the neurological effects I have already discussed, elevated lead levels in children are associated with many physiological defects, such as abnormal bone formation and bone weakness. Because lead is stored in the bones, and under normal conditions is released only when bone dissolves, it can remain in large concentrations in the bones throughout life. As we begin to age, our bones frequently break down, releasing not only calcium and phosphorus, but also lead and other metals that have been stored in them. Osteoporosis, an exaggerated process of bone destruction, releases large amounts of stored lead, as well as aluminum and fluoride, over a relatively short period of time. The released lead enters the blood stream, and then the nervous system where it proceeds to wreak havoc with the delicate cellular systems I described above.

This is akin to giving a person a single toxic dose of lead, but the osteoporosis patient and her doctor would not even begin to suspect complications caused by lead poisoning. In cases such as this one, physicians usually ask about recent exposure to hazardous materials and, if none is suspected, do not order a heavy metal screen for lead, mercury, aluminum, and cadmium.

The faster bones degenerate, the greater amounts of lead are released, and the higher the blood levels will be. People in nursing homes and shut-ins are at special risk, since their diets are usually poor, they receive no nutrient supplementation, and they get very little exercise.

The government, in all its wisdom, has decided that screening tests are not worth the expense unless recent exposure and ensuing toxicity can be easily pinpointed. What an absurd policy! In cases of metal toxicity, Medicare/Medicaid rules essentially say that a test can only be ordered if the diagnosis is already known: in order to obtain a blood lead level test, the doctor must have documented evidence that blood lead is elevated. It's a "Catch-22," bureaucratic socialized medicine at its best.

Clearing the Body of Lead

One of the problems with chelating lead is that during early stages of treatment, blood levels can actually increase due to release of lead from bone. Care must be taken to remove this newly released lead quickly so that it isn't redistributed to another organ or the nervous system. Furthermore, removal of toxic metals, especially from the nervous system is not an easy matter. Very exacting methods are required for proper chelation of each metal.

The most effective way to remove lead from the body is by DMSA chelation. Like mercury, DMSA binds very tightly to lead and allows the kidneys to flush it out into the urine, but the greatest difference between lead and mercury chelation is that mercury is not stored in the bone. An early consequence of lead chelation is the rebound effect, caused by lead leaving the bones once chelation has begun. With DMSA, after an initial drop, blood lead levels will rise and may be higher after chelation has begun than they were in the beginning.

As a result of this process, prolonged chelation is sometimes required, and is best accomplished in cycles. I suggest following the same precautions and follow-up studies I outlined at the end of chapter three. Once lead levels are sufficiently low—preferably undetectable—I suggest one additional twenty-four-hour provocative study, just to make sure your lead levels are not slowly creeping back up.

It must be remembered that the main goal in lead removal is to protect the brain. A recent study found that the use of DMSA was no more effective in removing brain lead levels than was a placebo.[177] This study was conducted on rhesus monkeys exposed both acutely and chronically to lead. Brain biopsies were taken from various brain regions both before and after chelation. Not only was DMSA ineffective in removing lead from the brain, but lead distribution in the brain was uneven, with levels in the following order from highest to lowest: prefrontal cortex, frontal lobe, hippocampus, and striatum.

The study also demonstrated that a single blood lead measurement was a poor predictor of brain lead levels, and that high brain levels can occur together with low blood levels. The problem with the study was that, in humans, considerable levels of lead can exist in the bones, acting as a continual source of the toxic metal. This is the value of DMSA, to remove lead deposits so that brain levels can decrease naturally. It has been shown that when sources of lead exposure are removed, brain lead levels will fall 34 percent in five weeks. In addition to chelation, then, it is obvious that you must isolate sources of lead exposure and eliminate them from your environment. *In particular, do not drink fluoridated water.*

Some have advocated intravenous EDTA to chelate lead, but one study demonstrated that high oral intakes of magnesium were superior to EDTA in elimination of lead.[178] In this study, researchers measured biochemical markers of lead toxicity such as protoporphyrin and delta-aminolevulinic acid, and found that magnesium treatment worked more slowly than EDTA but had a more profound effect on biochemical measures of lead toxicity.

Aluminum: The Insidious Toxin

Aluminum is the third most common element on earth, but is always found in chemical combination in nature. Our exposure to free aluminum or aluminum salts results from numerous industrial and household uses of the metal. It is not considered an essential element in biological systems and is found in only very small concentrations, or not at all, in populations of non-industrialized countries. For the most part, it can be considered a toxin whenever it is present in the body. Like so many of the toxic metals we have discussed so far, no one knows what constitutes a safe level.

Sources of Aluminum

In addition to fluoride, yet another additive—aluminum sulfate, used to treat public water supplies—is also very toxic. This compound is used widely to clarify water, and as a result, most municipal water systems contain significant amounts of aluminum. When combined with fluoride in even minute concentrations, this additive produces a compound that is very toxic to the brain, resulting in widespread brain-cell death.

Aluminum is also found naturally in many foods and beverages. In general, foods with the highest aluminum levels are acidic: tomatoes, cranberries, rhubarb, apricots, cabbage, and apples. Adding baking soda to these foods releases yet more aluminum. Major sources of aluminum include processed cheese, teas, some herbs, spices, and some commercial salt.

Aluminum utensils, cans, aluminum foil, and other aluminum containers all pose a risk for aluminum absorption into foods. It is known that dark-colored utensils contain more aluminum than do light ones, and the presence of sugar inhibits the corrosion of aluminum utensils. Aluminum colanders pose a risk for contamination of pasta. Cooking foods in aluminum foil leaches the aluminum out of the foil and into the foods, especially into meat gravies and tomato gravies. Baking potatoes in aluminum foil may encourage aluminum absorption in the skins of the potatoes.

Aluminum used in industry is obtained from bauxite ore. Those working in bauxite mines and aluminum smelting plants run a significant risk of developing high levels of brain aluminum, and as a result, suffer from severe neurological disorders. Synthetic zeolites, rocks which produce steam when heated, contain aluminum and are used in the paper industry and in concrete. Potassium aluminum sulfate, a dye-fixing chemical used in tanning, also contains aluminum.

Aluminum and the Brain

During the early 1970s, doctors working in the dialysis units of several hospitals noticed that a growing number of their patients were developing rather unusual symptoms, such as jerking muscles, hallucinations, and rapid-onset dementia. Several of these patients died before the culprit was discovered: high concentrations of aluminum in the water being used for dialysis. Ironically, this was ordinary tap water. Once aluminum was removed from the water, the dialysis dementia syndrome disappeared and patients improved significantly when chelated with a substance called deferoxamine, a medication that removes aluminum from body tissues. This was the first human demonstration that aluminum could cause dementia, somewhat similar to Alzheimer's dementia.

Like most of the toxic metals thus far discussed, aluminum is a significant brain toxin. It can reach the brain by several routes. Aluminum gases and dust can enter by way of the olfactory tracts in the mucous membranes of the nasal passages, pass directly along these tiny nerve filaments, and enter the olfactory parts of the brain where it is then distributed to other vital areas of the nervous system. There is also evidence that aluminum can pass along nerves in the limbs and travel to the spinal cord, in much the same way that mercury does.

When ingested—in medications, foods and beverages—aluminum is readily absorbed. Once in the blood stream, it is tightly bound by a special transport protein called transferrin, which is also the main carrier for iron and manganese. The brain cells themselves have special transferrin receptors that allow the aluminum to enter the cells easily. Recent evidence indicates that aluminum can also enter the body by other mechanisms as well.

Interestingly, some are of the opinion that when aluminum enters a neuron, the metal itself causes very little damage.[179] It appears that most of the damage is actually caused by increasing the concentration of iron within the cell. Remember that iron is a very powerful free-radical generator, and elevated levels of cellular iron have been observed in all neurode-generative diseases. Aluminum can also increase the oxidation power of several other pro-oxidant metals, including copper and chromium.[180] This means that elevated tissue aluminum levels will increase the destructive power of other types of metals.

You may recall that in chapter one I discussed the oxidative destruction of the fatty parts of cells (lipids), a process called lipid peroxidation. It is known that aluminum and iron both can significantly increase brain lipid peroxidation.[181] Studies have also indicated that aluminum has a special affinity for myelin, the fatty lining of nerve pathways. In one study, the presence of aluminum increased lipid peroxidation in myelin 72 percent.[182] This is especially important to persons with multiple sclerosis or any other myelin disorder. Both iron and aluminum can increase the oxidation of other parts of the cell, resulting in protein oxidation and/or DNA oxidation as well as lipid peroxidation. This can severely disrupt the function of the cells, and can eventually lead to their death.

Aluminum also acts on cell membrane function by binding to the parts of the membrane responsible for transduction, the relay of information signals within the cell. We know that calcium normally plays a vital part in this signaling process and that aluminum competes with calcium for its information receptors. When calcium levels are low, aluminum becomes significantly more toxic. The same is true for low magnesium levels.

Another way aluminum causes problems is by interfering with metal-dependent enzymes. Certain enzymes require the presence of a particular metal—such as zinc, iron, manganese, or magnesium—to work properly. Aluminum can displace these metals and cause those enzymes to function poorly or not at all.[183] Combined with citrate or malate, aluminum produces fewer adverse effects. This is how plants protect themselves from aluminum toxicity. Unfortunately, while citrate may block aluminum's ability to damage metal-dependent enzymes, it also significantly increases aluminum absorption and distribution.

Of equal concern is the enormous body of evidence collected over the past twenty years connecting glutamate accumulation to most of the neurodegenerative diseases, as well as to all other types of central nervous system injuries. The problem thus far has been determining how glutamate accumulates and why the brain's normal removal system cannot protect the brain from this excess glutamate. We may now have an answer.

Several studies have shown that aluminum forms a highly absorbable chemical complex with glutamate in the gastrointestinal tract. Not only will the aluminum-glutamate complex enter the blood stream in much higher concentrations than normal, it can also easily pass through the blood-brain barrier. These actions increase brain levels of aluminum, as well as glutamate levels in discrete areas of the brain. Several of these areas are involved in Alzheimer's disease and Parkinson's disease.

Why You Shouldn't Squeeze That Lemon in Your Tea!

It has been known for some time that organic acids, such as citrate from plants, can greatly increase the absorption of aluminum from the gastrointestinal tract. One test using eight normal men found that addition of citrate to the oral dose of aluminum hydroxide gel (found in most antacids) could increase aluminum absorption by as much as elevenfold.[184] This is important to remember when you are drinking tea, which can contain high levels of aluminum. If you squeeze a little lemon (high in citric acid) in your tea, you will greatly increase the aluminum absorption. The tap water you may use to make the tea can also contain significant levels of aluminum. As if that weren't bad enough, the tap water also contains fluoride, which forms toxic complexes and enhances aluminum absorption.[185]

Normally, absorption of aluminum from the gastrointestinal tract is rather low (0.1 percent) and excretion from the body is rather rapid following absorption. But, certain tissues, such as the brain, tend to gather the aluminum and hold onto it tightly. Also, people with poor kidney function are at special risk for aluminum toxicity, because their bodies cannot excrete ingested aluminum as efficiently as a person with normal kidneys. Because kidney function tends to decline as we age, the elderly are at special risk.

Several studies have shown that organic acids, such as citrate, not only enhance absorption of aluminum, but also enhance its passage into various tissues, including the brain.[186] It also promotes retention of aluminum in body tissues. Also, some flavonoids, such as gallic acid (found in pecans and berries) and chlorogenic acid (in apples), enhance entry of aluminum into tissues. This is an important factor when considering food combinations.

Teas, cheese, acidic vegetables, and soft drinks in aluminum cans can all be high in aluminum: avoid eating fruit or drinking fruit juice in combination with any of these. Cooking acidic produce in aluminum pans should also be avoided. Then there are the keg parties of college lore. Kegs are usually constructed of aluminum, and beer, which is naturally high in aluminum anyway, is also acidic—which can dissolve the lining of the keg and add even more aluminum to the mixture.

In a hospital where I once worked, the administration did all they could to please the doctors, from providing a refrigerator full of fruit juices and colas to keeping a big basket full of fresh fruit sitting on the coffee table. Day after day, unsuspecting medicos would sit around the table eating apples and oranges and swilling down solutions of diet cola and aluminum, never even considering how rapidly aluminum was being absorbed into their bodies, and poured into their brains, setting the stage for serious neurological damage later in life.

When you consider that, over the last two generations, consumption of beverages from aluminum cans and containers has begun at an increasingly early age, the average person will have absorbed enormous amounts of aluminum by the time he or she reaches age fifty. Is it any wonder we have seen such a dramatic increase in neurodegenerative diseases in the last twenty years?

Aluminum, ALS, Parkinson's Disease and Alzheimer's Dementia

One of the most-discussed environmental connections to disease is the relationship between aluminum exposure and Alzheimer's disease. In truth, the connection applies to most neurodegenerative disorders, including Parkinson's and ALS. While no absolute proof of causation currently exists, there is a lot of compelling circumstantial evidence, as well as laboratory evidence, for such a connection.

The epidemiological evidence comes from studies that looked at drinking water levels of aluminum and the incidence of Alzheimer's disease for large communities. Several of these studies demonstrated a close correlation. In one such study, eighty-eight counties in England and Wales were examined for incidence of Alzheimer's disease and its relation to aluminum levels in various districts. Researchers found that areas with high aluminum water levels had an Alzheimer's disease incidence 1.5 times higher than areas with low aluminum levels. While this study was criticized because of poor design, it did encourage other better studies.

Another such study involving 2,792 subjects found that populations of elderly people who drank water with higher aluminum levels (0.1 mg/l) demonstrated an incidence of Alzheimer's disease 4.5 times higher than populations whose drinking water had lower aluminum levels (0.01 mg/l). Most drinking water will test for aluminum between 0.01-0.15 mg/l of water. Some water systems have tested as high as 0.40 mg/l.

Supporting evidence comes from a study that indicated people who used aluminum-containing antiperspirants were at a modestly increased risk for developing Alzheimer's disease. Unfortunately, this study did not look at other sources of aluminum in the same population of people.

Another involuntary "experiment" involved the mining industry. It has long been known that aluminum can inhibit the toxic effects of silicosis, a condition that results in damage to the lungs from inhaling silicon. Armed with this bit of knowledge, mine owners from 1944 until 1979 designed an ingenious way to protect their miners: after each shift, miners would inhale aluminum dust from an "aluminum bomb" exploded in a common room. Years later, a scientific study confirmed what the miners and their families already knew. The aluminum dust had left them with severe mental difficulties in thinking and memory, as well as an assortment of other neurological disorders.

Analyzing the Brains of Alzheimer's Disease Patients

An early study in which the brains of Alzheimer's patients were analyzed for accumulation of aluminum indicated that 28 percent had aluminum levels three standard deviations above the normal control brains.[187] Of greater interest was the finding that these elevated levels of aluminum occurred in the areas of the Alzheimer's brains that had the most neurofibrillary tangles, the pathological hallmark of the disease.

Subsequent studies, using more accurate measuring techniques, did not find elevated levels of aluminum in Alzheimer's disease brains. Why the discrepancy? It appears that aluminum is not distributed in the brain evenly, and the studies that did not find elevated aluminum levels used large volumes of brain that diluted focal increases in aluminum, so-called "hot spots." Taking this into consideration, other researchers used much smaller volumes of brain, and using more advanced techniques, found focal elevations of aluminum in Alzheimer's brains when compared to normal control brains.[188]

Aluminum...

- increases release of free iron.
- increases free-radical production.
- increases lipid peroxidation.
- increases pro-oxidant copper and chromium effects.
- impairs membrane function.
- decreases total lipids, glycolipids, and phospholipids.
- impairs enzyme function.
  - enolase
  - myosin
  - calpain
  - proteinase K
  - phospholipase A2
  - argenase
- increases brain glutamate absorption.
- is neurotoxic when combined with fluoride.
- activates microglia.
- is associated with Parkinson's and Alzheimer's diseases.
- is active in formation of neurofibrillary tangles.
- depletes brain lipids.

TABLE 5.3

While this would seem to settle the controversy, it didn't. The picture was further clouded by yet more accurate analysis using highly sophisticated laser microprobe mass spectrometry (LMMA 500), which can analyze components of the neuron itself. Using this technique, no significant differences in aluminum were found between Alzheimer's brains and normal control brains.[189] That is, while the aluminum levels in the Alzheimer's brains were higher than controls, the difference was not statistically significant.

Does this throw the whole theory of aluminum's role in Alzheimer's disease into question? Not exactly! Remember that in the first three chapters we learned that a metal's toxic effects on the brain depend on numerous variables, such as strength of the antioxidant network, general nutrition, genetic weaknesses, enzyme competence, and the presence of other cellular protectors, such as growth factors. The degree of brain damage secondary to aging, primarily through free-radical damage, is also vitally important. What this means is that if a person has a favorable presence of all these factors, he or she unlikely to be affected by the same level of aluminum as someone who is less fortunate, and will eventually develop the disease. This is a universal rule of biology.

A more recent study using two highly sophisticated methods of analysis (SIMS and EDX) clearly demonstrated increased aluminum levels in the nuclei of neurons taken from the hippocampus of Alzheimer's patients, as compared to normal brains.[190] This reaffirmed the original study that reported elevated aluminum levels in Alzheimer's brains as compared to normal controls. This study was also important in that it showed a preference of aluminum for the nucleus of the neuron.

One of the pathological features of Alzheimer's disease is the neurofibrillary tangle, a dark staining clump found within degenerating brain cells in affected areas of the brain. These tangles are composed of twisted filaments (paired helical filaments) that normally occur in a very orderly arrangement. Several studies have shown that aluminum by itself can cause the formation of these filaments.[191] Of considerable interest was the finding that these neurofibrillary tangles could be reversed when the animals were treated with a drug that removes aluminum from the brain.[192] One clinical trial, using patients with Alzheimer's disease treated with a series of aluminum-chelating injections for two years, showed great promise in slowing the progression of the disease.

A final study helps to clarify the role of aluminum in dementing disorders of varying causes. Researchers examined the brains of patients with dementia secondary to Alzheimer's disease, due to repeated blows to the head—the so-called *dementia pugilistica* seen in boxers.[193] Using microprobe mass analysis to examine the brains, researchers found that in both types of dementia, aluminum and iron levels were increased in the hippocampus of the brain. The levels of these toxic metals were substantially higher in the boxers' brains.

The bulk of scientific evidence now available indicates that aluminum can enter the brain rather easily and is distributed to the parts of the brain known to be affected by Alzheimer's disease. Once inside the brain, aluminum is preferentially distributed within the neuron towards the nucleus, where it accumulates. By its interaction with DNA, it affects gene expression, primarily RNA synthesis, which controls numerous cell functions. It also appears that glial cells, which supply the neuron with much of its nurture and special molecules, are more vulnerable to aluminum toxicity than neurons themselves.[194]

Aluminum and ALS

Amyotrophic lateral sclerosis is a progressive neurological disorder that results in destruction of brain and spinal cord neurons that control motor movement of the limbs, as well as swallowing and facial muscle movements. Like other neurodegenerative diseases, its cause has long defied rational explanation, as well as treatment.

Researchers shortly after World War II discovered that the island of Guam had a very high incidence of ALS. The disease was unusual in that many patients also demonstrated dementia and Parkinson's–like symptoms. A careful and prolonged study disclosed several possible contributing factors. For example, on all areas of the island with dramatically elevated incidences of ALS, the inhabitants' diets consisted of large amounts of a flour called cycad, made from the sago palm plant. This plant contains a powerful excitotoxin that affects the same neurons that ALS does. Researchers also found that the soil in these same areas was low in calcium and magnesium, and high in aluminum and iron.

Several studies have demonstrated that low magnesium and calcium intake increases absorption of aluminum from the gastrointestinal tract and promotes its entry into the brain. Also, low levels of these ions make neurons more susceptible to aluminum, and other heavy metals, toxicity. In a study of thirty-seven thousand normal people in the United States, over 75 percent were shown to have a low intake of magnesium, putting them at a dramatically higher risk of developing aluminum toxicity.

One study conducted at the Wakayama Medical College in Japan, in which the spinal cords of patients with ALS were examined using a sophisticated x-ray emission spectrometry (PIXE), found that aluminum tended to accumulate inside the motor neuron around the cell's endoplasmic reticulum.[195]

Other studies using a laser microprobe mass spectrometer did not find abnormally elevated aluminum levels in the spinal motor neurons of ALS patients examined at autopsy.[196] What they did find was a 1.5- to 2-fold increase in iron and calcium levels in the nucleus and cytoplasm of ALS patients. More recent studies have confirmed elevated levels of aluminum in the spinal motor neurons of ALS patients.

Experimentally, there is a lot of evidence implicating aluminum as the cause of—or at least a contributor to—this horrifying disorder. In another Japanese study, aluminum was injected into the spinal fluid of New Zealand white rabbits.[197] This study demonstrated clinical and pathological changes that closely resembled human ALS. The rabbits exposed to aluminum developed progressive over-reactive reflexes (hyperreflexia), spastic limbs (hypertonia), loss of gait control, and eventual paralysis without signs of brain involvement (encephalopathy). Pathological examination of the spinal cords of these animals demonstrated changes similar to that seen in human cases of ALS. A more recent study confirms these findings.[198]

The effect of aluminum on mineral balance in the nervous system was recently demonstrated in experimental animals exposed to various degrees of mineral deficiency.[199] In this study, rats were fed either a standard diet, one low in calcium, one low in calcium and magnesium, or one low in calcium and magnesium and high in aluminum.

Animals fed diets low in calcium and magnesium were found to have elevated calcium levels and low magnesium levels in their spinal cord motor neurons. Animals given aluminum plus low-magnesium and low-calcium diets were found to have markedly lower magnesium neuron levels than were seen in all the other groups. Elevated calcium within the neuron is a powerful trigger for a whole set of destructive reactions, the principal one being free-radical generation. The destructive reactions are compounded by the presence of low spinal cord levels of magnesium.

An interesting observation cited in this study is that over twenty-eight cases of calcification of spinal ligaments were seen in ALS patients from the Kii Peninsula, an area in Japan with an incidence of ALS over one hundred times that of the United States. Why is this so astounding? Because only 120 cases of spinal ligament calcification have ever been reported *in the world*. When studied, these calcified ligaments were found to be very low in magnesium. These same individuals also had low bone-calcium content, again confirming the connection between low calcium and magnesium, and high aluminum in the soil, drinking water, and river water in areas reporting dramatically high ALS occurrence.

It should be recalled that mercury exposure, even in very small concentrations, can also produce conditions associated with ALS. Mercury is very toxic to the glutamate-transport proteins that normally remove the neurotransmitter glutamate from the outside of the neuron. Experimentally, drugs that paralyzed the glutamate transport protein produced an ALS-like disorder.

It has been established that a defect in this group of glutamate-transport proteins plays a critical role at least in the initiation of ALS. Until now, we did not know what could cause such an impairment of the carrier proteins. Mercury appears to be a likely candidate. Aluminum, by its ability to lower protective magnesium levels and raise intracellular calcium levels, greatly accelerates and magnifies this destructive process. We also know that a central part of the excitotoxic process is the production of enormous numbers of free radicals. Aluminum, iron, and mercury all increase free-radical generation in neurons. It is possible that their effect is synergistic, that is, greater than just the additive toxic effect.

Effects of Aluminum on Cell Function

Aluminum exercises a number of deleterious effects on cell function. For example, it has been shown that aluminum causes a significant decrease in the total lipid, glycolipid, and phospholipid content of the primate brain, all vital membrane fats.[200] Further, it has been shown that aluminum has a profound damaging effect on cell-membrane integrity, including a reduction in membrane-bound enzymes, which are vital to normal neuron function.

As we have seen, aluminum can have a profound damaging effect on numerous enzymes that utilize metals such as zinc, magnesium, and manganese. Aluminum has also been shown to inhibit several enzymes involved in glucose metabolism, such as glucose-6-phosphate dehydrogenase and hexokinase activity. High concentrations of magnesium can reverse this inhibition by aluminum. It also has been shown to inhibit acetyl-CoA, a vital mitochondrial energy-producing metabolic pathway.[201]

An early hypothesis about the cause of Alzheimer's disease suggested that onset was connected to impairment of the neurotransmitter, acetylcholine. We do know that brain levels of this neurotransmitter, which plays a major role in memory, are severely reduced in Alzheimer's brains. Of the enzymes important to acetylcholine production, attention has centered on choline acetyltransferase (which is also dramatically diminished in Alzheimer's disease), which is inhibited by aluminum. Also decreased is the enzyme acetyl-cholinesterase, which breaks down acetylcholine.[202] In severe cases, these enzymes can be reduced as much as 75-95 percent in selected parts of the brain.

While acetylcholine has gotten most of the attention in Alzheimer's dementia, studies have noted that several other neurotransmitters are also diminished, including dopamine, norepinephrine and serotonin.[203] all can be affected by the action of aluminum on key enzymes utilized in their production.

When aluminum combines with glutamate, it forms a compound that can pass through the blood-brain barrier easily, where it is distributed to several areas of the brain. In one study, this complex was found to increase levels of aluminum in the parts of the brain associated with Parkinson's disease (striatum) and Alzheimer's disease (hippocampus).[204]

The connection to Parkinson's disease was strengthened by a study that found aluminum enhanced lipid peroxidation in the presence of melanin.[205] This is an important finding because the part of the brain damaged by Parkinson's disease contains large amounts of melanin. When iron combines with melanin, large numbers of free radicals are produced, which can lead to lipid peroxidation and cell destruction. As the disease advances, the melanin-containing brain cells die off. Now we find that aluminum also promotes this destructive process in the same area of the brain. Autopsy studies of Parkinson's patients, using a microprobe analysis, confirm elevated levels of aluminum in these melanin-containing cells.

Not only do we see elevated levels of free radicals and lipid peroxidation with aluminum accumulation in the brain, but we also see a fall in several of the important components of the antioxidant network system. For example, in one study using rats, the antioxidant enzymes, catalase, SOD, and glutathione peroxidase were all decreased with aluminum exposure.[206]

Treating Aluminum Toxicity

Like most metal toxicities, treatment demands careful attention to numerous factors, such as antioxidant supplementation, chelation, prevention of redistribution of aluminum from the blood to the brain during chelation, and the use of special nutrients to protect the brain during treatment.

Step One: Stop Your Exposure

As with all toxic metal exposures, the most important step is to remove the metal from your world. This means you must check all food labels as well as other sources of exposure such as antiperspirants, medications, aluminum cans and containers, aluminum cookware and utensils, tap water containing aluminum, and aluminum-containing plant sources such as tea, condiments, and herbs. The safest containers are made of glass. (Plastic containers are not particularly safe as they can release PVCs, cadmium, and estrogenic substances.)

Never drink tea with lemon. Remember, citrate from fruits greatly increases aluminum absorption. You must also avoid all processed foods containing added glutamate in the form of monosodium glutamate (MSG), hydrolyzed vegetable proteins, soy protein extract, protein isolate, or any of the other disguised names for MSG. Glutamate binds with the aluminum and greatly increases absorption not only into the bloodstream, but also into the brain.

Most fast-food chains and restaurants use at least one of these forms of glutamate, which they use to enhance the taste of the food. Beware of antacids containing aluminum hydroxide gel, especially when taken in conjunction with citrus fruits or meals containing MSG. Many medications also contain aluminum.

Step Two: Increase Your Antioxidant Protection

Begin immediately. Most metal toxicities are associated with a dramatic increase in free-radical generation and lipid peroxidation, which can be reduced by increasing your intake of a variety of antioxidants. This should include:

Vitamin C (buffered form) 500 mg
This is the calcium or magnesium ascorbate form of vitamin C. Take one tablet three times a day on an empty stomach, and do not eat anything for forty-five minutes after taking it (because vitamin C greatly increases iron absorption).

Natural Vitamin E 800 IU
Take twice a day as either mixed tocopherols (natural form) or d-alpha tocopherol succinate. The natural form is probably best. Other forms of vitamin E, such as the acetate form, are poorly absorbed and do not enter the brain very well.

Tocotrienol 50 mg
Take one twice a day with vitamin E. This form of Vitamin E significantly enhances the antioxidant protection provided by the tocopherol form of vitamin E.

N-acetyl L-cysteine (NAC) 750 mg
Take one a day. Enhances production of one of the body's most important cellular antioxidants, glutathione.

Alpha-lipoic acid 100 mg
Take one twice a day. This powerful antioxidant also increases glutathione levels in cells and chelates mercury and cadmium.

Calcium pyruvate 500 mg
Take one twice a day. The calcium helps to counteract fluoride toxicity and the pyruvate binds aluminum, preventing its absorption. Pyruvate also blocks excitotoxicity.

Magnesium citramate with 150 mg magnesium
Take two capsules between meals and at bedtime with purified water.

Multivitamin/mineral
Take as directed.

6
The Vaccine Controversy

A Brief History of Vaccines

Vaccines have saved millions of lives over the last one hundred years, but less well-recognized is the impact of improved nutrition and sanitation methods in reducing diseases—often long before vaccine programs were implemented.

Infectious diseases, such as pneumonia, sepsis, and gangrene have killed more people throughout history than all wars combined. In the 1930s, the number one killer in the United States was infection; only after the widespread introduction of antibiotics and better sanitation did this statistic change. In underdeveloped countries, infection continues to be the single greatest killer. Once infectious diseases were brought under better control in the developed countries, other diseases began to command our attention, diseases such as cancer, heart disease, strokes, and diabetes.

Of particular concern among physicians and public health officials at the turn of the century was the terrible toll on young lives by a small group of infectious diseases: scarlet fever, measles, whooping cough (pertussis), diphtheria, polio, and tetanus. In fact, the four leading causes of death during the period 1911-1935 were diphtheria, pertussis, scarlet fever, and measles. Some of these microorganisms caused death and disability by direct infectious invasion of the body, while others did their damage by releasing toxins, as was the case for diphtheria.

Thanks to earlier work by medical giants like Edward Jenner, Louis Pasteur, Koch, and von Behring, a new method of preventing some infections was now available, which Pasteur named vaccination. In the eighteenth century, Jenner devised a way to protect people from the scourge of smallpox. As a humble country practitioner in the small town of Gloucestershire, England, he observed that by inoculating someone with the cowpox virus you could confer immunity against the more deadly smallpox virus. As a result of his discovery, which was initially rejected by the arrogant Royal Medical Society, millions of lives were saved every year thereafter.

The process was later refined by Louis Pasteur, who discovered that when bacteria were allowed to grow over a long period of time, they became less able to cause disease, a process we call attenuation. He demonstrated that, when injected, these weakened bacteria protected people from the fully virulent form of a disease. He also discovered that for diseases caused by bacteria-secreted toxins, inoculating a person with a diluted solution of the toxin would afford protection. This process has been applied to diphtheria and tetanus vaccinations.

In the case of viruses, a more complex procedure was needed to produce vaccines. This is because viruses are so difficult to grow outside a living organism. Researchers eventually learned that they could grow the viruses in chicken embryos and tissue cultures. These viruses, like their bacterial cousins, also seem to lose much of their disease-causing ability when passed through several cultures. The final non-disease-causing virus confers complete protection against the original pathogenic virus. This is how the polio-live virus vaccine was made. Unfortunately, the pharmaceutical company that produced the vaccine used kidney tissue from the African green monkey as a viral medium. More about this later.

At the time vaccines were first being made and widely used, scientists knew very little about the mechanism of their protection. Later we learned that it involved the immune system, but even today we do not fully understand how the immune system works and the effects of artificially stimulating the immune system by vaccination. Perhaps even more important, we do not fully understand the nature of the viruses we are injecting.

Early Problems with Vaccines

When Pasteur began inoculating children with the cowpox organism, he used pus from the udders of cows. He would scratch a place on the person's arm, take the pus, and wipe it into the wound. Unfortunately, the pus also contained other organisms, including bacteria, which often led to abscesses, or even worse, widespread infections.

With the widespread use of inoculations against a variety of diseases, doctors began to see unusual reactions in an increasing number of persons. Many of these reactions were life threatening or left the person severely neurologically injured. The latter reaction could cause a diffuse inflammation of the brain called postvaccinal encephalitis, which could result in blindness, deafness, writhing motor movements, mental retardation, and any number of neurological deficits. These children's brains, when examined at autopsy, resembled the brains of MS patients; that is, widespread stripping away of the fatty covering (myelin) of neuron pathways. This is because the vaccine triggers the immune system to attack the brain as if it were a foreign invader.

We now recognize that many viruses can adversely affect the immune system, either by depressing its function or causing it mistakenly to attack cells and tissues of the person exposed to the virus. The disorder is called autoimmunity, and the process, molecular mimicry. The measles virus is notorious for suppressing the immune system. Not uncommonly, it will also trigger autoimmune reactions. One of the most devastating autoimmune reactions to measles is called subacute sclerosing panencephalitis, a highly fatal disorder of young children.

Live viruses used in vaccines are also suspected to be associated with other disorders as well, such as multiple sclerosis, ALS, and autism. Particularly startling is the recent report of two cases of parkinsonism reported in young children who had been recently vaccinated with the MMR vaccine. It is important to remember that parkinsonism is *extremely* rare in children. In one of these cases, a five-year-old child developed a severe case of the disease that required continued drug treatment.

Dr. Andrew Wakefield has demonstrated by careful testing that autistic children suffering from unrelenting stomach problems frequently have live measles viruses growing within the cells lining their intestine. When observed through an endoscope, the intestinal lining looks like a tube filled with cobbled outgrowths that are beefy red from inflammation. These cobbled overgrowths are lymphoid patches in the wall of the intestine, infected with measles virus. When Dr. Wakefield tested these viruses, he found that they genetically matched the virus from the vaccine. The measles virus, both from vaccines and the naturally occurring virus, can also penetrate other organs, including the brain.

While vaccine proponents like to assure the public that these attenuated live-virus vaccines are safe, in truth no one knows what happens to the virus years or even decades after it sets up residence in the body. There is some suggestion, from people developing neurological disease after exposure to vaccinated children, that these latent viruses hide in the body and become active many years later.

Numerous neurological diseases have been examined to see if there is a relationship between the presence of these latent viruses and disease, and there is considerable suggestion that they may be causally related. Measles virus antibody titers are higher in persons with multiple sclerosis than those without the disease. Similar findings have been reported in some cases of ALS as well.

Another possibility is the contamination of the vaccines with other viruses. In fact, one of the most famous cases of this occurred with the polio vaccine. The virus was grown in kidney cells from the green monkey, the same monkey suspected as being the source of the HIV virus. Only years later were we to learn that the monkey cells were contaminated with the SV-40 virus, a virus that causes a very malignant tumor, called a sarcoma, in animals.

Vaccines...

- activate microglia.
- stimulate excitotoxicity.
- cause leaky gut syndrome.
- encourage release of neuroactive food components.
- promote yeast infections.
- deplete vital nutrients.
- precipitate abnormal brain-pathway development.
- destroy dendritic connections.
- deplete DHA.

TABLE 6.1

Approximately a hundred million Americans were vaccinated with this contaminated live-polio virus vaccine between 1955 and 1963.

Studies done by molecular pathologist Michael Carbone disclosed the presence of SV-40 viral genes and proteins in patients with bone cancers, lung cancers, and malignant brain tumors. This virus can remain in the body for a lifetime following vaccination.

The only way we ever even learned about the contamination of the polio vaccine was through a lawsuit. During discovery, the lawyers for the plaintiff pored through the Lederle pharmaceutical company's records and discovered that their scientists were having trouble separating numerous viruses found in the African green monkey kidney cells from the polio virus. Many of these contaminating viruses, some twenty-six in all, were known to cause disease in humans. Only later, in 1985, was it discovered that one of the contaminating viruses was the simian immunodeficiency virus SIV, very similar to the HIV virus. Even more shocking was the discovery that the FDA, as early as 1977, believed that retroviruses could have contaminated the vaccine. Yet, they released it for use on an unsuspecting public anyway.

Dr. John Martin discovered that the polio vaccine was also contaminated with another green monkey virus called cytomegalovirus. The unusual thing about this virus is that it has become fused with another virus found in humans, producing a hybrid with very dangerous properties. It seems that when animals were infected with this virus they lacked the usual inflammatory immune response normally seen with viral invasions. Dr. Martin labeled this a stealth virus, for its ability to evade the immune system.

These stealth viruses have been isolated from brain biopsies, blood cultures, spinal fluid, and even milk samples. Human studies have also demonstrated these elusive viruses in psychiatric disorders, brain tumors, and various neurological diseases. Because of the inability of the immune system to kill these viruses, no curative treatments are available. Intensive work is being done at the Center for Complex Diseases by Dr. John Martin and his group to devise newer, more effective treatments.

Another event that poses a real health hazard to those receiving vaccines contaminated by animal viruses was discovered by microbiologist Dr. Howard Urnovitz. He found that certain animal viruses could merge genetically with human viruses, producing a hybrid that was fully pathological in humans. These viruses, in an immunologically impaired host, could produce chronic immune responses either as autoimmune diseases or chronic viral infections, causing a lifetime of misery and disability.

There is also question as to contamination of these vaccines with another pathogenic virus linked to multiple sclerosis and chronic fatigue syndrome, called the human herpes virus-6 or HHV-6. There is even serious question as to HHV-6 being the major culprit in the AIDS syndrome, with HIV merely being a secondary invader.

It is interesting to note that no long-term studies have ever been done on vaccinated children to see if there are adverse effects occurring when they become adults. Almost all of the studies end within only a few days to two weeks following vaccinations—certainly not enough time to discover problems. Then again, with government regulators and their best-buddy owners of pharmaceutical companies footing the bills for such studies, why would they want to look?

Another problem the vaccine proponents were having was vaccine effectiveness. They sold the public on the absolute necessity of numerous vaccines to protect the public from deadly epidemics, but what they didn't tell us is that far too often vaccinated children were contracting these diseases despite being vaccinated. Or that children vaccinated with live viruses, such as the poliovirus, were actually spreading polio to unsuspecting parents and other children. In fact, following the widespread implementation of the polio vaccine program, the only reported cases of polio were those being caused by the vaccine.

What Really Caused the Disappearance of Infectious Epidemics?

Vaccine proponents love to display the dramatic successes that widespread vaccination had in eradicating many of the infectious diseases. While there is little question that vaccination programs were responsible for the eventual control of many of these diseases, most had already begun to decline drastically before widespread vaccination.

Neil Z. Miller, in a fascinating examination of the vaccine problem, discovered that most of the epidemic infectious diseases were declining drastically before mass inoculations were introduced.[207] For example, the measles death rate from 1915-1958 fell by 95 percent in both the US and the UK before the vaccine program was implemented. Pertussis death rates fell by 75 percent and diphtheria by 90 percent before immunization. Polio had fallen 47 percent in the US and 55 percent in the UK before 1953, the year the Salk vaccine was introduced.

Even more interesting was the finding that 58 percent of all measles cases were contracted by people who had been vaccinated, while only 42 percent of unvaccinated children contracted the disease. A similar finding was seen in those vaccinated against pertussis, with 46 percent of vaccinated children contracting the disease.

So what could account for the dramatic fall in infectious disease rates before vaccinations? It has been demonstrated numerous times that nutrition plays a vital role in susceptibility to infectious disease. Of particular importance is vitamin A status, which has been demonstrated numerous times. Nutrition, because of the widespread use of refrigeration and rapid delivery of fresh foods to the cities, was improving rapidly in the developed countries. Parallel with this were the improvements in public health measures, such as better sanitation, cleaner water supplies, and dissemination of public health information. You will recall that the same factors accounted for the dramatic fall in the incidence of cavities in children before the introduction of fluoride.

What vaccination did, at least in some people's minds, was to eliminate the remaining cases of the disease. Yet, as we have seen, it did not even do that, since the vaccines themselves caused many of the remaining infectious outbreaks. There is also evidence that children vaccinated with measles virus are actually more susceptible to complications than children who acquire the infection naturally. Children with a good nutritional status are far less likely to suffer complications than poorly nourished children, especially when vitamin A intake is adequate.

It was known that women who contract rubella (German measles) during pregnancy were more likely to deliver babies with serious birth deformities. To prevent this, health officials proposed a program to vaccinate everyone with the rubella vaccine, no matter their age.

Rubella is actually a very mild disease that rarely produces complications in children—that is, until they made it into a vaccine. Vaccination is associated with joint pains (arthralgias) and painful numbness in a significant number of people. Usually this subsides but can recur months later. The incidence of these complications is 10 percent in teenagers and 30 percent in older women.

Is it irrational for you to be concerned about the safety of this vaccine? Well, a survey taken among obstetricians found that 90 percent refused to take the rubella vaccine, and over two-thirds of pediatricians refused to take it.[208] Why? Because, according to the article that appeared in the *Journal of the American Medical Association (JAMA)*, they were afraid of unforeseen vaccine reactions.

The really upsetting thing about the rubella vaccine is that there is no evidence that it confers long-term immunity. In one rubella epidemic in Casper, Wyoming, 73 percent of the cases occurred in vaccinated children. Among army recruits in Melbourne, Australia, 80 percent of the vaccinated recruits contracted the disease during an epidemic. Miller points out that before the introduction of the vaccination, 85 percent of the population had natural immunity to rubella.

One of the most devastating complications associated with vaccination is encephalomyelitis, a diffuse inflammation of the brain that results in widespread destruction of brain structures. Michael Dye in his book, *Vaccinations: Deception and Tragedy*, cites a study from the National Childhood Encephalopathy Study conducted in Wales and Scotland of 1,182 children admitted to the hospital for acute neurological illness.[209] It was found that in a large number of cases, the DPT vaccine had been given from seventy-two hours to seven days before the onset of the disorder.

Examples of these tragedies go on and on, and are occurring in increasing numbers. For a masterly review of the problems associated with vaccinations, I refer the reader to two of the best books on the general subject, Michael Dye's *Vaccinations: Deception and Tragedy* available from Hallelujah Acres and Neil Z. Miller's *Vaccinations: Are they Really Safe and Effective? A Parent's Guide to Childhood Shots*. At the end of this book, I also have listed other excellent publications that address this topic.

The Effect of Poor Nutrition on Disease Virulence

One shocking study, which changed our way of looking at the relationship between microorganisms and nutrition, demonstrated that a person's nutritional status could change the virulence of a virus. Prior to this study, it was assumed that the connection between poor nutrition and increased severity and incidence of infectious diseases was secondary to impairment of a person's immune system. This seemed like common sense. But, it was found to be much more complicated than that.

The study was based on the observation in the 1930s that in certain regions of China a particular form of heart damage (referred to as Keshan cardiomyopathy) occurred in a significant number of people living in certain provinces. The disorder was characterized by progressive heart muscle failure with gross enlargement of the heart and abnormal rhythms of the heart beat. When the heart was examined at autopsy, it was found to have large areas of destruction of the muscle. This disorder is the most common one leading to heart transplantation in the United States.

Later, it was discovered that the disease occurred only in areas with low soil selenium levels, and dietary supplementation with selenium greatly reduced the incidence of this highly fatal disease. Still later, it was discovered that the disease was actually caused by a virus, called the coxsackievirus, one of a family of RNA-type viruses.

The connection was thought to be immune suppression caused by a deficiency of this critical element, which allowed the virus to invade the heart muscle. As with all viruses, most of the damage to the heart tissues was not due to the virus itself but rather to the immune system's attack on the virus, which triggered intense free-radical accumulation.

To find out why deficiencies in selenium, as well as vitamin E, increase the incidence and severity of the disease, scientists set up a unique experiment in which mice were fed various diets to simulate deficiencies in selenium and vitamin E. In the experiment they used two strains of the coxsackievirus, one that readily caused the disease and another that never caused the disease.[210]

What they found was that the animals on selenium- and vitamin-E-deficient diets not only suffered heart destruction when exposed to the virulent species, but also when exposed to the non-virulent virus that was not supposed to cause the disease. Even more shocking was the observation that the previously non-virulent virus could now produce heart destruction in the animals fed plenty of selenium and vitamin E. So, in essence, the healthy, nutritious mice were now being killed by a virus that was not supposed to cause the disease.

What was happening? A careful genetic analysis of the viruses disclosed that the previously non-virulent viruses were being altered genetically to become highly virulent viruses, all caused by nutritional deficiency in the group of mice without selenium or vitamin E. This was because the nutrient deficiency in the mice impaired their cellular defenses (T-cells and macrophages), and this allowed the previously non-pathogenic viruses to proliferate in the animal's heart muscle, which by itself would have only resulted in a mild case of heart inflammation (myocarditis).

The real problem developed as a result of the bombardment of the viruses during the immune system's attempt to attack these viruses. Since the white blood cells were not strong enough to actually kill the viruses, the attack continued for a very long time, releasing large amounts of free radicals. This flood of free radicals produced significant damage to the genes of the viruses, triggering a mutation that changed the benign, sleepy virus into a vicious killer.

This was the first time this phenomenon had ever been demonstrated, and the implications are mind boggling. It now appears that resistant organisms and highly virulent viruses can arise from a pool of previously non-virulent viruses, and the cause of this is poor nutrition in those who are infected! Meaning that those individuals walking around out there practicing poor nutrition, or who are the hapless victims of poor nutrition, may be endangering all of society by generating highly virulent organisms out of non-virulent species. They are acting as killer-virus generators.

The unanswered question then, is: what happens to attenuated viruses used in the vaccines over an extended period of time in an individual with poor nutritional habits? Remember, this is exactly what vaccinating large numbers of people with attenuated viruses does: it creates a large pool of viruses potentially susceptible to genetic damage. If the same genetic alteration occurs as we witnessed in the coxsackievirus experiment, then we have big problems, not only for the person vaccinated, but for society as a whole.

The mechanism responsible for the genetic conversion of non-virulent viruses to highly virulent forms was the bombardment of the genes of the virus by free radicals. When a child is vaccinated with a live virus, and the virus is not cleared by his or her immune system, it will continue to live in that person for the rest of his or her life. This means that the virus will be exposed to the very same free-radical attack as the coxsackieviruses in our experiment. This could potentially convert the virus into a completely different virus genetically, one that may trigger multiple sclerosis, autism, or other neurodegenerative diseases later in life. The reason we do not know the answer to this question is that no one is looking. I am convinced that both the government and private agencies involved do not want us to know.

Mercury in Vaccines: a Brainless Idea From the Very Beginning

Almost from the inception of vaccination programs, manufacturers added a mercury preservative called thimerosal to vaccines. The practice continued until recently, and was stopped only because of the outcry from thousands of concerned parents and numerous experts in the field. The American Academy of Pediatrics and the American Academy of Family Practice did not warn parents or pediatricians that the mercury was dangerous until they were forced to. That mercury was toxic to cells had been known for over sixty years, but manufacturers apparently were more worried about lawsuits stemming from bacterial contamination of vaccines than they were about the toxic effects of mercury in children. After all, mercury was a very effective antibacterial.

In 1999 studies began to surface showing that multi-dose vial vaccines, such as the MMR and hepatitis B vaccines, contained enough thimerosal to expose vaccinated children to 62.5 ug of mercury per visit to the pediatrician. This is one hundred times the dose considered safe by the Federal Environmental Protection Guidelines for infants! Worse yet, some infants will receive doses even higher; because thimerosal tends to settle in the vial. If it is not shaken up before being drawn, the first dose will contain low concentrations of mercury and the last dose will contain enormously high concentrations. If your baby is the unlucky one that gets the last dose, serious brain injury can result.

One problem in treating children, as well as adults, is that often we find either low or even undetectable levels of mercury on provocative testing of their urine, giving a false impression that the brain is free of mercury. I must admit that I fell into this trap early on. This may be because mercury in the nervous system is so difficult to remove that very little is chelated during a single test period. This would explain why autistic children improve with chelation even when their urine mercury levels are low. Hair mercury is also a poor measure of brain mercury levels: in such cases, one must go by clinical responses.

Studies of autistic children have frequently shown very high levels of mercury, with no other source but vaccines found for the exposure. These levels are equal to those seen in adults during toxic industrial exposures. Several autism clinics have found dramatic improvements in the behavior and social interactions in children from whom the mercury was chelated. Results depended on how soon the mercury was removed following exposure, but permanent damage can be caused if the metal is not chelated soon enough. Still, even in cases of severe damage, because of the infant brain's tremendous reparative ability, improvements are possible.

The problem of autism involves numerous body systems including the gastrointestinal, immune and nervous systems; as a result we see numerous infections and magnified effects of malnutrition. Intrepid workers in the shadows, that is outside the medial establishment, have worked many miracles with these children using a multidisciplinary scientific approach completely ignored by the orthodoxy. Some children have even experienced a return to complete physiological normalcy.

The only reason we even know about the mercury in vaccines and their devastating effects is the dedication of a handful of intrepid investigators who went public with what they had discovered. We can also thank the Internet for dissemination of this information to millions of concerned parents. Otherwise it would have remained buried in some obscure journal or newsletter. It is obvious that the major media would never have bothered to inform us of this very real danger.

Because of public outcry and congressional hearings stemming from it, the lethargic American Academy of Pediatric and American Academy of Family Practice finally came out in favor of removing mercury from vaccines. Incredibly, their proposed response for parents is beyond belief. Rather than calling for an all-out immediate ban on thimerosal-containing vaccines, they suggested that parents *continue* to have their children vaccinated with mercury-contaminated vaccines until new stocks of uncontaminated vaccine could be made available. Here are two doctors' unions that had to be beat over the head with an overwhelming amount of data that mercury-contaminated vaccines were harming children far worse than the actual diseases against which the vaccine was intended to protect them, only to have them suggest that parents continue to harm their children just to satisfy their vaccination obsession.

Are you surprised to discover that recent investigations have found that several doctor-members of vaccine boards were either receiving grants from vaccine manufacturers or held stock in the companies? They were willing to sacrifice the health of millions of children just to fill their pockets with cash. These people should be looking through bars, not serving on boards.

Why Removing Mercury Will Not Completely Solve the Problem

Many parents are convinced that removal of the mercury will correct the problem of vaccinations. Unfortunately, while it may help, it will not solve the problem. This is because much of the effect of today's vaccination policy is based on the idea that we can eliminate virtually every known infectious disease in the world if we can just force children to get enough vaccines.

Today, children are given as many as twenty-two doses of ten different vaccines by two years of age. Many of these inoculations are given at one time in the pediatrician's office. Some mothers have told me their child received as many as nine shots in one visit. This is incredible. I cannot conceive of how a trained physician can believe that subjecting a child's immune system to nine doses of microbial organism, enhanced with powerful immune adjuvants, would be safe. Only an idiot could believe such a thing.

The immune system at birth is still incompetent. This is why the baby depends on colostrum—loaded with immune components specifically designed to protect the baby during this critical gap in immunity—from the mother's milk for immune protection. Now here come the brilliant vaccination police insisting that newborns receive an inoculation against hepatitis B.

Keep in mind that many mothers today do not breast feed their babies, so that their babies continue to be immune deficient. Add to that the fact that their children are being forced to receive a powerful vaccine when their immune systems are not only immature, but also terribly dysfunctional. These vaccine programs are led by "evidence-based" doctors serving on vaccine boards in the Public Health Department. Where is their evidence that such a practice is safe? There is plenty of experimental, and even clinical, evidence that it is not safe, combined with growing evidence that thousands of babies have been irreparably harmed.

The proponents of mass inoculation of the population from the scourge of hepatitis B are mostly academic immunologists, pediatricians, and family practice professors. Why is no one listening to neuroscientists and neurologists, particularly when there is abundant medical and scientific literature on the harmful effects to the brain of overstimulating the immune system?

The brain's immune system depends largely on specialized cells called microglia. These cells are scattered throughout the brain, lying in wait for an attack. When stimulated by a foreign substance—and some local substances—the microglia are activated, secreting numerous chemicals and gearing up for a full-fledged immune attack. While normally fixed in the brain among other types of cells they can move about like amoebae when activated, spreading microbe-killing secretions anywhere they are needed.

Like other immune cells, microglia kill microorganisms by secreting free radicals. If the immune system is able to quickly subdue the invaders, the attack ends rapidly and the free radicals are either neutralized or carried off in the spinal fluid or blood stream. It is vital that such attacks in the nervous system are short-lived, since the released free radicals can severely damage the delicate cells and processes close by.

Recent evidence indicates that activated microglial cells can release large amounts of two nasty chemicals—quinolinic acid and glutamate, both excitotoxins. When these excitotoxins are allowed to build up, they begin to destroy synaptic connections, cause dendrites to dwindle, and eventually, they will kill numerous neurons. In other words, they produce widespread brain injury. With microglial activation, quinolinic acid secretion has been seen to increase as much as one-hundred-fold. Remember also that mercury activates microglia and blocks glutamate clearance.

While most of what I described above occurs within the brain itself, it is known that stimulation of the body's general immune system—as occurs with vaccinations—also can activate the brain's immune system.

Prolonged immune reactions, the most destructive type of attack, can be precipitated by the use of live virus vaccines, such as the MMR. It is known that the measles virus often suppresses the immune system, much like the HIV virus or HHV-6 virus. When I say "suppressed," I should make clear that not all of the immune system is suppressed; the component that kills viruses is suppressed, but the system that causes misdirected immune attack, called autoimmunity, is overactive.

When children are vaccinated using combined vaccines, such as DPaT and MMR, they are more likely to suffer immune suppression. This allows the measles virus to survive and inhabit the cells lining the gastrointestinal tract and even the nervous system. Now acting like a stealth virus, the measles organism can survive for a lifetime. Because the immune system continues to try unsuccessfully to rid the body and brain of the virus, much damage is done. It's a smoldering attack that never ends. Because of this process, the measles virus is suspected as a possible cause of multiple sclerosis and ALS, among many other diseases.

Based on scientific knowledge concerning the effects of overstimulation of the immune system, it is my belief that the biggest problem with today's immunization programs is that too many vaccines are being given too close together. I often tell parents that giving six vaccines at one sitting is like a child contracting six different diseases at the same time. As far as the immune system is concerned, that is exactly what has happened. How many of us would want to get measles, mumps, diphtheria, pertussis, and hepatitis all at the same time?

Lest you be skeptical, we do in fact have a shining example of just such an event occurring in adults as a result of the government's brilliant inoculation program perpetrated on soldiers serving in the Gulf War. These soldiers were required to take seventeen different vaccines over a short period of time, a massive assault on the immune system. As with the children and babies, many became ill and suffered debilitating disorders, many of which were neurological.

The Department of Defense recently admitted that there was a 200 percent increase in the incidence of ALS in Gulf War veterans. Knowing the connection between thimerosal neurotoxicity and microglial overactivation, one is not surprised to see such a result stemming from such an insane policy. There is also a possibility that the vaccines were contaminated with mycoplasmic organisms and possibly other viruses: we know that viruses and mycoplasma damage the nervous system by an excitotoxic mechanism.

In all these cases, the children, as well as the adults, are not only getting the viruses and bacteria as foreign antigens, they are also exposed to extremely powerful additives called immune adjuvants, chemicals designed to make the immune system react even more intensely than normal and assure a higher percentage of successful immunizations. Adjuvants include aluminum salts, which can also damage the brain. You see, one of the problems with any vaccination program is that a certain percentage of people will not be successfully immunized. In order to force a reaction, manufacturers add numerous adjuvants to vaccines.

Unfortunately, this means that the child who would react without the additive will over-react and be more likely to suffer vaccine-related damage. The genetically immune-impaired child, on the other hand, will be at even greater risk, because the portion of his or her immune system responsible for autoimmunity will also be overstimulated. As more and more vaccines are added, a greater number of adverse effects, especially those related to the nervous system, will occur. To convince those in positions of power that they are harming millions of children is nearly impossible. The only thing that will stop this insanity is an outcry from millions of parents and concerned scientists. If this doesn't work then lawyers must be called upon to do what they do best—force irresponsible people to act in the best interests of others.

What You Can Do

There are several steps you, as a parent, can take to protect your child. First and foremost, as I keep reiterating, good nutrition is vital. This means a diet that includes proper types of fats, proteins and carbohydrates and a proper assortment of vitamins, minerals, and occasionally, special nutritional supplements.

Step One: Reduce or Eliminate Vaccines

This step will depend on where you live, since vaccine laws vary from state to state. My state, Mississippi, has the most stringent vaccination laws in the country. There are no religious or philosophical exemptions allowed and medical exemptions are difficult to have approved. Even worse, combined vaccines cannot be broken up and given separately. This has nothing to do with anything medical: it is pure politics.

Your options in such a case are to: (1) move to another state, (2) home school your children and avoid day care centers, or (3) fight it in court. The easiest recourse is the second option.

If you are from a more friendly state, ask your pediatrician to give the mixed vaccines, such as the MMR and DPaT separately, spaced apart by at least six months. If possible, refuse any live-virus vaccines altogether. Spacing vaccines significantly reduces the risk of complications, even with live-virus vaccines. Do not pay any attention to your pediatrician's assurances that the vaccines are safe. They are just accepting the word of their medical unions, such as the American Academy of Pediatrics.

The live polio vaccine was finally voted out on June 20, 1996, and replaced with a killed virus vaccine. The only reason the live virus was ever used was pure politics. Jonas Salk, who invented the first polio vaccine, used a killed virus and warned that a live virus would cause problems, even the potential spread of polio. History proved him right, but it took over fifty years to convince the geniuses in charge of the vaccine program of the danger.

Refuse all vaccines, including flu vaccines, containing mercury (thimerosal). I always warn elderly patients against taking the flu vaccine. Instead, use nutritional supplementation and a healthy diet. It is much more effective and far less hazardous. Multiple studies have shown that the reason the elderly are so susceptible to the flu is because of age-related immune deficiencies, which I will discuss in chapter nine. At any rate, over 50 percent of the time, flu vaccines contain the wrong antigen and will not protect you, and a significant number of the vaccinated elderly actually *contract* flu because of the vaccine.

Elderly persons with pre-existing neurological illnesses, who have recently had surgery or who are recovering from an illness, should not have the vaccination. It will further lower immunity and can activate more serious latent viruses.

Step Two: Improve Nutrition During Pregnancy

You should take a good prenatal vitamin throughout your pregnancy. It should include 2,000 IU of vitamin A and 4,000 IU of beta-carotene. This will not only boost your immune system, but will ensure protection to your baby as well. These doses are not harmful to your baby.

During your pregnancy you should take DHA 300 mg a day along with vitamin E as mixed tocopherols 400 IU a day. Do not use either dl–alpha tocopherol form of vitamin E or dl or d-alpha tocopherol acetate. The acetate form is next to worthless. It is poorly absorbed, is a poor antioxidant, and may not enter the brain.

After your baby is born, and at least three weeks before the first vaccination, supplement your child's diet with a multivitamin, which should include 1,000 IU of vitamin A and all of the other vitamins in an appropriate dose. The vitamin should also contain zinc, selenium, and magnesium.

Step Three: Breast Feed

If at all possible, breast feed your baby. If for some reason you cannot breast feed, use a breast pump. If, for some reason, you are forced to bottle feed, add 50 mg of DHA to the bottle once a day and 50 IU of vitamin E. Unfortunately, American manufacturers of baby milk do not add DHA as European manufacturers do. There is a rumor that the American makers may start adding it. They're a little slow, to say the least.

Cow's milk should never be given to a newborn or young child since it has a much higher level of glutamate than human milk and also is *strongly* associated with juvenile diabetes. Do not feed your baby soy milk. Soy milk is high in glutamate and contains estrogenic plant compounds. In addition, soy significantly inhibits the thyroid gland, which is essential for proper growth, especially brain growth. If your child has an allergy to cow's milk, use goat's milk, which is closer to human milk in composition. But do not use raw goat's milk as it may contain numerous viruses.

Conclusion

While this chapter does not nearly cover the scope of the vaccine problem, I do want to alert parents that their children are in danger, and that they must speak out if their children and grandchildren are to be protected. The vaccine program is being led by irresponsible people wearing dollar-shaped blinders. They portray themselves as protectors of the nation's children while they have done more harm over the past thirty years to children than have all of the diseases they seek to eradicate. We live in an age of insanity.

Food Additives That Can Kill: The Taste That Kills

The subtitle of my first book on excitotoxic food additives was *The Taste That Kills*. Since publication of the book in 1997, a mountain of newer information has surfaced confirming the damaging effects of these additives. Because so many people have either read the book, seen me on a *700 Club* broadcast, or heard me interviewed on syndicated radio programs, awareness of the problem has grown significantly. The food industry has responded with feeble attempts to defend the continuing practice of adding such dangerous additives to our food.

In one of their more interesting attempts at self-justification, they were given an entire issue of a prestigious journal in which to expound the safety of MSG. The supposedly scientific articles mostly read like infomercials, with some even encouraging the elderly to eat more foods containing MSG! Interestingly, the Ajinomoto Company, primary manufacturer of MSG, funded every article in the journal. They *are* getting desperate.

Monosodium Glutamate

Those of you who have not read my previous book probably have never even heard the word excitotoxin, so I will provide a brief overview of the substance.

Monosodium glutamate is the sodium salt of glutamic acid, a form of glutamate, the (under normal circumstances) carefully regulated neurotransmitter I have already discussed. Glutamic acid is an amino acid that occurs naturally in many foods. In nature, it is bound by peptide linkages, which are broken down slowly during the digestive process, thereby preventing the sudden surges that are associated with the pure, processed additive, MSG.

The use of MSG as a food additive can be traced to Asian antiquity, when cooks used a variety of seaweed called sea tangle to make a starch used in traditional recipes. The connection between the flavor improvement produced by the seaweed and glutamate (which had been isolated as early as 1866) was discovered in 1908 at a Tokyo university. The Japanese began production immediately, and by the 1940s, MSG was being produced in North America from corn and wheat gluten.

The MSG added to food these days is produced by fermenting sugar beet molasses. The processed form is a fine white crystal that looks very much like salt or sugar. While it does not have its own taste, it is used as a ubiquitous flavor enhancer in virtually every canned, packaged, or otherwise processed food sold in stores. Because MSG fools the brain into thinking something tastes better than it actually does, manufacturers may use it in lieu of quality ingredients.

While MSG has been used as a flavor enhancer for a very long time, the discovery of its adverse physiological effects can be attributed to a chance discovery in 1957 by two British ophthalmologists, Lucas and Newhouse, who were studying a rare eye disorder.[211] They were attempting to improve the condition in test animals by feeding MSG, aspartate, and other metabolic products to mice, based on the idea that these substances can be used as fuel by some nerve cells.

What they found was that the mice who received glutamate and aspartate suffered severe destruction of the cells in the retina, and that the damage was worse in newborn animals than adult animals. The greatest damage occurred with exposure to glutamate.

Their report went virtually unnoticed, even though MSG had been added to processed foods in massive quantities since the late 1940s. In 1968 another research scientist, John Olney, repeated the experiment hoping to use the ability of MSG to destroy retinal cells to study neural connections dying within deep brain structures, a common technique in neuroscience.[212] What he found shocked him: the MSG not only destroyed retinal cells, it also killed vital neurons within the brain itself. On further study, Dr. Olney recognized that the MSG was killing neurons by exciting them to death. Based on this observation he named the process "excitotoxicity."

How the Brain Protects Itself Against Excitotoxicity

Glutamate only causes toxicity when it is found floating free outside a neuron, and the brain possesses several safety measures to protect itself. One is based on quickly removing glutamate once it is secreted from a synaptic terminal, whisking it away to be stored safely in a nearby cell called an astrocyte. The whisking away process is carried out by special carrier proteins, which can be thought of as escorts.[213]

A second safety measure is to protect the brain from glutamate floating free in the blood stream. Glutamate is normally found in many foods, including vegetables and meats. To prevent this glutamate from entering the brain and setting off destructive excitotoxicity, God created a special boundary called the blood-brain barrier that prevents most harmful substances in the blood from entering the interior of the brain. It can be thought of as a gatekeeper.

Under normal circumstances this gatekeeper is very efficient. Unfortunately, persistent manipulation of the foods we consume has endangered the balance necessary for this protective system to operate correctly. By artificially adding very high concentrations of free glutamate to food, blood glutamate levels in most people are far higher than were ever intended, taxing the ability of the protective gatekeeper. If blood levels remain high, the glutamate can gradually seep into the brain past the gatekeeper, creating havoc.[214]

Also, some areas of the brain—the circumventricular organs—are not protected by the blood-brain barrier. One area is the hypothalamus, which contains control systems for the endocrine glands, sleep-wake cycles, higher level control of the autonomic nervous system, and connections to the limbic system of emotional elaboration. Numerous studies have revealed that in every species of animal tested, high blood levels of glutamate occur after ingestion of glutamate, causing destruction of a vital group of cells in the hypothalamus called the arcuate nucleus.

It is now recognized that many conditions cause the blood-brain barrier to become defective. Hypertension, strokes (both major and silent), head injury, infections, Lyme disease, heat stroke, brain tumors, certain medications, autism, multiple sclerosis, Alzheimer's disease, lupus, and even aging itself have been shown to result in impairment of the blood-brain barrier.[215] From birth until two or three years of age, the barrier system is also deficient.

A
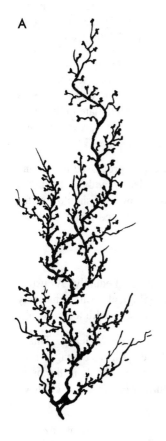

B
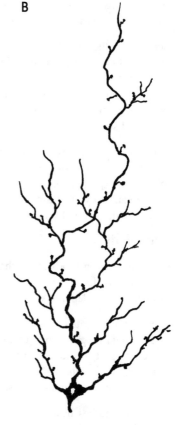

FIGURE 7.1   Demonstration of the effect of excitotoxins on nerve endings. "A" shows a normal dendrite with numerous synaptic connections. The nerve endings in the dendrite shown in "B" have been exposed to an excessive concentration of glutamate leading to widespread synapse loss.

Yet anyone suffering from any of these disorders almost certainly bears a substantial brain-glutamate burden.

It also should be appreciated that differing degrees of damage result from excessive buildup of excitotoxins. With very high doses, neurons swell and die within a few minutes. Slightly smaller doses produce a delayed death that takes approximately an hour to occur. All of the effects described so far can be seen with an ordinary light microscope: cells appear to shrivel and eventually disappear.

At still lower concentrations, neurons themselves do not die but their connections, called synapses, will shrivel and retract. This phenomenon may not be seen with a light microscope and may require electronmicroscopy. Defenders of glutamate safety frequently point to studies—albeit older ones—in which only light-microscope observations were used, and no examinations were done of the synaptic connections. Interestingly, the greatest damage in Alzheimer's disease is to the synaptic connections and not the cell bodies themselves.

Because of the effects of glutamate and aspartate on brain-cell excitation at even lower concentrations, it is even possible that no physical damage will occur on microscopic examination, yet brain functions may still be adversely affected. One of the more obvious effects of such exposure is the occurrence of seizures. We know that excess glutamate in the brain can precipitate seizures without causing physical changes in the brain, even though continued seizures can produce destruction of brain cells and its connections.[216]

This means that at lower doses, such as those easily attained by eating processed foods, one may feel confused or disoriented and have difficulty thinking clearly without having a seizure or experiencing obvious physical damage to your brain. However, should excitotoxic assault to your brain continue because you continue eating processed foods, physical damage will eventually result.

Sensitivity

If excitotoxins in foods cause these effects, why isn't everyone affected equally? As usual, the answer is that we are all individuals biochemically and physiologically, and sensitivity to such toxicity depends on numerous variables, as we have already seen with toxic metals.

There is an intimate connection between free-radical generation and excitotoxicity.[217] This is true not only for the brain but also for other cells in the body.[218] Free radicals damage virtually every part of the cell, including synaptic connections. Also, free radicals in the brain cause astrocyte cells and microglia to release their glutamate, further enhancing excitotoxicity. The cycle continues until severe damage occurs.

Numerous studies have shown that a high level of antioxidants and antioxidant enzymes powerfully protect against excitotoxicity. Vitamin E, at least in a culture of brain cells, can completely protect against excitotoxic destruction of the neurons. Persons who have high levels of antioxidant enzymes, or who consume antioxidant foods or supplements, are much less likely to suffer the severe effects of excitotoxins than those with low levels of antioxidants.

The presence and levels of antioxidant enzymes in a person depends on heredity as well as nutrition. If one eats a good diet and takes special supplements, the level of these enzymes will be high. Likewise, a diet high in antioxidants, or the use of a mixture of antioxidants, will offer significant protection. In addition, the antioxidants in our diets take a lot of pressure off the antioxidant enzymes so that they do not have to work so hard. Recent studies have shown that melatonin, the supplement that people take for sleep, not only is an excellent antioxidant for the brain, it also increases brain antioxidant enzyme levels.

One of the most important antioxidants in the brain is a substance called glutathione. Actually, it exists in every cell in the body. Several studies have shown that it is possible to predict the risk of degenerative diseases, even cancer, by the body's supply of glutathione.[219] Because the brain is the site of the greatest free-radical risk in the body, the presence of sufficient glutathione levels is critical. The level of glutathione is also important because it can neutralize certain types of free radicals not affected by other types of antioxidants, such as vitamins E and C or the carotenoids.

Recent studies have shown that glutathione levels are low in all of the neurodegenerative diseases, and that it falls to low levels long before the diseases become obvious.[220] What makes this connection even more convincing is that glutathione levels fall only in the types of neurons affected by a particular disease, yet unaffected areas nearby have normal levels of glutathione.

Another important protective factor is the amount of magnesium in the diet. Magnesium plays a major role in protecting the brain, especially against excitotoxicity, by dampening the glutamate excitation of brain cells. Experiments in which magnesium was denied demonstrated that under such conditions excitotoxicity was increased almost a hundredfold. This means that if one is deficient in magnesium, one will be infinitely more sensitive to glutamate damage than someone with an adequate intake. Magnesium deficiency is very common in industrialized countries.

It also should be appreciated that magnesium levels in the body are very difficult to measure accurately. Most doctors use blood levels to assess magnesium adequacy, but the problem with relying on blood levels is that magnesium is mostly an intracellular ion—meaning that normal blood levels will tell nothing of tissue levels. On the one hand, if the blood level is low the tissue levels will be even lower, but if the blood level is normal there still could be a severe tissue deficiency. This is also true when attempting to gauge brain magnesium levels based on blood levels.

Energy production by brain cells is also closely linked to toxicity of glutamate and the other excitotoxins.[221] Experiments have shown that when the brain's energy levels are low, excitotoxic damage is greatly magnified.[222] In Alzheimer's disease, the brain's ability to generate energy is depleted in selected areas of the brain at least a decade before any symptoms develop. The same is also true with Parkinson's disease.

Brain energy levels fall for many reasons. A good example of this occurs when diabetics overshoot their insulin needs. Recent studies have shown, especially in children with diabetes, that repeated episodes of hypoglycemia lead to atrophy of the brain.[223] Also, excessive exercise during periods of poor glycogen storage can lead to profound hypoglycemia. Glycogen, the stored form of glucose, is the first storage site to be tapped during extreme exercise. When someone experiences hypoglycemia, the brain has essentially no glycogen on which to operate.

In children, hypoglycemia can occur with the use of aspirin or other drugs. Certain amino acids, such as leucine, isoleucine, and proline also can stimulate profound hypoglycemia. Furthermore, about a third of the population suffers from a condition called reactive hypoglycemia, which occurs when consumption of simple sugars—especially as liquids—precipitates an overstimulation of pancreatic insulin release that in turn drives the blood sugar to dangerously low levels.

During these spells, the brain is operating on a very low glucose supply and the brain secretes increasing amounts of glutamate and aspartate. This is why one feels so hyperactive, and even angry, when hungry. Mothers of hypoglycemic children can attest to the dramatic improvement in their children's behavior once they have eaten. Numerous experiments have shown that increasing the brain's energy supply can significantly reduce excitotoxic damage.[224]

All of these factors play a role in excitotoxicity and determine who will be severely affected and who will suffer only minor damage. Unfortunately, most of us are unknowingly injured every day by a high intake of foods containing additives such as glutamate and aspartate. Those of us with the fewest protective factors—low energy supply, magnesium levels, antioxidant defenses, and glutathione levels—will be the ones who eventually develop a neurodegenerative disease.

Developing Children

Unlike other organs, the brain undergoes it greatest growth and organization during the last trimester of pregnancy and during the first two years after birth, even though it is the first system to begin development. This process of brain organization and development continues throughout the teen years.

As the brain begins to develop and organize its trillions of connections, it actually overproduces its circuits and synaptic connections. In a miracle beyond man's understanding, a choice is made as to which circuits and synapses will remain and which will be destroyed. The means by which this is done seems to depend on fluctuations in glutamate levels.[225]

At intrinsically programmed times, glutamate levels in the brain suddenly rise, shearing off unneeded connections and synapses. And as suddenly as it began, glutamate levels fall rapidly so as to preserve the newly selected connections and circuits. The timing of this rise and fall in glutamate is so critical that too little glutamate during the pruning period can result in too many circuits, leading to jumbled messages.[226] This may be the problem in such disorders as Down's syndrome and tuberous sclerosis.

If too much glutamate is present during the pruning period, or if elevated levels extend past the normal pruning period, too many circuits will be lost and those that aren't may be misguided, making improper connections.

Several experiments in which pregnant animals were fed MSG found that offspring were adversely affected by the substance. One of the most impressive was a two-part study conducted on pregnant mice, which investigated behavioral and neurochemical brain changes.[227]

Researchers found that feeding MSG to the mothers produced no obvious effects on learning in the offspring. Well, not exactly. When learning behaviors were divided into simple and complex learning tasks, the offspring could perform a simple task without difficulty, but their performance on complex tasks indicated cognitive impairment. In humans, this is comparable to a child seeming intellectually normal from infancy through early childhood, but then demonstrating a severe impairment once he begins school, seemingly unable to grasp complicated subjects. A chemical dumbing-down of children.

The second part of the experiment focused on finding an explanation for *why* the mice were functioning as if mentally retarded. Researchers removed their brains and examined major neurotransmitters used for various functions. They found the major learning and memory neurotransmitter acetylcholine was decreased 80 percent, and the neurotransmitter that allows attention-focusing, norepinephrine, had also fallen significantly. These vital brain chemicals remained low while the animals were young, and later began to return to normal. If MSG produces the same neurochemical changes in humans, the implication of this experiment is that children are being denied the tools (essential neurotransmitters) necessary to learn during the most critical time of life.

Most children today start life gorging on junk foods filled with excitotoxins. Unfortunately, many of their mothers also ate badly during pregnancy. And junk foods have replaced the pacifier: many mothers will give their children bags of MSG-laced chips and sit them on the couch to watch cartoons. Without fail, thirty minutes later they are screaming and throwing things all over the room. Why? Because the MSG in the unhealthy treat intensely stimulates the child's brain, which is four times more sensitive to the additive than an adult's brain.[228]

Other studies have described similar findings on brain development and function. In one study mice exposed to MSG soon after birth demonstrated significant difficulties in adapting to stress and to new environments,[229] similar to behaviors seen in autistic children. A more recent study found that mice exposed to MSG have greater difficulty performing a non-spatial water-escape task. Examinations of the brains of animals exposed to MSG have shown injury to the hippocampus of the brain, an area vital for learning and memory, as well as emotional development.

Another recent study found that when pregnant mice consume MSG, the amount of gluta-mate entering the baby's circulatory system is twice as high as the mother's.[230] Newborns were significantly more likely to have seizures, and later in life the exposed mice had diffi-culty completing a maze.

A recent comprehensive study of MSG disclosed that infant formulas frequently contain glutamate levels that are equal to those causing brain lesions in experimental animals.[231] Levels of free glutamate are especially high in formulas that contain casein hydrosylates, which is made from cow's milk. Because many of these formulas are also devoid of DHA, it is no wonder that we are seeing widespread, intractable developmental and behavioral problems in the children of this country.

Of special concern are soy-based formulas, since they too are high in free glutamate as well as phytoestrogens.

One of MSG's more alarming properties is its affect on anger. Researchers who injected MSG in microscopic concentrations into the hypothalami of test animals' brains were able to produce intense rage reactions in the subjects[232]—a not-unexpected effect since the hypothalamus is an integral part of the brain's limbic system, the complex of nuclei concerned with emotional elaboration. Glutamate is the major neurotransmitter in the hypothalamus, as well as the amygdala—a large nucleus tucked deep within the temporal lobe of the brain—that is concerned with more elaborate expressions of emotion, including fear and anger.

We are now witnessing the effects of a decades-long manipulation of the human brain. As more and more brain-altering drugs—both legal and illegal—come into use, especially combined with widespread exposure to food-based excitotoxins and Ritalin, we will witness a growing number of neurological diseases and neuropsychiatric disorders. Many of these drugs act on brain systems responsible for our highest level of thinking, especially as it relates to emotional sophistication. These drugs and food additives can induce states of apathy, rage, disordered thinking, perceptional distortion, and states of increased suggestibility.[233]

It is also interesting to note that in virtually all of the school shootings, the kids responsible for the violence were taking SSRI medications, which are known to produce suicidal and homicidal side effects. It is also known that these medications increase brain levels of the neurotransmitter serotonin, which in high concentrations can also act as an excitotoxin.

Cocaine destroys brain cells in the limbic system by an excitotoxic mechanism, as does methamphetamine.[234] Amphetamine drugs are being given to millions of children to control ADHD at the insistence of school counselors and the public health Gestapo. Furthermore, few in the medical profession have concerned themselves with the effects of mixing numerous brain-altering drugs and food additives, especially in children and adults with poor nutritional habits. Yet without good nutrition to protect the brain, these drugs and food additives can have a profound negative affect on brain function.

Obesity

Over the last decade, the United States has witnessed an explosion in childhood obesity that has gone unexplained. *Newsweek* carried a picture of an obese child eating an ice cream cone with a subtitle that read, "Fat for Life? Six Million Kids are Seriously Overweight." On closer inspection, there are actually several clues as to the cause for this alarming increase in childhood obesity.

Let us travel back to 1968 when Dr. Olney was conducting his experiments on mice fed MSG. (Mice are frequently used as test animals because they react most like humans to MSG.) Obsessed with the microscopic changes in the brains of the mice he overlooked something quite dramatic first noticed by his assistant. She pointed out to him that all of the mice were grossly obese. At first he thought it was just a fluke, but as the experiment progressed he noticed that indeed all the mice fed MSG became grossly obese.

Since his early observation, other studies have confirmed that MSG causes gross obesity in animals.[235] At an international neuroscience meeting, Dr. Olney was asked if he thought the reason Americans were so obese was, in fact, due to their high consumption of MSG additives. The question was never answered, but since that conference in the 1970s, America has undergone this virtual epidemic of gross obesity, especially among its youth.

While most will attribute the problem to children's couch-potato lifestyles or diets high in sugar and other forms of carbohydrate and fat, other research has been conducted that sheds further light on the theory of MSG-induced obesity. One study discovered that animals fed MSG soon after birth preferred foods that were high in carbohydrates and low in nutritional value.[236] They also ate less, but ate rapidly. In other words, they were eating like teenagers.

Researchers also found that this fat could not be exercised off and was extremely difficult to remove through dieting, no matter how stringent.[237] Again, this is reminiscent of the problem in our population. Today, most processed foods contain significant amounts of glutamate, enough to produce injuries to our children's brains similar to those seen in exper-imental animals. This is extremely important when you consider that, of all the mammals, humans are the most susceptible to physical damage from ingested MSG. We possess a sensitivity five times greater than the mouse and *twenty* times greater than the rhesus monkey.

With this enormous consumption of foods laced with MSG additives, it is no wonder that we have an obesity problem in this country, especially when combined with the hypothal-amic lesion caused by MSG to the high-fat and -carbohydrate diets of young people. Of particular concern is the suggestion that MSG ingested by pregnant women may actually cause this lesion in children while they are still in the womb.

One of the worst offenders is pizza, especially commercial pizza. The tomato sauce alone is high in naturally derived free glutamate. When you add this to a liberal helping of MSG, you have a very neurotoxic mix. Add to that a twenty-ounce diet drink and you can see why we are having problems with obesity. Our children have become lab rats.

Juvenile Diabetes and MSG Intake

One of the most devastating things that can happen to a child is to develop diabetes early in life. These children are insulin-dependent, and often spend much of their lives in an emergency room or hospital bed. Numerous complications are associated with juvenile diabetes, including frequent infections, early onset atherosclerosis, hypertension, brain atrophy, and early onset heart attack.

It is known that these children are genetically susceptible, but that the disease develops only when an unknown environmental trigger sets the disease in motion. Some have proposed a viral trigger, caused by a common childhood virus.

It has been known for some time that a particular strain of mice is also susceptible to diabetes, and that they, too, require an environmental trigger before developing the full-blown disease. Interestingly, MSG is a powerful trigger in these mice.[238] Despite this startling finding, no one has bothered to see if MSG can trigger diabetes in human children!

There is also another trigger for juvenile diabetes—early exposure to cow's milk.[239] Several studies have demonstrated that a protein in cow's milk closely resembles the molecular structure of the cells in the pancreas that produce insulin, called islet cells. Because the immune system confuses the two, it begins to attack the islet cells by mistake, leading to their destruction.

Although proof of this connection appeared in one of the most prestigious diabetes journals, the general public is still not aware of the risk. Why? Because of the power of the milk producers. It seems the media would rather have tens of thousands of children suffer a life of diabetes than anger one of their biggest financial contributors. I would also point out that cow's milk has significantly higher levels of glutamate than human milk.

Type II Diabetes and Insulin Resistance

The incidence of type II diabetes has increased some 600 percent over the last thirty years. Historically a disease of overweight, middle-aged people, it is not unusual today to see children as young as ten who have developed this devastating disorder. Overall, incidence of type II in the teenage population has increased 16 percent over the last decade alone.

Many theories have attempted to explain why we are now seeing such an explosion of type II diabetes, but none really meet all the observations associated with the condition.[240] While children and teenagers are eating a lot of junk food and exercising little, the situation is not that different than when I was a teenager. What is different are the huge amounts of MSG and similar excitotoxic food additives children are consuming. The amounts of these additives has doubled every decade since their introduction in 1948.[241]

This also means that, while pregnant, mothers of diabetic children also consumed very large amounts of these excitotoxin-containing foods. Likewise, many parents feed their babies table food from an early age—food often laced with large amounts of MSG. In addition, large numbers of babies are fed formula, and many formulas are known to be high in excitotoxins such as caseinate. I have already cited studies showing that gross obesity is frequently linked to excessive MSG consumption in test animals. In addition, genetically susceptible mice exposed to MSG developed juvenile-onset diabetes. Several independent studies have shown that MSG causes significant increases in insulin secretion, just as we see in cases of type II diabetes.

Yet, in studies, animals without the gene for type I (insulin-dependent) diabetes still became grossly obese. This MSG-induced obesity was characterized by a preference for carbohydrates and an aversion for more nutritious foods, just as we are now witnessing in our youth. Also, excess weight was extremely difficult to exercise off or diet off in these experimental animals.

These experiments showed that damage occurred in the hypothalamus of the brain. As far back as 1940, it was known that stereotactic lesions to a particular part of the hypothalamus could produce grossly obese mice, exactly like those seen with MSG exposure. Because the FDA has refused to address this issue, we are more likely to see an unchecked increase in childhood obesity and type II diabetes.

Also characteristic of MSG exposure is an increase in insulin release from the pancreas. As we have seen, the pancreas contains numerous glutamate type receptors, and glutamate in the diet can induce as much as a threefold increase in insulin release from the pancreas. In addition, experiments in animals have demonstrated that MSG can induce insulin resistance, exactly as we see in type II diabetes in humans.

Now that we have experimental evidence that dietary MSG can cause insulin resistance, it is ludicrous to allow the food processors to add increasing amounts of MSG to our food. In addition to type II diabetes, MSG also causes abnormal lipid profiles, hypertension, and abnormal adrenal responses. With our children consuming tons of this toxic additive, we can expect things to get worse.

The major contributing factors related to type II diabetes include: obesity; overeating refined carbohydrates and fats, both polyunsaturated and saturated; a lack of omega-3-type fats in the membranes of cells; chromium deficiency; and a lack of soluble fiber and phytochemicals.

The final common cause is a defect in the insulin receptor on cell membranes, most often caused by an abnormal composition of fats in the membranes. Diets high in saturated fats, trans fatty acids and omega-6 type fats contribute to this diabetes-related membrane malfunction. It may be that food-borne excitotoxins are the final common denominator.

Excitotoxicity and Illegal Drugs

Recent studies indicate that many of the damaging effects produced by illegal drugs is caused by excitotoxicity within specific brain circuits. Most teenagers and adults using these drugs think that the only harmful effect is the risk of being punished by the law. Unfortunately, it's more serious than that.

For example, cocaine and methamphetamine stimulate the release of excess glutamate in the same part of the brain responsible for Parkinson's and Huntington's disease. Both drugs are also capable of producing serious long-term injury to the brain. After repeated use, millions of brain cells and synaptic connections are destroyed.

Because of the tremendous overlap and excessive number of synaptic connections at this age, the obvious effects of neurological damage in most young people will be minimal. But, because these drugs dramatically increase free-radical production in the brain, neurons and synaptic connections begin to die off in greater and greater numbers, essentially aging the brain at a greatly accelerated rate.

Recall that accumulated attrition of brain cells and their connections accounts for brain aging and degenerative diseases. What this means for chronic users of powerful drugs is an elevated risk for developing Parkinson's or Alzheimer's at forty or even thirty, rather than sixty. Not surprisingly, this is exactly what we are seeing today. The age at which people are developing degenerative diseases of the brain has been sliding steadily toward a younger age group. Also, there has been a dramatic rise in the total incidence of these brain diseases over the last several decades.

When you consider that this is also the age group that consumes the highest amount of excitotoxic foods, you can see we have a real predicament on our hands. Our biggest problem in the future may be where to put all these brain-injured people. At one time our mental institutions were filled to overflowing with cases of neurosyphilis. Tomorrow, it could be victims of the drug culture.

Let's say a teenager smokes some marijuana and has a few hits of crack at a party (not at all unusual these days, unfortunately), then dances for hours to the point of sheer exhaustion. By this time, his body core temperature is extremely high, his blood-brain barrier resembles a sieve (which means any glutamate in his blood will pass directly into his brain), and all of his tissues are being assaulted by wave after wave of free radicals secondary to a massive increase in metabolism brought on by exertion. In this weakened physical state, any further assault (taking more drugs, getting hurt in a fight, falling and hitting his head) will cause damage to his body tissues and brain far worse than in a sober, rested state.

While this scenario may seem unrealistic and apocalyptic, the truth is that for growing numbers of this country's youth, this kind of behavior has become a lifestyle, not just an isolated incident from which their bodies can recover with rest and good diet. Many young people repeat this damaging cycle every week, sometimes several times a week, and let's not forget that a lot of teenagers practically subsist on junk food—meaning their level of antioxidant protection is virtually nonexistent, even before engaging in other unhealthy behaviors such as taking illicit drugs.

Parents often convince themselves their child is going through a phase and will eventually outgrow the strange behavior. Despite the recurring signs of drug abuse (slurred speech, difficulty paying attention or completing sentences in some of the worst cases) and the fact that their child may suffer serious, permanent brain damage, many parents don't even consider the possibility that drugs could be involved.

Unfortunately, many kids are also doing multiple drugs, and we simply don't know how these substances interact chemically within the body. Further, there have been no careful evaluations of how particular drugs are actually being used by our youth; that is, most studies look at the effects of one drug at a time. Still, some good work has been done recently on the effects of a single drug.

For example, a recent study of the effect of the drug ecstasy, in which regular users were followed for one year, found significant impairment of participants' ability to think. What makes the study results very interesting is that, to eliminate the immediate effect of the drug itself, participants were not allowed to use the drug for two weeks prior to each test that was performed during the study period. In other words, this designer drug was producing long-term damage in the brain, which most likely will be permanent.

At this young age, the brain is still undergoing maturation, some growth, and significant fine-tuning. We know that even by the teenage years, the prefrontal areas of the brain, responsible for social control and complex learning, are not fully developed.[242] Many drugs alter this process, resulting in brains that interpret reality in bizarre ways, or produce emotional cripples unable to cope in society. Several studies have shown a direct connection between juvenile crime and drug use, especially violent crimes, which is not surprising.

The glutamate neurotransmitter plays a major role in the parts of the brain controlling emotion. Of particular importance are parts of the limbic system known as the amygdala and hypothalamus, both of which contain many glutamate receptors. Animal experiments where injury was caused to those parts of the brain demonstrate that intense, purposeful attacks of rage could be elicited using glutamate. Mice with these lesions could be made to attack cats.

Cardiovascular Disease

It has been discovered recently that the nerve bundles and neurons in the heart contain an abundant supply of glutamate receptors.[243] This may explain why some people suddenly die after consuming foods containing large amounts of MSG. Many reports tell of people who eat out at restaurants and an hour later develop crushing chest pain and shortness of breath. Despite all the signs and symptoms of a major heart attack, when they are taken to the emergency room, the ECG may indicate minor abnormalities or, in some cases, severe abnormal heart beats (arrthythmias), but angiograms reveal no problems with the coronary arteries.

By overstimulating the nerves of the heart, MSG could very well induce symptoms similar to a heart attack. Most likely, people suffering from this effect also have low magnesium levels, which would not only make the heart muscle more irritable, but could throw the coronary arteries into spasm, producing a full blown fatal heart attack. Like the brain, magnesium in the heart prevents the glutamate receptors from over reacting.

Experiments have shown that when animals are fed low magnesium diets and then given a sudden fright, many will die, whereas those fed normal magnesium diets are much more resistant to such sudden death.[244] This may explain many of the deaths seen in people caused by sudden shocking events or stress, especially when low magnesium is combined with a high intake of MSG.

Besides the acute danger faced when eating meals high in MSG, another less obvious danger exists. Recent studies have found that animals exposed to MSG soon after birth show markedly elevated levels of triglycerides and the very low-density lipoproteins (VLDL) that persist throughout life.[245] The values were higher in males than females. It is now accepted that elevated serum oxidized lipids are associated with an increased risk of heart attack and stroke.

Interestingly, glucose levels in the MSG-treated rats were also markedly elevated, as were insulin levels. This combination—high insulin level along with elevated glucose levels (hyperinsulinemia)—is also found in non-insulin dependent diabetes (type II) in humans. Several studies have confirmed these findings of hyperinsulinemia with MSG exposure.[246] Like gross obesity, type II diabetes is also increasing astronomically in children—the very ones who consume the most MSG-containing foods.

High insulin levels combined with hyperinsulinemia, high triglycerides, and hypertension are all symptoms of a newly described disorder called Metabolic Syndrome, a condition that constitutes major risk factors for atherosclerosis, heart attacks, and strokes. So we see that, if the same effects found in test animals also occur in humans, a diet high in MSG-containing foods and snacks would greatly increase the likelihood of a child developing early-onset diabetes and cardiovascular disease—*exactly* what we are seeing today.

Recent studies have also demonstrated the existence of glutamate receptors on the cells lining arteries in the brain, called endothelial cells, which control calcium entry into the cells. Abnormal functioning of these cells, triggered by excess calcium entry into their interior, is thought to be the central event in the early stages of atherosclerosis. Excess glutamate, derived from the diet, could trigger such calcium flow into the endothelial cell, initiating the events leading up to plaque buildup. Unfortunately, no one has looked at this possibility. If it turns out to be true in humans, MSG in the food supply could be a major contributing factor in atherosclerosis, and so heart attacks, strokes, and peripheral vascular disease.

Fibromyalgia

Many years ago, while working on my first book, I came across some early experiments that indicated MSG could stimulate muscle contractions. At the time, in my practice, I was seeing a large number of patients suffering from muscle aches, pains, and spasms, as well as various other nondescript complaints. In those days we called it myofascial pains. The condition is now known as fibromyalgia.

As with most medical problems for which the medical profession cannot find a ready cause, it was classified as a psychiatric problem secondary to stress and depression. This is the same route they took with chronic fatigue syndrome, even though brain lesions were being seen on MRI scans. I was convinced at the time that the tremendous increase in this disorder was in some way related to the large amounts of food excitotoxins being ingested.

A recent clinical study by Dr. J. D. Smith and his co-workers found that complete or near-complete relief could be attained by removing all MSG- and aspartame-containing foods and

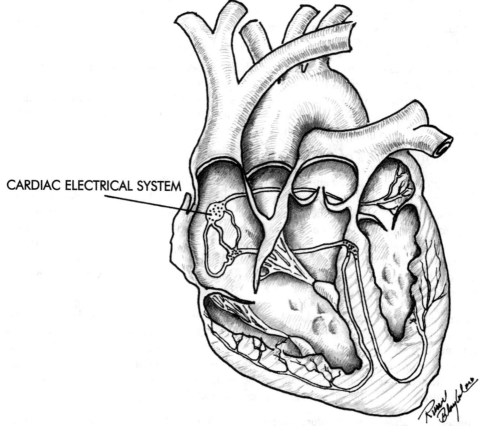

CARDIAC ELECTRICAL SYSTEM

FIGURE 7.2 The heart's electrical system contains numerous glutamate receptors, making the heart very susceptible to injury by food-based excitotoxins such as MSG and aspartate. This may explain the rising incidence of congestive heart failure and sudden cardiac death following ingestion of meals containing high concentrations of monosodium glutamate.

drinks from the diet of fibromyalgia sufferers.[247] What makes the study impressive is that these patients had suffered from the disorder for two to seventeen years, and despite numerous treatment attempts were no better until they removed excitotoxins from their diets.

The observation linking excitotoxins to fibromyalgia is further strengthened by the known relationship between exercise and fibromyalgia symptoms. Most physicians treating the disorder have noted that fibromyalgia patients get some relief with regular exercise. It was originally assumed that the release of endorphins from the brain during exercise relieved the pain; after all, it was like getting a shot of morphine daily. But it is also known that exercise plays a major role in clearing glutamate from the blood stream and tissues, and it may be this mechanism that accounts for the improvement caused by exercise.

Recent studies have shown that glutamate receptors also play a role in pain.[248] It makes sense that diets high in glutamate would greatly increase pain from whatever cause. You can only wonder how many people suffer from intractable spinal pain or chronic pains from injuries made worse because of excitotoxins in their diet.

In addition to the fascinating discovery that the heart has glutamate receptors, we now know that multiple tissues contain these receptors, including the lungs, kidney, ovary, testes, and endocrine cells.[249] This indicates that high consumption of MSG and other excitotoxins in the diet could produce widespread problems in numerous organs. Of special concern is the effect of excitotoxins on the endocrine system.

Endocrine Effects of MSG

The brain destruction of test animals first observed by Dr. Olney in 1969 was localized in a small group of cells in the hypothalamus called the arcuate nucleus, a tiny group of neurons that controls the release of the regulating factor for growth hormone, and may also be responsible for other pituitary hormones. Animals fed MSG not only produced less growth hormone, they also lacked the normal release pattern seen in all other mammals, including humans.[250] Normally the pituitary gland secretes growth-regulating hormone in spurts, with an extra blast occurring when we fall asleep or take a nap, one reason why it is so important for children to get plenty of sleep.

Later studies found that this nucleus connected to all the other nuclei of the hypothalamus, and was therefore given a special status. We have also learned that the most important neurotransmitter in the hypothalamus is glutamate.[251] As a result, high doses of glutamate given to newborn animals could damage several of the important nuclei in the hypothalamus. This was reflected in observations that many of the regulating hormones secreted by the pituitary, and controlled by the hypothalamus, were deficient in these animals.

Numerous studies using immature mice have shown that LH, FSH and prolactin (the reproductive hormones), HGH (growth hormone), ACTH (adrenal regulating hormone), and TSH (thyroid regulating hormone) were all decreased following exposure to MSG.[252] These hormone deficiencies were reflected in the animals by small size, low reproductive ability, gross obesity, and low metabolism.

Other studies have confirmed these earlier findings.[253] In males, one sees atrophy of the testes and lower levels of testosterone. In females, we see significantly lower LH, FSH and estradiol-17beta, the main form of estrogen hormone. In fact, the level of these hormones fell 68 percent following MSG treatment, which accounts for the decrease in the size of the ovaries and uterus.

There is some evidence that lower doses of glutamate can cause the early onset of puberty.[254] Therefore, it is not surprising to learn that young girls are now undergoing early breast development and premature onset of menses in large numbers. Could this be the result of excess glutamate in the diet? We may never know since no one is looking. One problem is the widespread promotion and use of soy products. Soy is not only high in glutamate, it is also a source of phytoestrogens. The effect of this combination on the developing hypothalamus is anyone's guess.

A fairly recent series of studies found that infant animals treated with MSG have higher cortisone levels than normal mice, and following stress it takes longer for the high levels to normalize.[255] This same process occurs in the elderly, and is known to endanger the brain. High levels of cortisone, especially over a long period of time, can destroy neurons in the hippocampus, a part of the brain damaged in Alzheimer's disease. Some have proposed that the elevated levels of cortisol and slow clearance following stress eventually lead to Alzheimer's dementia. That our children may be constantly exposed to high cortisone levels from early childhood is a frightening prospect.

Cancer

With the widespread effects of MSG on numerous tissues, is it possible that high consumption could trigger the development of a cancer? It is known that MSG does have an effect on selective gene activation, but it has not been determined to be mutagenic.[256] (Substances that are mutagenic are frequently carcinogenic as well.)

I am unaware of any studies looking for mutagenicity, yet numerous studies have shown that MSG, free glutamate and other excitotoxins produce enormous amounts of free radicals in tissues—which are a major cause of cancer induction in tissues and organs. By consuming foods on a daily basis that are high in excitotoxic additives, we would certainly expect high levels of free radicals and lipid peroxidation in numerous tissues. Again, no one has looked at the possible association.

We know that constant bombardment of the DNA by free radicals leads to the eventual activation of cancer genes (oncogenes). Once these genes are activated, cancer is inevitable. As with nervous system disease, cancer risk in the face of high MSG and aspartame consumption would be highest in persons possessing a genetic propensity for cancer. For example, a women with a strong family history of breast cancer or ovarian cancer would be at a much higher risk than a women with no such history. (Interestingly, the ovaries also contain glutamate receptors.)

MSG consumption, then, would pose a special danger to the cancer patient, since increased inflammation and free-radical production can promote tumor growth as well as invasiveness and metastasis of cancerous tumors. This is also demonstrated in the experiments using carrageenan, a very powerful inflammatory substance and food additive (used as a thickener). When even small amounts of carrageenan are injected near developing tumors in animals, tumor growth, and eventual metastasis, increases dramatically.[257] Carrageenan is usually found in baked goods, some breads, and ice cream.

The scientific evidence that free radicals play a major role in cancer induction and growth is so powerful it would be foolhardy to encourage millions of at-risk people to consume a substance that we know does just that—produces free radicals. But I suppose it is hardly surprising that no one is advising cancer patients to avoid excitotoxic food additives, since health care professionals and the media are telling them little else about cancer and diet anyway.

A significant number of cancer patients suffer from intractable pain. It is known that glutamate receptors in the spinal cord play a major role in pain perception, and there is some evidence that drugs that block glutamate receptors also reduce pain. Conversely, a diet high in MSG and other excitotoxins could certainly be expected to greatly increase pain. Despite the scientific evidence making this connection to pain, cancer patients are not being informed of this risk, and no work is being done by medical researchers to see if patients improve on excitotoxin-free diets.

One recent study provides very strong evidence that even mildly elevated levels of glutamate in the brain can cause tumors in experimental animals to develop more aggressively and become more malignant.[258] Blocking the glutamate receptors on these tumors was shown to reduce their growth. Excess brain glutamate levels will also increase brain swelling around the tumor and increase the risk and severity of seizures (frequently associated with brain tumors). For these reasons alone, anyone with a brain tumor should avoid all foods containing MSG.

Immunity is one of our most important weapons against cancer. It is widely known in the oncology world that immunosuppressed transplant patients have a significantly higher cancer rate than those with normal immune systems. This is thought to be secondary to a loss of the body's normal immune surveillance system, which seeks out cells transforming into cancer cells and destroys them.

Over fifteen years ago scientists found that exposing animals to MSG could produce a significant loss of delayed type immunity, and that this immune defect would persist for a lifetime.[259] This inhibition involved both humoral and cellular immunity, the most important for fighting tumors. While it is known that lesions to the hypothalamus can cause immune suppression, in this experiment, the effect was unexplained. It may be that glutamate also directly affects white blood cells (lymphocytes and macrophages).

At this point, you must be asking yourself: why are the medical profession and scientific world not pursuing this idea? In most cases, it is because there is little money available for such research—and most researchers are afraid of being attacked by the glutamate industry if they do. I find it amazing that so much research can point to the connection between human disease and excitotoxic food additives, but scientists seem unwilling to take that final step. Fear of professional ridicule and criticism renders impotent so many good researchers.

Eye Diseases

As you will recall, the discovery of the neurotoxic effects of MSG were first demonstrated on the retinas of animals in 1957. Since that original discovery, much research has been conducted on the connection between excitotoxins and diseases of the eye. One of the most startling discoveries was that much of the destruction caused by glaucoma is not a direct result of elevated pressure inside the eyeball, as was assumed, but rather was the result of a buildup of glutamate in the retina.[260] This glutamate arises from the retinal eye cells themselves.

The question has to be asked: how much greater damage is produced by high levels of glutamate in the food? We know that glutamate from the diet does enter the retina. There is evidence that by blocking glutamate receptors, or lowering the glutamate level in the eye, one may be able to prevent a loss of vision, a common complication of glaucoma. So why do we tolerate an industry that loads our food up with this destructive compound?

Now that we know that excessive glutamate in the eye can cause damage to the retina, what about other eye disorders, such as retinal detachment, inflammatory diseases of the eye, trauma, macular degeneration, infectious diseases of the eye and cataract? Cataracts are the result of free-radical damage to the proteins in the lens, and so would be susceptible to excitotoxic damage.

One recent study found that the concentration of glutamate in the retina increases 40 percent when an animal is made diabetic.[261] In addition, this study showed that the elevated glutamate increased free radicals and lipid peroxidation in the retina by 100 percent. By using antioxidants, glutamate levels were lowered to normal, and free-radical and lipid-peroxidation damage were abolished. This is critical for the diabetic to know, since diabetic retinopathy is a leading cause of blindness and may be prevented by avoiding excitotoxin-containing foods and beverages, and by increasing the intake of antioxidants.

This study may also explain why diabetics who drink large amounts of aspartame-sweetened drinks are more likely to go blind. Aspartame is composed of the excitotoxin, aspartic acid, as well as methanol (also a known eye toxin) and the amino acid, phenylalanine. Given this evidence, why, then, do the American Diabetes Association, and thousands of doctors encourage their diabetic patients to use aspartame? At least where the American Diabetes Association is concerned, it may have something to do with the fact that the organization has received large monetary contributions from Monsanto—maker of NutraSweet®!

Another interesting observation, reported several years ago, is that patients with Alzheimer's disease have a significant loss of retinal neurons, even more than would be normally expected given the ages of the subjects.[262] Could this be related to dietary excitotoxins destroying retinal cells? Although not proven, it is certainly possible given that the type of cell loss in these patients is consistent with excitotoxic destruction.

Degenerative Brain Diseases

In *Excitotoxins, The Taste That Kills*, I made it clear that there was no evidence that the excitotoxins found in foods are themselves the primary cause of neurodegenerative disorders such as Parkinson's and Alzheimer's disease, but one frightening possibility is that there may be a link between the widespread excitotoxic contamination of our food supply and the heretofore-unexplained dramatic increase in neurodegenerative diseases—which have also begun to occur on average at an earlier age. While these diseases existed long before the introduction of excitotoxic food additives, this does not mean that certain food additives

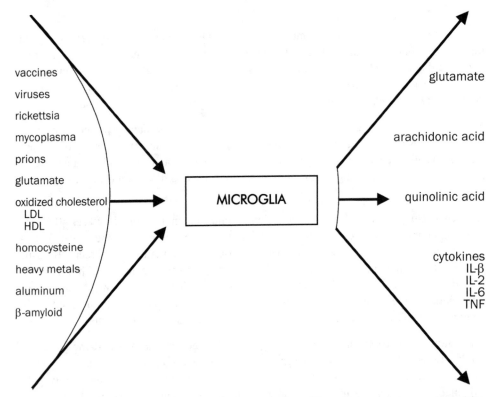

vaccines
viruses
rickettsia
mycoplasma
prions
glutamate
oxidized cholesterol
   LDL
   HDL
homocysteine
heavy metals
aluminum
β-amyloid

MICROGLIA

glutamate

arachidonic acid

quinolinic acid

cytokines
   IL-β
   IL-2
   IL-6
   TNF

FIGURE 7.3 On the left are numerous substances and conditions that can induce excitotoxicity, activating the brain's immune system. Once triggered, microglia secrete large concentrations of arachidonic acid, which promotes inflammation, as well as inflammatory cytokines.

cannot increase the likelihood that a person with a genetic weakness for the disorders will develop the disease.[263]

We know, for example, that people carrying the apoE4 gene have a significant risk of eventually developing Alzheimer's disease. Now if you happen to carry the apoE4 gene and consume foods high in excitotoxins, your risk of developing the disease will, most likely, be much greater than a person who eats unadulterated foods. Why? Because having the apoE4 gene indicates that you do not have the same level of antioxidant protection as someone without the gene. Excitotoxins significantly increase the brain's exposure to free radicals.

High consumption of excitotoxin-containing foods would increase your risk not only of developing one of these diseases, but could also augment the risk of early onset and severity of the disease.[264] I am shocked when I see patients with Alzheimer's or Parkinson's disease consuming foods high in these brain-toxic additives. Hospitals can be the world's worst in this regard, and most doctors haven't a clue as to the danger.

I have seen neurological patients with strokes, head injuries, and degenerative brain diseases being fed liquid diets in hospitals that contained as much as five to ten grams of excito-toxins—a huge amount of these toxic substances! Remember, brain disorders are most often accompanied by defects in the gatekeeper mechanism, the blood-brain barrier, and stress and poor nutrition further increase the defects in this protective system.

As a neurosurgery resident in the 1970s, I saw only one case of amyotrophic lateral sclerosis in five years. The head of the neurology department also stated that he rarely saw such cases. Today, ALS cases are not at all infrequent. While many factors may account for this dramatic rise, I believe that the massive addition of excitotoxins to our food supply plays a major role in this increase. Other toxins, such as pesticides, herbicides, industrial chemicals, mercury, fluoride, lead, and viral infections, may also make a contribution. But, it should be recalled, many of these environmental toxins share central mechanisms of action-excitotox-icity and free-radical injury in the diseases I have discussed.

Excitotoxins and the Elderly

While we are never completely safe from excitotoxic damage at any age, the two periods when we are most vulnerable are infancy/early childhood, and during our elderly years.

There is overwhelming evidence that aging is the result of destruction caused by free radicals, which damage cell membranes, DNA, and proteins. Of particular importance is damage to proteins, which make up enzymes, structural proteins, information molecules, and cell membranes. Damage to enzymes interferes with metabolism, particularly energy production, and growing evidence suggests that damage to DNA-repair enzymes increases risk for developing numerous degenerative diseases including cancer.

Injury to the membranes of the cell is particularly important as well, especially those that surround the mitochondria. These membranes are more than coverings used to contain the contents of the cell: they are very active metabolically, shifting information in and out of the cell and its many components. Loss of the membrane's natural fluid quality is associated with aging, and means that information molecules embedded in the membranes can no longer function efficiently. In addition, the various channels that normally control the flow of ions in and out of the cell are also sluggish.

In the case of the mitochondria, a loss of membrane fluidity means that the cell can no longer generate the energy it needs. As a result, the cell's many metabolic and functional processes that depend heavily on this energy begin to slow down or even fail. This is the basic process of aging. As we have seen earlier, when energy supplies fail in the brain, glutamate begins to accumulate outside the neurons. This initiates excitotoxicity, with a rapid, sustained flow of calcium into the cell, which then triggers numerous destructive reactions.

Once the calcium channel gets stuck open, the cell is in real danger. Free radicals of every sort begin to accumulate inside and outside the cell, triggering the release of even more glutamate. Recent evidence indicates that when glutamate begins to accumulate outside the cell, the brain's immune system is activated. The brain's immune cells, microglia, then begin to secrete a host of immune-activating chemicals called cytokines, which stimulate inflammation of the brain, in turn generating more free radicals and a greater release of glutamate.

As if this were not enough, the microglia secrete two excitotoxins, glutamate and quinolinic acid.[265] The whole process speeds up, and we have a brain that's in real trouble. This is the probable scenario of Alzheimer's disease, Parkinson's disease, Lou Gehrig's disease, and possibly autism. Early on in this process, one sees damage to the mitochondria with reduced cellular energy production.[266] The more glutamate, the greater the damage, and the more rapid the progression to severe dementia.

When the elderly eat foods containing excitotoxic food additives, they increase their brain levels of glutamate.[267] But, what about the protection afforded by the blood-brain barrier, you say? In the last decade, we have learned that one effect of aging is a gradual loss of the gatekeeper's ability to keep harmful substances out of the brain. In addition, many elderly have been exposed to one or more conditions known to impair the barrier, such as hypertension, head injuries, certain medications, diabetes, autoimmune diseases (lupus and rheumatoid arthritis), strokes, and chronic infections.

In fact, there is evidence that glutamate and free radicals can themselves impair the blood-brain barrier. Stress is also another common cause of barrier breakdown. So we see that as we age our brain is less and less protected from what we eat. If we consume diets high in free glutamate or aspartate, we risk serious brain damage. And if we happen to carry the gene for a high risk of Alzheimer's disease, elevated levels of blood glutamate from a bad diet may be just the trigger that is needed to initiate the disease. The same is true for Parkinson's disease and ALS.

Aging makes us susceptible to other threats, as well. Our brain depends on a steady supply of glucose to function. While it can use other fuels to a limited extent, glucose is its main fuel. Unfortunately, glucose cannot just enter the brain, it has to get past the blood brain barrier. To control its glucose supply, the brain has a special carrier molecule sitting at the blood-brain barrier whose job it is to escort glucose into the brain. So why have an escort system? Because in high concentrations glucose is toxic to the brain, especially when the brain is injured.

This glucose carrier system begins to fail as we age, making it difficult to control glucose entry.[268] As a result, the brain becomes starved for glucose, creating a very strange situation where blood can have high levels of glucose while the brain is starved for it. The result is an isolated hypoglycemic brain. If you suffer from this condition, a doctor testing your blood would find normal or possibly elevated glucose levels. As a result, the doctor would assure you that all was well, and that your memory loss is just the result of normal aging. It has been noted that Alzheimer's disease resembles hypoglycemia in many ways, the only difference being that you cannot recover by eating something sweet.[269]

As a result of all these problems, we see that the neurons in the brain are unable to make enough energy from what little glucose they can get. Because of this unrelenting damage, the brain begins generating a product, called beta-amyloid protein, that slowly condenses, forming an insoluble lump outside the cell.

This lump is quite caustic and can generate some nasty free radicals of its own, in particular, hydrogen peroxide. This further aggravates the damage already started in the brain. It is so irritating that it will also activate microglial immune cells in the brain, which significantly increases the inflammation within the parts already affected by Alzheimer's disease, such as the frontal, temporal, and inferior parietal lobes. These areas of the brain control attention, concentration, recent memory, and our orientation in the world: damage to the inferior parietal lobe causes Grandpa to get lost on the way to the store.

Inflammation is known to play a major role in Alzheimer's disease.[270] In fact, people who regularly take arthritis medication significantly decrease their risk of developing Alzheimer's. Interestingly, the types of cells destroyed with Alzheimer's disease are not only glutamate-type neurons but are also the only ones having the COX-II enzymes associated with inflammation. It is this enzyme that arthritis medications inhibit to block inflammation, thereby protecting these neurons from degenerating.

This same central mechanism explains the relationship to other features of Alzheimer's disease. For example, elevations of brain iron, mercury, and aluminum, combined with low magnesium levels, all act to increase free-radical generation, activation of the COX-II enzyme, and activation of the brain's immune system by way of the microglia. They also all increase the level of glutamate in the extracellular space.

The final piece of the puzzle is another microscopic change in the brains of Alzheimer's patients, the neurofibrillary tangle. This intracellular clump of tangled material appears to be the remnant of neurofibrils, a special conducting system within neurons. The neurofibrillary tangle is a twisted structure composed of tau proteins, and develops when the tau binds with too many phosphate molecules (excessively phosphorylated). Many substances can contribute to the creation of these tangles: one is a lipid-peroxidation product called 4-hydroxynonenal, others are mercury, aluminum, and MSG.

It has also been noted that the brains of Alzheimer's victims are severely deficient in many essential antioxidants, including carotenoids, vitamin C, magnesium, and glutathione.[271] It may be that people with these particular antioxidant deficiencies early in life are the ones most at risk for developing the disease later, especially if combined with free-radical-generating factors, such as excessive iron, mercury, aluminum and MSG in their systems.

As I mentioned before, low levels of magnesium in tissues can dramatically increase free-radical generation, reduce energy production, and enhance excitotoxicity. Several studies have found that people with Alzheimer's disease also have low brain magnesium levels, but only in the parts of the brain affected by the disease.

It has also been determined that people with this dementing disorder have very low levels of vitamin B_6 (pyridoxine), folate, and vitamin B_{12} (methylcobalamin) in their tissues as well. Vitamin B_6 plays a major role in protecting the brain against excitotoxicity. Methylcobalamin can directly block excitotoxicity, and folate plays a critical role in the production of acetylcholine, brain phospholipids, and DNA.

One of the metabolic products produced in the series of reactions utilizing these vitamins is called S-adenosyl methionine (SAMe), the molecule that actually performs all of the functions attributed to these vitamins. Not too surprisingly, studies have shown that Alzheimer's brains have very low levels of s-adenosylmethionine.

In the past, doctors frequently gave their elderly patients a B_{12} shot to boost their energy. Soon, we became too scientifically sophisticated to do such a stupid and wasteful thing. After all, large studies had been conducted on the elderly demonstrating that very few healthy elderly people were deficient in this vitamin.

Unfortunately, these studies were based on measuring blood levels of vitamin B_{12}, and recent research has shown that this is not an accurate measure for this substance. One such study compared the blood levels of vitamin B_6, folate, and B_{12} in groups of healthy and hospitalized elderly, matched for all the variables. At the same time, researchers also drew metabolic studies that more accurately determined if the vitamins were actually in the tissues doing their job. What they found was shocking.

Using only blood levels, it appeared that only 8-9 percent of the healthy elderly, and 19 percent of the hospitalized, had low vitamin levels for one or more of the vitamins. Yet metabolic studies demonstrated that 43 percent of the healthy elderly and 86 percent of the hospitalized elderly had low levels of one or more of the vitamins! It would seem that if we continue to listen to leaders in the medical establishment, a great number of us will end up very sick. Obviously, much evidence-based medicine isn't concentrating on the right evidence.

It is very likely that the "unscientific" doctors of the past, who routinely gave their patients B$_{12}$ shots, saved millions of older people from lives in nursing homes or early deaths from cancer. Our evidence-based leaders have learned nothing: they continue to snub their noses at nutrition-based doctors who are saving lives.

Heart Disease

I should say a word concerning heart disease and excitotoxins. Most experts in the field of cardiology have commented on the dramatic increase in heart failure in this country, yet like most such observations, no one seems to have a clue about the real cause of the problem.

We do know that nerves in the heart begin to die as we age. For example, by age 75 about 90 percent of the cell bodies in the nerve ganglion (sinus node) of the heart are dead.[272] This could explain the huge number of people in this age group with cardiac arrhythmia, and eventual heart failure. But, it doesn't tell us *why* the cells are lost in such huge numbers. The discovery that heart nerves contain numerous fully functional glutamate receptors may give us an answer.

As we saw previously, overstimulation of these nerves can produce sudden spells of irregular heartbeats and even sudden cardiac death. It is also reasonable to assume that a lifetime of excessive stimulation of these glutamate-sensitive nerves could produce a gradual loss of the nerves in the heart, accounting for their virtual disappearance by age seventy-five. In addition, high glutamate levels in the elderly would increase free-radical generation in the heart muscle itself and the arteries supplying the heart.

A young person who is very active can clear a significant amount of glutamate from his or her blood. This is because glutamate—especially as its metabolic precursor, glutamine—can be used as a fuel for muscle. And intense exercise has been shown to increase clearance of glutamate significantly, but this should not be construed as a justification for continued consumption of diets high in glutamate additives.

As we age, we begin to slow down. Some people slow down so much that they are barely moving, much less spending any time exercising. Muscles also become less efficient at removing and utilizing glutamate. As a result, a greater percentage of glutamate will remain in the blood to stimulate not only brain glutamate receptors, but also those in the heart and other organs. Remember also that many of the elderly are deficient in antioxidants, magnesium, and intake of basic foods. This obviously puts the elderly at much greater risk than the young.

While this final connection is pure speculation at this stage, the explanation certainly fits very well with what we know about heart failure and nerve loss in the heart. Because of the enormous implications of such a connection, it certainly demands further examination.

Other Additives to Avoid

Aspartame (NutraSweet®, Equal®):

This particularly nasty substance should have never even been approved for human use. In fact, had it not been for some fancy footwork by those in power in the FDA, it never would have. Early experiments using low, medium, and high doses with aspartame all found dramatic tumor increases in test animals. These included brain, pancreas, and breast tumors, and tumors of the testes, thyroid, and prostate. Experiments also demonstrated a direct correlation between intake quantity and tumor incidence.

Several possibilities explain the high rate of cancer in these animals. One is that aspartame breaks down in the body into a substance called diketopiperizine or DKP, which chemically closely resembles a group of cancer-causing chemicals. Aspartame also contains methanol, which breaks down in the body into formaldehyde and formic acid. Formaldehyde has been shown to accumulate near DNA, causing serious damage that is accumulative. That means that drinking even one diet cola a day can cause formaldehyde buildup in cells, so that the amount of the toxin increases daily.

There is also evidence that aspartame can worsen depression in those already suffering from the condition, may cause weight gain and insomnia, worsen diabetic control, aggravate multiple sclerosis and other neurological diseases, precipitate migraine headaches, trigger seizures, cause blindness, and may also damage a fetus' developing brain. One component of aspartame is aspartic acid, a known excitotoxin. Even small concentrations in gum have been shown to precipitate headaches.

I strongly suggest avoiding all products containing aspartame, including NutraSweet® and Equal®, as well as any other artificial-sweetener brands that include aspartame.

Carrageenan

Carrageenan is a rather new additive. It is a complex polysaccharide extract made from seaweed, and is used as a binding agent. Experimentally, carrageenan is used as an agent to induce intense inflammation in experimental animals. A recent study found that when carrageenan was injected in animals along with a cancer-causing chemical, tumors appeared more rapidly and in significantly higher numbers than in control animals injected with carcinogen alone. The same was seen when human breast cancers were implanted in animals along with carrageenan: the combination made the tumors grow faster and spread more widely than in control animals. As a result, carrageenan is classified as a tumor promoter.

Many foods contain carrageenan, and the number continues to grow. It is commonly found in baked goods, ice cream, candies, and breads. It is particularly hazardous for those either at risk for colon cancer and those who already have or have had colon cancer, since carrageenan comes into direct contact with colon cells. It is also suspected to worsen inflammatory bowel conditions such as ulcerative colitis.

So What Can I Do?

Step One: Stop Ingesting Excitotoxins

Obviously, the first step is to stop consuming foods containing excitotoxic additives, which basically means you have to stop eating all processed foods (canned, bagged, boxed) and foods prepared in restaurants. Our obsession with taste has become so consuming that no one in the food processing or restaurant business wants to lose out by not adding these substances to our food. As a society, we have become so used to the overwhelming, artificial tastes of our packaged foods that anything untreated strikes us as bland and unpalatable. After all, MSG and its cousins do only one thing: enhance the taste of foods. And MSG makes them taste delicious, scrumptious, and irresistible.

This competitive race for taste has escalated to the point that food processors are adding MSG to foods at a rate that doubles every ten years. Some foods can have three or more types of excitotoxins in a single package or can. This is especially dangerous since experiments have shown that excitotoxins act synergistically, meaning that adding numerous subtoxic (below toxic levels) concentrations together is equivalent to a fully toxic dose.

As the featured speaker at a convention in Chicago soon after my book on excitotoxins came out, I was waiting to give a second speech when a grossly overweight man with a W.C. Fields nose and plethoric look waddled over to me. He introduced himself as an owner of one of the nation's largest food additive businesses, then proceeded to ask me about my strong objections to MSG. I politely explained, but could tell that he wasn't really listening. He twiddled the tip of his bulbous nose, staring at me over a pair of bifocals and said, "It doesn't matter what you say or do, we will figure out some way to put these additives in the foods."

I have come to learn that he was telling the truth. Food manufacturers have used every name in the book to disguise high-glutamate additives. And, as always, they have used their power in Congress to have laws enacted to help them in this cover-up. FDA regulations now say that manufacturers do not have to put the term "monosodium glutamate" on the label as long as a particular ingredient doesn't contain more than 99 percent pure product. What this means is that you will have to learn all the disguised names and become an obsessive label reader.

Two intrepid workers in this area are Dr. Adrienne Samuels and her husband Jack, who started the organization, Truth in Labeling. Dr. Samuels is expert in the design and analysis of scientific studies and has spent an immense amount of time poring through MSG studies. As a result of their work, we now know that the food industry will stop at nothing— including influencing scientific studies that fraudulently portray MSG as safe—to continue the practice of adding excitotoxins to our food.

In truth, the only way to protect yourself and your family is to eat only fresh foods that have no additives. If enough people do this, in time, the industry will yield to the demands of the public. All they are looking for is a market large enough to justify changing their methods. We must give them the incentive.

Step Two: Increase Your Defenses

Increasing your body's defenses will include supplementing your diet with: vitamins E and C; the carotenoids; basic minerals, such as selenium, zinc, copper, and magnesium; and the trace elements, boron, molybdenum, manganese, and chromium.

Your main antioxidant defense should come from a high intake of fruits and vegetables, especially vegetables. These plants contain about ten thousand phytochemicals, five thousand of which are flavonoids, which are the most powerful and versatile antioxidants known.

As we have seen, pyridoxine (vitamin B_6) lowers both blood and brain levels of glutamate, thereby reducing the risk of excitotoxic damage. Methylcobalamin (vitamin B_{12}) directly blocks the glutamate receptor, as do Ginkgo biloba and pycnogenol.[273] Pyruvate and malate, products of metabolism, have also been shown to block glutamate toxicity and increase brain energy production at the same time.[274] All of these are available as supplements without a prescription.

Anything that increases brain energy production will reduce excitotoxicity. This includes alpha-lipoic acid, CoQ10, niacinamide, all of the B vitamins, acetyl-L-carnitine, and creatine monohydrate.[275]

A combination of CoQ10 and niacinamide has been shown to completely protect the brain areas affected by Parkinson's disease against excitotoxicity.[276] Magnesium not only increases energy production, but also plays a major, direct role in protecting the brain against excitotoxicity.

The omega-3 fatty acid DHA also plays a major role in brain protection by improving the health of mitochondria and cell membranes, and increasing the supply of serotonin in the brain. It also directly blocks excitotoxicity.

It is also known that estrone, one of the estrogenic female hormones, strongly protects the brain, especially the hippocampus.[277] The adrenal hormone precursor DHEA is protective of brain cells. For both men and women, testosterone has been found to protect the brain against age-related injury. These hormones should be used only after careful testing, to prevent oversupplementation.

Recommendations for Protection Against Excitotoxicity

Natural Vitamin E (Unique E) 400 to 800 IU
Take twice a day.

Vitamin C (buffered) 500 mg
Take three times a day on an empty stomach.

Extend Core (multivitamin/mineral)
Take one three times a day with meals.

DHA 100 mg
Take two twice a day. (Keep refrigerated)

In addition, take the following supplements if you are at a high risk of neurological disease or have a neurological disease.

Pyruvate 500 mg
Take twice a day.

Methylcobalamin 1,000 ug
Take one twice a day.

CoQ10 100 mg
Take one twice a day.

DHA 100 mg
Take two twice a day. (Keep refrigerated)

Alpha-lipoic acid 100 mg
If you are using alpha-lipoic acid take 50 mg twice a day after lunch and dinner. If you are using R-lipoic acid, cut the dose to one 25 mg capsule to be taken just before your biggest meal of the day.

Acetyl-L-carnitine 500 mg
Take one twice a day.

Curcumin 250-500 mg
Take one twice a day. Curcumin is an oil soluble substance that is poorly absorbed if taken as a capsule or dry powder. Empty the contents of the capsule into one tablespoon of extra virgin olive oil or fish oil and mix well. This will greatly increase absorption.

Quercetin 500 mg
One to two capsules twice a day. Like curcumin, quercetin is oil soluble. Some forms are specially compounded to be water soluble, if not, also mix with oils as described for the curcumin.

This flavonoid not only protects the brain against free-radical damage, but is also a rather potent antihistamine substance. This is good not only for sinusitis, but has been shown to reduce neuron damage caused by histamine enhancement of excitotoxicity.[278] Special brain cells can produce abundant amounts of histamine in the brain.[279]

Ginkgo Biloba 120 mg
Take one twice a day. (Do not take with aspirin, arthritis medications, or other anticoagulants.)

Phosphotidylserine 100 mg
Take one two times a day.

Phosphotidylcholine (with other phospholipids) 750 mg

Take one twice a day.

8
Pesticides and Other Chemicals in Our World

As we have seen, major questions have not been answered about the toxic effects of aspartame and monosodium glutamate on the human brain, yet neither the government, nor the industries that use these chemicals, are doing anything to satisfy our right to know. We have witnessed the same blindness with fluoride, vaccinations, and other toxins forced on the public.

It has been observed that of the over sixty-five thousand chemicals in the EPA's registry, the vast majority have not been tested adequately for potentially toxic nervous-system effects, especially higher cortical functions, such as memory, cognitive ability, and executive functions of the brain. Because we come into contact with them every day, food additives and cosmetics ingredients pose a particular concern.

For example, in earlier centuries, face powder contained white lead. Hundreds of incidences of lead-poisoning cases later, cosmetics containing the harmful component were removed from the market. In 1955 AETT (acetylethyl tetramethyl tetralin), a fragrance component of many cosmetics, was being used by millions of women until it was discovered that the compound caused degeneration of neurons in animals, as well as marked behavioral changes, including aggressiveness and irritability. It was removed from the market twenty-three years later. What was the fate of women exposed to AETT? No one knows and no one seemed to care.

Anyone who has tried to decipher ingredient labels on food packages knows they pretty much all read like organic chemistry texts. Most of us just assume the unidentifiable ingredients must be safe, or the FDA would have recalled them. We also blithely imagine that each must have been carefully tested or our regulatory agencies wouldn't let food processors use them in the first place. Wrong! The vast majority of these ingredients have never been tested for long-term neurological effects. You and your family get to be the guinea pigs.

When it comes to food additives, the vast majority have never been tested for long-term effects on the brain. Even those that have been tested for effects on body tissues have never been tested in combination with other toxins. For instance, what happens when you combine the two food additives, linalyl isovalerate and benzyl phenylacetate, in the body? I don't know. Nobody knows. And that's the real problem.

It has been estimated that more than nine million people come into regular contact with known neurotoxins in the workplace, and tens of millions of us must live with these chemicals in our own homes. Most are not even aware that these commonly used chemicals can damage the nervous system. We assume that if they were really dangerous, the FDA or EPA, or some other alphabet organization would have told us so. We put our trust in those who should not be trusted.

The EPA and FDA simply ignore neurotoxicity when they can, and in some instances, as we saw with Dr. Phyllis Mullenix's treatment by the NIH, bureaucrats go out of their way actually to *protect* the offending industries. Those who blow the whistle can expect the full wrath of the system to fall on them.

I cannot overstate the scope of this problem. It is already enormous, and continues to grow unchecked. More than a thousand new compounds are added every year to the existing stock of sixty-five thousand chemicals. Additionally, there are some two million mixtures, blends and other formulations already in use by industry. Of these compounds, about three to five percent are known to be neurotoxic, meaning that over sixty thousand are known to damage the nervous system! And since most registered substances have never been tested, the number actually may be much greater.

Among these chemicals are thirty-four thousand pesticides registered by the EPA, many of which are neurotoxic. We can appreciate the scope of this problem when we learn that, on average, 1.1 billion pounds of these pesticides are being used every year. Worldwide, four billion pounds are used annually. In the United States alone these pesticides are being spread over 900,000 farms, equal to millions of acres. In addition, 70 percent of livestock are also treated with pesticides.

In the past, pesticides allowed us to grow the enormous amounts of food necessary to literally feed the world. There is little question that millions of lives were saved by the use of pesticides, yet things have improved on the bug-war front as well. Newer, natural methods of controlling insects have been devised but never implemented on a wide scale. Corporate farms did not want to cut profits for the sake of safety, and smaller family farmers have been brainwashed into believing in the safety of these noxious chemicals.

One telling fact is that, of cancer cases, especially lymphomas and leukemias, the highest incidence in the population occurs in people who work on farms. The same is true for Parkinson's disease. Lured into believing these powerful chemicals were safe, farmers drenched everything in pesticides, herbicides, and fungicides—including themselves and their families.

In the course of my nutritional practice, I saw a number of people who grew up on farms, especially along the Mississippi Delta—cotton country. One of my patients, who is suffering from a neurological disorder, told of crop dusters flying over her family's house when she was a child, releasing a virtual rain of pesticides over everything. The children would run out in the yard and smell the pungent odor of the chemicals. Soon it would be all over their hands and clothes. Her father thought nothing of it because the farm agent had told them it was safe as spring water.

If you think you're safe because you don't live on a farm, think again. Because of our national obsession with bug-free homes and perfect lawns, these same chemicals are saturating city neighborhoods as well. In my old neighborhood I would see a lawn treatment truck going from yard to yard, spraying a heavy layer of herbicides and weed-control toxins over the grass. We had to hide in our house until the vapor settled and warn our children not to play in yards that had been treated.

Several studies have shown that children, and even pets, who play in such yards have a significantly higher incidence of leukemia than those not exposed to these toxins. Most parents we talked to about the dangers of lawn chemicals just laughed and said they were sure the lawn companies would have told them if it was dangerous.

Here in Mississippi one of our greatest health scandals was a pesticide case in the late 1980s. It seems an enterprising fellow and his buds decided to open a cut-rate pesticide treatment company. To save on costs, they used cotton poison to debug the homes of their hapless clients. Once discovered, the men were sent to Parchman prison and their clients' homes had to be torn down. Unfortunately for many, even licensed pesticide companies can leave your home uninhabitable.

Now let us look at some of the more important risks caused by our society's ever-increasing reliance on untested chemicals.

Pesticides and Herbicides

The most commonly used pesticides are organophosphates, chlorinated hydrocarbons, and carbamates, and include products like Malathion, Diazinon, Sevin, and DDT. All of these pesticides employ a neurotoxic mechanism to kill insects. Furthermore, most pesticides and herbicides are easily absorbed through the skin and lungs. This is why you see warnings on the label to wash all spills off your skin with copious amounts of soap and water— IMMEDIATELY!

The EPA estimates that sixty-nine million families in the U.S. alone store and use these readily available pesticides. It is not surprising then, to find that there are sixty to seventy thousand poisonings a year from organophosphate pesticides alone.[280] As staggering as this number is, it is most likely grossly understated because many people who experience symptoms of poisoning will never see a physician.

Dr. David Hartman, author of the textbook, *Neuropsychological Toxicology*, points out that when you consider the magnitude of the potential exposure to these toxins it is incredible that fewer neuropsychological studies are done on these products than on almost any other neurotoxic substances in use.[281] It is estimated that 150,000-500,000 pesticide-related illnesses are reported every year, with two hundred people dying from this exposure.[282]

When we consider the magnitude of exposure from indoor bug and termite treatments, our pesticide-herbicide exposure from foods is actually pretty small. I know people who buy vegetable wash and religiously scrub all their fruits and vegetables to remove pesticides, and then just as religiously have a pesticide service treat their home inside and out every month. Because they don't see any lingering vapors, they assume the pesticide, and therefore their homes, are safe.

Organophosphate pesticides kill bugs by inhibiting a special enzyme, also found in humans, called cholinesterase. Under normal circumstances, this naturally occurring enzyme deactivates acetylcholine to prevent overstimulation of muscles and central neural pathways. When cholinesterase is deactivated, acetylcholine overstimulates muscles, resulting in an inability to control movements. Heavy exposures can cause rapid death from respiratory paralysis.

While it has been assumed that the toxic effects of organophosphates are caused solely by cholinesterase inhibition, recent studies have shown that another mechanism may also be involved.[283] In fact, low-concentration exposure can produce lasting neurological problems, such as memory defects, impaired vigilance, and a reduced ability to concentrate. Even workers exposed to these pesticides over a long period of time with no obvious neurological effects demonstrate abnormal EEG (brain wave) patterns,[284] clearly indicating that their brains are not functioning properly.

Dr. Hartman tells of a physician who, following exposure to Dursban® in a basement exercise room, suffered from persistent abnormalities in memory, word-finding, and visual perception. Other reports recount similar effects.

Another disturbing effect of the organophosphate, Dursban®, is the finding of a high incidence of auto-antibodies to myelin and the nucleus of cells (ANA antibodies).[285] These are the types of autoimmune antibodies found in autism, lupus, and allergic encephalitis. Persons exposed to this particular pesticide have reported muscle pains, fatigue, flu-like symptoms, and defects in tests of rapid visual identification and decision-making. In addition, they demonstrate difficulties with problem-solving and complex processing of information.

Carbamates are widely used as herbicides, pesticides, and fungicides. Like organophosphates, they are easily absorbed through the skin, producing rapid toxicity. Exposure can cause acute memory loss, vertigo, numbness in the hands and feet, increased sensitivity to light, fatigue, and visual impairment that can last over a year. In some instances, these symptoms are permanent.

Chlorinated cyclodienes are the most highly toxic of any of the organochlorine pesticides. These include chlordane, heptachlor, aldrin, endrin, and endosulfan. Excessive exposure can cause seizures, continuous muscle spasms (fasciculations), a loss of coordination, brain swelling, and liver failure. Fortunately, chlordane was banned in 1988, but not before 200 million pounds had been spread throughout American homes and businesses.

One ongoing problem with chlordane is that it can persist in the soil twenty years, and in homes fifteen years after application.[286] According to the EPA, over 19.5 million homes were treated with chlordane before the ban went into effect. This means that some fifty-two million people are still at risk. Another problem is that it is also fat-soluble, meaning that the toxin is stored in the body for a long time. Humans are much more sensitive to chlordane's toxicity than animals are.

GABA

The organochlorine group of pesticides (lindane, dieldrin, and bicucullinne) kills bugs by interfering with GABA receptors, making them convulse to death. GABA is a neurotransmitter that calms the nervous system by inhibiting excitatory neurons. The brain becomes overexcited when GABA is deficient.

The importance of the GABA system is emphasized by the fact that it is one of the earliest systems to develop in the fetal brain, usually by seven weeks. The number of GABA receptors increases sharply between eight and eleven weeks of development. It is known that drugs that target these receptors can cause long-lasting behavioral changes. Human studies involving children exposed to organochlorine pesticides have also shown similar long-term behavioral changes.[287]

Those with neurological diseases, especially disorders related to excitotoxicity, are especially vulnerable to these pesticides, since GABA is essential in preventing overexcitation of the nervous system. Of particular concern is a person with ALS, the excitotoxic disorder of the spinal cord.

Organochlorine-type pesticides are accumulating in our foods, and in our bodies as well. Significant levels of these compounds have been measured in human breast milk,[288] and can pass easily through the placenta.

What About Residues on Fruits and Vegetables?

While our main source of exposure to these neurotoxins may be from products we use in our homes, this by no means obviates the danger from chemical residues on our food. With over 1.2 billion pounds of pesticides and herbicides used in this country alone, we do have a problem. Because many pesticides—including DDT, aldrin, dieldrin, endrin, and heptachlor—have demonstrated major toxicity and carcinogenicity, they have been banned in the United States. But we are still at risk from many of these banned pesticides because they are being used in developing countries. Mexico, for example, supplies an increasing amount of our produce and that country's farmers legally use many of these banned pesticides.

Of the six hundred pesticides in current use, the EPA has identified sixty-four with cancer-causing potential.[289] A study by the National Research Council found that of these, thirteen widely used pesticides pose the greatest danger. These include 0-phenylphenol, metiram, zeneb, folpet captafol, thalonil, benomyl, linuron, chlordimeform, captan, maneb, ancozeb, and permethrin.

The highest concentrations of these pesticides can be found in the following foods (listed in decreasing order of concentrations): tomatoes, beef, potatoes, oranges, lettuce, apples, peaches, pork, wheat, soybeans, beans, carrots, chicken, corn, and grapes.

Many of us are further comforted by government and food-industry pronouncements that our food supply is carefully checked by both federal and state agencies for dangerous pesticide residues. A review of this process has shown that only 1 percent of the food supply is even examined, and then not for all pesticides. Surprisingly, the FDA does not prevent food processors from marketing foods that contain illegal residues.

Pesticide poisoning is not at all uncommon. One particularly alarming incident occurred in 1985, following the use of a systemic pesticide, called aldicarb, on watermelons. A systemic pesticide is one that permeates the entire plant, not just the outside. Approximately one thousand people were poisoned by eating these tainted watermelons. Symptoms varied from nausea and vomiting to seizures, nerve damage, and blurred vision.

It should also be appreciated that combinations of pesticides are being used on produce. Seventy different pesticides are used on bell peppers, 110 on apples and 50 on broccoli. Industry spokesmen respond by pointing out that most pesticides are water-soluble and can be washed off or removed by peeling fruits. But some fruits and vegetables, such as bell peppers, peaches, cucumbers, oranges, apples, avocados, and eggplants, are waxed to slow spoilage. Often, pesticides that cannot be washed off with water are added to these waxes.

Recent studies have shown fifty to seventy chemical residues present in the fatty tissue of ordinary Americans. Multiple studies have shown pesticide residues in breast milk,[290] yet no long-term studies have been conducted to determine the effects of pesticide and herbicide combinations. Considering that many are fat-soluble, we should be *very* concerned about this lack of knowledge.

In the brain, many of these powerful chemicals alter neurotransmission, receptor function, and membrane physiology. Of special concern is the recent finding that many of these chemicals can have specific localized effects on the nervous system.[291] For example, some preferentially alter the brain's immune system, while others mainly affect the vascular supply to the brain, and still others destroy specific parts of the brain such as the substantia nigra responsible for Parkinson's disease.

Most people assume that if they experience no symptoms at the time they are exposed, they haven't been affected. This is a dangerous presumption. The effects of early exposure to many of these chemicals may not appear until much later in life. We know that most neurological disorders do not develop clinically until 80 percent of the neurons in a particular area of the brain have been destroyed. With aging there is a natural attrition of these cells, and injury early in life will greatly increase risk of later loss of these neurons, and at an earlier age.

The Minamata mercury spill I discussed in chapter three demonstrates this principle of delayed effects very well. Investigators initially assumed those exposed had suffered few toxic effects, but the unfortunate victims later developed full-blown symptoms, even long after the mercury had been eliminated from the environment.

Examination of the distribution of Parkinson's disease in the population has demonstrated that this devastating disorder is over twice as common in farmers as city dwellers.[292] Normally, about 5-7 percent of the neurons of the substantia nigra, the part of the brain primarily affected by the disease, die every decade. Exposure to neurotoxic chemicals increases the rate to 10-15 percent per decade, substantially raising our risk of developing the disease. Add a diet laden with excitotoxins and the danger is even higher, especially since many pesticides are capable of opening the blood-brain barrier.

One particular set of cases is very instructive. A report that appeared in the prestigious journal, *Neurology*, described five cases of acute onset of parkinsonism following exposure to organophosphate pesticides.[293] In the most remarkable case, a sixty-four-year-old woman developed a rapid and severe onset of parkinsonism after fumigating her home with bug spray daily for ten days. She was admitted to the hospital and slowly improved on medications for parkinsonism.

All her symptoms reappeared within a day of returning to her contaminated home, and progressed to the point that she was bedridden and unable to swallow. Increasing her parkinsonism medications did not help. Again, after transfer to the hospital, she recovered rapidly.

This time her family scrubbed her house thoroughly with soap and water. Yet, when she returned, her symptoms returned. Exasperated, she moved to a new residence, where her symptoms finally resolved. For two years she had no symptoms. Then she had her family bring clothes from the other house. On wearing these clothes, her parkinsonism returned. The symptoms disappeared when she purchased new clothes.

It is important to note that no one else in the contaminated house developed symptoms, indicating that she had an unusual sensitivity to organophosphate pesticides. We do not know why. It is possible she had a defective detoxification mechanism that made her more susceptible. The case also demonstrates that even minute concentrations of pesticide can produce devastating disorders of the nervous system, even years after original contamination. This is especially true for genetically susceptible people.

Another study, this one from the Rochester Medical Center, demonstrated an equally frightening scenario.[294] Researchers found that exposing rats to a mixture of the herbicide, paraquat, and the fungicide, maneb, could produce parkinsonism in the animals. Yet, neither compound alone could cause the disorder. It seems the combination opened the blood-brain barrier, allowing paraquat to produce the brain lesion responsible for parkinsonism.

Both of these chemicals are sprayed on tomatoes, potatoes, corn, lettuce, and many other crops. Since the EPA does not test for chemical interactions, this problem would never have been discovered by our watchdog government agency.

Effect of Pesticide Exposure on the Developing Baby

While pesticide exposure may not be as great from eating treated foods, the cumulative effects can be significant, especially considering that exposure begins even before birth.[295]

The brain is one of the first systems to arise in the embryo, and its development continues long after birth, putting the organ at an extreme disadvantage during the nine-month period in the womb. Most injuries to the brain during the early phase of development are fatal before birth; of greatest concern are those that occur later in the pregnancy and do not kill the fetus, but may cause serious defects in the child.

Most pesticides kill bugs either by interfering with neurotransmission or by altering neuron function. Unfortunately, these substances also affect humans in the same way. The governing theory behind using these dangerous substances as bug killers is based on the idea of differential toxicity: bugs are smaller than humans, so killing them requires a proportionately smaller dose. My concern is with sublethal doses, concentrations that do not kill but rather alter cellular functions.

PCBs

Another contaminant of concern is polychlorinated biphenyls (PCB), which was banned for general use in the 1970s. This oily substance was used in the electrical industry, in die- and machine-cutting oils, as heat-exchange fluids, and in materials such as paints, plastics, and sealants. Like many other neurotoxic compounds, it is highly fat-soluble (lipophilic). Remember that the brain is composed of 60 percent fat, and readily accumulates these toxins.

Normally, the liver detoxifies these lipophilic substances by making them water-soluble, thus increasing their excretion from the body; however, PCBs inhibit the liver enzyme necessary to accomplish this task. As a result, toxins may linger in the body for a very long time. In fact, PCB's half-life is 8.4 years, meaning that after 8.4 years, only half the PCB in your body will have been eliminated.

Studies of women poisoned during two major accidents involving PCB consumption, one in Japan and one in Taiwan, found that their babies were very small, had skin and nail deformities, and suffered psychomotor impairment.[296] Much of the transfer of the poison was via breast milk.

Again, don't be overcomforted by reports that PCB-use has been severely restricted. As with many of these long-lasting compounds, PCBs bioconcentrate in the food chain. With time, overall environmental concentrations increase because plants and animals extract the toxin from the environment; it is then concentrated in their tissues. This is also a major problem with the addition of fluoride to water.

One disturbing article that appeared in *Neurotoxicology* reported that children exposed to pesticides developed hypersensitive reactions to these or similar pesticides as adults.[297] This may explain some cases of multiple chemical sensitivity. Cross-reaction among chemical toxicants is increasingly recognized in the medical literature. For example, exposure to formaldehyde makes one overly sensitive to cocaine. With the enormous number of powerful chemicals entering our environment, we can only expect that occurrences of such interactions will increase.

How to Protect Yourself

First, and most important, remove as many toxins from your immediate environment as possible. This means no further pesticide treatments (including bug bombs and contracted pesticide services) inside your house, no bug sprays used indoors on plants, and using only safe, natural insecticides outdoors. It also means canceling your lawn service, if you have one. The fewer of these chemicals you use and are exposed to, the better.

As for foods, you should avoid canned, packaged, and other forms of processed foods. Prepare as many of your meals as possible from fresh ingredients. Resort to canning and other forms of safe food storage. When you buy vegetables and fruits, buy organic. Even better, grow your own vegetables and fruits. If that is impossible, buy them from a farmer's market. Be sure to ask about their use of pesticides and herbicides.

For non-vegetarians, buy meat locally from people you know. If that is not possible, buy minimally processed meats, and avoid the meat of animals that were injected with antibiotics and hormones or that were fed animal feces. I was shocked to learn that on some of the big corporate farms, chickens are fed pig feces: this is one of the most disgusting forms of recycling I have ever heard of.

Meat from wild game is probably the safest to eat. It is low in fat, and because game animals graze on grasses, berries, and other plants containing healthy omega-3 fatty acids, it is also naturally higher in omega-3 fatty acids than commercial meats are. Some smaller farms still graze their cattle.

By now, everyone has probably heard of "mad cow disease," a disease with a 100 percent fatality rate whose cause is unknown. There are two major theories as to its origin: that it is spread by a tiny virus-like protein particle, called a prion, that lacks nuclear material; or that the disease is triggered by pesticide exposure.[298] The latter of these seems to have the best circumstantial evidence.

The theory is based on the fact that the normal prion, a complex protein wound in a particular three-dimensional conformation in the brain, becomes unwound; as the process spreads through the brain, brain cells are slowly destroyed, leaving behind a swiss-cheese brain.

Prion proteins are normally found near synapses and function as an antioxidant system to protect the delicate connections to other neurons. As they unwind, the protein loses its protective ability, and the result is destruction of the brain caused by a combination of excitotoxicity and free-radical accumulation at the synapse. It has been shown that certain pesticides can trigger this unwinding process.

Theoretically, ingesting "infected" tissues of dead animals can spread mad cow disease. Several cases have been diagnosed in England and across Europe, and as a result, hundreds of thousands of cattle have been killed and their carcasses burned. Gelatin vitamin capsules, glandular supplements, and supplements containing cow parts have also become suspect. Vitamin manufacturers are switching to vegetable capsules and people are avoiding animal-based products.

We have known for a long time that people with powerful detoxification systems can tolerate exposures to many toxins that make people with weak detoxification systems very sick. We saw in the chapter on mercury poisoning that people with higher selenium and zinc levels were far less likely to suffer toxicity.

Detoxification systems exist in most cells, but the body's major detoxification apparatus is the liver. Basically, it consists of two parts. The first part, called the phase I system or MFO system (mixed function oxidases), utilizes a p-450 enzyme system to alter normally lipid-soluble toxins to a water-soluble form that can be easily excreted in the urine. The phase II system uses various molecules, primarily glutathione, to bind these altered toxins so they can be safely excreted.

This cleansing system depends on a good supply of detoxification chemicals, such as sulfur, glutathione, taurine, and selenium to successfully accomplish its task. Several plant flavonoids and vitamins have also been shown to possess a remarkable ability to stimulate both phase I and II detoxification. This is especially true for the carotenoids, indole-3-carbinol (from broccoli), and curcumin.

Milk thistle plant extract significantly improves liver cell function and is a powerful antioxidant, protecting liver cells from free-radical and lipid-peroxidation damage. The flavonoid, curcumin, also protects the liver, and improves the flow of bile as well. A combination of alpha-lipoic acid, selenium, and milk thistle has demonstrated remarkable success in regenerating liver function in cases of viral and alcoholic hepatitis.

Rather than guess about your liver's detoxification ability, I would suggest a test for detoxification capacity. Presently, I recommend the detoxification profile by the Great Smokies Diagnostic Laboratory. With this test, you are given caffeine, aspirin, and acetaminophen tablets—detoxification test products. The test breaks down your detoxification into its various components, so that corrective steps can be directed at the problem. I always tested my patients, rather than guess. I often found things I never would have suspected, such as yeast overgrowth of the bowel, heavy metal toxicities, and malabsorption problems.

In addition to detoxification, you also need to protect your cells, especially brain cells, from excitotoxicity, free-radical damage, and lipid peroxidation. This means that you will need to enhance your dietary antioxidants, such as vitamins, minerals, and flavonoids. The B vitamins improve cell metabolism and energy production, which, we have seen, protect us from excitotoxicity.

Of particular importance is the protection of cellular, especially mitochondrial, membranes. These membranes play a major role in energy production as well as other cellular functions. Cell membranes are made of complex phospholipids obtained from the diet (such as phosphotidylcholine, phosphotidylserine, phosphotidylethanolamine, and phosphotidylinositol), as well as gangliosides and cerebrosides in the brain.

It is also important to have good immune function, since many toxic metals and pesticides can suppress the immune system, but I would not recommend the average person to overstimulate his or her immune system with products like echinacea and IP-6. Simply maintaining an adequate vitamin, mineral, and flavonoid intake will keep your immune system well up to par.

For special toxin exposures, you might need a different set of supplements. For example, Thorne Research company has formulated several compound supplements for specific toxicities, such as solvent exposure, formaldehyde toxicity (which would also be good for aspartame toxicity), and pesticide exposure. They also make a basic detoxification supplement that covers exposure to various industrial chemicals.

It should be noted that certain vitamin deficiencies are particularly common with chemical toxicities. For example, vitamin B_6 deficiency has been observed in 60 percent of all chemically sensitive individuals. When B_6 is low, taurine is also deficient. Taurine plays a major role in detoxification and deficiencies result in extreme sensitivities to chlorine, hypochlorite (bleach), aldehydes, alcohols, solvents, and ammonia. It is preferable to take pyridoxal 5-phosphate than pyridoxine, since the former is the active coenzyme form. Those with chronic disease or extreme toxicities cannot metabolically convert pyridoxine to its active form.

Riboflavin also plays a major role in detoxification, as it is a component in the phase I detoxification process. Riboflavin is especially important in detoxifying Azo dyes, which are known to produce cancer.

Magnesium deficiency is very common with heavy metal toxicity and toxic chemical exposure. Both of these toxicities cause increased excretion of magnesium in the urine. Magnesium deficiency impairs the phase I detoxification process and has been shown to decrease hydroxylation of aniline and demethylation of aminopyrine, both carcinogenic compounds. Magnesium supplementation reverses this effect.

To increase liver detoxification I suggest the following:

Milk Thistle Extract 200 mg
Take twice a day for three weeks, then once a day thereafter.

Aged garlic extract 600 mg
This extract supplies sulfur compounds for the detoxification process. Take 600 mg three times a day.

Curcumin 500 mg
This flavonoid is a powerful antioxidant and anti-inflammatory, and enhances immune function as well as liver detoxification. Take one capsule two times a day, mixed with one teaspoon of extra virgin olive oil or fish oil.

Alpha-lipoic acid
Take 50 mg twice a day with meals. If using R-lipoic acid, take 25 mg just before the biggest meal of the day. This is a powerful antioxidant, energy generator, and metal chelator that protects the liver and encourages regeneration of damaged liver cells. It also significantly enhances cellular glutathione levels. Take one twice a day.

Phosphotidylcholine 750 mg
Take one twice a day. This phospholipid combination protects the liver and all cells.

Thiamine 200 mg
Take once a day.

Vitamin E succinate
Take 400 IU a day.

Preventing the Golden Years from Tarnishing

Section II

Introduction

Everything that lives undergoes a series of physiologic changes that we call aging. In basic terms, aging is a progressive breakdown of cellular and tissue structures. When the process reaches a stage beyond which cells can no longer function, life ends. Presumably, each of us would like to live a full life, free of diseases. No one wants to become a crippled old person, wracked with pain, unable to care for oneself, and a burden to children and loved ones. The good news is that while our bodies may be pre-programmed for aging and death, we also do have choices—but we must begin to exercise them early enough in our lives so that we can avoid many of the worst aspects we associate with aging.

Although the mystery of aging remains unsolved, we *are* getting close to understanding the mechanical processes that contribute to the changes we experience as our bodies grow older. Theories of aging have abounded in the last few decades. An early hypothesis posited that our cells are programmed for a set number of divisions, and once we reach that limit, we will die. Studies examining the ability of human cells to reproduce in culture dishes have lent substantial credibility to this idea. In the early 1960s Leonard Hayflick, a prominent gerontologist, discovered that human cells can divide at most about fifty times. After fifty divisions, no matter how well cells are cared for and nurtured, they will die. This has been called the Hayflick Limit. Furthermore, by studying other species, he was able to show that all animals' cells possess limits on the maximum number of divisions before dying. For example, the Galapagos tortoise is known to live as long as 175 years, and its cells can reproduce at most 90 to 120 times. Mice, who live only two or three years, have cells that can reproduce only fourteen to twenty-eight times before dying.

Not all cells are programmed this way, though. Highly malignant cancer cells, strangely enough, are immortal. In fact, cancer cells removed in 1951 from one patient, Henrietta Lacks, continue to grow and reproduce—five decades after her death! Called HeLa cells, these specimens are still used in cancer experiments all over the world.

Research scientists have also theorized that aging may be due to the introduction of small errors in DNA during cell reproduction. With time, according to this theory, errors accumulate, leading to fatal errors in the genes after a certain number of cell divisions. The problem with this theory is that some cells which are most vulnerable to the aging process, such as neurons in the brain, do not divide at all.

The neuroendocrine theory of aging proposed that eventual failure of the endocrine system leads to gradual systemic failure of the body. Basically, the theory states that the hypothalamus and pituitary—control centers for much of the endocrine system—begin to fail, leading to disruptions in immunity, metabolism, and other physiological functions. But, while it is true that many people's endocrine systems begin to fail with age, it is more likely that progressive endocrine failure is a *product* of the aging process itself, rather than its cause. After all, the hypothalamus and pituitary age right along with the rest of the brain.

Telomeres and Aging

Recent studies have helped to clarify the mechanics of aging. Our best evidence right now points to two closely related processes, telomere shortening and free-radical damage, that play a central role in aging.

Telomeres (from the Greek *telos* "end" and *meros* "part") are terminal caps located at the ends of chromosomes, discovered and named in 1938 by biologist Hans Muller. In the early 1970s, two scientists working independently—a Russian named Alexei Olovnikov, and the Nobel-Prize winner, James Watson—proposed that telomere caps shorten with each cell division, and concluded that this progressive shortening process might be a cellular clock for aging. Subsequent research has confirmed that idea.

Unlike all other human cells, we know that germ cells (those that form sperm and ova) do not age. In 1986 Howard Cook and his co-workers discovered that germ cells have significantly longer telomeres than other cells. In addition to a lengthened telomere, germ cells contain an enzyme, telomerase, which continuously replaces the telomere fragment that is lost during cell division. No other cells possess this enzyme.

Despite this extraordinary finding, it does not appear that aging and death result solely from telomere loss. Cells taken from a centenarian will still divide, yet they will reproduce fewer times than younger cells before finally dying. As ancient cells reach the Hayflick limit, their divisions slow, apparently in an attempt to preserve whatever telomere length is left. It is also important to note that cells divide at different rates, thus reaching their Hayflick limit at different times.

The Free-Radical Theory of Aging

While rates of free-radical production vary widely among individuals, they are an unavoidable hazard of life itself, from conception until the moment of death. As we saw in chapter one, free radicals can damage virtually all parts of the cell: membranes, DNA, proteins, and complex carbohydrates.

Since generation of free radicals occurs near membranes, such as those covering the mitochondria, damage to cell membranes is a major component of aging. Normal cell membranes are extremely fluid, allowing the numerous molecular structures—such as ion channels (antenna-like molecular chains that poke into and out of the cell), enzymes, and information-transcription molecules—to float freely. With time, a constant free-radical barrage initiates a chain reaction that spreads through the membrane in all directions, altering its consistency and eventually making it stiff to the point of rigidity. Once this happens, the membrane can no longer function properly: signals are no longer transmitted from the outside of the cell to the structures inside, ions have difficulty passing through the microscopic channels, energy enzymes no longer function properly, and the cell, in essence, becomes sick. This process is part of the aging effect.

In addition, free radicals attack all the proteins within a cell. Proteins perform three major functions. They provide structural support, create molecular signals, and provide numerous enzymes for initiating reactions from energy production to the creation of other molecules. Each type of protein has a special three-dimensional shape that is critical to its function, and even a slight alteration can have deleterious effects on performance.

With age, an increasing number of these free-radical-altered proteins, called protein carbonyl products, accumulate in the body. The number of these altered proteins increases dramatically in neurodegenerative diseases, diabetes, and autoimmune diseases (such as lupus and rheumatoid arthritis). While the amount of protein carbonyl products in extremely old people who do not have one of these diseases is substantially lower than in someone with, for example, Alzheimer's disease, these proteins do significantly affect how cells—and hence bodies—function past a certain age.

The third cellular component affected by accumulated free-radical damage is DNA. Remember that mitochondria have their own DNA, allowing them to reproduce themselves based on energy demands. Therefore, weightlifters and exercise enthusiasts have a far greater number of muscle mitochondria than couch potatoes. Likewise, those who exercise their minds possess more mitochondria in their brain neurons than people who sit and watch sitcoms all day.

We know that the vulnerability of our DNA (both cellular and mitochondrial) to free-radical damage increases with aging. This also means that the telomere is at greater risk of being shortened. DNA contains the codes that control literally millions of operations in our cells, every second of our lives. It is known that cellular DNA of older people oxidizes five times faster than that of younger people, and that mitochondrial DNA is oxidized ten times faster. This means that not only will a cell's operational instructions as a whole be damaged, its ability to produce vital energy will also be significantly impaired. A loss of cellular energy-generating capability is one of the central features of aging.

Virtually every cell process requires energy—and a lot of it. This is especially true for brain cells. In fact, the brain consumes 25 percent of the body's glucose and 20 percent of its oxygen, even though it makes up only 2 percent of the body's mass in the average person. Even in the deepest drug-induced sleep or anesthesia, the brain continues to consume at least 50 percent of its normal oxygen supply. The reason we feel sleepy when blood sugar falls, which happens in reactive hypoglycemia, is that the brain becomes starved for energy-giving glucose. Normal aging of the brain only slightly lowers the energy production of the brain. In Alzheimer's disease, energy production in specific parts of the brain is drastically lowered. The same is true with Parkinson's disease.

So, anything that damages mitochondrial DNA impairs energy production. Because free radicals easily damage DNA, cells have numerous forms of built-in protection, including antioxidant nutrients, special antioxidant enzymes, and DNA repair enzymes. Unfortunately, mitochondrial DNA possess few repair enzymes as compared to nuclear DNA. This means that mitochondria rely greatly on antioxidants and special antioxidant molecules (such as glutathione) which are nutrition-dependent.

DNA damage caused by free radicals is continuously fixed by a series of repair enzymes, but in cases where free-radical production is unusually intense (as with chronic illness), these repair processes cannot keep up with the damage. Eventually, the system begins to break down and the entire body starts to fall apart.

While the worst damage by free radicals occurs inside cells, damage also occurs outside the cell in tissues and blood. Here, free radicals weaken connective tissue, the fibrous tissue that normally holds everything together, including muscles, ligaments, joints, organs, blood vessels, and skin. As age-related, free-radical damage mounts, we begin to suffer from frequent injuries and inflamed joints, tendons, and muscles. In addition, we become weak as our muscles atrophy, and our immune and endocrine systems begin to fail.

Free radicals in the blood oxidize the cholesterol-carrying lipoproteins called LDL and HDL. Once oxidized, they can damage blood vessel walls which leads to atherosclerosis and all of its related complications, including heart attacks, strokes, and peripheral vascular disease. In the blood stream, albumin, flavonoids from fruits and vegetables, minerals, and vitamins act as powerful antioxidants. In fact, these antioxidants work in concert, possibly synergistically, to prevent oxidation of lipoproteins and other tissues outside cells.

All told, a lifetime of accumulated free-radical damage can lead to varying degrees of impaired cellular function. If you avoid the hazards I discussed in the first part of this book, and maintain a diet high in fruits and vegetables, low in sugar, low in omega-6-type fats and higher in omega-3-type fats, and avoid food additives that can damage cells, you will suffer far less cellular damage than someone who does just the opposite. Unfortunately, we have far more meat-and-potato eaters than fruit-and-vegetable eaters.

One activity far too many Americans engage in, and that significantly increases aging of all the body's tissues and organs, is smoking. Some studies have shown that smokers age at a rate twenty years beyond their chronological age. People living in developed countries also suffer from chronic, unrelieved stress, which significantly increases free-radical generation and lipid peroxidation in virtually every area of the brain, another process that dramatically increases aging.

The bottom line is that, over a lifetime, our bodies endure a continual assault of free radicals and other cellular toxins. While our bodies attempt to repair as much of this damage as possible, there is always some injury that goes unrepaired or is repaired incorrectly. This unrepaired damage accumulates over a lifetime, leading to major disruptions in cell function later in life—the seemingly inevitable process of aging. When our bodies produce a lot of free radicals, or we do things that increase our sensitivity to free-radical injury (e.g., consume too many simple sugars), the accumulated damage is greater and cell malfunction occurs sooner, and is more severe. In other words, we age faster.

Now let us look at some specific diseases and conditions associated with human aging.

9
Atherosclerosis: Hardening of the Arteries

The adult human body contains a complex circulatory system composed of about 100,000 miles of blood vessels, of which there are three types: arteries, veins, and capillaries. Arteries carry oxygen- and nutrient-rich blood away from the heart and to cells; capillaries connect arteries to veins and facilitate the exchange of oxygen and carbon dioxide, and veins carry oxygen-depleted blood back to the heart. A robust blood supply is therefore vital to good health. Of all the organs, the brain and the heart are most vulnerable to impaired circulatory function. Under most circumstances, the brain can survive only thirty minutes of interrupted blood supply. Heart muscle is slightly more resistant, mainly because it can use a wider variety of energy fuels to support its metabolism than the brain can, which depends solely on glucose.

Atherosclerosis (more generally known as arteriosclerosis), often called hardening of the arteries, is this country's number-one killer, leading to approximately one million deaths every year. The human and economic costs are staggering. Over forty million Americans suffer from cardiovascular disease alone, with associated costs for treatment estimated to be about $259 billion annually. More than 500,000 coronary bypass operations are performed every year, each costing between $50,000 and $100,000. And strokes and peripheral vascular disease affecting arteries to the legs and kidneys account for billions more in medical expenses. Those who survive the complications of atherosclerosis are frequently physically impaired, and many are no longer able to work or enjoy life.

Millions of people are completely unaware that their blood vessels are 80, or even 90, percent occluded, and, of the 1.5 million heart attacks that occur each year, one-third of those are the first sign most people have of a vascular problem. In cases of such high degrees of occlusion, some form of ill health is inevitable, and short of a heart attack or stroke, other warning problems may manifest. Occluded heart arteries can lead to coronary artery pain (angina), which manifests as chest pain, shortness of breath, or pain radiating into the left arm or jaw that lasts for seconds or minutes. When obstruction occurs in arteries supplying blood to the brain, symptoms may include short periods of weakness or numbness on one side of the body. If vessels on the left side are affected, brief periods of speech difficulty, stammering for words, or inability to understand what someone else is saying may result. These spells are called transient ischemic attacks or TIAs. "Ischemia" means reduced blood supply to a tissue or organ. All these conditions are symptoms of a larger problem, and may eventually lead to a catastrophic event such as a stroke or heart attack.

Over the years, doctors have identified many factors that increase stroke and heart-attack risk. These include: obesity, diabetes, smoking, heavy drinking, chronic stress, chronic illness, a diet high in saturated fats (especially trans fatty acids, mainly the products of partial hydrogenation of vegetable oils), hypothyroidism, hypertension, and the use of oral contraceptives. Recently, the medical profession has begun to realize that certain infectious organisms may also play a role in atherosclerosis.

Progression of Atherosclerosis

An artery is tough on the outside and smooth on the inside; it actually has three layers: an outer tissue layer, an elastic muscular middle that is very strong, and an inner layer of endothelial cells. The endothelium is very smooth so that blood can flow easily through the lumen (hollow vascular channel through which blood flows) with no obstacles in its path.

Interestingly, the process whereby we develop atherosclerosis begins while we are babies. Autopsy studies have shown that early vascular changes associated with atherosclerosis begin in infancy, and obvious fatty streaks are evident in the major arteries by early childhood. These changes occur in 50 percent of children between the ages of ten and fourteen years of age.

In time, these fatty streaks continue to grow, eventually collecting fatty debris, overgrown smooth muscle cells, and connective tissue within the wall of the blood vessel. These streaks and fibrous plaques form mainly at arterial stress areas, such as where an artery branches, or where a large vessel sharply curves. Although these fibrous plaques are plainly visible by the time we reach our twenties, blood flow is not significantly impaired until 60-70 percent of the lumen is obstructed.

While we still do not completely understand why debris begins to collect in blood vessels, we do know quite a bit about the ensuing inflammatory process. The central event in atherosclerosis appears to be an interruption of the normal function of endothelial cells lining blood vessels. More than just a protective covering, this layer is a very active player in blood vessel reaction and function. Numerous metabolic events take place within these cells every moment of the day.

In brief, the endothelium's job is to make sure blood flows smoothly, and when more blood is needed to an area, endothelial cells signal the underlying smooth muscle cells to contract or dilate as needed. Under normal conditions, the endothelium also controls blood viscosity (sluggishness), preventing it from coagulating within the lumen.

Once the lining of an artery is injured, cholesterol can enter the blood vessel wall where it is easily oxidized. Cholesterol is a waxy substance essential for functions throughout the body: it is used in cells for membrane repair, steroid synthesis, and other functions. Cell membranes contain a significant amount of this fatty substance, and the brain is especially rich in cholesterol. Like other fats, it cannot dissolve in blood, and must be transported to and from cells by special carriers called lipoproteins. However, oxidized cholesterol is very irritating, triggering an inflammatory response involving numerous chemicals and immune cells.

When this occurs, the wall of the blood vessel can attract specialized white blood cells called macrophages. Normally these cells slide right over the lining of the blood vessel, but when endothelial cells are not working properly, these immune cells can attach to the endothelium, enter, and interact with the oxidized cholesterol. A series of complex events is then triggered leading to a localized, intense inflammatory reaction. More white blood cells are drawn to the area of macrophage attachment, reacting as they would to a virus or other foreign body.

When infections occur, white blood cells flow to the site of an invasion and attempt to kill the invader by spraying it with a barrage of destructive free radicals. The same series of immunological events occurs along the lining of our blood vessels. Blood flowing past areas of intense inflammation causes LDL-cholesterol to enter the wall of the blood vessel. Another type of fatty molecule called HDL, or high-density lipoprotein, also carries cholesterol, but in general, it is removing cholesterol that has accumulated in the blood as a result of cell breakdown.

When LDL cholesterol enters the site of a macrophage attack, it too comes under attack by free radicals, and is oxidized, magnifying inflammation in the blood-vessel wall. In an effort to contain this irritation, the macrophages gobble up the oxidized LDL cholesterol and soon look like cells filled with foam—hence the apt designation, foam cell. As more oxidized cholesterol accumulates, the inflammatory reaction becomes more intense.

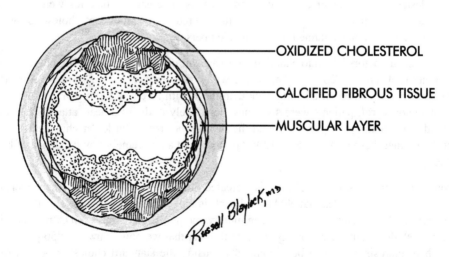

OXIDIZED CHOLESTEROL

CALCIFIED FIBROUS TISSUE

MUSCULAR LAYER

FIGURE 9.1 Cross-section of an artery showing the changes caused by atherosclerosis. The oxidized cholesterol has induced an inflammatory response that produced a build-up of calcified fibrous tissue, partially obstructing the lumen.

In an effort to contain the fire, the body attempts to wall off the inflamed area with scar tissue. The smooth muscle cells under the endothelium react by overgrowing, further aggravating the problem. The inflammation soon grows from a small fatty streak to a thick, crusty overgrowth that protrudes into the lumen. We call this thickened crud a plaque. In time, calcium can enter the plaque, further weakening the wall of the blood vessel.

Not infrequently, an ulcer crater forms in the center of the plaque. This can trigger clotting of the blood that is flowing by, resulting in either a sudden occlusion of the vessel, as occurs in a stroke or heart attack, or the clot can break free and travel to a smaller artery further down the line, causing an embolism. Sometimes a shower of emboli produce numerous smaller blood vessel occlusions. If this occurs in the carotid artery in the neck, this torrent of clots can enter the tiny arteries of the eye, resulting in a loss of vision on the side of the arterial plaque.

The ultimate cause of a heart attack or stroke is the development of unstable plaques, which either have roofs that rupture, spilling toxic fats into the blood vessel, or that are stripped of their endothelial lining. Both events cause blood clots to develop at the site. The crud itself rarely totally blocks off the artery.

Cholesterol

Most of us know that eating the wrong kinds of fats can increase our risk of developing atherosclerosis, but few are aware of just how important *types* of fats really are in this process. During the late 1940s and early 1950s, scientists believed that a high consumption of cholesterol was a major cause of atherosclerosis. The earliest theories were based on information collected by pathologists, who discovered large amounts of cholesterol within atherosclerotic plaques obtained from autopsied persons.

Next, clinical doctors began to examine their vascular disease patients for high blood levels of cholesterol. They discovered that people with cholesterol levels at 240 mg/dl were four times more likely to die of a heart attack than those with levels at 220 mg/dl. At 260 mg/dl of total cholesterol, patients were six times more likely to die of a heart attack. They then looked at populations of people around the world who had much lower cholesterol levels and found that those with levels of 120-160 mg/dl had an extremely low incidence of heart disease.

From these early observations, scientists created the cholesterol theory of atherosclerosis, which is based on the idea that cholesterol itself is the cause of the disease. This theory has been repeated so often to the medical community and public that it has been extremely difficult to dislodge from their thinking, despite the fact that we now know only 50 percent of all atherosclerosis cases can be accounted for using the standard cholesterol-based risk-factor index built up over the last several decades. It's interesting to note that, even in the earliest years of research, leading cardiologists strongly resisted the idea that cholesterol was solely responsible for atherosclerosis.

At this same time, the pharmaceutical industry, always looking for a way to expand profits based on new discoveries, began a crash program to develop cholesterol-lowering drugs. In the meantime, clinical doctors began to call for lowering cholesterol in diets. A chief recommendation was to switch from saturated fats—which are found mostly in animal products—to polyunsaturated vegetable oils. Among these "healthy oils," corn oil (and margarine made from corn oil) was hailed as the solution for our society's vascular problems. Manufacturers of vegetable oils and margarine launched extensive advertising campaigns, touting endorsements from the American Heart Association. Suddenly, America was on a cholesterol-lowering binge. Food manufacturers inundated the public with guarantees that their foods were "low in cholesterol" and "heart healthy."

Despite this frenzied enthusiasm for lowering cholesterol, there existed an unheeded rumbling in the medical community, raising serious questions about the validity of the theory. In fact, if we look at all the conventional risk factors combined—hypertension, diabetes, smoking, alcohol abuse, and elevated cholesterol—only half of all atherosclerosis cases can be explained. Other factors *must* be at work, and their impact is being largely ignored. For example, if elevated cholesterol is the true cause of atherosclerosis in mammals, what about hibernating animals, such as bears, whose cholesterol levels hover around four hundred, and who rarely show signs of atherosclerosis? The same is true in humans.

This is not to say that fats do not play a significant role in atherosclerosis, but it also seems obvious that they do not act alone to produce vascular occlusions. The process actually appears to involve a complex interplay of metabolic events and environmental factors—discussions of which are not nearly as conducive to fifteen-second sound bytes on the evening news, or multi-million dollar day-glo ad campaigns.

It is important to note that medically "acceptable" cholesterol levels are lowered almost every year. Today, most doctors seek levels that are below 200 mg/dl. This is based on the famous Framingham study that found people with cholesterol levels below 175 mg/dl had half the number of heart-attack deaths as those with levels from 250-275 mg/dl. These two extremes were then used to justify a vigorous attack on cholesterol.

One of the biggest problems with the cholesterol theory is that its proponents ignore contributing factors that always seem to accompany high cholesterol. For example, when populations of people known to have low incidences of atherosclerotic-associated diseases (strokes, heart attacks, peripheral vascular disease) are examined, most studies ignore the fact that such groups not only consume fewer cholesterol-containing foods, they also eat more foods high in plant phytochemicals, antioxidant vitamins, minerals, and fiber. Such populations also consume considerably less sugar than people with high rates of atherosclerosis, a consideration I will discuss later in this chapter.

Problems with the Cholesterol Theory

Obviously, there are a few problems with the cholesterol theory, not the least of which is the fact that half of all people who end up having a heart attack or stroke have no conventional risk factors. Unfortunately, modern science, when faced with a paradigm that may endanger funding considerations, tends to ignore such anomalies; yet, investigation of such anomalies in the past has led to radical breakthroughs in our understanding of various diseases. *The most glaring problem with the cholesterol theory centers around the fact that all early studies on cholesterol-lowing drugs found no statistical evidence linking reduced cholesterol levels to fewer heart-attack deaths.*

The only newer studies that have shown a drug-based reduction in cardiac mortality used cholesterol-lowering drugs that were also antioxidants. It has been hypothesized that the antioxidant effect, not the lowered cholesterol, actually accounts for the enhanced protection. In addition, they have platelet inhibiting properties, which when combined with their antioxidant effects, explains the reduction in heart attacks and strokes. As I will discuss later, there are much safer antioxidants than those you can get in a prescription medication.

One of the biggest secrets in the medical world is the connection between cholesterol drugs and cancer. In a paper that appeared in the *Journal of the American Medical Association* in 1996, Drs. T.B. Newman and S.B. Hulley discussed the long-term implications of twenty-six million people taking these drugs.[299] First, they observed that no long-term studies have been done in humans to determine safety: the millions of people currently taking these drugs are essentially test subjects.

They also point out that a meta-analysis (a composition of many studies) indicated cholesterol-lowering drugs may increase mortality rates caused by other conditions. A review of the available research indicated that all cholesterol-lowering drugs cause cancer in rodents, and that the dose of the drug used in test animals was comparable to that used in humans. This important information is conveniently omitted from the *Physicians' Desk Reference* (published by Medical Economics Company), which your doctor uses to determine drug risk.

While studies have found that cholestyramine and probucol are not directly carcinogenic, these drugs do act as co-carcinogens, enhancing the carcinogenicity of other chemicals. It is important to stress that all known human carcinogens are also carcinogenic in mice or rats. Given this evidence, and for safety's sake, it seems wise to assume the opposite is true—that animal carcinogens are human carcinogens—unless good experimental evidence to the contrary can be produced.

According to Dr. L.S. Gold and co-workers, of a list of eighty possible carcinogenic hazards to humans, the average cholesterol-lowering drug was ranked second.[300] According to FDA safety guidelines, a medication must not produce cancer in test animals at doses twenty-five times the usual dose. The lipid-lowering drugs produce cancer in doses far below this. In addition, some of these drugs also have been shown to damage nerves in the brain stem.

Cardiologists, in a widely covered press release, have recently suggested that even more people should be on lipid-lowering drugs. This is ludicrous, since mild cholesterol elevations can be controlled easily by dietary changes and special supplementation.

Another theory suggests that lipoprotein(a), not LDL cholesterol, is the actual culprit. A recent study found that this special protein is a stronger predictor than cholesterol of heart attack risk.[301] It is very sticky and tends to attach to arterial walls. In fact, those with high levels of lipoprotein(a) are 70 percent more likely to have a heart attack than those with lower levels, and people with elevated lipoprotein(a) have ten times the risk as those with elevated LDL cholesterol.

Unlike LDL cholesterol, lipoprotein(a) is not affected by diet, smoking, or other risk factors. It is purely hereditary—but vitamins will reduce levels in your body. Nicotinamide (as inositol hexaniacinate) and vitamin C are especially effective, and a combination of these two can lower levels over 36 percent. Two amino acids, lysine and proline, have also been shown to reduce lipoprotein(a)'s stickiness. Lysine is preferable, since proline can act as a neurotoxin. Five hundred milligrams of lysine three times a day should suffice. Your doctor can track lipoprotein(a) levels to determine dosage adjustments.

Most doctors, even some cardiologists, tell their patients that a high LDL-cholesterol value is bad. What most patients aren't told is that recent evidence indicates that there are actually two forms of the LDL molecule: one small and one large. Because it is easily oxidized, only the small one appears to be harmful. In fact, the larger LDL-cholesterol molecule may be just as protective against atherosclerosis as HDL-cholesterol, the so-called "good" cholesterol.

What this means is that if you get a cholesterol test that doesn't differentiate the two types of LDL, you will not know if your risk is high or not, since most of the LDL may, in fact, be the "good" type. Only a few laboratories test for this difference.

It is also important to know the difference because a higher intake of omega-3 fatty acid can actually increase LDL-cholesterol levels, but it is thought that only the good form is raised by omega-3. This would explain why diets high in omega-3 significantly reduce heart attack and stroke rates, despite raising LDL-cholesterol levels.

While the matter is far from settled, I would caution the reader not to be taken in by the shrill hype over cholesterol. A high intake of a variety of antioxidants, a balance of proper fats, and the use of special supplements will protect most of us from coronary heart disease and stroke.

Chronic Infection as a Cause of Atherosclerosis

The idea that chronic infections within arteries might cause atherosclerosis first arose when doctors observed that people with even high normal levels of c-reactive protein, a marker for inflammation, had much higher rates of coronary heart disease and stroke than those with lower levels. The natural question then arose: What infectious organism was responsible for the inflammation?

The first suggestion came in 1988 when Dr. Pekka Saikku and his co-workers reported a study of Finnish men infected during an epidemic of mild pneumonia caused by the organism *Chlamydia pneumonia*. They found that men who tested positive for the organism were more likely to have a heart attack than those who tested negative. Later, the Helsinki Heart Study found that patients seropositive for *C. pneumonia* were 2.6 times more likely to have cardiovascular disease than those who were seronegative for the organism. It is interesting to note that *C. pneumonia* antibodies are present in about 50 percent of the adult population, often without any clinical symptoms. Exposure to the bacteria in early childhood, combined with the difficulty of eradicating the organism from the body, permits its continued presence in the body long after initial infection or exposure.

Allan Shor, a South African investigator, first demonstrated the presence of the organism within the atherosclerotic plaque itself using electronmicrographs. This was later confirmed by Dr. Joseph Muhlestein and his co-workers when they examined the atherosclerotic crud removed from ninety patients during surgery.[302] Using an immunofluorescence technique, they found that 70 percent of the specimens contained the *Chlamydia* organism. Similar results have been confirmed using a variety of sophisticated techniques, including electron microscopy, immunocytochemistry, direct immunofluorescence, polymerase chain reaction, and in one patient, by direct culture.

All very impressive, but the possibility still existed that it could just be an inactive coincidental organism that had nothing to do with the atherosclerotic process. In other words, *C. pneumonia* could simply be a free rider. Final proof depended on the ability to experimentally produce atherosclerosis in animals by infecting them with the *Chlamydia* organism.

Initial attempts did produce mild atherosclerotic lesions, but overall, the results were not very impressive. Dr. Muhlestein then wondered if there could be an interplay between high cholesterol levels and the infection. He repeated the experiment using rabbits, this time feeding the animals a diet high in cholesterol before infecting them with the organism. The combination produced significantly accelerated atherosclerosis. It should be noted that these animals were infected in the same way that humans would be, by entry of the bacteria into the body through the nose.

As persuasive as the evidence was, the real question remained: could eradicating the organism help prevent atherosclerosis in people? The idea was tested in sixty male patients with stable coronary heart disease. Twenty patients were used as placebos and forty were given an antibiotic known to kill *Chlamydia*. At the end of the study, those receiving the antibiotics had significantly fewer episodes of heart ischemia than did the controls. This study was repeated with similar results in 202 patients in Buenos Aires.

Chlamydia is a very unusual organism. Unlike conventional organisms, it can exist outside the cell in a spore-like form part of the time and then enter the cell, change form, and take over the cell's metabolism. When it is within the cell it can again change form, become inactive, and in this form effectively hide from the immune system, as well as become resistant to antibiotics. In this state it is called a persistent body.

It is for this latter reason that *Chlamydia* is so hard to treat. First, we do not know if antibiotics can penetrate deep enough into the plaque to kill the organism, and second, we do not know how long we should treat someone to assure that all the organisms have been killed. After all, we have to wait for the dormant organisms to reactivate before they can be killed.

Other infectious organisms are also suspect. One of the most obvious is the cytomegalovirus, a member of the herpes virus family. Many people carry this virus silently within their cells. When the immune system is impaired, the virus can activate and cause significant illness and even result in death. On some occasions, the virus can, instead of causing an acute illness with fever, chills, and muscle aches, result in a chronic infection that produces slow pathological changes in tissues, such as we see with atherosclerosis.

The strongest evidence comes from cardiac transplant patients, who frequently develop a rapidly progressive occlusion of their coronary arteries. Furthermore, patients who receive hearts from persons infected with the virus are more likely to reject the transplanted heart and to develop rapid atherosclerotic occlusion.

One study looked at patients with coronary heart disease and found that these patients were positive for the virus in 90 percent of cases, versus 60 percent in controls. Finally, chickens infected with a cancer-causing herpes virus were also found to have profound atherosclerosis throughout all their blood vessels.[303]

Scientists are now looking at several other organisms as possible causes of atherosclerosis. For example, the *Helicobacter pylori* organism is now known to be the causative organism in most cases of gastric ulcer and a particular form of stomach cancer. Another bacterium, *Nanobacterium sanguineum*, is smaller than many viruses, can change shape with ease, and appears to be involved in the calcification of arterial walls and heart valves. Incredibly, this bacterium can coat itself with calcium and embed itself deep within the arterial wall. In such a state, it cannot be killed by antibiotics or the immune system, and is even resistant to hydrochloric acid and formaldehyde. There is mounting evidence that it is also associated with renal stones, dental stones, plaque, and even brain calcification. Several laboratories can now test for the presence of the organism.

The bottom line is that while infection of the blood-vessel wall may not itself cause severe atherosclerosis, when combined with one or more of the other risk factors mentioned, it may greatly accelerate the process. This makes sense, because the immune attack against these organisms initiates the release of tremendous amounts of free radicals from macrophages, which in turn oxidize the LDL cholesterol. Because the infection persists for such a long period of time, the destruction is extensive. We see a similar process in the nervous system with neurodegenerative diseases.

This mechanism might also explain the effectiveness of flavonoids, vitamins, and garlic in reducing the incidence of heart attacks and strokes, and in preventing atherosclerosis in general. All of these nutraceuticals, especially vitamin C and garlic extract, have antibacterial and antiviral properties. By taking them daily, you keep your blood and tissue levels high, which kills and inhibits the growth of these viruses and bacteria over a prolonged period of time.

It has been shown that, unlike antibiotics, bacteria never become resistant to products such as garlic. In addition, not only are there far fewer side effects with natural products, they help your body in numerous other ways. For example, vitamins C and E and garlic all improve immune activity, protect against oxidation, and improve cellular function.

Processed Foods and Sugar

Current rates of vascular disease are peculiar to modern societies, and a careful examination of the contributing reasons for this sudden explosion of cardiovascular and cerebrovascular diseases indicates that the introduction of processed foods at the turn of the century has played a major role. This is not to say that the trend was all bad. Processing foods was initially a two-edged sword: it did improve the nutrition of millions of city dwellers, who, prior to refrigeration and food processing, did not have access to a wide variety of fruits and vegetables.

The problem is that over the years, large numbers of people have begun to depend totally on processed foods for nutrition—while the nutritional quality of processed food has fallen dramatically. These foods contain more sugar, more oxidized oils and fewer essential nutrients than ever before. More recently, food processors have engaged in the genetic manipulation of foods, creating a set of problems never before faced by man. And if that were not enough, processors also add enormous quantities of food additives, many of which have never been tested for human safety.

Sugar consumption in this country has increased over 2,500 percent since the turn of the century! In fact, there is a better correlation between excess consumption of refined sugar and heart disease than there is with cholesterol consumption. Excess sugar consumption also increases blood triglycerides, produces disease-causing cross-links in proteins, inhibits immune function, and interferes with vitamin C transport.

Protein cross-linking, a process that interferes with protein function in cells, is a particularly dangerous result of excess sugar consumption. Many of the affected proteins are enzymes essential to proper energy generation and metabolic function within cells. Sugar also interacts with proteins and DNA bases (resulting in advanced glycation end products or AGEs), greatly increasing the risk of oxidation: one of the most damaging events associated with diabetes.

In addition, high glucose intake stimulates insulin release, which activates a set of substances (eicosanoids) that promote inflammation in tissues, including arteries. And we already know that chronic inflammation within arteries is a major cause of atherosclerosis. Because high-sugar diets interfere with vitamin C absorption, antioxidant defenses are lowered, increasing the likelihood that LDL cholesterol, as well as triglycerides, will oxidize.

So you can see that there is a lot more to atherosclerosis than merely eating too much cholesterol-containing food. Cholesterol blood levels will increase from eating foods high in cholesterol in only one in five hundred people. The rest of us are protected genetically. Of course, this does not mean that you should gobble up all the high cholesterol foods you can, since such foods can produce other deleterious effects.

Fruits, Vegetables, and Atherosclerosis

Dr. Barry Halliwell and his co-workers, some years ago, examined the advanced atherosclerotic plaques from autopsied persons and measured their free-radical content using sophisticated methods. They found that the "crud" from these arteries contained high levels of iron and copper, both of which are powerful free-radical generators, in addition to other oxidation substances. In other words, the crud was a hot spot of free-radical activity. The question that arose was: is this a late event, or did these free radicals play a part in the process itself? Examination of very early atherosclerotic lesions (fatty streaks) yielded the same findings.

One of the main culprits associated with hardening of the arteries is high levels of *oxidized* LDL cholesterol. It is impossible to overstate how important this concept is: high levels of oxidized LDL cholesterol are dangerous, but *unoxidized* LDL cholesterol appears to be harmless, even if levels are high. The real reason that high LDL cholesterol is associated with heart disease is simply that the more LDL cholesterol you have floating around in your blood stream, the higher the likelihood that some of it will become oxidized.

LDL cholesterol has its own internal antioxidant protection system. Key to this protection is vitamin E, a very powerful and efficient antioxidant, especially in protecting fats from oxidation. Normally, there are six molecules of vitamin E incorporated in LDL's molecular structure. But, the LDL molecule contains other antioxidants that also play a significant role in protecting it from oxidizing. These include vitamin C, the carotenoids and plant-based flavonoids. Early in the 1930s, it was shown that individuals with high intakes of vitamin C had significantly lower risk of heart attacks. This observation has stood the test of time. Vitamin C probably protects against atherosclerosis, at least in part, by regenerating vitamin E's antioxidant capability.

Plants contain thousands of antioxidants, mostly in the form of complex chemicals called flavonoids. The carotenoids in particular play a vital part in protecting us from LDL cholesterol oxidation. You may have heard of beta-carotene, but others such as alpha carotene, lutein, lycopene, canthoxanthin, zeaxanthin, and cryptoxanthin are also important.

Studies testing the ability of individual phytochemicals to inhibit LDL oxidation have shown either minor effects or no effect at all. One thing we have learned recently is that antioxidants when combined have a much greater effect than when tested individually, a property called synergy (the sum is greater than its parts). By combining a little of each, we have tremendous protection against the oxidative process associated with atherosclerosis. Those whose diets are composed of French fries, red meat, diet sodas, and junk foods are severely deficient in these vital protective molecules.

The Nurses' Health Study, which involved seventy-five thousand women ages thirty-four to fifty-nine followed for fourteen years (beginning in 1976), found that one serving a day of cruciferous vegetables (broccoli, cauliflower, brussels sprouts, and cabbage) reduced stroke incidence by 32 percent.[304] I have already said that anything less than five servings of fruits and vegetables a day provides no health benefits, and it is important to note that this study focused on the most nutrient-dense vegetables. Other studies—which have not produced such impressive results—have not discriminated among low- and high-nutrient vegetables (French fries, for instance, provide almost no nutritional value). The Nurses' study also found that leafy green vegetables, citrus fruits, and fruit juices provided protection.

Omega-3 Fatty Acids

One of the most interesting relationships between diet and vascular disease is the effect of omega-3 fatty acids on atherosclerosis. It was observed many years ago that Eskimos have a very low incidence of atherosclerosis, despite the fact that their traditional diet is extremely high in fats and devoid of fruits and vegetables. They also do not suffer from autoimmune diseases, such as rheumatoid arthritis and lupus. However, when they adopt a typical Western diet, they develop all of the diseases we do, and at the same statistical rate within the population.

Omega-3 fatty acids in the Eskimo diet come mainly from fish and whale blubber, and studies on this form of fat have indicated several remarkable properties: it is a mild blood anticoagulant, reduces inflammation by changing eicosanoid balance, and alters immunity, all things that potentially could reduce atherosclerosis. This finding led researchers and clinicians to test the results of adding omega-3 fatty acids to the diets of other populations. They found that omega-3 fatty acids eventually replaced the bad fats in cells and tissues of test subjects.

Some early studies seemed to indicate omega-3 fatty acids had a protective effect against heart attacks and strokes, but different studies produced conflicting results. Some demonstrated a dramatic reduction in heart attacks and strokes, others a minor effect, and some no effect at all. One of the problems with the negative studies was that olive oil was used as a control. Even at that time, it was known that olive oil has slight anticoagulant properties. Thus the control was not a placebo control at all: it is physiologically active, as are many such placebos.

One extremely large study involving 22,070 male physicians between the ages of forty and eighty-four years of age found that eating one fish per week reduced the incidence of sudden cardiac death by 52 percent.[305] This is a dramatic reduction when you consider 250,000 people die of a sudden cardiac arrest every year, and that 55 percent of those people have had no previous history of heart disease. Most will die before reaching the hospital, and the survival rate is a dismal 30 percent for those who do make it to a hospital alive.

Interestingly, researchers found that the number of heart attacks was not reduced among test participants who consumed fish, but the incidence of sudden death associated with the event was lowered dramatically. They hypothesized that sudden death was caused by arrhythmia, which is powerfully inhibited by omega-3 fatty acids even at low concentrations.[306] But some scientists have questioned the hypothesis that the main benefit provided by omega-3 fatty acids is related to arrhythmia reduction: in the study, the men who experienced the greatest benefits from increased omega-3 consumption also had the highest pre-existing incidences of hypertension, higher cholesterol levels, and a family history of heart disease. In other words, since they were already at significantly greater risk of coronary heart disease, the individual benefit was statistically greater than that reflected in the reported results.

Another stronger bit of information supporting the broader benefits of omega-3 fatty acid consumption comes from the Western Electric Study, which looked at the relation between fish consumption and coronary heart deaths among 1,822 men followed for thirty years.[307] This study looked at heart failure, rather than sudden death, and found that participants with the highest fish consumption were the least likely to suffer coronary heart failure.

Analysis of the effects of consuming large amounts of omega-3 fatty acids in persons with high triglyceride levels demonstrates that the fish oils can significantly lower these levels, as well as significantly improve blood flow (by reducing blood viscosity) and raising HDL levels.[308]

A more recent analysis demonstrated that the two components of fish oils, EPA (eicosapentaenoic acid) and DHA (docosahexaenoic acid), have important differential effects.[309] While this study found no difference in the respective capacities of the two fatty acid components to lower total cholesterol, only DHA was shown to raise a particular type of HDL cholesterol—a subfraction called HDL_2—which is protective against atherosclerotic vascular disease. In fact, DHA consumption increased HDL_2 levels by 29 percent.

DHA also increased the levels of the larger LDL particle. This is important because recent studies have found that the size of the LDL particle is very important in atherosclerosis. Small LDL particles increase atherosclerosis and large ones may actually be protective. Unfortunately, doctors rarely order the test that differentiates the two forms of LDL cholesterol.

Other important differences were discovered over the course of the study. For example, one of the drawbacks of high omega-3 fatty acid intake is its effect on glucose tolerance, especially in type II diabetes. Some studies have shown that high intake of fish oils can impair glucose control, worsening this form of diabetes. This study has shown the effect occurs only with EPA, and not DHA. Interestingly, even with EPA, this negative effect on glucose control can be avoided by *moderate* exercise. I should emphasize that EPA does not cause problems with glucose control in normal individuals, only type II diabetics.

There is also some evidence that EPA reduces platelet adhesiveness, which is advantageous since platelet clumping is linked to an increased risk of sudden heart attack or stroke. Still, I recommend patients supplement their diets either with DHA only or with low EPA/DHA fish oils. This is because the Western Electric Study cited above also demonstrated that about 9 percent of DHA is metabolized back to EPA in amounts normally found in the body, providing exactly the right balance of EPA's clot-inhibiting effects. Therefore, DHA alone has all the properties that we desire from omega-3 fatty acids, such as beneficial anti-inflammatory, immune-modulating, antidepressant, and anticancer effects, as well as brain protection.

After reviewing the scientific literature, I think DHA-supplementation is an acceptable practice, and a safer alternative to food-source omega-3 fatty acids. Vegetarians will certainly appreciate this fact since DHA is derived from an algae, and not from fish. In fact, fish get their DHA from algae.

Some studies have shown that flaxseed oil provides the same benefits as fish oils.[310] But, while some people, especially young healthy individuals, may derive the same benefits from either source, this is not true for everyone. Because flaxseed oil is high in alpha-linolenic acid, a fatty-acid precursor of EPA and DHA, it must first be converted to omega-3 fatty acid by the enzyme, delta-6 desaturase, which is naturally deficient in the very young, in the elderly, and in those with chronic illnesses. EPA has also been shown to interfere with delta-6 desaturase's ability to convert alpha-linolenic acid to omega-3.

Not All Exercise Is Good Exercise

It seems to make sense that exercise would reduce the risk of heart attack and stroke, but this actually depends on a variety of factors. The truth is that extreme exercise is fraught with dangers: exercising vigorously can actually cause an aneurysm to burst or even cause a fragile, atherosclerotic blood vessel to rupture. Furthermore, if done improperly, intense exercise can actually worsen atherosclerosis by increasing free-radical generation and lipid peroxidation.

As you will recall in our discussion from chapter one, the main source of free radicals— those angry little molecular particles that attempt to destroy everything in our cells, DNA, membranes, and proteins—is metabolism itself. When we exercise, we increase our metabolism. And intense exercise increases metabolism dramatically and for many hours afterward, which can do a lot of damage to our cell membranes, metabolic enzymes, and DNA. Remember, while we can repair a lot of this damage, the unrepaired portion accumulates.

Numerous studies have shown that extreme exercise can depress the immune system and dramatically increase free-radical injury to all organs and tissues, increasing the risk of degenerative diseases. In females, extreme exercise can suppress reproductive hormones, leading to amenorrhea–absence of menstruation. We also know that exercise causes the brain to release special neurohormones called endorphins. Like their cousin, morphine, they reduce pain, elevate mood—and are addictive.

Long-distance runners who are forced to stop exercising suddenly can experience the same symptoms as addicts withdrawing from morphine or other opiates. They can have stomach cramping, severe depression, irritability, and difficulty thinking. Their craving for the "fix" of exercise is so powerful that they will run even when injured. Many extreme athletes have noticed that when they are forced to quit their exercise program they acquire numerous aches and pains that they never experienced before. This is because endorphins killed the pain during their intense exercise and for many hours afterwards. Once the endorphins are removed, all of the injuries that were sustained during the years of exercise become obvious.

There are also several cases of marathon runners developing rapidly advancing Parkinson's disease and even sudden death from heart attacks. Most of us have noticed that long distance joggers and marathon runners often look haggard and older than their chronological age. This is because of accumulated free-radical damage.

The Good News

But don't get the idea that because intense exercise can cause damage, you shouldn't exercise at all. Studies examining levels of physical fitness and physical activity indicate that for both men and women, sedentary lifestyle is associated with increased mortality from cardiovascular disease.[311] When comparing physical fitness, dramatic differences are seen between mortality rates of fit men and women and the more sedentary.

The least fit men are six times more likely to die from coronary heart disease than the most fit, while the least fit women have five times the risk. Interestingly, studies comparing physical activity (low, moderate, or high) in women found higher mortality in those engaged in high activity than those at moderate activity. In essence, what was important was being fit, and fitness can be obtained by moderate exercise.

More recently, the association between physical activity and fitness, and mortality from all causes, was confirmed in a study using twins.[312] The value of the twin study was to reduce the influence of genetics in determining mortality, since identical twins share the same chromosomal pattern. In this study, the twins who exercised vigorously demonstrated significantly lower mortality from all causes than did their more sedentary matched twins. This was true even when all other possible contributing factors were considered, such as smoking, alcohol use, and occupation.

It should be noted that in this study vigorous exercise was defined as exercising at least six times a month for a mean duration of thirty minutes. Activities included vigorous walking or jogging. There is no evidence that intense aerobic exercise is necessary for good cardio-vascular health, and in my opinion, should be avoided, especially after age forty.

It has been known for some time that Seventh Day Adventists, who strictly adhere to a health-promoting vegetarian diet, have the lowest mortality rates of any population group studied.[313] Their program disallows smoking, alcohol, and coffee. In addition, those who added moderate to high-level physical activity have an even greater increase in longevity.[314] It's important to note that what this study defined as "high-level activity" was actually moderate exercise.

Based on this information, we can draw some conclusions about appropriate levels of exercise. One important thing to remember is to tailor your exercise to your age and overall health. While young people can exercise for two to three hours daily without any untoward effects, after age thirty, you must slow down the pace. One hour of moderately strenuous exercise every other day (or daily, depending on your conditioning), is highly beneficial without being damaging. After age forty, most people find one hour every other day suffi-cient for health conditioning. The elderly should temper their exercise program to their conditioning. Some are able to follow the same exercise program as forty-year-olds. Others, especially if they have a restricting medical condition, will need to have a lower level program, such as brisk walking, stationary-bike riding, or light weightlifting.

Now let us look at some specific conditions associated with atherosclerosis, and ways in which you can prevent or treat them.

10
Stroke and Heart Attack: Are They Really Inevitable?

Stroke is a general term used to describe any brain injury caused when blood supply to the brain is interrupted, resulting in tissue loss and temporary or permanent impairment of function. It is the third leading cause of death in developed countries, and may result from a variety of factors, including atherosclerosis, heart disease, connective-tissue diseases (lupus, arthritis, etc.), and drug use.

Ninety percent of all strokes are ischemic (dry). An ischemic stroke results when blood flow to the arteries that feed the brain is interrupted. This type of stroke may be caused by a clot that arises within the arteries of the brain itself (thrombus), or a blood clot, plaque, or other blood-borne material that travels from another part of the body into the brain (embolus). Thrombosis is generally attributed to atherosclerosis, while embolisms are linked to heart disease and arrhythmia.

Hemorrhagic strokes account for 10 percent of all strokes and are caused when arteries within the brain form a balloon (aneurysm) that then explodes, or by the rupture of a weakened blood vessel. Apoplexy, or bleeding within the brain, is caused by hemorrhagic stroke. This type of stroke is usually caused by a combination of atherosclerosis and hypertension.

The effect of any kind of stroke depends on what part of the brain is affected, how large a volume of brain tissue is involved, and the overall health of the brain at the time of the stroke. Not all strokes are clinically evident: silent strokes affect parts of the brain that do not produce paralysis or obvious cognitive problems. In fact, a person may suffer many silent strokes before neurological problems occur.

Dry Strokes: Papa Can't Speak

Occlusion of blood vessels to the brain involves either the large blood vessels that feed the brain (two carotid arteries and two vertebral arteries) located in the neck, or a smaller vessel located within the brain itself. The effect of the occlusion depends on the side of the brain affected and the specific functional part of the brain most involved. For example, when the left carotid artery is occluded, the person often suffers from varying degrees of paralysis on the right side of the body, and impaired speech.

Blockage of the right carotid artery, on the other hand, causes a loss of movement on the left side of the body, but does not affect speech. Both types of strokes can also cause a loss of sensation on the affected side of the body. The severity of movement and sensory loss depends on the size of the stroke, and where in the brain it occurs. In general, large strokes can produce complete paralysis that persists indefinitely, whereas smaller strokes may allow full recovery of affected functions. However, some very small strokes, located in brain areas packed tightly with critical neural pathways, can produce severe paralysis, a loss of speech, or other equally devastating effects. Much larger strokes in "silent areas" of the brain may not produce any obvious loss of function.

Not infrequently, a person will suffer from numerous small strokes in "silent areas" of the brain and not even be aware of it. With time, these small strokes (called mini-strokes) accumulate so much damage that the person develops dementia, speech loss, or varying degrees of weakness in the arms and legs. Many such patients are simply labeled Alzheimer's disease, and, as a result, the person is relegated to a life in a total care facility.

It should be remembered that the same process that produces hardening of the arteries in other areas of the body is also responsible for atherosclerosis of the arteries feeding the brain. The really strange thing about atherosclerosis of brain arteries is that it can occur diffusely in all of the blood vessels or can be quite localized, affecting only one or two vessels. Sometimes we see severe arteriosclerotic narrowing of the main arteries in the neck, the carotid arteries, and completely normal arteries in the head itself. Other times, it is just the opposite: the neck arteries are normal and the smaller vessels in the brain are severely affected.

Not all strokes produce paralysis; some may only affect vision or speech. A loss of speech almost always means a stroke has occurred in the left side of the brain, even in left-handed individuals. The loss may be temporary and mild or severe and permanent. Speech is a very complex proposition, involving many areas of the brain. The motor speech area (called Broca's area) is located in the left frontal lobe, while the sensory speech area (Wernicke's area) is located in an area comprising the back part of the temporal lobe and the lower part of the parietal lobe of the brain.

Strokes affecting the motor speech area can result in difficulty saying words, even though you know what you want to say. Strokes in the sensory speech area make it difficult or impossible to understand what someone else says to you. Strangely enough, you may not even know there is a problem. In such cases, the person jabbers away in nonsense syllables that no one can understand, a condition called jargon speech.

Some of the more bizarre effects of strokes include an inability to recognize the face of someone familiar, or an inability to tell the right hand from the left. A particular combination of symptoms—loss of the ability to name objects (anomia), recognize your own arm or leg on one side as being yours (apraxia), and an inability to do math (acalcula)—is called Gerstman's syndrome.

Strokes involving the brain stem can cause a number of complex clinical disorders involving the cranial nerves, motor pathways, autonomic system, and sensory pathways. Severe occlusions of the blood vessels feeding the brain stem can result in a strange state called the "locked-in syndrome." In this disorder, the person is essentially paralyzed from the chin down, unable to speak or swallow, yet they remain fully conscious and can communicate by blinking their eyes. Fortunately, most that survive a brain stem stroke eventually improve.

With most strokes there are warning signs, especially when larger arteries in the neck are involved. Initial symptoms may include brief spells of being unable to speak, or being unable to understand what someone says to you. In other cases, numbness, usually starting in the extremities and ascending towards the body, appears in brief spells. Weakness or even temporary paralysis can also occur, with a complete recovery between spells. These spells of neurological symptoms, called transient ischemic attacks or TIAs, can occur many times a day or may occur only once before the main stroke hits. Usually, these spells are brief, passing in a few seconds or minutes.

TIAs are warning signs and should not be ignored! But, human nature being the way it is, especially in men, we tend to ignore the spell and trust that it will eventually go away. Several factors—especially allowing oneself to become dehydrated—can precipitate the final event. Most of us do not drink enough water and as a result, our blood becomes more viscous, increasing the likelihood that a clot will suddenly form at the site of a plaque formation.

A very common cause of sudden clotting of the blood in these partially occluded vessels is eating a fatty meal. When fat floods the blood stream following such a meal, a hormone called thromboxane is released, which causes the arteries to constrict and clot more easily. This is why both heart attacks and strokes frequently follow a big meal. When you combine viscous blood with a fatty meal, your risk increases.

Some have proposed taking a single aspirin in the event of a TIA. This can stave off a stroke in many cases, but if a stroke occurs anyway, taking aspirin may convert a simple stroke into a catastrophic cerebral hemorrhage, where there is bleeding deep in the brain. The risk is probably less than the stroke, but it should be considered.

Appearances Can Be Deceiving

When a blood vessel feeding the brain is closed off, the cells fed by that artery begin to lower their metabolism. On the border zone between the territory of the blocked artery and the normal brain, changes begin to take place. Here the brain cells have not been denied blood, but their supply is less than optimal. In response, these neurons and astrocytes begin to release glutamate.

As you will recall, glutamate is a powerful brain toxin when released in higher concentrations than the brain can utilize. Glutamate levels around these neurons rise quickly, and they begin to fire impulses very rapidly, exhausting themselves and eventually dying. Glutamate from these dead and dying neurons and astrocytes seeps into the surrounding normal brain, causing more brain cells to die. Soon, the area of brain death is many times larger than the zone supplied by the artery. The only reason the process doesn't continue to spread is that in areas with normal blood flow the excess glutamate is carried away.

When released in large concentrations, glutamate greatly increases free-radical production leading to further injury to the brain, blood vessels, and the blood-brain barrier. The blood-brain barrier keeps excess glutamate from the blood stream out of the brain, and this is especially critical during a stroke or any brain injury.

Because of this injury to the blood-brain barrier, any increase in blood glutamate or aspartate will increase the likelihood of greater damage to the part of the brain injured by stroke. Many of the liquid nutritional diets given to hospitalized stroke patients contain substantial levels of free glutamate and/or aspartate. Even as they start to recover, stroke patients are often fed foods containing the additive MSG. This not only increases the likelihood for increased brain injury, but also increases the likelihood of a seizure.

Because of brain swelling caused by the stroke or pre-existing hypertension, many of these patients are given powerful diuretics. To combat swelling, neurosurgeons and neurologists will also resort to the use of steroids. Both diuretics and steroids lower brain levels of magnesium. This, in turn, increases the likelihood of blood vessel spasm and damage to the brain by glutamate and other excitotoxins. Magnesium, as we have seen before, plays a vital role in protecting the brain from glutamate toxicity.

So, the amount of brain killed by a lack of blood supply is actually much smaller than the volume of brain killed during the stroke. Although you may not think so, this is good news, because it means something can be done to reverse the process.

Another phenomenon associated with ischemic strokes is the ischemia/reperfusion effect. Experiments on animals have shown that inducing ischemia by clamping a vessel supplying blood to any tissue, and then opening the blood vessel back up within thirty minutes (reperfusion), actually makes the damage worse, not better. Recent studies have provided an explanation for this anti-intuitive phenomenon.

Sometimes, especially in medicine, what seems logical just isn't so. It would make sense that when you shut off the blood supply to a part of the brain, the cells fed by that blood vessel would die from a lack of oxygen and fuel. And, if that were true, there would be little you could do to improve the situation following a stroke. After all, cells cannot live without oxygen for more than thirty minutes. Fortunately, it is a lot more complicated than that.

When the vessel is shut off, the changes I described in the first part of this section begin to take place. However, once the blood vessel is opened back up, the sudden rush of oxygen-containing blood dramatically increases free-radical production. These free radicals are very destructive and begin to severely damage or even kill cells within the affected tissue.

The reason this is so important is that we now have a way to open up blood vessels following a stroke or a heart attack using digestive enzymes, such as urokinase. But this only works if done within four hours of a stroke, and doctors must be very careful not to make the patient worse by flooding the stroked area of brain with free radicals. To prevent this, we use powerful antioxidants, at least experimentally.

Although some people will experience TIAs days or weeks before a stroke, most people do not experience any warning signs. This is why it is vital to keep your antioxidant defenses strong at all times. First of all, if you keep your antioxidants high, you are unlikely to have a stroke in the first place. If it does happen, your stroke will be much milder and you will most likely make a good recovery with few, if any, neurological deficits.

In fact in one experiment, when antioxidants were combined with excitotoxin-blocking agents, protection was even greater.[315] Animal experiments, in which the powerful antioxidant alpha-lipoic acid was given several hours before stroke was induced, demonstrate that damage is dramatically reduced. But, the secret with alpha-lipoic acid is that it has to be given *before* the stroke. This is because alpha-lipoic acid itself is not an antioxidant, but once in the tissues it is quickly converted into the form, DHLA (dehydrolipoic acid), that is a very powerful and versatile antioxidant.

The same is true for magnesium. Several studies have shown that by elevating magnesium levels you can reduce the volume of brain injury caused by a stroke by close to 50 percent.

Because we often get little warning of these impending disasters, good nutrition is essential to a good outcome. Numerous studies have shown the value of nutritional supplementation and a healthy diet in not only preventing strokes of all kinds, but also in reducing their severity. The longer you utilize a program of good nutrition, the greater your protection against all manner of disease.

Wet Strokes: Something Just Popped in My Head

A rupture of an artery in the head happens suddenly—without the possible warning signs associated with ischemic stroke—and is usually catastrophic. The unfortunate person grabs his or her head, cries out, and falls to the ground unconscious. Frequently, he or she will develop a sudden, excruciating headache that builds unrelentingly over the next several minutes. Some say later they felt something "pop" in their heads. Gradually, they develop weakness on one side of the body, followed quickly by a deepening loss of consciousness. Within hours, they stop breathing and if nothing is done to relieve the pressure caused by hemorrhaging within the brain, they die.

Several conditions can cause ruptured blood vessels in the head. One of the most common is breakage of a blood vessel weakened by long-standing atherosclerosis. Usually, but not always, this is complicated, or even precipitated, by high blood pressure. The pressure of the blood pounding against the weakened wall of the blood vessels eventually breaks through, spilling blood, under great pressure, into the brain.

Usually the broken blood vessels are one of a series of tiny arteries located deep in the white matter of the brain (called lenticulostriate arteries). The reason these arteries are so prone to break is that they arise straight off the first branches of the carotid arteries, just as they enter the base of the skull. This means that they receive the full pressure of the pumping heart. Hemorrhages from these arteries are usually devastating, because they dissect deep into the center portions of the brain hemispheres. In the case of large hemorrhages, only emergency surgery can save the life of the person afflicted. Smaller hemorrhages can be treated without surgery, and patients generally make a good recovery.

One of the problems seen in those who make good recoveries from such hemorrhages is that most will hemorrhage again within several years of the original bleeding episode. This is because nothing has been done to strengthen these arteries, or in far too many cases, to reverse the high blood pressure. Nutritionally, both of these goals can be reached in a majority of cases.

A second common cause for sudden brain hemorrhages is a ruptured aneurysm. An aneurysm is a bulging artery at a site where a blood vessel has thinned. The mechanism is much like a tire blowout. The tire has a weak spot that begins to bulge out, then grows, getting thinner and thinner, until it finally explodes with a loud pop.

Brain aneurysms may exist from birth, follow an injury to the head, or be the result of an infection. Most are considered to be congenital weak spots on brain arteries. Over time, constant pounding of the blood against the weak spot causes it to bulge and eventually to rupture. Like the arteriosclerotic rupture of blood vessels, aneurysms can also be strengthened nutritionally, so that at least we may be able to reduce their chances of rupture.

The rupture of an aneurysm is a catastrophic event. Several patients I have treated say they felt something pop in their head, followed by the worst headache they had ever experienced. Within a short period of time they experience a stiff neck and, like the arteriosclerotic rupture, they may experience a loss of consciousness. Treatment may involve surgical clipping of the aneurysm, or occlusion with a radiographically guided balloon. Unfortunately, about 30 percent of people who suffer such a rupture die before reaching the hospital.

One of the big problems seen by neurosurgeons in treating aneurysms is the development of spasms of the blood vessels containing the aneurysm. In some instances, all of the blood vessels in the brain go into severe spasms (vasospasm). This is the leading cause of death in aneurysm patients.

During my neurosurgical practice, I found that early treatment of aneurysm patients with high-dose magnesium significantly reduced the incidence and severity of this dreaded complication. Magnesium deficiency is linked to the incidence of these fatal spasms: those with the most severe deficiency are likely to suffer the most intense and widespread spasm.

I have also found, and this has been confirmed in the neurosurgical scientific literature, that antioxidants reduce blood-vessel spasm following hemorrhage. One of the most useful antioxidants, alpha-lipoic acid, was quite successful in preventing spasms of blood vessel, and reducing brain swelling, another severe complication of ruptured aneurysms.

Several drugs have been developed by the pharmaceutical companies to combat vasospasm. They are all very expensive and work no better than magnesium, which is very inexpensive and has few complications. Both work by the same mechanism: blocking calcium entry into endothelial cells. Magnesium blocks the glutamate receptor, which is one of the mechanisms used to control calcium entry into cells.

Abnormally functioning mitochondria also play a role in vasospasm, since mitochondria play such an important role in calcium control once it enters the cell. Acetyl-L-carnitine, alpha-lipoic acid, and other mitochondrial nutritional factors also enhance calcium control, and hence reduce vasospasm.

It has been known for some time that the reason so many surviving aneurysm patients do so poorly is the high incidence of brain infarctions (strokes) caused by the spasm, virtually shutting down the blood supply to critical areas of the brain. As we shall see, these micro-strokes can also be prevented or their severity reduced by nutritional means. The same principles are true for multiple small strokes as with strokes caused by atherosclerosis.

Thinning the Blood to Prevent a Stroke

Many doctors place their high-risk patients on anticoagulants. Various anti-clotting drugs are used, such as Plavix or Persantine. Unfortunately, these drugs also have some major complications including aplastic anemia, extreme fatigue, and even leukemia. Aspirin is safer than these prescription drugs, but it is associated with gastrointestinal hemorrhages, ulcer activation, and kidney damage.

Of greater concern is the risk of hemorrhagic strokes in persons who take aspirin regularly. One of the largest stroke-prevention studies using aspirin, the Physicians' Health Study, involved 22,000 physicians and found that patients taking aspirin had twice as many brain hemorrhages as those who did not take aspirin.

Another double-blind, randomized study involving one hundred people with TIAs, showed that those on vitamin E (400 IU) and aspirin at the same time experienced a significant reduction in strokes as compared to those on aspirin alone.[316] Also, the number of hemor-rhages in those on the vitamin E/aspirin combination was no higher than in patients taking aspirin alone.

The problem with taking aspirin alone to prevent either a heart attack or stroke is that aspirin does nothing to strengthen the blood vessel itself. And, weakened blood vessels usually accompany atherosclerosis, especially in smokers. With the blood thinned and the wall of the vessel weakened, you have the perfect set-up for a brain hemorrhage. So what should you do?

We know that several natural products thin the blood and strengthen blood-vessel walls. One of the most useful is the herb, Ginkgo biloba. Several components in the Ginkgo extract inhibit platelet-activating factor (PAF) in the same way that aspirin does.[317] Unlike aspirin, Ginkgo also contains numerous flavonoids that protect the weakened vessel from further damage by free radicals. In addition, it directly strengthens the collagen and elastin in the blood vessel walls.[318]

Other natural products have the same effect. Pycnogenol and grape-seed extract, bind tightly to the collagen in blood vessels, protecting it from further damage both by free radicals and an enzyme called collagenase. These products have also have been shown to inhibit stress and smoking-related platelet activation, that is, clotting of the blood at sites of blood vessel injury. At a dose of 100 mg, pycnogenol was found to be extremely effective in preventing platelet activation, but did not increase bleeding, as was seen with aspirin.

Pycnogenol and grape-seed extract have the added advantage of powerfully inhibiting gluta-mate-induced excitotoxicity, which as we have seen, plays a major role in the brain injury caused by strokes. In addition, pycnogenol produces relaxation of the smooth muscle in blood vessels, thereby increasing blood flow.

The flavonoids quercetin and curcumin protect blood vessels by neutralizing free radicals, chelating iron, and inhibiting inflammation. Several studies suggest that these flavonoids may be more effective than vitamins in protecting and strengthening blood vessels. Flavonoids also have the added advantage of being powerful anti-carcinogens.

Magnesium also plays a vital role in endothelial cell function. When magnesium levels are low, cells lining the blood vessels malfunction, setting the stage for atherosclerosis. Magnesium also prevents dangerous artery spasms, which can cause strokes directly.[319]

Copper and zinc are also essential for maintaining the strength of blood vessels. Research has shown that animals deficient in copper develop very fragile blood vessels. Recent studies have shown that copper is important in preventing the microvessels from leaking abnormally, and in maintaining normal smooth muscle reaction in blood vessels.[320] The same is true for zinc, a major nutrient needed for collagen strength. Excess copper is harmful, since, like iron, it is a major generator of free radicals. This, again, emphasizes the impor-tance of laboratory testing of blood levels to safely correct these imbalances.

The types of fats present in the body play a major role in protection against atherosclerosis. Several studies have shown that supplementing the diet with omega-3 fatty acids can reduce the incidence of ischemic strokes. The Eskimo-population study I cited above showed that members of this group rarely experience ischemic strokes, yet, like those who take an aspirin a day, they have the highest incidence of hemorrhagic strokes in the world. This should not be surprising because, while Eskimos eat a lot of healthy omega-3 fatty acids, which contain the clotting inhibitor, EPA, they also eat very few vegetables or fruits. Therefore, their bodies are deficient in necessary flavonoids and blood-vessel-strengthening vitamins and minerals.

The amino acid, taurine, may also play a vital role in preventing thrombosis. One study found that taurine supplementation significantly reduced thrombosis associated with heart attacks, and improved the effectiveness of thrombolytic enzymes (urokinase) in opening up coronary arteries following a heart attack.

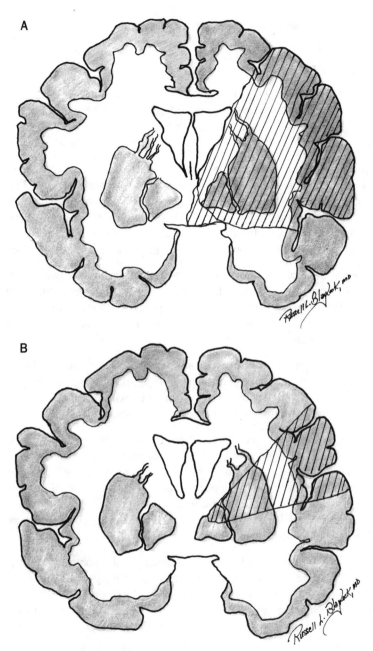

FIGURE 10.1 Cross-section demonstrating the dramatic effect of magnesium and antioxidants on the volume of brain destroyed by a stroke. "A" shows a stroke resulting in a subject deficient in magnesium and/or antioxidants. "B" shows the same stroke model in a subject given additional magnesium and/or antioxidants. Note that the amount of brain tissue destroyed by the stroke is over 50% smaller in the subject receiving magnesium and/or antioxidants.

If You Have a Stroke ...

In case of a stroke, it is vital that the brain has DHA for repair. Also needed are the phospho-lipids, such as phosphotidylcholine, phosphotidylserine and phosphotidylethanolamine. Several studies have shown that supplementing brain-injured animals and humans with these phospholipids improves recovery time and the degree of recovery.

The dose will depend on response. Since phosphotidylcholine also is converted to the neuro-transmitter, acetylcholine, it can affect muscles as well as the brain. To begin, I suggest two 750 mg capsules, twice a day (3,000 mg). Increase to two capsules three times (4,500 mg) a day as tolerated, but you may experience muscle spasms if you take more than your body needs. If that happens, cut back the dose to one or two capsules. Choline itself will also increase brain acetylcholine levels, but you will not have the benefit of the phospholipids.

One fairly recent study from Poland found that a complex made of silymarin and lecithin had very powerful anti-atherosclerotic effects in experimental animals, more so than when each was given alone. The supplement complex also improved liver detoxification, normal-ized lipid metabolism, and corrected histologic changes in the animals' aortas. Further tests are being conducted on this complex.

Another supplement associated with acetylcholine levels in the brain is DMAE. Problems with muscle cramping are greater with this supplement. I would suggest no more than one 150 mg capsule twice a day (300 mg daily) when taken with the phosphotidylcholine. If muscle spasms become a problem, drop the DMAE completely.

Garlic is also an extremely important natural product that can produce important health benefits for those suffering from atherosclerosis. Interestingly, garlic extract is one of the few substances we know of that not only is capable of arresting atherosclerosis, but actually reversing it! The benefits of garlic are numerous and include: dilation of coronary arteries (by stimulating the production of nitric oxide), by acting as an antibiotic, lowering choles-terol, and as an antioxidant. It also improves endothelial cell function, which as we have seen, is vital to normal blood flow to organs and tissues.

Two supplements, nicotinamide and acetyl-L-carnitine, hold much promise in preventing stroke damage. An Italian study demonstrated that stroke damage in experimental animals was significantly reduced by giving dogs acetyl-L-carnitine shortly after blood flow to the animals' brains was interrupted and then restarted. This occlusion-reperfusion process normally produces increased damage secondary to a dramatic increase in free radicals and lipid peroxidation.[321]

Another study, by Harvard Medical School neurosurgical researchers, found that giving rats nicotinamide even two hours after tying off one of the brain's major arteries dramatically reduced the size of damaged brain.[322] The fact that the supplement worked two hours after occlusion makes it more useful for patients, since most experience at least a one hour delay before being seen by a medical professional.

For a comprehensive list of recommended supplements, see the special section on supplements under the heading Stroke Prevention and Treatment at the end of this chapter.

Other Things of Importance for Stroke Patients

You must maintain a low-fat diet in terms of omega-6 type fats (corn oil, safflower oil, sunflower oil, peanut oil, and canola oil). High intake of these oils inhibits the enzyme that converts alpha-linolenic acid into the omega-3 fatty acid components, EPA and DHA. They also promote inflammation and immune suppression, as well as free-radical production and lipid peroxidation.

Avoid pesticides, herbicides, fluoride, aluminum, and other toxic metals. If you have dental amalgams, especially if they are new, you should be checked for mercury levels. It is also important that you have gastrointestinal functional studies to assure adequate digestion, absorption, and the proper distribution and amounts of "friendly" bacteria in your colon. Yeast overgrowth in the colon can produce serious problems and must be attended to.

Your diet must consist of at least seven servings of fruits and vegetables daily, especially vegetables. Concentrate on eating as many nutrient-dense vegetables as possible. If you do not have a yeast overgrowth, you can also eat less sweet fruits, such as apples, blueberries, strawberries, and blackberries. Avoid over-ripe bananas, since they contain mostly simple sugars.

The injured brain does not tolerate excess sugar very well. Several studies of brain-trauma patients have shown that hyperglycemia can actually increase brain injury. In addition, high sugar intake depresses immunity and increases the formation of glycated cell components, which can increase free-radical injury.

Persons who already have had a stroke should avoid brain stimulants such as caffeine, MSG, and aspartame, all of which can increase the likelihood of a seizure. Smoking—which dramatically increases free-radical generation, reduces blood oxygenation, raises carbon monoxide levels, depresses immunity, and dramatically lowers vitamin C levels—should also be avoided at all costs.

Fruit juices, carbonated beverages, and tap water should also be avoided. Water should either be filtered by reverse osmosis or distilled. If you use reverse osmosis, you will need to change the filter every three months, since fluoride is so caustic that it will quickly erode the filter. In addition, if you distill your own water, you should also run it through a carbon-based filter to remove dissolved industrial chemicals, which can pass with the vapor.

Cardiovascular Disease: Great Killer of an Affluent Society

Cardiovascular disease is responsible for over 900,000 deaths a year, and remains the number one killer of Americans. In addition, over 1.5 million people had a heart attack this past year, and sixty million Americans have high blood pressure. All told, forty million Americans suffer from cardiovascular disease, and many times that number are unaware they are at severe risk of cardiovascular disease.

The same process that causes ischemic strokes also causes heart attacks (called myocardial infarctions or MI in medical lingo)—that is, atherosclerosis. In this case, one or more of the arteries supplying blood to the heart muscle become occluded to the point that a sudden blockage can occur by the formation of a blood clot at the site of the narrowing. Before an MI occurs, the person may experience episodes of sudden pain radiating either down the left arm or into the jaw, much like the warning attacks we see with strokes.

The pain usually lasts for only a few seconds or minutes, but many spells of pain may occur together. The more frequent the painful spells occur, the more likely an impending full-blown heart attack is to develop. As the artery becomes occluded, the person may experience crushing chest pains, shortness of breath, or even sensations similar to indigestion. Occasionally, there is no pain or shortness of breath, something referred to as a silent heart attack, again similar to the silent stroke.

When blockage of the blood supply to the heart muscle occurs, events take place much like those seen in the person having a stroke. The greatest damage to the heart muscle occurs closest to the territory of the blood vessel involved, sort of in a cone-like shape with the tip of the cone at the site of vessel obstruction. Surrounding this core of severely damaged heart tissue is another zone of less damaged heart muscle, also called a penumbra.

As in the case of injured brain during a stroke, damaged heart muscle also begins to release large amounts of free radicals, magnesium levels in the affected muscle falls, and calcium levels in the heart-muscle cells increase. The calcium flowing into the muscle cell triggers numerous destructive reactions including lipid peroxidation.

The low magnesium in the surrounding area next to the damage (called the penumbra area) makes the heart muscle very irritable. This can lead to one of the most common side effects of a heart attack, and one that is the most frequent cause of sudden death, called an arrhythmia (a heart seizure). Supplying extra magnesium immediately after a heart attack can reduce this dangerous side effect.[323] Most likely, those with higher levels of magnesium in their diets, and hence tissues, have less chance of sudden death following a heart attack.

The effects of a heart attack depend on several factors, such as which artery is occluded, how large an area of heart muscle is affected, the nutritional state of the heart muscle before the occlusion, and the state of one's antioxidant defenses. Large heart infarctions are, of course, more likely to result in severe disability or death than smaller infarcts. Yet, sometimes, even small infarcts can cause significant problems to the heart and its owner. A series of nerves courses deep within the heart muscle that regulate the heart beat. If the infarct involves either one or the other of these nerve bundles it can interfere with the heart's ability to beat regularly. We call these "bundle branch blocks."

Like the stroked brain, free radicals accumulating within the heart muscle after a heart attack further damage the heart muscle, long after the blockage has occurred. It has been shown experimentally that by giving an animal high doses of antioxidant vitamins, the amount of heart muscle that is damaged can be substantially reduced.[324] The same is true with magnesium. In fact, both antioxidants and magnesium can reduce the severity of a heart attack injury by almost 50 percent. This can mean the difference between sudden death and surviving with minimal long-term disability.

Protecting the Pump: Heart Failure

The heart works extremely hard. Normally it beats about 100,000 times a day, pumping over 2,000 gallons of blood over tens of thousands of miles of blood vessels throughout the body. This is equal to going around the world twice. When large volumes of heart muscle are damaged by a heart attack, or even a series of smaller heart attacks, the ability of the heart to pump blood is impaired. The heart as a pump may fail for other reasons as well, such as is seen in viral infections of the heart (cardiomyopathy) and as a result of aging changes, or as a result of prolonged hypertension. A study presented at the American College of Cardiology in Detroit of 26,000 people followed over a ten-year period found that the incidence of heart failure was increasing significantly. In fact, since 1989, the number of heart failure cases has doubled! An examination of heart clinics throughout the United States reveals the same dramatic rise in heart failure.

As a result of pump failure, many organs are forced to work with reduced oxygen and nutrient supplies, leading to such problems as shortness of breath with mild exertion, impaired kidney function, and overall fatigue. Gradually the heart begins to enlarge, a condition called congestive heart failure. Because the rest of the body and organs are denied adequate blood supply, free-radical generation increases within these tissues as well. This leads to accelerated aging of the entire body, not just the heart. In time, these organs begin to break down as well, as is seen with kidney failure associated with heart muscle decompensation.

Because the heart has to work so hard, it requires an increased supply of antioxidants and energy supplies. It has been found that falling levels of CoQ10, L-carnitine, and magnesium accompany heart failure. In fact, heart muscle biopsies of cardiac disease patients have shown a CoQ10 deficiency in 50-75 percent of cases, with the levels decreasing greatest with increasing severity of the heart disease.[325] Other studies have shown this energy-supplying coenzyme to be deficient in numerous cardiac disorders such as mitral valve stenosis, angina, cardiomyopathy, and congenital heart defects. Supplementation with CoQ10 and L-carnitine, as well as the other B vitamins, often significantly improves heart muscle contraction and so heart function. This in turn improves the oxygen supply to the other tissues and organs.

Numerous experimental studies have shown the benefits of CoQ10 for strengthening heart muscle. A considerable number of human studies have also shown the benefit of this supplement in improving congestive heart failure. For example, in one study of twenty patients with congestive heart failure who were treated with 30 mg of CoQ10 per day, 55 percent demonstrated improvement in symptoms after two months.[326] Thirty percent of the patients showed a dramatic reduction in fluid buildup in the lungs, a major complication of congestive heart failure.

Some might criticize that more objective testing of heart function would be needed to confirm that the supplement was actually improving heart muscle function. Indeed, examinations measuring stroke volume, cardiac output, ejection fraction, and cardiac index have confirmed that the effect was more than subjective.[327]

In another large study involving multiple medical centers in Italy, 2,664 patients with mild to moderate congestive heart failure were given CoQ10 in doses ranging from 50-150 mg per day. Most (78 percent) received 100 mg per day. Following three months of therapy, the vast majority improved in terms of swelling of extremities, shortness of breath, arrhythmia, heart palpitations, and nighttime urination.[328]

While the most consistent improvements in cardiac function were associated with mild to moderate heart failure, even severe, advanced heart failure patients have responded to this treatment. For example, in one study involving thirty-four patients with highly advanced congestive heart failure, in which cardiologists gave the patients 100 mg per day of CoQ10, 82 percent of the patients showed improved heart function. Equally impressive was the finding that the survival rate two years later was 62 percent—compared to less than 25 percent survival for patients treated with conventional therapy.

CoQ10 has also been shown to reduce significantly the oxidation of LDL cholesterol, a leading culprit in cardiovascular and cerebrovascular disease. In a study done on human volunteers given 300 mg of CoQ10 daily for eleven days, researchers found a fourfold increase in the level of CoQ10 in the blood, and more importantly, within the LDL cholesterol itself.[329] This was found to reduce significantly the risk of the LDL cholesterol becoming oxidized.

So what about the studies that show no effect for CoQ10? (These studies are carried around in the pockets of some skeptical cardiologists.) In most such studies, CoQ10 was given alone. As we have seen throughout this book, nothing in human biology works alone, especially with respect to disease. Congestive heart patients, both because of their disease and the numerous medications given by their doctors, suffer numerous nutritional deficiencies, especially of magnesium. In these studies, little attempt is made to identify these deficiencies, much less to correct them.

In addition, few doctors doing clinical research understand the intricacies of nutritional supplementation. For example, CoQ10 is a fat-soluble substance. Giving it with water results in poor absorption. It must be given with fats, such as phospholipids or extra-virgin olive oil. Dosing is also important. The best results are obtained with higher doses, such as 300-600 mg a day. And finally, if the heart is severely depleted of numerous nutrients, especially L-carnitine, providing CoQ10 will provide far less benefit. Remember these things the next time your cardiologist starts waving his negative study in your face.

It should be appreciated that most cholesterol-lowering drugs also dramatically lower CoQ10 levels. Dr. Karl Folkers, of the University of Texas at Austin, addressed this problem in the journal, *Proceedings of the National Academy of Sciences*, in which he cautioned that as a result of this drug-induced deficiency, patients may experience life-threatening deterioration of heart function.[330] Unfortunately, his warning has gone unheeded.

One patient I was seeing for a heart problem wanted to know if CoQ10 would help her ninety-five-year-old mother, who was also suffering from heart failure. I answered that, in conjunction with other nutrients, it certainly would. She then told me that her cardiologist had told her to be sure not to give her mother CoQ10.

I thought the statement was a little strange, but on the outside chance the cardiologist might have known of some rare complication occurring in ninety-five-year-olds taking CoQ10, I asked her why he said that. She replied, "He said that studies showed it didn't work." I had to laugh. The medical profession writes millions of prescriptions every year that do not work, yet they never bat an eye to fill their patients' hands full of them.

I recall a pediatrician telling me that he routinely wrote antibiotic prescriptions for viral illnesses in children because the parents wanted an antibiotic for them, and if he didn't prescribe it, they would just take the kid to another pediatrician who would. He didn't want to lose the business, so he gave them a useless and dangerous antibiotic. I hear the same refrain about Ritalin from pediatricians: hypocrisy at its best.

L-carnitine

Another metabolic fuel needed by the heart is L-carnitine. It is known that animals have forty times higher levels of L-carnitine in their heart muscles than in their blood. The same is suspected to be true in humans. Because of this huge difference between blood and heart-muscle levels, it is suspected that the heart has a special transport mechanism to push L-carnitine into the heart muscle.[331]

So what does L-carnitine do? Basically, it allows our cells to metabolize fats (mainly long-chained fatty acids) for energy. In fact, fats supply most of the heart muscle's fuel. It does this by allowing fats to enter the mitochondria, where it is converted into energy—and lots of it.

Studies on children suffering from a certain form of heart failure have shown that their heart-muscle L-carnitine levels were drastically low.[332] Surprisingly, many others have blood levels of L-carnitine that are either normal or slightly elevated. The problem appears to be in the mechanism that pushes L-carnitine into the heart muscle. Untreated, these children's hearts progressively enlarge until they fail altogether. By giving very high doses of L-carnitine to these children, doctors have been able to reverse this otherwise fatal condition.

Then, what about adults? We know that there is a virtual epidemic of congestive heart failure in this country, and that the incidence is continually rising. Severe depletion of carnitine from the hearts of patients with congestive heart failure has been demonstrated in numerous studies.[333] Several double-blind studies have shown that giving patients with congestive heart failure large doses of L-carnitine significantly improved cardiac function in most,[334] and the beneficial effect increased the longer they took the supplement.

Magnesium and the Heart Muscle

It is ironic that doctors prescribe drugs that cost thousands of dollars to treat the complications of heart disease, yet rarely pay attention to one of the most versatile, powerful, and least expensive weapons in their arsenal: magnesium.

Magnesium plays a vital role as a coenzyme (helper) in over three hundred enzyme reactions, many of which control energy production. Numerous studies have shown the value of maintaining normal magnesium levels in persons having cardiovascular disease. For example, one study found that congestive heart disease patients having normal blood levels of magnesium had almost twice the survival rate as those with lower levels.[335]

Next to potassium, magnesium is the most abundant cation in the body. The body contains 1,000 mM of magnesium, with over 50 percent in the bones, slightly less than 50 percent in the soft tissues (such as muscle, skin, ligaments, and organs), and less than 1 percent in the blood. This is why blood levels of magnesium are so notoriously inaccurate for estimating tissue magnesium levels. The heart muscle normally has one of the highest magnesium levels of any organ.

While many patients with cardiovascular disease have normal blood levels of magnesium, a significant number of these patients will have low *tissue* levels. Animal studies have shown that chronic depletion of magnesium can significantly worsen elevated levels of triglycerides and cholesterol, and can lower the good type of cholesterol—HDL.[336] And, as we have seen previously, dogs on a magnesium-free diet subjected to coronary artery occlusion (a heart attack) have heart muscle destruction involving areas twice as large as those on a normal magnesium diet.[337]

Patients who have sudden heart attacks frequently experience a precipitous fall in magnesium concentration in their blood, with the lowest levels occurring twelve to twenty hours after hospital admission. This is because of the massive release of catecholamines (adrenaline) released after the heart attack, in conjunction with the associated release of fatty acids, that binds the magnesium. Other forms of severe stress have also been shown to cause a significant, sudden drop in magnesium levels, including major burns, infections, trauma, alcohol withdrawal, hypothermia, and during cardiac surgery.

It is also important because of the widespread occurrence of magnesium deficiency based on poor diets. Younger generations are especially at risk because of their dependence on carbonated drinks, junk foods, and diets devoid of the main dietary source of magnesium—vegetables.

One frightening condition associated with low magnesium levels is sudden cardiac death. Experimentally, it is known that if you feed animals a diet deficient in magnesium and then frighten the animals, a significant number will die suddenly. The same is true of humans with low tissue magnesium levels; that is, those who have a diet deficient in magnesium. A combined study of a number of heart attack patients found that magnesium infusions could lower mortality rates by 54 percent compared to patients who did not receive magnesium treatment.[338]

One effect of magnesium is to increase blood flow through the coronary arteries, which occurs because magnesium is a calcium-channel blocker and dilates blood vessels. This is especially important in cases of sudden cardiac death in young people, and frequently a cause of death in athletes, in which a segment of the coronary artery is hyperactive and goes into spasm. Magnesium can counteract this spasm.[339]

Another frequent cause of death following a heart attack is the development of uncontrollable irregular heartbeats called an arrhythmia. In one study, ten of thirteen patients who had had a heart attack as well as low magnesium levels, developed arrhythmia afterwards.[340] While not all doctors agree that magnesium supplementation can prevent arrthythmias, most agree that it can reduce the incidence of difficult-to-control arrthythmias.

One type of arrhythmia, atrial fibrillation, may be controlled with magnesium supplementation. Supplementation can also reduce the incidence of digitalis-induced atrial tachycardia, a condition in which the heart's atria beat too quickly. We also know that low potassium levels are associated with increased risk for arrhythmia: less well known is the fact that low magnesium also lowers potassium levels. In fact, patients with low potassium often have significant difficulty correcting their potassium deficit until the magnesium deficiency is corrected.

Because it is a slight anti-coagulant, magnesium also helps to reduce heart-attack incidence by thinning the blood.[341] This is especially important in individuals who have high fibrinogen levels, a condition that increases blood coagulation. Elevated fibrinogen levels are an independent risk factor for heart attacks and strokes: that means that even if all other studies—triglycerides, LDL cholesterol, and total cholesterol—are normal, you are still at increased risk of having a heart attack.

Not only can magnesium be used to effectively treat people who have already had a heart attack, it can also significantly reduce the incidence of arteriosclerosis. More recent studies have shown that magnesium improves endothelial cell function, reduces entry of cholesterol into the wall of the blood vessel, and acts as an antioxidant.[342] Magnesium deficiency has been shown to double free-radical production in cells of various types. These deficient cells are also twice as likely to die under stress as cells grown in a magnesium-containing medium. Cellular glutathione levels are significantly lower in cells made magnesium deficient. Recall that glutathione is one of the most important antioxidant systems in cells, including endothelial cells lining our arteries.

On top of all these benefits, magnesium also plays a major role in protecting the brain, improves blood flow to the kidneys, and improves lung function. These benefits are particularly important to the heart-attack patient, since impaired cardiac function impairs blood flow to all of the organs of the body, especially the brain.

As Benjamin Franklin said over two hundred years ago, "An ounce of prevention is worth a pound of cure." The time to correct low tissue magnesium levels is not after you have heart disease, but before. It will significantly lessen your risk of developing heart disease in the first place. And if you *do* have a heart attack, sufficient magnesium intake will greatly improve your chances of survival and recovery.

Angina (Oh! My Aching Heart)

When one or more blood vessels to the heart narrow enough to rob the heart muscle of sufficient amounts of blood flow (without actually killing the heart muscle), we experience episodes of intense pain—either in the chest, down into the left arm, or to left side of the neck and jaw. Like TIAs with stroke, this condition is a warning sign of an impending full-blown heart attack. Depending on the degree of vessel obstruction, you may experience these attacks only occasionally or quite frequently.

These attacks of pain are frequently precipitated by exercise, stress, or following a fatty meal. Some people are so fragile that even teeth-brushing can induce anginal pain. An episode may also be precipitated by a meal high in glutamate (MSG).

Not surprisingly, given its success with treating heart attacks, several studies have demonstrated that CoQ10 can significantly reduce the number and severity of anginal attacks. In one double-blind crossover trial using twelve patients with stable angina, doctors gave the patients either a placebo or 150 mg of CoQ10 a day.[343] To measure response, patients were required to run on a treadmill until they began to experience chest pain and before an EEG demonstrated heart muscle ischemia.

Compared with the patients taking the placebo, those who received CoQ10 experienced a 53 percent reduction in episodes of anginal attacks and a 54 percent reduction in the number of nitroglycerine tablets needed. While CoQ10 reduced the number and severity of anginal attacks, it is not a definitive treatment for coronary heart disease. That is, it will not open up clogged arteries.

Other supplements—including garlic, magnesium, arginine, Ginkgo biloba, and hawthorn berry extract—can also improve coronary artery flow and reduce the incidence of anginal attacks.

The amino acid, arginine, and garlic dilate blood vessels by increasing production of nitric oxide. One of the effects of aging of arteries is a loss of the ability of the endothelial cells to produce nitric oxide. Proper nutritional supplementation can regenerate this ability.

Ginkgo Biloba

Ginkgo is the oldest living species of tree. Many nutritionists take this to mean that because it is so hardy, it may pass its elixir of life on to us. Strangely, this may be true! Unlike many things in life, Ginkgo biloba extract deserves its sterling reputation. Testing has shown that it is both safe and useful in preventing and treating various diseases.

Probably the most extensively studied herb, Ginkgo biloba contains numerous beneficial substances, some with powerful pharmacological properties. It is an incredible substance, capable of significantly increasing blood flow through arteries in all organs and tissues, including the brain and heart muscle. It is composed of special alkaloids (ginkaloids) in combination with a multitude of antioxidant flavonoids making Ginkgo extract a very powerful tool against numerous disorders, especially those associated with degenerative aging and impaired microvessel blood flow.[344]

We know that Ginkgo improves blood flow through the brain, mainly in very small blood vessels (microvessels) that actually supply the brain with oxygen and glucose.[345] This is especially important in people with poor blood supply to their brain (cerebrovascular insufficiency). Several clinical tests using the herb have even shown a significant improvement in people with cerebrovascular disease.[346]

The flavonoids found in the Ginkgo extract powerfully inhibit free-radical damage in numerous tissues and organs. But, of special interest is their ability to prevent oxidation of LDL cholesterol, since this plays a key role in the atherosclerotic process. These flavonoids also have antibiotic effects as well.

Another property of the Ginkgo extract is its ability to inhibit arrhythmia in heart muscle. As we have seen, arrthythmias constitute a major cause of death following heart attacks, especially in smokers. (Smokers have low magnesium levels.) In essence, we have in this one extract the ability to suppress arrthythmias, improve coronary blood flow, reduce blood viscosity and hypercoagulability, and reduce the damage by free radicals.

The tremendous ability of this extract to prevent and treat disease seems to be frightening pharmaceutical companies to death, since widespread use of the extract would significantly reduce the need for their expensive, and often dangerous, medications. To stem enthusiasm for Ginkgo biloba, stories have mysteriously appeared concerning the "extreme danger" of Ginkgo biloba. The smear campaigners implant stories about sudden hemorrhaging, and dangers during surgery: one reported case described a subdural hematoma occurring in an elderly man taking Ginkgo biloba.

The problem with this report is that Ginkgo biloba has about the same anticoagulating effect as one aspirin. Why is it that the doctors who issue these shrill warnings do not hesitate to put millions of elderly patients on an aspirin a day, or even more dangerous platelet-inhibiting drugs? It is estimated that the use of aspirin to prevent strokes or heart attack accounts for one in one thousand brain hemorrhages.[347] When you consider that approximately five million people are taking aspirin, that number can be quite significant. I have never seen a national warning for people to stop taking their aspirin a day before surgery. In fact, I have operated on hundreds of patients who have taken their doctor's prescribed aspirin the day before surgery—not because they were not warned to stop the aspirin, but because they forgot. Bleeding was never made uncontrollable.

Of course, it *would* be folly to combine anticoagulant drugs and anticoagulant herbs. If you take Ginkgo biloba, you should not take an aspirin or any other medication or product known to thin the blood. In fact, those on more powerful anticoagulation medications should avoid Ginkgo biloba altogether. If you are taking Ginkgo biloba there is no need to take an aspirin a day, since you will get all the beneficial effects of aspirin plus a whole lot more. Unfortunately, the public has been so brainwashed by the media concerning the miraculous effects of taking an aspirin a day that most people are reluctant to stop taking it. Most doctors will know little or nothing of Ginkgo biloba, if they have heard of it at all.

Hawthorn Extract (Crateagus oxacantha)

This plant extract has been shown to increase the strength of heart contractions (ejection fraction), dilate blood vessels (which lowers blood pressure and improves blood flow through the coronary arteries), and acts as a powerful antioxidant.[348] I have found it to be especially effective with patients who have hypertension, since it blocks the angiotensin-converting enzyme responsible for elevating blood pressure. The extract also contains a group of flavonoids called procyanidins and luteolin that powerfully neutralize several types of free radicals. This may reduce the risk of developing atherosclerosis.

This extract has a wide margin of safety, but when combined with other heart medications could potentially magnify their effects. Long-term experience with the extract has not shown specific problems, and even extremely high doses of the extract in animals have shown minimal toxicity. Despite this, you should inform your doctor that you are taking hawthorn extract. Pregnant women should avoid hawthorn extract since no studies have been done on toxicity to unborn babies.

In Germany, hawthorn is approved for use in cases of stage I and II heart disease (New York Heart Association classification), which is characterized by being comfortable at rest but experiencing fatigue, shortness of breath, and limitations during physical activity. A study examining patients with advanced heart failure found that those taking 600 mg of hawthorn extract a day experienced a 50 percent improvement in symptoms, and ability to ride an exercise bicycle.[349]

The usual recommended dose is 120 mg three times a day. Higher doses should be monitored by a physician knowledgeable in the use of such extracts. Adverse reactions include fatigue, nausea, and sweating. Because of its ability to lower blood pressure, it should not be used with prescription medications that also lower blood pressure. Those taking heart medications should also get clearance from their cardiologist before using this extract.

What Tests Will I Need?

After examining several laboratories, I would suggest the Great Smokies Diagnostic Laboratory for most of my cardiovascular testing. They offer a series of tests that measures markers for cardiovascular disease risk. Each of these tests indicates either an independent risk or a combined risk. For example, if both your LDL cholesterol and C-reactive protein are increased, you have a much greater risk of heart disease than if either one was elevated alone. All of these tests are available with the Comprehensive Cardiovascular Assessment.

Blood Lipids

This test measures the circulating levels of the major lipid (fats) in the blood stream. This portion of the test includes:

Total Cholesterol

While the numbers do not directly relate to heart-attack risk, it can indicate the presence of a problem. Total cholesterol is a combination of LDL, HDL, and VLDL cholesterol levels. While this study is suggestive, there are many other factors involved as well, such as dietary differences in the two groups, exercise levels, and overall healthier lifestyle of the lower cholesterol group.

LDL Cholesterol Levels

Numerous studies have shown that the level of LDL cholesterol correlates better with coronary-death risk than does total cholesterol. And, as we have seen, even more important is the size of the LDL particle. Unfortunately, most labs do not differentiate for particle size. LDL is subclassified into small dense (LDL_{SD}) and large buoyant types. The LDL_{SD} is the only one associated with increased risk. The large buoyant type may actually reduce risk.

HDL Cholesterol Levels

In the lay press, HDL cholesterol is known as good cholesterol. Its function is to remove cholesterol from the tissues and blood stream, but it should be recognized that even oxidized HDL can contribute to atherosclerosis. Fortunately, it is more difficult to oxidize than LDL. Higher levels of HDL appear to be protective.

Triglycerides

These are esterified fatty oils. High levels of triglycerides also act as an independent risk factor separate from all other factors. Some studies have shown that triglyceride levels are a good measure of the severity of coronary artery disease. Diets high in some saturated fats (especially myristic and laurel fats) may increase triglycerides, but in most cases, it is a high sugar and carbohydrate diet that elevates triglycerides.

Homocysteine

As we have seen, elevations in homocysteine are independently associated with coronary heart disease. That is, even if all other studies are normal, high homocysteine levels put you at substantial risk of atherosclerosis.

Lipoprotein (a)

This is a special transport molecule bound to the LDL molecule. When elevated, it is an accurate measure of coronary-artery-disease risk, even when all other tests are normal. Elevations in this lipoprotein are mostly hereditary, but can be controlled nutritionally.

A diet high in vegetables and low in hydrogenated oils lowers lipoprotein(a) levels, as do steps that increase HDL levels. Inositol hexaniacinate, L-lysine, vitamin C, and proline (an amino acid) also lowers levels of this factor. Diabetics and those with low thyroid function often have elevated levels of this factor.

Apolipoprotein A-1
This molecule is major constituent of HDL. Higher levels of this factor predict a lower risk of coronary artery disease.

Apolipoprotein B
This is a primary molecule in LDL structure. Elevated levels are associated with increased cardiovascular disease risk.

Ratio of Apo B/Apo A-1
A high ratio has been associated with a high incidence of coronary artery disease. Several studies have shown that this ratio is particularly valuable in predicting a family history of coronary artery disease.

Fibrinogen
This is a globulin associated with blood coagulation. Studies have shown an important link between high levels of fibrinogen and death from strokes. It also plays a critical role in the mechanism of atherosclerosis of all vessels. Levels are increased by smoking, oral contraceptives, chronic inflammation and with aging.

C-reactive protein
C-reactive protein is a marker for inflammation, which is accompanied by release of special chemicals called cytokines. These chemicals encourage coagulation of the blood, and promote atherosclerosis. A high C-reactive protein indicates a significant risk of heart attack or stroke. It also raises suspicion of a possible infection by *Chlamydia pneumonia* or *Helicobacter pylori*, both associated with atherosclerosis.

Program for Vascular Health

Fruits and Vegetables

Numerous studies have shown that people whose diets consist of the greatest quantity of fruits and vegetables have the lowest incidence of heart attacks and strokes. In fact, many earlier studies reporting significant benefits from high intakes of vitamin C or beta-carotene concentrated on people who maintained diets high in a variety of fruits and vegetables. Researchers just assumed that because fruits and vegetables were high in beta-carotene or vitamin C, these particular vitamins were responsible for the beneficial health effects that study participants were enjoying. Now we know that these same fruits and vegetables contain over *10,000* complex chemicals, many of which are very powerful and versatile antioxidants against numerous types of free radicals.

There is growing evidence that it is the *combined* effects of these complex nutrients—not single nutrients—that provide us with such remarkable health benefits. Remember, there are dozens of types of free radicals, each operating in different areas of the body and cells. Some antioxidants act against a small number of these free radicals and not against others. For example, beta-carotene appears to have no affect on oxidation of DNA, but is an excellent antioxidant in preventing oxidation of cell membranes and neutralizing free radicals in the cytoplasm of cells. Many other flavonoids, on the other hand, are very powerful at protecting the DNA from oxidation.

One of the best studies ever done on the relationship between diet and cardiovascular-disease rates was the Seven Countries Study,[350] which examined the diet and health outcomes of sixteen groups of people residing in seven countries of Northern Europe, Japan, and the Mediterranean countries over a thirty-eight-year period. It was found that people residing on the island of Crete had the lowest cardiovascular disease rate when compared to populations in the other seven countries. They also lived longer. Despite being heavy smokers, they had lung cancer rates lower than those of northern European countries.

So what accounts for this remarkable health affect on the island of Crete? Analysis of their diets demonstrated a very high intake of extra virgin olive oil, and of fruits and vegetables. In fact, they had the highest intake of antioxidants in their diet than any other group—including the Japanese. Despite the fact that Japanese consumed fewer saturated fats and more omega-3 fatty acids as fish, the people on Crete had lower coronary heart disease.

When intakes of vitamins C and E in various countries were analyzed, researchers found that the highest dietary amounts of both vitamins was in the Crete population. As we shall see later, extra virgin olive oil (which is actually a vegetable extract) contains numerous antioxidant flavonoids as well as health-promoting monounsaturated oils. By combining a high intake of fruits and vegetables with high intakes of extra virgin olive oil, the people living on the island of Crete have significantly lowered their risk of heart attacks and cancer, despite having the highest incidence of smoking in the world! They have even outdone the Japanese, the next-healthiest population in the world.

A recent study has also demonstrated that a diet rich in potassium, magnesium, calcium, and fiber was protective against stroke fatality among men.[351] The greatest benefits were experienced by hypertensive men, but these nutrients also protected study participants who had normal blood pressure.

We can draw some conclusions from this study, based on what we already know about each of these nutrients. Potassium and magnesium can both lower blood pressure, and magnesium, as we have seen, can independently inhibit atherosclerosis. Magnesium also protects the brain and the heart from the effects of a lack of blood supply (ischemia).

Lowering blood pressure, the number one risk for a stroke, by just 9 mm systolic and 5 mm diastolic can reduce risk of coronary heart disease by 20 percent and stroke by 34 percent. When we are talking about such a widespread disease—one which affects over a million people a year—even small improvements in the percentage of the population affected translates into saving a lot of lives.

There appears to be a close association between vitamin C and high blood pressure, another risk factor. Some have hypothesized that as we age our vitamin C intake falls, resulting in the higher incidence of hypertension with aging. There is some evidence for this idea. In several studies, having a combined population of greater than ten thousand people, a strong correlation was found between low vitamin C intakes and high blood pressure.[352] Several other studies have shown that giving 1,000 mg of vitamin C to mildly hypertensive women reduced both their systolic and diastolic blood pressure. Smokers are known to have drastically low vitamin C levels and a high incidence of hypertension.

A fruit-and-vegetable diet has been experimentally tested and found to achieve these very goals. The DASH (Dietary Approaches to Stop Hypertension) diet is based on findings from the National Institutes of Health clinical study, and is designed to be high in fruits and vegetables and low-fat dairy products. I disagree with the choice of dairy products, since consumption of even low-fat ones increased incidence of heart disease and prostate cancer in men in other studies.[353] With this in mind, it is important to note that DASH may have been even more impressive if dairy products had been eliminated altogether.

Another study, in which British vegetarians were followed over a ten-year period, found a significantly lower incidence of coronary heart disease than among non-vegetarians.[354] This finding conforms to the data on Seventh Day Adventists that demonstrated a positive relationship between eating meat and coronary heart disease. Vegetarians were also found to have lower cholesterol levels, and a lower incidence of hypertension than non-vegetarians. A more recent study, using the Framingham Study group, found a significant relationship between a high intake of fruits and vegetables and a lower incidence of strokes in men.[355]

In these various studies, the amount of fruits and vegetables in participants' diets made all the difference in the world. Eating two servings a day provided very little protection, if any. In fact, protection was not seen until five servings of fruits and vegetables a day. Ten servings were even better. It should also be appreciated that not all studies found this positive effect. The problem with the negative studies is that, in most, no consideration was given to the quality of the vegetables: not all vegetables are created equal in terms of nutrient density and quality.

Vegetables with the highest concentrations of nutrients include cruciferous vegetables, such as broccoli, brussels sprouts, cauliflower, cabbage, and kale. All these vegetables are high on the ORAC (oxygen radical absorbency capacity) scale, which measures a food's overall antioxidant capacity. Developed by Dr. Guohua Cao, a food scientist at the USDA, the system's greatest advantage is that for any food the synergistic effects of many antioxidants are taken into account—factors that would be easily overlooked in attempting to evaluate the effects of each antioxidant, and then merely adding the results together.

These nutrient-dense plants play the greatest role in preventing disease. In most of the reported studies, no effort is made to determine the number of high-quality vegetables that are being consumed. It's as if researchers simply assume a vegetable is a vegetable: in fact, some studies classify french fries as a vegetable, which they are—but only technically. I, for one, hardly think a high-carbohydrate vegetable saturated with unhealthy fats can be considered equivalent to a nutrient-dense vegetable such as broccoli.

One interesting study, in which 34,492 postmenopausal women were studied over a ten-year period, found that broccoli intake correlated strongly with a reduction in coronary heart disease death.[356] The women with the highest broccoli intake had a 38 percent reduction in heart attack deaths.

How fruits and vegetables are prepared is also important. In the South, most vegetables are combined with fatback (chunks of animal fat), and broccoli is served smothered with cheese. Fruits are often dipped in sugary concoctions or covered in ice cream. Such combinations significantly blunt the beneficial effects of otherwise healthy food. In most studies, no consideration is made for such culinary practices.

A study of Finnish men and women found that coronary mortality and the incidence of coronary heart disease was significantly reduced in those with the highest intakes of flavonoid-containing foods such as fruits and vegetables.[357] In this study, women who ate the most fruits and vegetables reduced their risk of coronary heart disease by 31 percent and the risk of dying from a heart attack by 46 percent. The men reduced coronary heart disease risk by 25 percent and the risk of dying from a heart attack by 33 percent. The study was adjusted for blood pressure, age, smoking, cholesterol levels, and body size to remove the effect of other factors that might influence the results.

These findings are consistent with a Japanese study, which found that the greatest influence in reducing coronary disease risk was a high intake of flavonoids, not soy products.[358] This study is important because many are expounding the virtues of a diet high in soy products to reduce coronary disease risk. There are significant hazards to a high intake of soy products, including hormonal effects on babies and children, high glutamate levels, and thyroid suppression.

Interestingly, a high intake of fruits and vegetables not only can help protect us by preventing atherosclerosis in the first place, but in case of a heart attack or stroke, they can significantly reduce the damaging effects of the attack. This was dramatically demonstrated in a study involving over four hundred persons suffering from an acute heart attack.[359] These patients were divided into two groups for comparison. One group was put on a diet high in nutrient-rich fruits and vegetables starting twenty-four to forty-eight hours after admission, and the other group received a routine hospital diet. At the end of the study, those on the high fruit and vegetable diet showed a significant decrease in mortality and a greater improvement in measures of heart function than those on the routine hospital diet.

Of special interest was the finding that when these patients were examined one year later they were found to have significantly improved LDL levels, lower total cholesterol levels, improved glucose utilization, and normal blood pressure: their risk of having another heart attack was significantly reduced. It should also be emphasized that the difference in mortality between the groups while they were in the hospital was dramatic. For example, in the hospital-diet group, twenty-five died whereas only six in the fruit-and-vegetable group died. Patients in the two groups were matched for severity of coronary disease and other variables.

There are multiple reasons why a high intake of fruits and vegetables protect us from heart disease. As we have seen, in addition to phytochemicals, fruits and vegetables are high in magnesium, potassium, calcium, and fiber—all of which have been associated with improvement of risk factors. In addition, plants are an excellent source of folate, which is necessary to prevent the accumulation of homocysteine in the blood and tissues. Homocysteine even in high normal concentrations is a significant independent risk factor for atherosclerosis.

As a good source of numerous nutrients, fruits and vegetables strengthen all of the tissues of the body, assure efficient energy production, improve the body's ability to detoxify, and protect us from free-radical damage. Fiber from plants helps control blood sugar levels, removes toxins from the digestive tract, may lower blood pressure, encourages a proper balance of colon bacteria, and improves elimination of colon contents. And if that is not enough, plant-based foods also contain complex carbohydrates and carbohydrate-protein complexes that stimulate the immune system for maximum efficiency.

Dietary Recommendations

Your diet should consist of seven to ten servings of fresh fruits and vegetables a day, with as many as possible in raw form. I have found that most people who say they eat a lot of fruits and vegetables actually eat only one or two types of vegetables—and then at most only one or two servings a day. Everyone should eat close to ten servings of fruits and vegetables every day: for densely packed fruits and vegetables, such as apples and broccoli, a serving is equal to one-half cup. One cup is considered a serving size for looser vegetables, such as lettuce and spinach. In general, your body needs *at least* five servings of fruits and vegetables a day to benefit from their disease-inhibiting effects. Most studies show that smaller quantities offer little, if any, protection against disease.

Unlike animal cells, plant cells contain a wall that we cannot digest, and therefore must be mechanically cracked open to get to the phytochemicals. We do this by chewing. Unfortunately, most of us do not chew our vegetables until they are a mush—which is the optimal state for nutrient absorption in our bodies—but you can blenderize them to achieve the same effect.

Cooking can destroy some vitamins, but it also releases vital flavonoids and other health-promoting phytochemicals from some fruits and vegetables, making them more available for absorption. If you do want to cook your vegetables, use distilled water for boiling or steaming. When you use fluoridated water for cooking, the fluoride becomes progressively more concentrated as the water evaporates. This is very dangerous, since fluoride cannot be washed off foods.

If you're unable to prepare ten servings of fruits and vegetables a day, I highly recommend using a blender to make up a liquid supply. If you eat whole vegetables, your body can absorb only about 30 percent of the available nutrients, whereas juicing or blenderizing allows up to 90 percent absorption.

Even if you are extremely busy, find one day a week that you can spend blenderizing foods. I have found that the high-powered Vita-Mix processor is excellent for breaking down the plant-cell wall and releasing nutrients from fruits and vegetables. Whatever method you use, make a large amount of the fruit and vegetable mix described below, reserve enough to last the week, and freeze the rest. That way you can carry some with you in a thermos bottle and have plenty in the freezer to thaw and use later.

Purists will scream heresy because they think vegetables or their juices must be consumed fresh to take full advantage of their nutritious enzymes, but blending is certainly preferable to the alternative: a junk-food diet, completely devoid of *any* form of fruits and vegetables.

The vegan diet—which disallows *all* animal products, including eggs and milk—is one of the healthier diets you can follow. In particular, the Hallelujah Diet, developed by George Malkmus, contains an excellent blend of fruits and vegetables that has been shown to significantly reduce disease rates, and in some cases, produce dramatic improvements in some very serious diseases.

The only problem with the vegan diet is the potential for vitamin B_{12} deficiency. A recent study found that the overall healthiest diet is vegan-vegetarian, which is mostly fruits and vegetables with a little fish thrown in for additional nutrients. Since we've already seen that seafood contains mercury and pesticides, that leaves us with a vegetarian diet plus nutrient supplements. If meat is included in the diet, it should always be from a trusted organic source (e.g., grass-fed cows and free-range poultry that have not been pumped full of antibiotics and other drugs).

One mistake people often make, especially those who juice, is to eat only their favorite fruits or vegetables, often overlooking nutrient-dense vegetables, such as kale, cabbage, celery, or broccoli. In general, you should use more vegetables than fruits, and if you have cancer, diabetes or *Candida* yeast infection, it is wise to avoid fruits altogether.

Following is a list of highly nutritious fruits and vegetables that you should include in your diet—whether or not you are making a blended mix. For blenderizing, pick at least four fruits and four vegetables from the following lists (a "+" means nutrients are destroyed by heat).

Drink at least twelve ounces twice a day of your blend. At first, this may provide too much fiber, and may cause diarrhea. In that case, dilute the blend by half with distilled water. Once you adjust to that, gradually increase the amount of blend and reduce the amount of water. It may take a couple weeks to accomplish this.

Some of you will ask: is that one glass *each* of fruit blend and vegetable blend? I prefer to mix the two together. This adds a little sweetness to the vegetable blend. I suggest mixing

Fruits	*Vegetables*
currants (black or red)	kale
oranges and tangerines	broccoli
Macintosh apples+	brussels sprouts
blueberries	tomatoes
blackberries	cauliflower+
raspberries	cabbage (purple or red)+
strawberries	cilantro
cranberries	parsley
grapes (only if fluoride-free)	beets+
prunes	rhubarb
sweet-and-sour cherries	spinach
pineapple+	

four ounces of fruit mix to eight ounces of vegetable mix. Drink this twice a day. If you prefer to drink them separately, I suggest six ounces of fruit mix and one full twelve-ounce serving of vegetable mix.

Fats

As we have seen, the modern diet is full of omega-6 fatty acids—such as those found in corn, safflower, sunflower, peanut, and canola oils—but very low in omega-3 fatty acids. We have also seen that increasing omega-3 intake can improve blood flow, reduce the risk of heart attack and stroke, improve brain function, reduce inflammation, improve the immune system, and inhibit the formation of cancer.

While most studies have shown that eating fish even once a week reduces heart attack and stroke risk, there are serious drawbacks to eating fish containing large amounts of omega-3 fatty acids. The main danger is that fish with the highest omega-3 fatty acid content also have the highest methylmercury levels. Serious accumulations of mercury can occur from eating these types of fish regularly.

Another concern is pesticide and herbicide residue in seafood. We know that fish tend to accumulate and retain these poisons for long periods of time, and that bottom-feeding animals (shrimp, oysters, crabs, and lobsters) present the greatest risk. In the case of seafood from the Gulf coast, the problem is that all of the giant industries, refineries, aluminum plants, and fertilizer plants dump their waste into the Mississippi River, which empties out into the Gulf. All of these bottom-feeding creatures contain significant levels of mercury, lead, and other heavy metals as well.

As I mentioned in the discussion on omega-3 fatty acids, I recommend taking a high-DHA and low EPA supplement instead of high EPA oils, since DHA is responsible for most of the benefits attributed to omega-3 oils. Many of the fish-oil capsules you find in health food stores contain only 30 percent omega-3 oils,[360] which would require you to take twenty to thirty capsules a day to get the necessary amount of these healthy oils. Unfortunately, pure, high-quality omega-3 fatty acid capsules are rather expensive, but the expense is worth it, and several brands of extremely high quality can be found that contain 50-98 percent pure omega-3 oils.

If you do decide to take omega-3 fatty acids, do not buy cheap brands. Many contain numerous contaminants, including mercury and pesticides. If, when you take a fish-oil capsule, you taste something like rotten fish, you have definitely gotten a very cheap brand. The capsule should be crystal clear when held up to the light, and contain no white specks when placed in the refrigerator. Note that *all* supplements that contain oil should be kept in the refrigerator.

Use only small amounts of butter, and certainly no margarine. If you do use butter, make sure it has high purity rating. I prefer to use extra virgin olive oil in place of either margarine or butter.

As far as salad dressings go, all commercial brands contain unhealthy oils, including Paul Newman's Olive Oil Dressing, which, in my opinion, is the best of the commercial salad dressings. If you read labels, you will quickly discover that they all contain canola, corn, safflower, or some other vegetable oil. Many people have asked me about canola oil, since it is marketed as being very safe and healthy. Few people realize that canola oil is produced from very toxic rapeseed oil. To make it fit for consumption, processors attempt to remove the toxic components, but serious questions have been raised recently as to the success of the purification process. I advise avoiding canola oil at this time, until the issue is settled.

I recommend that you make your own salad dressing. The base oil should be extra virgin olive oil extracted by the cold press method. Add about two to three teaspoons of balsamic vinegar and spices of your choice. Play around with the formula until it suits your taste. Some people like more salt or more vinegar than others.

When eating out, avoid dishes made with butter or margarine, and salad dressings made with oils other than olive. Most such dressings, especially thousand island and ranch dressings, contain significant amounts of monosodium glutamate or hydrolyzed proteins, both of which are excitotoxins.

In general, your intake of "bad" oils should not exceed 10-15 percent of your caloric intake. The remainder of your essential oil needs can be met by using extra virgin olive oil and increasing your intake of vegetables, all of which contain small amounts of omega-3 fatty acids.

Meat

There is a direct connection between meat consumption and atherosclerotic diseases, such as heart attacks and strokes—a correlation that is especially strong with heavy meats such as beef and pork. Part of the problem is that they not only contain high levels of saturated fats, but also high concentrations of iron. Some vegetables, such as broccoli have iron levels as high as beef, but the iron in plants is poorly absorbed (less than 5 percent), whereas the iron from beef is highly absorbed (about 60 percent). This is because plants contain iron-binding flavonoids.

As if the problems with atherosclerosis weren't bad enough, meat consumption has also been linked to cancer. One of the most common diseases of cattle is cancer, primarily lymphoma and leukemia.[361] Studies have proven these two forms of cancer are caused by viruses—in both animals and humans. According to USDA rules, slaughterhouses can use meat from cancer-afflicted cattle as long as the tumors are thrown away. The problem with this practice is that the cancer-causing virus is disseminated throughout the animal. While cooking may partially destroy the organisms, people who like their steaks rare are really taking chances. While there is no proof that these cancer-causing viruses can cause cancer in humans, there is compelling circumstantial evidence.

Several studies have found that cancer rates in slaughterhouse workers are not only higher than average, but many of these cancers are of the same type found in cattle. In addition, the food consumption most associated with cancer in humans is milk. Not surprisingly, lymphomas and leukemias are the cancers most often seen in such cases.

There is some suggestion that carcinogenic viruses in animals can be transmitted to humans. This doesn't even approach the "mad cow disease," which may not even be an infectious disease, but rather one caused by a particular pesticide within the meat. This would explain why even intense heat can't stop the disease from spreading.

A recent study found that Iowa farmers had a significantly higher mortality from cancer, especially of the prostate and colon, than nonfarmers, even though they smoked less and drank less alcohol.[362] Surprisingly, the farmers in this study ate more meat and fewer fruits and vegetables than nonfarmers.

For people unwilling to do without their processed packaged meats, hot dogs, and frozen dinners, all I can say is, be prepared for a life fraught with illness and heartache. A high intake of fruits and vegetables will lessen the damaging impact of your chosen diet, but you will still be at significant increased risk of disease. It's like bailing water out of a boat with a hole in the bottom instead of just plugging the hole and then bailing the water out.

The more a food is processed, the fewer nutrients are left in the end product—and the more likely harmful additives and fats will be added to salvage taste. This is especially true with low-fat foods. Most processors add considerable amounts of MSG, hydrolyzed proteins, or other excitotoxic food additives to boost the tastes of these supposedly healthy foods. They also contain other chemicals for texture, as well as preservatives. If you read labels, you already know that most of them look more like ingredients for industrial cleaners and solvents than something you would eat.

For decades, food scientists and cancer specialists have known that nitrates and nitrites were converted in the human stomach into powerful cancer-causing substances called nitrosamines. Yet, tons of these preservatives are still added to luncheon meats, hot dogs, bacon, and other processed meats. The only reason we are not up to our ears in cases of stomach cancer is that vitamin C significantly inhibits the formation of the powerful nitrosamines. Most studies agree that the fall in stomach cancer over the past three decades is due to increased consumption of vitamin C. In fact, recent research indicates that certain flavonoids commonly found in green vegetables and fruits may inhibit these carcinogenic substances up to three hundred times better than vitamin C. Praise the Lord! He has saved us from ourselves again.

You should also appreciate that many food additives have never been adequately tested and none have been tested to see what affect adding them together has on the body. Reassuring, isn't it? That hot dog you love so much is made from lips, jowls, and body parts that a slaughterhouse otherwise could not sell. And a few grams of fly parts and feces to spice it up. In addition, processors add a good helping of excitotoxic taste additives.

If you feel you cannot live without bacon, do this first. Fill a bowl with distilled water, place the strips of bacon loosely in the water and cook in a microwave for forty-five seconds, or on the stove for two minutes. Stir the water and let it sit for about two more minutes. Then pour off the water and repeat the process. You'll notice the bacon has become very bland after all this cooking. This is because sodium nitrite has a salty taste and is water-soluble. All you have to do is add a little sea salt, free of aluminum, to bring back the taste.

I also advise cooking bacon in extra virgin olive oil. Just pour a thin layer over the bottom of the pan and sprinkle with turmeric, which will dissolve in the oil and give your bacon a nice bright yellow color. The flavonoid curcumin in the turmeric is a powerful cancer-inhibiting substance, and will protect the meat from forming dangerous heterocyclic amines (cancer-causing chemicals formed when meat is seared) in your body. In addition, curcumin is an antibacterial substance and a powerful antioxidant. It is interesting to note that many spices have antibacterial properties.

Do not eat more than six ounces of meat with each meal. Dr. Barry Sears, author of a series of diet and nutrition books, has a good rule of thumb. He recommends limiting per-meal protein intake to the amount that will fit in the palm of your hand. While I've seen some Mississippi farmers who could fit a rack of ribs in their palm, for most of us, a palm-sized serving is a reasonable amount.

For the non-vegan, try to limit yourself to minimally processed turkey, chicken, pork, or ostrich. The problem with chickens is that they are often loaded up with antibiotics and hormones, and are often fed on the feces of other animals. Not a pretty visual I know, but reality.

If you insist on frying your chicken, fry it in extra virgin olive oil with turmeric or extra virgin coconut oil with turmeric and use unprocessed flour. Many people say they cannot eat turkey night after night, and want some variety in their cooking. If so, introduce chicken, but eat it no more than once a week.

At this point, let me clarify my position on this issue for my vegetarian friends. While I don't think there is anything wrong with eating organic meats it must be balanced with an increased consumption of high-nutrient-dense vegetables and some fruits. There is no question that most people on a vegetarian diet feel much better, and many of their aches and pains disappear. But, I do have to admit, if you are afflicted with hypoglycemia, it will be very difficult for you to be a full vegetarian.

Eggs and Dairy

Now, what about eggs and dairy? The solution is simple: avoid all dairy products from cows, save a small amount of butter. That means no cheese, milk, or ice cream. A few of my patients have actually stopped coming to me when I recommended cutting ice cream from their diets, but the truth is that humans were never meant to consume cow's milk. I know the celebrity with the milk mustache told you that your kids won't grow and your bones will snap if you don't drink a quart of the moo juice a day, but it's a lie, pure and simple. Think about it for a minute: why would humans be the only mammals on the face of earth that need to drink milk after weaning? Especially another animal's milk? Elephants, who reach a healthy weight of five tons without snapping in two, manage to avoid milk. So do giraffes and rhinos.

In fact, milk is very harmful to most of us. It has even been discovered that exposing small children to milk before age two is a major cause of juvenile diabetes.[363] The reason for this seems to be that milk proteins closely resemble the protein in the pancreatic island of Langerhans, which is responsible for manufacturing insulin. The body mistakenly attacks not only the milk protein but also the insulin cells as well—a condition we call molecular mimicry.

Despite the fact that several scientific journals have reported this finding—one as recently as 1999—there have been no media announcements to the mothers of the world to avoid giving their young children cow's milk. Why? Because of the power and influence of milk producers, the same guys who created the milk-mustache ads.

There is also evidence that milk-drinking increases incidence of heart attacks and possibly strokes,[364] a relationship that seems to hold true whether the milk is whole or low fat. In fact, the heart-attack rate was higher with low-fat milk. Also, a recent study reported in a peer-reviewed medical journal found that men who drank milk had a higher incidence of prostate cancer. With twenty-five thousand men a year dying of prostate cancer you would think that the media hounds, who love to report phony stories about vitamin C, would headline this story. The silence is deafening. The lesson is: don't depend on the media when your life is at stake.

Remember the cancer-causing viruses common to cattle I mention above? Well, they also end up in cows' milk and are spread to nursing calves.[365] We call this vertical transmission. When you drink the milk, these cancer-causing viruses end up in you as well. Do they cause cancer in humans? While there has never been a direct connection, mainly because it would be difficult to test experimentally (combined with the fact that no one has looked very hard) there is suggestive evidence. We know that of all foods, ingestion of milk and milk products has the highest association to the very types of cancer found in cattle.

Does pasteurization kill viruses? The dairy industry would like you to think it does, but the answer is a resounding no! When you put that carton of milk in the refrigerator and go for a drink a week later, only to find a stinking clabber-looking mess, it's because bacteria have curdled the milk. The bacteria didn't come from the refrigerator, they were already in the milk. Government regulations actually allow so many pus cells per cubic centimeter of milk, cells that often contain live bacteria and viruses. With time they begin to grow and fill the milk with that putrid odor we all love. This is why ultrapasteurized milk can be left on the shelf for very long periods of time without spoiling. The high heat kills everything. Even after it is opened it, it will last much longer than regular milk.

Sugar

For their first visit, I usually ask my nutrition patients to bring a journal outlining a typical three-day diet. I am appalled at what people will eat for breakfast. Many women have a cup of black coffee only. Men either eat no breakfast or have toast with margarine and jelly, while some have pancakes, bacon or sausage, and a big glass of bovine extract (milk) to wash it all down. Professional people usually have at least two cups of caffeinated coffee to get their motor started.

Doctors are the world's worst. They drink coffee as if it were the elixir of life. The only time I see them without a styrofoam cup in their hand is when they are operating. Being sleep-deprived most of their professional lives, they feel they need the caffeine to keep going: not a very good plan. A department head at the medical university where I trained fell to the floor one afternoon with a full-blown grand mal seizure. We later learned that he drank about twenty cups of coffee a day. Most people are not aware that high caffeine intake can actually precipitate seizures in otherwise normal people.

We have seen throughout this book that sugar can be a very toxic substance. It can form attachments to proteins that interfere with their function and significantly increase the risk of oxidation, which makes them vulnerable to free-radical injury and causes rapid advances in aging. This is a major problem with diabetes.

High sugar intake is also known to suppress the immune system, increasing the likelihood of bacterial and yeast infections, chronic viral illnesses, and even cancer. We know that cancer's major fuel is glucose (sugar). So anyone who has cancer should avoid sugar as much as possible—which is hard to do since food processors add it to virtually everything, including salt.

High-sugar diets also increase insulin release. In high doses, insulin causes increased production of inflammatory chemicals in the body and interferes with several enzymes, one of which converts alpha-linolenic acid (flaxseed oil) into omega-3 fatty acid components EPA and DHA.

It is estimated that about 20 percent of Americans have a condition called reactive hypoglycemia: an over-reaction of insulin secretion when glucose is absorbed from the gut. I believe the incidence of the disorder is actually much higher. Those of us with a genetic predisposition for reactive hypoglycemia can be conditioned, through diet, to become hypoglycemics—simply by eating too many simple sugars early in life. With so many youngsters drinking such large volumes of soft drinks, the problem can only grow worse. If the pancreas is continually stressed for a long enough period of time, it will simply exhaust itself and stop producing insulin. At that point, we will need insulin by injection: a condition known as diabetes.

Carbohydrates

In general, your carbohydrate choices should be based on the glycemic index, which rates foods on a scale of 1 to 100 based on how quickly they affect blood sugar levels. The index is designed so that the most desirable foods are rated below fifty. Also, the more refined a food is, the higher it will be on the glycemic index. For example, foods that release their sugar slowly, such as kidney beans, are rated at 27, while highly refined foods, such as pasta, are rated in the low nineties. While the index is not perfect, it is a good guide. As you begin to notice the effects of different foods, you will be able to determine which ones to avoid.

Black beans have been shown to slow the absorption of glucose significantly. So, try to stick with whole-grain rice and cereals rather than highly refined grains.

Food Additives

If you check labels on packaged foods, you will find a list of names that reads like a chemistry-textbook index. Many of these chemicals have not been adequately tested, but a few are definitely known to adversely affect humans. Among these to be avoided at all costs are: monosodium glutamate (also known as MSG and various other aliases), aspartame (found in many artificial sweeteners and diet drinks), and carrageenan. See chapter seven for a comprehensive discussion of food additives.

What to Drink

Most people have developed a obsession with drinking some form of sweetened colored liquid to satisfy their thirst: cola, tea, coffee, fruit juice, or Kool-Aid-like drinks. Few people in this country drink water. This is both good and bad.

It is good, since tap water in most areas is polluted with fluoride, arsenic, aluminum, pesticides, herbicides, and other organic chemicals. As we saw in chapter seven, the presence of fluoride in the water increases lead content as well. The more you drink, the worse is the pollution of your body. Many of these pollutants are fat-soluble, meaning that they will be with you for a long time, and they will accumulate in the nervous system.

You should drink pure water, either distilled or filtered through a reverse osmosis type filter. Only these two methods of water purification can remove fluoride. If you decide on reverse osmosis, you will have to change the filter every three months, because the fluoride eats little holes in the filter, destroying its effectiveness. After you filter your water through the reverse osmosis filter you will also need to filter it once again through a regular filter. Isn't it nice that the government has made you go to all this trouble and expense just to have a drink of pure water?

Several studies have found that adults just don't drink enough water. This situation is particularly bad for the elderly, for two reasons. Not only is dehydration in older people particularly dangerous (elderly patients have told me they don't drink liquids after five in the afternoon so they won't have to get up all night and urinate!), if they're not drinking enough water, it means they're not moving around much.

The problem with this philosophy is that most of us, and practically all of the elderly, are chronically dehydrated, which increases blood viscosity, slows circulation through the arterioles and capillaries, reduces toxin disposal, and increases the likelihood of a sudden stroke or heart attack. Remember, this thickened blood is trying to flow over rough atherosclerotic vessel walls and through narrow openings caused by atherosclerosis. Staying well-hydrated improves blood flow, especially through these smaller vessels.

One area in which good hydration is especially important is in the brain. With aging and progressive atherosclerosis, millions of tiny arteries begin to narrow and lose their elasticity. Periodically, several of these small arterioles will shut down, producing a very tiny stroke that may go completely unnoticed. Gradually, the number of these small strokes begins to accumulate, until we start to lose our ability to think clearly and become forgetful. One form of Alzheimer's disease is associated with these strokes and widespread atherosclerosis. Even in the absence of Alzheimer's disease, people suffering from this process often become demented, a condition called vascular dementia. Staying well-hydrated will help to prevent these small vessels from closing off.

What about fruit juices? Fruit juice provides many health benefits, since juicing releases numerous flavonoids and health-promoting phytochemicals. The problem is that many commercial brands are made with water containing fluoride, and some, like grape juice, may have extremely high levels of fluoride. Juices are also high in sugar, and many industrial processors will add extra sugar to satisfy the kiddies. Some products have other ingredients that may do harm, but since they have been inadequately tested, we may never know. It is best to make your own orange juice or other fruit juices. The makers of Vita-Mix have a recipe book filled with all kinds of juice concoctions. Just ignore the parts suggesting adding honey or sugar.

Tea Is Superior to Coffee

Tea can also have a beneficial effect on reducing atherosclerosis. Several studies have shown that the flavonoid components of tea can significantly reduce oxidation of tissues. Green tea contains high levels of the powerful antioxidant, quercetin, as well as special flavonoids, including epicatechin and epigallocatechin 3-gallate. These flavonoids not only reduce oxidation of LDL cholesterol, but have powerful anticancer effects as well.[366]

In one interesting study, calcification of the aorta, as seen on x-ray, was used to follow progression of atherosclerosis in a group of men and postmenopausal women.[367] Careful analysis showed that those drinking one to two cups of tea a day reduced their risk of severe aortic atherosclerosis by 46 percent, and those drinking four cups a day reduced their risk by 69 percent.

One drawback of tea consumption is that it contains high levels of aluminum. Recent studies using human volunteers found that despite this fact, aluminum was not well-absorbed, most likely because it was bound by the flavonoids in the tea. I do caution though: never add lemon to your tea because citrate in the lemon dramatically increases aluminum absorption. In human studies, it increased absorption as much as elevenfold. One way to counteract aluminum toxicity is to take malate as a supplement. It binds to the aluminum, preventing absorption and rendering it nontoxic in tissues and cells. Because fluoride can be high in teas, especially in black tea and less so green tea, I recommend white tea, which has very low levels. White tea has the highest antioxidant levels.

An additional benefit of tea is that the epicatechin flavonoids have been shown to bind tightly to the collagen in tissues, including in blood vessels, protecting the collagen against destruction. This improves blood vessel strength.

Coffee has several drawbacks, but a few benefits. The coffee bean itself does contain some flavonoids and helpful minerals, including zinc and magnesium. But it also contains caffeine, which can raise blood pressure and contribute to cardiac muscle irritability. Coffee drinkers also have significantly higher homocysteine levels.

What about decaffeinated coffee? Unfortunately, it contains rather large amounts of hydrogen peroxide that can add to your body's free-radical burden. Hydrogen peroxide is broken down into the powerful and destructive hydroxyl radical. Still, an occasional cup won't hurt, especially if you keep your antioxidant reserve high.

Red Wine

In 1993 Dr. E. N. Frankel and his co-workers discovered a possible explanation for the so-called "French paradox."[368] The French paradox is based on the observation that the French, who eat high-fat foods, smoke heavily, and exercise little, have lower cardiovascular disease rates than Americans with similar habits. The one difference is that the French, per capita, consume more wine than any other population in the world. Dr. Frankel discovered in laboratory studies that wine contained special flavonoids that powerfully inhibited the oxidation of LDL lipoproteins.

In fact, even when diluted to a concentration of 1:1,000 red wine still inhibited LDL oxidation. White wine was much less effective, with about one-tenth the benefits of red wine. While this seems to explain the phenomenon, little was known about how well wine flavonoids worked in humans. Using human volunteers, he found that supplying 400 mg of red wine a day for two weeks to these happy guinea pigs, significantly reduced the ability of LDL to be oxidized in the presence of copper, a standard measure of LDL oxidizability.[369] Other studies did not reproduce this effect.[370] In fact, this same study found that white wine actually increased the risk of oxidizing LDL.

Another way red wine may reduce atherosclerosis is by the action of flavonoids, such as catechin, epicatechin, and quercetin, to bind free iron. In humans, drinking red wine, especially with bread, significantly inhibits iron absorption.[371] This is an important property since as we age we absorb and retain more iron in our tissues, which leads to increased free-radical injury. In addition to iron chelation, quercetin—which is also found in apples, onions, and tea—has been shown to stimulate relaxation of the muscle layer (smooth muscle) in blood vessels, thus improving blood flow.[372]

Other explanations have been proposed to explain this phenomenon. For example, some have proposed that the weak estrogenic effects of flavonoids in the wine actually reduce the risk of cardiovascular disease.[373] Estrogens may reduce the risk of LDL oxidation.

While most of us would like to think that red wine is a magic elixir, the French paradox may have very little to do with wine at all. In all the excitement over red wine, epidemiologists somehow forgot to mention that the French also have a very high intake of fruits and vegetables, which as we have seen, contain numerous substances (including fiber, flavonoids, plant sterols, magnesium, potassium, and folate) that inhibit atherosclerosis.[374]

I remember one lecture on disease prevention in which, when I mentioned the health effects of wine, someone in the audience let out a whoop of joy and applauded loudly. Now, he thought, he could get healthy *and* imbibe a little fruit of the vine at the same time. Then I dropped the bomb: there are other substances in wine that should give us pause.

California wines, especially, are problematic since grapes from that state contain rather high levels of fluoride. Apparently, vineyards there use fluoride as a pesticide—in addition to watering with fluoridated water. As one of the most reactive chemicals in the periodic chart, fluoride binds tightly to the plant proteins and cannot be removed. Most grape products in fact, especially juices, contain high levels of fluoride and should be avoided.

Another problem with wines is that they all contain sulfites. While some people are highly allergic to sulfites, that is not my major concern. Recent studies have shown that sulfites enhance the excitotoxicity of glutamate and aspartate, and may increase our risk of developing a neurodegenerative disease. Sulfites are also added to other processed foods, such as jams, fruit juices, cheese, dried fruits, and raisins.

In general eat foods that you prepare yourself. The fresher and less processed the food, the better it is for you. You will feel better and have far less risk of disease. Eat fresh or frozen fruits and vegetables, and meats that have no additives. Raising your own foods is best. Organic foods are next best.

Other Precautions

Outside of vascular considerations, and to improve your overall health, do not use fluoride toothpaste, fluoride mouthwashes, or have fluoride treatments by your dentist. Also, if you have dental amalgams ("silver" fillings) or crowns with amalgam underneath, you should be tested for mercury, and undergo chelation therapy if necessary. Have amalgam fillings removed by a dentist trained in the approved removal methods (see appendix) and replaced with ceramic.

Exercise

Most of us are aware that exercise reduces our risk of having a heart attack, but it does much more than that. It has been shown to improve immune function, reduce atherosclerosis, increase antioxidant-enzyme levels, improve lung function, increase muscle tone and strength, relieve pain, improve cognitive function, increase blood flow through thousands of miles of small blood vessels, and relieve depression. The real unknown is just how much exercise is needed, and how vigorously it must be done to achieve these effects.

Unfortunately, too much attention has been focused on aerobic exercise. A commonly held belief is that unless you maintain a specified heart rate for a particular period of time, little good comes of the effort. As a result, many people just give up after a brief foray into the fitness jungle and resume a sedentary lifestyle. Fortunately, growing evidence indicates that moderate exercise, such as brisk walking or a moderate workout with an exercise machine, can impart the most healthful benefits. The most important consideration is that, whatever exercise you choose, it must be done on a regular basis and for at least forty-five minutes per session.

The important thing to remember is that the number of free radicals generated during exercise depends on the intensity of the exercise and its duration. Recent studies on intensely training athletes have demonstrated a remarkable increase in free-radical generation and lipid peroxidation. Fortunately, these harmful effects can be reduced by increasing antioxidant intakes. It seems the reason more athletes do not develop severe diseases and advanced degeneration of tissues is that exercise also increases antioxidant enzymes, such as glutathione peroxidase and catalase, but it is not enough to protect the extreme athlete or chronic aerobic exerciser fully.

Unless antioxidants in the diet are proportionately increased, intense exercise can actually do more harm than good. In fact, a regular program of intense exercise will use up the body's existing supply of antioxidants, and then start draining fixed antioxidants, such as glutathione, in cells. Why is this important? Because glutathione is one of the most versatile and powerful antioxidants in our bodies. It is critical to health and life itself.

The good news is that glutathione can be increased in our cells by nutrition. When other antioxidants, such as vitamins C and E, the flavonoids, and alpha-lipoic acid are in plentiful supply, glutathione is preserved. Supplements such as alpha-lipoic acid and NAC actually increase the supply of glutathione, and do so rather dramatically.

It is probably not a good idea to take large doses of glutathione alone. This is because even though most cells in the body can absorb glutathione from the blood, brain cells cannot. As a result, the glutathione is broken down. One of its components is cysteine, a fairly powerful excitotoxin. In fact, very little glutathione is absorbed from the intestine, most is broken down by digestive enzymes.

Another very important effect of exercise is improved glucose control. Previously I discussed the deleterious effects of elevated levels of glucose on cells and tissues and the connection to cross-linking and advanced glycation end products (AGEs). Exercise significantly improves glucose regulation, even in lean young people.[375] The effect is especially important in obese people with diabetes, and works no matter the age. By reducing excess glucose, one also reduces glycation, and as a result, free-radical damage.

In general, depending on your age, exercise at least three times a week, for forty-five minutes to one hour, at a moderate pace. I discourage long-distance running and intense aerobic exercises.

For the elderly, I advise a weight program to keep muscles toned and prevent muscle-wasting. Resistance exercises also strengthen the bones and helps prevent osteoporosis. When weather permits, exercise outdoors, to harvest the benefits of sunshine and fresh air. Many studies on the elderly have found significant vitamin D deficiencies due to confinement in the darkness of their houses. Air conditioning, although a wonderful invention, has the drawback of encouraging us to stay indoors to avoid the sweltering heat of summer. As a result, many elderly rarely feel the sun on their skin. Being outdoors also allows us time to appreciate God's creations, relax mentally and thereby reduce the stresses of the day.

Relaxation and Prayer

Our society is too hurried and fast-paced. We get too little quality sleep, and combined with our poor nutrition, we place ourselves at very high risk for all kinds of degenerative diseases, including cancer. We need to have a quiet time every day that allows us to escape our problems and demanding schedules.

While many suggest relaxation of any sort, as a Christian, I suggest prayer. Not only is it relaxing but, as a believer, I feel it realigns my life so that I can spend time communing with God, praising Him and asking for His help and guidance. Everything else should take second place to this special time. God gave us a day of rest and we should observe it.

Vitamins and Vascular Disease

As I stated earlier, one of the earliest observations, somewhere around the early 1930s, was that persons with the highest intakes of vitamin C had the lowest incidences of heart attacks and strokes. The more we learn about vitamin C, the more we can begin to appreciate its almost miraculous health effects. This water-soluble vitamin does a lot more than just strengthen collagen tissue and act as an antioxidant, it also plays a vital role in immunity, controls brain levels of neurotransmitters, acts as an energy source, protects the nervous system from glutamate toxicity, and has antiviral and antibacterial properties. Its role in building collagen tissue is also very important in protecting our blood vessels, since collagen gives them their strength.

A recent news story created quite a stir because it suggested the possibility that vitamin C caused atherosclerosis. Unfortunately, the news media got the facts all wrong. The article reported a study using male smokers that used ultrasound to measure the thickness of the arterial wall. Results demonstrated that subjects placed on vitamin C developed a thickening of their arteries.

There are several problems with this study. Most glaring is the fact that smokers have extremely low vitamin C levels, and as a result, develop thinning of the arterial wall caused by a loss of collagen. Because vitamin C thickened these weakened vessels, the test subjects actually reduced their risk of atherosclerosis. Furthermore, researchers did not measure atherosclerotic plaque formation or blood flow, both of which can be measured by this same technique. In fact numerous, better-controlled clinical and laboratory studies have shown that vitamin C slows the development of atherosclerosis.[376]

For example, one recent study followed 520 smoking and non-smoking men and postmenopausal women for three years and examined them for progression of atherosclerotic disease using an ultrasonogram to make the measurement objective.[377] Researchers found that men given a combination of vitamins C and E experienced a 74 percent reduction in atherosclerosis. Other studies have shown that vitamin C improves the function of the endothelial cells within blood vessels, which greatly improves blood flow.[378]

Clinical studies have shown that vitamin C supplementation can reduce coronary heart disease mortality by as much as 42 percent.[379] It has also been shown to be effective in cases of chronic heart failure by improving the strength and elasticity of blood vessels.

B Vitamins

Several B vitamins have also shown effectiveness in reducing atherosclerosis. A recent article in *Annals of Vascular Surgery* reported that vitamin B_1 (thiamine) protects against the early causes of atherosclerosis in cases of diabetes, a condition which is also associated with an extremely high incidence of atherosclerosis.[380]

One of the best-studied connections between vitamin deficiencies and atherosclerosis is with three of the B vitamins: folic acid (folate), vitamin B_{12} (methylcobalamin), and vitamin B_6

(pyridoxine). These three vitamins are cofactors in the metabolism of methionine. If one or more of these vitamins is deficient, blood and tissue levels of homocysteine will rise. Several recent studies have shown that even modest elevation of homocysteine, even within the normal range, can significantly increase the risk of a heart attack, stroke, or peripheral vascular disease.[381] Smoking, obesity, inactivity and stress can all increase homocysteine levels. Homocysteine is an independent risk factor, possibly having more importance than cholesterol levels.

Deficiencies of these three vitamins are very common in the elderly, reaching an incidence as high as 80 percent in carefully done studies of normal elderly.[382] One of these three vitamins may have an additional benefit in preventing atherosclerosis, long before the first pathological signs begin to appear. In 1949 two researchers named Rinehart and Greenberg found they could reproduce atherosclerosis in monkeys simply by maintaining them on a diet deficient in vitamin B_6 for two-and-a-half years. Unfortunately, since scientists at that time were unable to explain why this could result in atherosclerosis, they did what leading scientists have always done: they simply ignored it. Besides, cholesterol had just arrived on the scene and seemed to offer a far more direct connection.

In the early 1980s Dr. C. I. Levene, a pathologist with the Department of Pathology, University of Cambridge, England, read the 1949 study and found a possible explanation of the effect.[383] He already knew that atherosclerosis tends to occur at places of maximum stress in arteries, and discovered that a weakness occurred at these stress points because collagen and elastin had not developed properly.

It seems that the strength of collagen and elastin, the substances that gives strength and elasticity to blood vessels, requires a cross-linking process for full development. This molecular bridging utilizes an enzyme, lysyl oxidase, that requires vitamin B_6 for it activity. A B_6 (pyridoxine) deficiency leads to a weakening in the blood vessels so that increased stress at arterial branching points and sharp curves leads to small tears in the wall of the vessel. This increases the likelihood of accumulation of oxidized LDL cholesterol, and explains why atherosclerosis is more severe at places of high-flow stress. It also explains why people with hypertension have higher rates of atherosclerosis.

Dr. Levine noted that during pregnancy, the physiological requirements for vitamin B_6 increase greatly, leading to a high incidence of vitamin B_6 deficiency in the mother as well as the child. This would explain the presence of early changes of atherosclerosis found in infants and small children. Deficiency in pyridoxine has also been shown to interfere with the conversion of alpha-linolenic acid (flaxseed oil) to EPA and DHA, especially affecting DHA production. These oils play a major role in preventing atherosclerosis.

Deficiencies in vital antioxidants, and an increase in free radicals and lipid peroxidation products, have been found to worsen as the damage to the heart increases. One study of twenty patients with heart failure found that as heart-failure rates increase, the levels of markers for lipid peroxidation and the superoxide radical also increased significantly. At the same time, critical antioxidant enzymes, such as catalase, glutathione reductase, and superoxide dismutase (SOD) decreased. This creates a very dangerous situation that will eventually lead to a heart attack or stroke. When a group of these heart failure patients were given vitamin B_6, all of these factors markedly improved.

The Role of Garlic

Millions of Americans are gobbling down garlic pills in an effort to prevent the occurrence of a heart attack or stroke. Just how much scientific evidence is there for this practice? In truth, quite a lot. When endothelial cells are exposed to either garlic extract or one of its major compounds (S-allylcysteine), we see significant protection against oxidation and cell-membrane damage.[384] Recall that malfunction of endothelial cells initiates and promotes atherosclerosis.

Another potential way garlic may help prevent heart attacks, strokes, and peripheral vascular disease is by reducing blood coagulability. Sudden coagulation in the vicinity of atherosclerotic crud (plaque) is the precursor for dramatic onset of a heart attack or stroke. These plaques have rough surfaces that activate platelets, causing them to clump together. This then causes the activation of fibrinogen, leading to clotting of the blood.

All this is well and good when doing experiments in test tubes, but what about effects in humans? A recent study of the affects of garlic on platelet function in men with high blood-cholesterol levels found that those taking aged garlic supplements over a ten-month period showed a significant reduction in platelet clumping (adhesion) and activation by various stimulants commonly seen in clinical conditions, such as epinephrine release and exposure to collagen.[385] Subjects taking the garlic also showed less oxidation of their LDL cholesterol. In addition, the garlic reduced the adhesion of the platelets to fibrinogen, an early event in heart attacks and strokes.

In another recent study, thirty patients with coronary artery disease were given garlic capsules and thirty were given a placebo.[386] Those given the garlic capsules experienced a significant fall in total cholesterol and triglyceride levels, and a significant increase in HDL cholesterol levels. Researchers also found a decrease in blood coagulability.

One of the more impressive studies found that garlic extract not only prevents atherosclerosis, it actually seemed to cause the crud in the arteries to regress![387] The study was extended over a forty-eight-month period, which means with longer treatment even further removal of the plaque would have occurred.

Because of garlic extract's anticoagulant effect, it should not be combined with other anticoagulants, such as coumadin and warfarin. There is no evidence that combining garlic with other anticoagulant supplements, such as Ginkgo biloba or omega-3 oils, causes bleeding problems, but there is a potential risk. In my medical practice, I have used them together for many years and never observed a bleeding problem.

Anecdotal reports crop up in the medical journals periodically, claiming a link between taking certain supplements and spontaneous bleeding. As I discussed in the section on

Ginkgo biloba, most of these reports are dubious at best. Yet, I do believe it may present a problem for certain people who are more susceptible to spontaneous bleeding or trauma related bleeding (usually elderly persons). I have found that in most such cases the patient had a pre-existing problem with fragile blood vessels, most often due to poor nutrition. Vitamin C, bioflavonoids, zinc, and special phytochemicals can significantly strengthen these fragile vessels.

Another very important effect of garlic extract is that it stimulates nitric oxide formation within cells lining the blood vessels.[388] This mechanism explains how garlic lowers high blood pressure, but its benefits go beyond that: by stimulating nitric oxide production within blood vessels, garlic significantly improves blood flow through the vessels, and therefore, improves the health of the organs and tissues supplied by these blood vessels.

Grape Seed Extract

This extract was at one time very popular as a powerful antioxidant. In fact, several studies indicated that it was twenty times more potent than vitamin C and fifty times more potent than vitamin E. Later studies indicated that it was an excellent free-radical neutralizer and could powerfully inhibit lipid peroxidation. Like many of the flavonoids, it also could bind iron, thereby preventing free-radical generation.

Grape seed extract contains various flavonoids, classified as either oligomeric or polymeric. The oligomeric are called procyanidins and the polymeric, condensed tannins. Oligomeric procyanidins (OPCs for short) are extracted in typical grape seed extract. About 20-30 percent of the flavonoids are found in the skin of the grape, and 60-70 percent within the seeds.[389]

Grape seed extract has been used in Europe for many years to treat capillary fragility and vascular insufficiency. It has been especially helpful in preventing vascular damage to the eyes caused by diabetes. In fact, grape seed extract has been used successfully for numerous vascular conditions, including varicose veins, hypertensive retinopathy, cerebral and peripheral vascular insufficiency, and "leaky vessels."

In animal studies, grape seed extract has been shown to protect the interior of blood vessels against powerful caustic agents.[390] The extract protects blood vessels by several mechanisms, but primarily by protecting them from destructive enzymes, such as collogenase and elastase.

Several human studies have shown a significant improvement in cases of poor blood supply to the legs, with improvement in symptoms varying from 74 percent for tingling and numbness to 67 percent for night cramps.[391]

As we have seen, strengthening of the blood vessels is critical in many vascular conditions, especially in preventing atherosclerosis and its related problems, such as strokes, heart attacks and peripheral vascular disease. It is especially important to strengthen the small arteries in the brain, since these are the vessels that, when ruptured, lead to bleeding into the brain in cases of high blood pressure (hypertensive intracranial bleeding). Strong blood vessel walls are also important in preventing the formation of aneurysms and in preventing existing aneurysms from rupturing.

One group especially vulnerable to blood vessel diseases of all sorts is the diabetic. Several studies have shown that grape seed extract significantly improves the blood vessel injury seen in diabetics, especially vascular problems within the eye.[392]

When buying grape seed extract, be sure to get a brand that says "guaranteed potency with 85 percent proanthocyanidins." Most studies used doses from 150 to 300 mg a day. To maintain good blood vessel strength, I recommend 100 mg a day minimum.

In general I divide supplements into those needed for maintenance and those used to treat an existing disease. While the vegetarian diet supplies most of the nutrients, some people will need to be boosted for added protection. Follow the program below that best fits your health needs.

Essential Basic Supplementation

Multivitamin/mineral capsule

In general, I prefer an encapsulated vitamin that contains loose powder. This assures maximum absorption. Some hard tablets contain so many binders used to hold the tablet together during shipping that the thing will not dissolve in the GI tract. I have one patient that is wonderful for evaluating supplements: she has an ileostomy bag that connects to her small intestine. She told me one brand of hard-tablet multivitamin came out of her ileostomy bag just like it went into her mouth.

If you don't have an ileostomy bag, a quick test is to put one teaspoon of vinegar in a six-ounce glass of water and plop the suspect vitamin in it. It should dissolve in less than a minute. If it remains intact, toss it and go for the encapsulated form.

The multiple vitamin/mineral capsule should provide a total of 25-50 mg each of the B vitamins, such as thiamine (B_1), riboflavin (B_2), and pyridoxine (B_6), and 100 mg of niacinamide, etc. The mineral portion of your multivitamin should contain no iron, and either no or very small quantities of copper.

Vitamin E 400 to 800 IU

What we refer to as vitamin E is not really one substance in its natural state, but rather four different molecules, called tocopherols. They are named alpha, beta, gamma, and delta. Each form has a different function. Most assays look for antioxidant power. The most powerful antioxidant form is alpha-tocopherol. Gamma is suspected to play a role in preventing atherosclerosis, but the amounts are naturally lower than the alpha form.

When buying supplements, you will find several forms of vitamin E, some called dl-alpha tocopherol acetate or d-alpha tocopherol acetate and others referred to as mixed tocopherols. The latter of these is the kind found in nature. Dl-alpha tocopherol acetate is the least active form of the vitamin. It is poorly absorbed, does not seem to enter the brain, and is a poor antioxidant. In addition, it has been shown to have little or no effectiveness in inhibiting cancer. The same is true of the d-alpha tocopherol acetate. The addition of the acetate group actually reduces its effectiveness.

The most powerful cancer-inhibiting form of the vitamin is d-alpha tocopheryl succinate. It also appears to have greater antioxidant power than other forms. Next in line is the natural form, or mixed tocopherols. The only problem I have with the mixed tocopherols is that many are dissolved in vegetable oil. Unique E is pure natural vitamin E without vegetable oil. There is also a question about the gelatin capsule and the risk of "mad cow" disease. While risk appears to be very low, when you are dealing with a disease reported to have 100 percent mortality, it is a major concern.

The d-alpha tocopherol succinate form comes as a dry powder. It is often referred to as "dry E." Most manufacturers use a vegetable-based capsule rather than a gelatin capsule, because of the concern about mad cow disease. This form of vitamin E is also the most powerful antioxidant form, and powerfully inhibits the development and growth of cancer. It also enters the brain very easily, where it provides maximum protection against free radicals and lipid peroxidation.

Vitamin C (ascorbate)
Take 500-1,500 mg a day in three divided doses. For instance, either 250 mg or 500 mg twice to three times a day. *Never take vitamin C as ascorbic acid.* It is far too acidic for general use and will, in many individuals, produce acidosis of the tissues, and can lead to activation of herpetic mouth ulcers.

To prevent this complication, always use either the calcium or magnesium ascorbate, preferably magnesium ascorbate. It is probably best to take the vitamin C on an empty stomach, since it is a very powerful enhancer of iron absorption when combined with foods containing iron. Taking time-release forms of the vitamin can present a problem because it constantly releases ascorbate, even during meals.

This brings us to a precaution when using vitamin C. Because of the tremendous enhancement of iron absorption caused by the vitamin it should never be taken by people who have hemochromatosis, sideroblastic anemia, or thallisemia major, all conditions associated with tissue iron excess.

Unfortunately, not everyone knows whether or not they have hemochromatosis. It can be a silent disorder until advanced liver destruction has taken place. For this reason, you should have a complete series of iron tests that includes iron levels, iron-binding capacity, ferritin levels, and iron saturation before starting on high-dose vitamin C supplements.

Several studies have shown that vitamin C absorption is limited to 200 mg, and that doses higher than this are excreted in the urine or feces. So far, we do not have a final word on this controversy. There is some suggestion that the equilibrium with the tissues occurs so rapidly that blood levels do not truly reflect total absorption. This view is held by those endorsing megadoses of vitamin C to treat disease. No one, at this stage, can definitively say if they are wrong.

We do know that smokers have a defect in vitamin C absorption. This has been confirmed in several carefully conducted human studies. A more recent study found that even those who breathe second-hand smoke have this problem. Even supplementation with higher than RDA levels of ascorbate will not return blood levels to normal. In most studies it takes 200 mg of vitamin C to reach even low-normal ascorbate blood levels. Most likely, it will take much higher concentrations of the vitamin to reach adequate tissue levels. Several investigators have proposed a direct connection between low vitamin C levels and the high level of atherosclerotic disease in smokers.

Garlic Extract 300 mg of standardized extract 0.8 percent allicin
Numerous studies have shown that garlic lowers total cholesterol as well as LDL cholesterol and raises HDL cholesterol. In addition, it will lower triglycerides, thin the blood, and act as an antibacterial. And, as we have seen before, it is one of the few supplements that can actually reverse atherosclerosis. You should take two capsules twice a day with a meal. Selenium-enhanced garlic is even better.

Methylcobalamin 1,000 ug
This comes as a sublingual tablet. Dissolve under the tongue twice a day. Do not use cheaper cyanocobalamin forms of vitamin B_{12}. These are made by chemically binding cobalamin (the B_{12} portion) to cyanide. This gives stability to the molecule. The problem is that it also requires enzymatic removal of the cyanide before the vitamin can be utilized. Some people's systems are unable to do this, making the vitamin useless. Methylcobalamin is the form of vitamin B_{12} normally used by the body. It is very well absorbed and utilized.

Antioxidants for Preventing Atherosclerosis

Alpha-lipoic acid 50 mg
This is the basic daily dose. For greater protection, you can go up to 100 mg two or three times a day. Doses higher than 50 mg a day and the more potent R-lipoic acid can induce hypoglycemia and precipitate migraine headaches in those with a migraine history.

Coenzyme Q10 100 mg
Take once a day. For maximum protection, go to 100 mg three times a day, to 600 mg a day in divided doses. CoQ10 is a powerful antioxidant that has been shown to reduce oxidation of LDL cholesterol.

Quercetin 500 mg
Take one twice to three times a day. This flavonoid, found in high concentrations in teas, apples and onions, is a powerful antioxidant both on a cellular level and in preventing LDL cholesterol oxidation in blood vessel walls.

Curcumin 500 mg

This flavonoid is a powerful antioxidant against numerous types of free radicals and has very potent anti-inflammatory properties as well. It will reduce the inflammatory response within blood vessel walls, thus reducing atherosclerosis.

Vitamin E (as succinate or mixed tocopherols) 800 IU a day

Vitamin E is the major antioxidant found within the structure of LDL. It also improves blood flow and protects other organs and tissues from free-radical damage.

Vitamin C (as calcium or magnesium ascorbate) 250-500 mg, three times a day

Some may wish to go to 1,000 mg three times a day. Again, take it on an empty stomach. It works in conjunction with vitamin E, as well as other antioxidants.

N-acetyl L-cysteine (NAC) 700 mg

Take one a day. This supplement is metabolized efficiently to form glutathione in all cells. Glutathione is one of the most important antioxidants in the body. I would not recommend taking glutathione directly. It is poorly absorbed and cannot enter brain cells. As a result, it is broken down into its constituent parts, one of which is cysteine, an excitatory amino acid that can damage brain cells. NAC, because it has an acetyl group, is not excitotoxic in the brain. It is taken up into the cell before the cysteine group is removed.

DHA 100 mg

This is not to be confused with DHEA, the hormone precursor. DHA is a fatty acid, part of the omega-3 fatty acids. Take two capsules two times a day. Vitamin E should always be taken with DHA because DHA is highly unsaturated, making it susceptible to oxidation. Keep this and all other oils in the refrigerator.

Because of the expense of these supplements, they should be reserved for those at high risk of atherosclerosis—or those who just have a lot of money.

Reducing Elevated Cholesterol or Triglycerides

Guggulipid

This product is extracted from the Indian Bdellium tree, which is in the same genus as myrrh mentioned in the Bible. Its effectiveness will depend on the purity of the brand you are using. It should be standardized to 25 mg of gugulsterone per 500 mg capsule. Take one capsule a day. The longer you take the supplement, the more effective it is, so do not expect immediate results. Usually within two to three months you should have maximum effectiveness.

Guggulipid also has powerful anti-inflammatory activity, and has been shown to be as effective as tetracycline in treating cystic acne. This antibiotic effect also may account for some of its ability to inhibit atherosclerosis.

Safety note. Clinical trials have shown it to be generally safe. Some will have gastric upset, headache, mild nausea and hiccups. It also can stimulate thyroid activity and should be used with caution when taking thyroid medications. It is contraindicated for those with hyper-thyroidism.

Interactions with other medications. It can interfere with the effectiveness of propranolol (Inderol) and diltiazem (Cardizem) and may interfere with thyroid therapies. (*Natural Medicines Comprehensive Database, 2001*)

Inositol hexaniacinate

This is a special formulation of the basic vitamin niacin that avoids the flushing of conventional niacin and has fewer serious side effects. It has been used in Europe for the past thirty years to lower cholesterol. Inositol is related to the B group of vitamins and is used to improve nerve function in diabetics. Because of its role in cell-membrane function, it has also shown beneficial effects for depression and general neurological function. The dose is 500 mg taken three times a day with meals. Like guggulipid, full effectiveness will take four to five months. Human studies have shown that by twenty-six weeks LDL cholesterol was lowered 23 percent and HDL cholesterol was elevated 33 percent. This equals or exceeds that of prescription drugs, and has a much better margin of safety.

While it is much safer than niacin, there is still some risk of liver toxicity. It should be used with caution, especially in those with a history of hepatitis, alcohol abuse and other liver disorders. It is a good idea to obtain a baseline liver function test and to repeat these after three weeks of therapy. The risk of liver toxicity is extremely low.

Garlic Extract

Should contain 10 mg of 0.8 percent alliin or a total of 4,000 ug of allicin potential for the total daily dose. Always buy quality brands.

Vitamin C (as ascorbate) 250-500 mg a day in divided doses on an empty stomach

Vitamin C has been shown to lower total cholesterol and triglycerides, and increase HDL. For each 1 percent rise in HDL the risk of heart attack drops by 4 percent.

Artichoke Extract (leaf, stem, or root) 1-4 g three times a day

This extract has shown a capacity to lower cholesterol and contains high levels of luteolin, a powerful anticancer and antioxidant flavonoid. Do not take if you have gallbladder disease. There are no known interactions with medications. (*Natural Medicines Comprehensive Database, 2001*)

Lysine 1,500 mg a day in three divided doses

Five hundred milligrams of lysine three times a day should suffice. Your doctor can track lipoprotein(a) levels to determine dosage adjustments.

Methods of Lowering Homocysteine

Do not smoke. Smoking dramatically increases homocysteine levels as well as increasing free-radical generation in all organs of the body. It also lowers vitamin C levels dramatically.

Do not consume foods or drinks that contain caffeine. Caffeine not only increases homocysteine levels, it also increases the irritability of the heart.

Folic acid (folate) 400 ug
Take twice a day. This enzyme cofactor plays a major role in converting homocysteine to methionine. Elevated homocysteine levels are also associated with Alzheimer's disease and birth defects.

Vitamin B$_{12}$ (methylcobalamin) 1,000 ug
Take sublingually (dissolve under the tongue) twice a day. This vitamin also plays a major role in the conversion of homocysteine to methionine.

Vitamin B$_6$ (pyridoxine)
You guessed it; this vitamin is also involved in the homocysteine conversion to methionine reaction. Take 50- to 100 mg a day. Doses over 500 mg a day have been associated with nerve damage. Some people, especially the elderly, can have difficulty converting pyridoxine to its active form, pyrodoxyl-5 phosphate. In that case they will need to take pyridoxal-5 phosphate directly. It is available and should be taken in doses one-third those of vitamin B$_6$ itself.

Trimethyglycine
Also called TMG or betaine. This is a metabolic product that helps to lower homocysteine in cases that are resistant to the triple vitamin therapy mentioned above. It does so as a methyl donor, which converts homocysteine to methionine. In studies it lowered homocysteine levels 20-30 percent. It is a very safe nutrient.

The dose is three grams taken twice daily for adults. Higher doses will lower homocysteine levels even more. The product does not interact with prescription drugs and has a high margin of safety.

Avoid excess stress, since stress has been shown to increase homocysteine levels. This will require getting at least eight hours of sleep every night.

Stroke Prevention and Treatment

Vinpocetine
Vinpocetine is an indole alkaloid derived from the periwinkle plant. It has been shown to increase blood supply, oxygen utilization, and energy production in the brain. It also increases serotonin levels in the brain (decreased serotonin also plays a role in depression and violence). The recommended dose is two 5 mg tablets three times a day (30 mg total) for one month and then switch to one tablet three times a day (15 mg total).

On rare occasions, people have experienced a brief drop in blood pressure, or a fast heart rate. Lowering the dose usually corrects this problem. Doses greater than 10 mg the first day can cause headache. Start with the lower dose and increase gradually.

Acetyl-L-carnitine 500 mg
This supplement is a substance used by the brain for fatty acid metabolism as well as numerous other functions, including iron chelation, energy production, generation of brain acetylcholine, and protection of the mitochondria. Several studies have shown it signifi-

cantly reduces the effects of aging on the brain. One of the ways it does this is by improving the function of the mitochondria, returning them more to the way they were when you were twenty. I suggest taking a 500 mg capsule twice to three times a day (1,500 mg total).

Alpha-lipoic acid

This component is found naturally in the body, and is quickly converted to dehydrolipoic acid. In this form it is a very powerful and versatile antioxidant and iron chelator, and has been shown to increase mitochondrial energy production. In my neurosurgical experience I have found it to be very protective of the injured brain. In large doses, 600 mg or more, it can lower blood sugar. I suggest 200 mg a day in two divided doses.

Vitamin E succinate 400 IU

This is considered to be the most powerful antioxidant form of vitamin E, as well as the most potent against cancer growth. It penetrates the brain well and protects the many cell membranes in neurons and other cells. It also protects the blood vessels feeding the brain. The dose is one 400 IU capsule twice a day (800 IU total).

Vitamin C

The brain has one of the highest levels of vitamin C found in the body, exceeded only by the adrenal glands. In the brain, the highest concentration is in the hippocampus, an area that plays a major role in memory acquisition and emotional elaboration. There is evidence that it plays an important role in regulating glutamate in the brain, protecting neurons against excitotoxicity. In conjunction with flavonoids and vitamin E, it protects the brain against numerous free radicals as well. I would suggest 500 mg of buffered vitamin C three times a day on an empty stomach.

Multivitamin/mineral

The brain utilizes large amounts of B vitamins, especially thiamine, riboflavin, pyridoxine, B_{12}, folate, and niacinamide. It is best to buy multivitamins in a powdered form, either as a loose powder or in capsules. The vitamins should be in sufficient doses to be effective. For example, thiamine, pyridoxine, and riboflavin should be in 25-50 mg doses, niacinamide in 100-500 mg doses, folate in 400 ug doses, and vitamin B_{12}, as methylcobalamin, in 1,000 ug doses. They should have 100-200 ug of selenium (as selenomethionine or selenium enhanced garlic extract) and 200 ug of chromium picolinate, as well as all the other trace elements and essential minerals. It is unusual to find a vitamin that contains all of these components in the proper doses, which may require you to take them individually. *Do not purchase multiminerals that contain iron.*

One experiment conducted by neuroscientists at Massachusetts General Hospital and Harvard Medical School found that nicotinamide (niacinamide), a precursor of an energy-forming molecule in the brain (NAD), when given to rats with an occluded cerebral artery, could dramatically reduce the size of the stroke.[393] In fact, the supplement worked even when given two hours after the vessel was tied off.

Ginkgo Biloba

Ginkgo contains alkaloids that improve brain oxygenation and blood flow, and protect blood vessels and neurons against free-radical injury. Because of the risk of hemorrhage (again, no more than is associated with taking aspirin), limit intake to 120-240 mg a day. Also, take blood-vessel strengthening supplements for one month before starting the Ginkgo if possible. If you wish to be assured that anticoagulation is not excessive, have bleeding and clotting studies done three weeks after starting the Ginkgo. Generally, this is not necessary.

With hypertensive hemorrhages, I would use only a low dose of Ginkgo biloba—60 mg— and then check bleeding and clotting time three weeks after beginning supplementation.

Methylcobalamin (Vitamin B_{12})

I suggest taking methylcobalamin as 1,000 ug three times a day, and the folate no more than 800 ug a day.

Strengthening the Heart Muscle

Coenzyme Q10 (CoQ10)

Most patient studies used at least 100 mg of the extract. For those with congestive heart failure, the dose begins at 300 mg a day and goes up to 600 mg a day in three divided doses, that is take 200 mg three times a day. CoQ10 is a fat-soluble substance and will require that you either take it with a meal containing fats (extra virgin olive oil) or take it with your DHA supplement.

Cholesterol-lowering drugs all deplete CoQ10. This is because the enzyme that generates cholesterol, HMG CoA reductase, is also responsible for the production of CoQ10. The Cholestyramine drugs (Questran, LoCHOLEST and Prevalite) also lower beta-carotene, folic acid, and vitamins A, D, E, and K by inhibiting absorption. The drug, Colestid, inhibits absorption of beta-carotene, folic acid, and vitamins A, D, and E. (Source: *Natural Medicines Comprehensive Database, 2001*).

L-carnitine

The dose varies from 500-1,500 mg a day. The major side effect is diarrhea at the higher doses. If you develop diarrhea and dose reduction does not help, I suggest switching to acetyl-L-carnitine which is less likely to cause this side effect and has the added advantage of entering the brain more easily, where it improves brain-cell function and memory and chelates excess iron from the brain. The dose is the same, but it is much more expensive than L-carnitine.

Ginkgo Biloba Extract

Take 120-240 mg a day. This extract has been shown to improve blood flow through all tissues, especially the heart and brain. It also contains numerous antioxidant flavonoids and special substances called ginkgolides, which have been shown to reduce blood viscosity and improve blood flow through the microvessels. There is also evidence that it reduces the irritability of the heart muscle (arrhythmia). It should not be taken with anticoagulants, aspirin, or non-steroidal anti-inflammatory medications.

Hawthorn Extract

This extract should contain both the flower and leaf of the plant. The dose is 200-500 mg three times daily. Not only does it improve heart contractions, but in patients with stage II heart failure, it has been shown to improve exercise tolerance and reduce symptoms such as angina, fatigue, and palpitations. In addition, it can lower blood pressure in hypertensive patients.

Safety precautions. Hawthorn extract can cause agitation, insomnia, GI complaints, and headaches. It should not be used with cardiac glycoside medications, since it can potentially increase toxicity. Some herbs—such as digitalis leaf, figwort, motherwort, and lily of the valley roots—also contain cardiac glycosides. Do not use with fenugreek, ginger, Panax ginseng, parsley, devil's claw, or coltsfoot.

In general, it should not be used with drugs that cause vasodilation, act as CNS depressants, or be used with digoxin. You will need to ask you doctor about these drugs. (*Natural Medicines Comprehensive Database, 2001*).

11
Other Disorders of Aging

Adult-Onset Diabetes: A Growing Epidemic

From six to twelve million people in the United States suffer from adult-onset diabetes, making it one of this country's largest health problems. Of the two types of the disorder, type II diabetes accounts for an astounding 95 percent of all cases. Worse, incidence of the disease continues to rise, and is nearing epidemic proportions. While we know that there is a genetic propensity to develop this form of diabetes, poor nutrition seems to play the major role in its precipitation.

Most of us automatically think of diabetes as a disease in which the body is unable to produce insulin—a condition which is universally true for type I (juvenile-onset) diabetes. With type II diabetes, however, the opposite frequently occurs; sometimes, the body produces more insulin than the body can use. In reality, type II diabetes is characterized as the body's inability to *properly* use the hormone insulin to move glucose into cells. Therefore, sugar, starches and other food cannot be adequately converted to the energy needed for daily life. The condition occurs when insulin receptors, found on the surface of cells throughout the body, stop responding to insulin, a condition called insulin resistance. Blockage of the insulin receptor prevents the hormone from escorting glucose into cells, and leads to increased insulin secretion. Since the pancreas rightly assumes that cells need more glucose and is unaware that the insulin it is sending is malfunctioning, it just keeps sending more.

Numerous complications result from type II diabetes because several major problems are occurring at once: insulin and blood-glucose levels are too high at the same time that cells are starving for glucose. As a result, the body's metabolism is seriously disrupted, leading to significantly increased free-radical generation and lipid peroxidation. This in turn damages every part of the cell, including mitochondria and its DNA, further impairing energy production.

As soon as a person develops insulin resistance, free-radical generation and lipid peroxidation begin to rise. This explains not only the enormous increase in general complications, but also the high incidence of degenerative disorders associated with diabetes. See Table 11.1 for a list of common health problems; note that every one of the complications is associated with free-radical damage. In addition, life expectancy for diabetics is reduced five to ten years.

One interesting study found that diabetics have significantly lower serum DHEA and DHEA-sulfate levels, precursors of reproductive hormones, than normal aged-matched controls.[394] In fact, researchers concluded that DHEA in type II diabetes is significantly and maximally suppressed. How this ultimately affects someone with diabetes is unclear, but a deficiency would certainly alter reproductive hormones, which could explain some cases of diabetes-related impotence.

A Complex Metabolic Disease

It is unfortunate that so many diabetics, and some doctors, do not understand that diabetes entails a lot more than elevated blood sugar. In truth, it is an extremely complex disorder involving numerous metabolic pathways. This is why so many organs and tissues are involved in the disease: eyes, blood vessels, nervous system, kidneys, and heart. Interestingly, the disease exercises a profoundly negative sffect on the vascular system.

We have known for a long time that diabetics have a much higher incidence of heart attacks and strokes than the rest of the population.[395] This appears to be linked to an increased risk of LDL cholesterol oxidizing in their vessels, which means a greatly increased risk of atherosclerosis affecting virtually every blood vessel in the body, especially microscopic vessels.[396] Alteration of these microvessels leads to diabetic retinopathy (blindness) and kidney damage.

As we have seen, oxidized LDL cholesterol beneath the endothelium intensely irritates the artery, which responds by thickening its muscle layer and sending fibroblast cells to wall off the inflammation to prevent further damage. The result is a narrowed lumen that significantly slows the flow of blood through the affected artery.

This is the simplified version of a very complex process that involves biochemical reactions involving special enzymes, eicosanoids, cell-adhesion molecules, growth-promoting molecules and metabolic intermediates. What *you* need to know is that many natural substances have been found to block these destructive reactions and correct various metabolic malfunctions.

Take vitamins C and E and the carotenoids, for example. LDL contains, deep in its core, six vitamin E molecules, which act as built-in protection against oxidation. Normally, this is a very effective mechanism. Vitamin E, for example, can scavenge a powerful free radical called peroxyl ten thousand times more powerfully than it can fat molecules. But, there is a problem. The inner core of the LDL molecule is liquid and can contain free radicals that escape the fat-soluble vitamin E. This is where water-soluble vitamins come into play: vitamin C and carotenoids, both water soluble, can enter this area and neutralize these free radicals, preventing the vitamin E from being oxidized. Once again, this process demonstrates the importance of the antioxidant network, and why you should take all of the antioxidants, not just one or two.

Vitamin E also helps diabetics in other ways. A recent study of diabetics showed that two important metabolic products become elevated when blood glucose levels are high, diacyglycerol (DAG) and protein kinase-Cß (PKC-ß), both of which are associated with severe

---

Diabetics are...

- two to four times more likely to have a heart attack.
- two to four times more likely to have a stroke.
- four times more likely to go blind.
- eight times more likely to develop cataracts and/or glaucoma.
- two to four times more likely to suffer kidney failure.
- five times more likely to be impotent.
- more likely to experience pregnancy complications.

TABLE 11.1

---

damage to microvessels in the kidneys. In experimental studies, vitamin E has been shown to correct both of these defects and return kidney function to normal in diabetic rats.

Another way vitamin E helps is by binding to the wall of the smooth muscle cells in the blood vessel wall, where it increases the formation of a chemical (the eicosanoid called PGI_2) which prevents damage to the vessels. In addition, by inhibiting the enzyme protein kinase-C, vitamin E reduces inflammation in the blood vessel, a major cause of atherosclerosis. Other studies have shown that vitamin E inhibits an enzyme in platelets called thromboxane A2, which reduces the risk of thrombosis.[397] Flavonoids from fruits and vegetables also powerfully inhibit these enzymes, and may explain their protective effects against atherosclerosis.[398]

Numerous human and experimental studies have demonstrated that vitamin C, especially when combined with vitamin E, dramatically reduces the risk of heart attack and strokes, anywhere from a 43 percent to a 75 percent reduction. This finding is especially significant for diabetics.

A fairly recent article that appeared in the *Journal of the American College of Nutrition* reported a study in which vitamin C was used in patients with type II diabetes.[399] This was a placebo-controlled, double-blind, randomized, crossover study (to satisfy all the skeptics) involving forty patients. Researchers found a significant decline in insulin levels, glycosylated hemoglobin (Hb-A_{1c}), total and LDL cholesterol, and apolipoprotein B concentrations, as well as improved insulin action and glucose metabolism. The dose of vitamin C used in the study was 1,000 mg in a divided dose.

Another study, comparing the effect of a combination of vitamins E and C and beta-carotene in non-diabetic and diabetic men, found that the vitamin combination significantly lowered LDL cholesterol oxidation, and also reduced uptake of LDL by macrophages.[400] Combined with numerous other epidemiological studies, this study confirms that a combination of antioxidants can significantly reduce risk of having a heart attack or stroke. This becomes especially important in the case of diabetics.

Recent studies have found that, in addition to other benefits, some flavonoids potently protect LDL from becoming oxidized. For example, the flavonoids in pycnogenol, mainly catechins, have been shown to inhibit inflammation by blocking a group of powerful inflammatory chemicals called leukotrienes.[401] In addition, it strongly inhibited stress- and smoking-related platelet aggregation, a process that can lead to sudden clotting of the blood, as is seen with heart attacks and strokes.

The beauty of pycnogenol is that it was equal to aspirin in blocking platelet overactivity, but did not prolong bleeding time. This is particularly important when one is facing surgery or has a condition associated with a high risk of brain hemorrhage, such as hypertension. In human studies, a dose as small as 100 mg gave adequate protection against heart attacks and strokes. Some people may prefer grape seed extract to pycnogenol: both contain similar flavonoids.

Quercetin is another flavonoid that has shown great promise in preventing cardiovascular disease. It is the most abundant flavonoid in foods, with the highest levels occurring in onions, tea, cranberries, kale, and apples. Several large epidemiological studies have shown a strong correlation between flavonoid intake and a reduction in heart attacks and strokes.

The most well known of these studies, the Zutphen Elderly Study, which involved 552 middle-aged Dutch men, found that men who consumed the highest amount of fruits and vegetables had a stroke rate one-third that of those eating few fruits and vegetables.[402] The most common flavonoid in these foods was quercetin.

Other flavonoids found to reduce the risk of cardiovascular disease include rutin, luteolin, and curcumin.[403] Rutin is found in cherries and other fruits, luteolin is high in artichokes and celery, and curcumin is high in turmeric. Curcumin, quercetin, and apigenin (also in celery) all inhibit the enzyme protein kinase-C, that causes much of the microvascular damage associated with diabetes.

Finally, a series of studies has shown that diabetic patients have significantly elevated homocysteine levels, and that at the same time, they developed kidney damage.[404] As we have seen, elevated homocysteine levels are associated with rapid and extensive atherosclerosis. The studies found that diabetics with the earliest age of onset and poorest metabolic control had the highest homocysteine levels.

Diabetics also have problems with recurring infections and poor wound healing. The flavonoid curcumin (extracted from turmeric) remarkably enhances immunity, and promotes white blood cell proliferation and wound-healing.[405] Vitamin C, zinc, and the B vitamins also play a role in wound healing, especially in the diabetic.

An enormous amount of this evidence was presented at the American Diabetes Association Research Symposium on the Role of Oxidants and Antioxidant Therapy on Diabetic Complications held in Orlando, Florida, in November 1996.[406] The information furnished at this symposium was published in the journal, *Diabetes Care*. Unfortunately, it has had little impact on doctors who treat diabetes.

Throughout all my years of practice, I have never seen a diabetic patient who was put on vitamin E, much less any other vitamin. I once had a patient who suffered from multiple diabetic complications, who came to me from another doctor specializing in diabetic patients. I discovered that the physician had never recommended a single nutritional supplement, despite the patient's medical problems.

My response was to place her on supplements known to improve diabetic complications— only to have the other doctor stop them when the patient returned for her next visit. I asked why. The patient told me the diabetic doctor said they would do no good, and would just be a waste of money. Incredible! Here was a doctor specializing in diabetes, with no clue as to the connection between nutrition and a metabolic disorder of this magnitude. More evidence-based medicine.

Diabetes and Neurological Problems

One of the more debilitating problems associated with diabetes is nerve injury, so-called diabetic polyneuropathy. This condition generally involves nerves supplying sensation to the feet, with resulting numbness, and occasionally an intense burning sensation. Many patients describe the sensation as "walking on cotton."

The cause of this nerve damage is still being debated, with some arguing that it is caused by microvascular damage to the fibers in the nerve and others attributing it to metabolic derangement within the nerves. Most likely, it is a combination of both.

During early studies, researchers found that diabetics suffered from an inositol deficiency and posited a link between this shortage and nerve damage. It was found that supplementing diabetics with inositol did improve their neuropathy.[407] Recent studies have also found that omega-3 fatty acids, especially the DHA (docosahexiaonic acid) component, improve nerve function. Vitamin E is also beneficial and should always be taken with DHA because DHA is a highly unsaturated, making it susceptible to oxidation.

One study of twenty-one type II diabetics given 900 mg of vitamin E for six months found a significant improvement in the nerve conduction velocity test (NCV), which evaluates damage or disease in peripheral nerves. Histological evidence of nerve fiber regrowth was also seen in a large number of the patients. Those given a placebo did not improve.[408]

All nerves require B vitamins for normal function. Folate, vitamin B_{12}, pyridoxine (B_6), riboflavin (B_2), and thiamine (B_1) are especially important. Supplementation should also include biotin, pantothenic acid, vitamins D, K, and C, and minerals. Iron, because it is a powerful free-radical generator, should be excluded from the supplements, unless a severe deficiency exists.

Because of the continual increased production of free radicals and lipid peroxidation in diabetics, it is vital to increase the body's supply of glutathione. Oral glutathione is poorly absorbed and is better supplied by taking N-acetyl L-cysteine (NAC). Alpha-lipoic acid also increases glutathione levels in cells, including brain cells. In addition, alpha-lipoic acid increases energy production and removes excess iron from the tissues (by chelation).

Experimentally, N-acetyl L-cysteine was shown to improve results of nerve conduction velocity studies significantly, and significantly reduced the number of nerve fibers that suffered myelin loss.[409] NAC also reduced lipid peroxide formation, which can increase tissue destruction and produce fatigue commonly seen in diabetics.

Alpha-lipoic acid is found naturally in all cells, and exists in two forms: an oxidized form called alpha-lipoic acid, and a reduced form known as dehydrolipoic acid or DHLA. The latter is the most powerful antioxidant form. Following ingestion, alpha-lipoic acid form is quickly converted to DHLA, which is not only a powerful and very versatile antioxidant, but can regenerate other antioxidants, increase cellular glutathione levels, and force glucose into cells without the aid of insulin. I have used it in both type I and II diabetics with good success. In the type I diabetic, glucose levels often improve dramatically, usually significantly lowering their insulin requirements. A dose of 600 mg a day is required to attain these beneficial effects.

Alpha-lipoic acid is also one of the most useful supplements in treating and preventing peripheral neuropathy associated with diabetes.[410] Several studies have shown that it can improve electrical conduction in affected nerves and dramatically improve symptoms. The degree of improvement depends on the length of time the problem has existed. The sooner the supplement is begun, the better the results.

Devastating problems can also be caused when autonomic nerves are affected. This set of nerves controls numerous activities that do not require conscious control, such as swallowing, intestinal contraction, cardiac regulation, and blood-pressure control. Severe damage to autonomic nerves can cause such serious problems as acute gastric pain, intestinal paralysis, extremely low blood pressure, and cardiac irregularities.

One study of diabetics with cardiac nerve problems due to autonomic nerve injury demonstrated that alpha-lipoic acid in high concentrations could slightly improve heart function.[411] Unfortunately, test participants in this study had advanced injuries; better results probably would have been obtained with earlier treatment of the condition.

Folic acid (folate), thiamin, riboflavin, pyridoxine, and vitamin B_{12} all play prominent roles in nerve function, and many diabetics are deficient in these vitamins. Loss of these vitamins is directly tied to carbohydrate consumption, especially refined sugar. Diabetics typically have diets high in sugary foods before becoming diabetic, and as a result are very deficient in these vitamins when the disease finally manifests. Folate should never be given alone, since it may mask serious vitamin B_{12} deficiencies. The only form of vitamin B_{12} that should be taken is methylcobalamin, the form naturally found in the body.

There is some evidence that high doses of these vitamins may be needed for them to work properly. It is important to know that all vitamins, and many minerals, act as coenzymes, assisting enzymes in their functions. Free-radical injury over many years damages these enzymes, making them less efficient, but we know that we can sometimes force these sluggish enzymes to work more efficiently by supplying larger concentrations of the coenzymes—higher doses of vitamins and minerals. Unfortunately, most doctors do not know this, and tell their patients, with condescending grins, that taking "all those vitamins" is just a waste of money.

Making Insulin Receptors Work

The easiest way to correct diabetes-related disorders is to fix the main problem, insulin resistance. It has been found that regular exercise and a carefully constructed diet can actually correct most cases of insulin resistance.[412] However, to achieve any benefit, such a program must be strictly followed: unfortunately, diabetics cannot afford the occasional lapses that someone with a normally functioning metabolism can.

Exercise increases glucose entry into muscles, and also lowers glucose levels. It also improves blood flow through tissues and organs, including the brain. Regular exercise can also reduce levels of tumor necrosis factor-alpha (TNF-alpha), a powerful inflammatory cytokine in the muscles, remarkably improving muscle function and reducing muscle pain and weakness. There is some suspicion that TNF-alpha is increased in diabetics and may play a role in insulin resistance.[413] N-acetyl L-cysteine, used to increase cellular glutathione levels, also decreases TNF-alpha levels, which may explain in part why diabetics show such significant improvement on NAC supplementation.

When tested in thirty-nine diabetics, CoQ10 lowered blood glucose levels by 30-31 percent and ketone bodies from 30-59 percent, which demonstrate significantly improved metabolism. The supplement was especially effective in one patient who was poorly controlled on sixty units of insulin a day before receiving the CoQ10. The dose used in this study was 120 mg a day. It is important to stress that the benefits of CoQ10 go far beyond correcting elevated glucose levels, since it also powerfully stimulates energy production, is a robust antioxidant, and is capable of increasing cellular glutathione levels.

Lowering levels of fats and simple sugars also improves insulin receptor function. N-6-type fats (omega-6) worsen diabetes, and N-3 fats (omega-3) improve diabetes. The N-6 fats include vegetable oils such as corn oil, safflower oil, sunflower oil, and peanut oil. Fish and flaxseed oils comprise the N-3 fat group. A cautionary note about flaxseed oil: in order to be converted to its healthy oil components, EPA and DHA, it must be converted by an enzyme called delta-desaturase. Some people lack a sufficient amount of this enzyme to make the conversion. High insulin levels also inhibit the enzyme.

A major defect found in diabetics is an abnormal fat content in cell membranes.[414] One recent study of over 575 diabetics found a defect in their ability to incorporate polyunsaturated fatty acids into their cell membranes, especially omega-3-type fats. Human studies have shown that a high content of saturated fat in cell membranes significantly increases insulin resistance.

Gamma linolenic acid (GLA) and omega-3 fatty acids have been shown to partially correct this membrane defect and improve insulin receptor function. We already know that GLA levels are low in diabetics, and recent studies indicate that supplementation is helpful for relieving peripheral neuropathy. GLA-rich primrose oil has shown promise in relieving diabetic neuropathy. Ounce for ounce, borage oil contains more GLA than primrose, and is less expensive, but studies have shown that it is not as effective as primrose for relieving diabetic neuropathy.

Chromium deficiency is linked to impaired glucose metabolism, impaired glucose clearance, a decrease in the number of insulin receptors, and a reduction in binding of glucose to those receptors. In addition, we see lowered HDL (the good cholesterol) levels, and an increase in total cholesterol and triglycerides—all factors that increase atherosclerosis. There is good evidence that chromium supplementation improves carbohydrate metabolism in diabetics.[415] It is especially effective when there is a significant deficiency of the mineral.

We know that a diet high in refined grains and sugars increases chromium depletion. In fact, with high sugar intake, chromium loss in the urine can be increased by as much as 300 percent. Strenuous exercise, aging, pregnancy, poor absorption, infection, chronic steroid use, and trauma can all increase chromium loss.

Most commercial brands are available as chromium picolinate, even though the body uses a form called GTF-chromium. (GTF stands for glucose tolerance factor.) A debate rages over which form is the best. Personally, I favor the GTF form, since it is found naturally in our bodies, but good studies exist that support the efficacy of the picolinate form as well.

For example, one double-blind study conducted in China on three test groups with Type II diabetes found that those who took 500 ug of chromium twice daily for four months had lower blood sugars, and nearly normal glycosylated hemoglobin as compared to those on the placebo. Total cholesterol and insulin levels also fell.[416]

Other minerals also play an important role in the prevention and treatment of diabetes. For example, low dietary intake of copper in experimental animals can cause the pancreas to shrink (atrophy) and reduce insulin secretion.[417] Another mineral, vanadium, has also been shown to act in many ways like insulin.[418] The only problem with vanadium is that beneficial effects have been observed only near the toxic dose.

Zinc plays a major role in the synthesis, storage, release, and stability of insulin. Not surprisingly, zinc deficiency is very common in diabetics. When zinc intake is improved we see corresponding improvements in glucose levels and insulin function. Zinc is also a powerful inhibitor of free radicals and lipid peroxidation.[419]

Another area of interest is the hypoglycemic properties of many herbs and flavonoids. One review found that of the 295 traditionally used plants screened for anti-diabetic effects, 81 percent were found to be useful for this purpose. Over two hundred phytochemicals are known to produce a fall in blood sugar. Unfortunately, many of these are also toxic.

A methylhydroxy chalcone polymer of cinnamon extract has been shown to increase glucose metabolism by cells twenty times, while also improving capillary function. Other plant extracts with hypoglycemic effects include juniper berries, izui, Siberian and panax ginseng, cumin, curcumin, cucumber, garlic, and bottle gourd.

One of the more useful plants is Gymnema sylvestre (Gumar) which stimulates insulin secretion and lowers cholesterol and triglycerides with minimal side effects. A test on twenty-two type II diabetics found 400 mg per day to be superior to prescription medications for long-term blood-sugar stabilization and an overall sense of well-being.[420]

Korean ginseng (Panax), given at 200 mg per day for eight weeks to type II diabetics, improved mood, increased physical activity, and lowered fasting blood sugar as well as glycosated hemoglobin levels.[421] The last effect is especially important, since glycosation of tissues is the leading cause of damage associated with diabetes. Onion and garlic extracts have also been shown to lower blood sugar, which may be due to the presence of thiosulfinates and dially disulfide.

Fiber and Diabetes

Fiber, especially soluble fiber, lowers elevated blood sugar levels. Fruits, vegetables, and some seeds, such as pectins, gums, and mucilages are good sources of soluble fiber. Flaxseed has one of the highest levels of both soluble and insoluble fiber known for any food. It also contains a substance called lignan, which inhibits breast and prostate cancer.

One test of non-diabetics demonstrated that taking fifty grams of water plus flaxseed mucilage reduced by 27 percent normally elevated blood sugar levels following a high-glucose meal.[422] Fenugreek seed, which contains about 50 percent fiber, is another good source of soluble fiber. Similar tests in diabetic patients have found a significant reduction in blood glucose levels.[423] Another advantage of increasing fiber intake to control diabetes is that it significantly reduces cell glycation. Remember, this process is responsible for much diabetes-related damage. In addition, a high-fiber diet removes dietary toxins, improves bowel elimination, and reduces the risk of colon cancer.

For a very interesting discussion of the nutritional treatment of diabetes, I suggest a 1997 article by Dr. C. Leigh Broadhurst in the journal, *Alternative Medicine Review*.[424]

Conclusion

You should not take all of the herbs and supplements I have listed above, but selected supplements *can* dramatically reduce insulin needs for type I diabetics and improve insulin function in type II diabetes.

When combined with a diet low in sugar, high in cruciferous vegetables, moderate in fruits and complex carbohydrates, and low in saturated fats, these supplements can significantly improve glucose control, prevent diabetic complications and improve your sense of well-being. Remember that to gain the most benefit from these recommendations, you *must* strictly adhere to a lifelong program of diabetes control, which includes a healthy diet, moderate exercise, proper supplementation, and toxin-avoidance—especially aspartame and MSG—in your diet.

Dem Bones: Preventing and Treating Osteoporosis

Bones are not what many of us imagine: a rigid nonliving frame. They are dynamic, ever-changing tissues just like all the other body's tissues. As people age, they tend to shrink, and many end up with spines that twist like pretzels, their bones often snapping with little effort. Is this just a side-effect of aging—like wrinkles—or can we actually do something to prevent it?

Today, osteoporosis affects some twenty million people, and millions of women take tons of calcium every day out of a fear of developing this mysterious disorder that makes bones brittle and skeletons dwindle. Visions of broken hips and spinal fractures hold many in a grip of panic. So where did this craze get started, and can gulping down Tums really prevent this debilitating disease?

The term osteoporosis literally means "porous bone." While outer (cortical) bone is relatively unchanged, internal, trabecular bone is weakened though demineralization, that is, a loss of calcium and other minerals, such as magnesium and zinc. Trabecular bone resembles the support structures on a radio tower: if these support structures are weakened, the tower breaks and falls. Fractures that result from such simple actions as getting out of bed or trying to lift a window are common in osteoporosis sufferers. Such injuries are more common at points of maximum stress—the neck of the femur, the lower spine, and the radius bone of the forearm.

Osteoporosis is responsible for 1.2 million fractures a year, which can be fatal in the elderly. It has been estimated that as many as 20 percent of hip fractures in the elderly are fatal, and that over 50 percent of survivors never leave the nursing home. Obviously, we should both respect the impact and dread the onset of osteoporosis.

Normally, bone mass peaks around age thirty and gradually falls thereafter. The rate of bone loss, especially in some women, is much faster after estrogen levels begin to decline.

Women who have had their ovaries removed before menopause often develop osteoporosis early. Hormone replacement has been shown to reduce the incidence of osteoporosis.

Yet, taking large amounts of calcium has been shown to play only a minor role, if any, in remineralizing osteoporotic bones or reducing fractures. This is because osteoporosis is far more complex than a simple calcium deficiency. Magnesium, zinc, boron, and vitamins K and D3 deficiencies, as well as improper fatty acid balance, also contribute to the course of the disease. One study I found most shocking examined over nine thousand women with high calcium intake. Researchers found that women currently using calcium had an increase in hip and vertebral fractures, and that women who took Tums had an increased risk of fractures of the humerus—the upper arm bone.[425] Adding vitamin D did not improve the protection.

Osteoporosis is essentially unknown in societies whose diets include little or no meat. Studies of American vegetarians have shown a very low incidence of osteoporosis as well. This is because high-protein diets are very acidic. In addition to its supporting function, bone also acts as a major buffering system. If blood is too acidic, calcium is mobilized to neutralize the acid. If acidity is chronic due to a long-term, high-protein diet, the buffering process continues until bones are severely weakened.

It has been estimated that by the time 30 percent of the calcium in bones has been mobilized, the bone itself becomes so weakened it will break very easily. The process occurs far more rapidly when blood-acid content is high.

One way to prevent acidity is to buffer the blood through good nutritional practices. A recent review found that of all the factors associated with reducing osteoporosis, the most effective was maintaining a diet high in fruits and vegetables,[426] which contain large amounts of magnesium and potassium, both of which are strong buffers. When such buffers are present, calcium in the blood actually moves back *into* bone. In addition, flavonoids in plants also prevent bone loss.[427] Edible plants also contain numerous other vitamins and minerals— including boron, zinc, magnesium, vitamin K, and some omega-3 fatty acids—that play a role in strengthening bones. Recent studies have found that omega-3 fatty acids inhibit osteoporosis.

You're probably wondering exactly how much fruits and vegetables are necessary to prevent osteoporosis. In general, plant foods—especially vegetables—should comprise the majority of your diet. This means at least seven to ten servings a day. That's a lot of plants, but blending makes it a lot easier since you can drink your fruits and veggies. (See the Program for Vascular Health in chapter ten for a comprehensive discussion of diet.)

Studies have shown that vegetarians do not necessarily have *stronger* bones than omnivores during the third to fifth decades of life, but bone loss in this population is much slower, or even nonexistent, after age fifty compared to omnivores.[428] Besides magnesium and potassium, high levels of boron and vitamin K in leafy green vegetables are also important. Boron significantly reduces calcium loss, and vitamin K has been shown to enhance the active form of osteocalcin in the bone, which forms the anchor for calcium.[429] Tums and other calcium supplements do not contain these vital components.

Of all forms of calcium, the most absorbable is calcium citrate. Also, all forms of calcium derived from previously living organisms—such as dolomite and oyster shells—should be avoided since many contain lead and/or mercury.[430]

One characteristic of osteoporosis is that bone-construction cells, the osteoblast, are normal, but bone-dissolving cells, called osteoclast, are overactive.[431] The disorder is much more common in women than men and usually follows menopause. This has led to the speculation that estrogen plays a major role in preventing bone loss.

Early studies indicated that isoflavones, a family of phytoestrogens found chiefly in soybeans, could reduce bone loss in cases of osteoporosis, but of some concern was a report of abnormalities in white blood cell function in some people taking the supplement. One of these products, a soy extract called ipriflavone, was shown to reduce significantly a biochemical marker for bone loss.[432] I am opposed to soy products in general because of concerns about high glutamate levels and other adverse effects including increased risk of breast cancer. Highly purified products, devoid of glutamate, may be useful.

This brings us to a new connection to excitotoxins in food. Recent research has disclosed that multiple tissues, including the nervous system, contain glutamate receptors that seem to behave just like those in the brain. That is, they increase calcium content in cells and act as triggers for cell activity or cell death when levels are too high.

A recent study reported that glutamate receptors were detected on both osteoblast and osteoclast bone cells. At this stage, we do not know what these receptors do, but if excess glutamate in the blood overstimulates the osteoclast, one might see accelerated osteoporosis. Possibly, overstimulation may cause the death of both types of cells, leading to a situation where bone cannot repair itself efficiently. More research is badly needed in this area.

I have one particular concern about all the calcium being consumed in the name of staving off osteoporosis. As we age, we lose our ability to keep calcium out of our cells, a process called calcium homeostasis, which leads to cellular damage to DNA, mitochondria, and cell membranes, by increasing free-radical generation and lipid peroxidation. In the brain, it may trigger excess glutamate release, leading to neurodegeneration. Flooding tissues with calcium may accelerate these destructive processes and contribute to neurodegenerative disease.[433] In addition, increased calcium within arterial endothelial cells is a powerful trigger for atherosclerosis. In all of these instances, the main effects of excessive intracellular calcium are increased inflammation and increased free-radical generation.

The other side of this coin is the affect of fluoride on calcium balance. Fluoride lowers tissue calcium levels rather dramatically. In fact, this is how acute fluoride toxicity kills. One of the largest lawsuit awards in this country involved the death of a little boy who swallowed a mouthful of fluoride treatment solution at the dentist's office. He died several hours later of cardiovascular collapse, secondary to severe calcium depletion. While calcium may be the antidote for acute fluoride poisoning, it will not protect against chronic poisoning.

With the amount of fluoride significantly increasing in our environment due to biomagnification, calcium depletion may become an even greater problem. One effect of fluoride overdosing, as we saw in chapter four, is osteoporosis. Fluoride poisons the osteoblast cells that normally build and repair bone.

Diagnosing Osteoporosis

What to do? I suggest, first of all, to have a complete skeletal survey for osteoporosis. If you have normal values, do not take additional calcium. If you have a strong family history of osteoporosis, combined with a survey that indicates osteoporosis, you may want to take additional calcium, but not alone. You should take a complete supplement with all the factors we talked about, including magnesium, zinc, vitamin K, DHA, vitamins C and D_3, and boron.

There are many ways to diagnose osteoporosis, some very accurate and some of questionable value. Dual-energy x-ray absorptiometry, also called DXA or DEXA, is the most accurate. Not only can it diagnose full-blown osteoporosis, but it can identify those at high risk before the disorder manifests. Of great value is its ability to measure density of bones that are most at risk for osteoporosis, such as the hip, lower spine and bones of the forearm. Other methods, such as simple x-ray absorption and SXA (single-energy x-ray absorptiometry) have little value, except as a screening tool for follow-up.

Urine tests are available as well. Biochemical evaluation of bone loss has been shown to be very accurate in pinpointing those at the greatest risk of osteoporosis and for following patients' progress. Pyridinium and deoxypyridinium crosslink excretion are based on the release of collagen, mainly from bone, with disease states such as osteoporosis and other bone disorders. Pyridinium crosslink excretion can also increase with osteoarthritis and rheumatoid arthritis, while deoxypyridinium is increased primarily in bone disorders.

The urine test can be used as a screening test and for follow-ups, while the more sophisticated DXA should be used for more accurate assessment.

The Role of Exercise in Protecting Your Skeleton

The skeleton undergoes a lifelong process of constant restructuring, a process determined mainly by stress forces at the attachment points of ligaments and tendons. When increased force is applied to a stress point, the bone responds by depositing more calcium-containing matrix at that site. Otherwise, the bone might snap. This principle may explain why heavier women are less likely to suffer from osteoporosis than skinny women: heavier women's bones are always under stress.

Because of the mechanics of bone stress, bone strengthening depends on type and duration of exercise. For example, walking produces a different restructuring effect than weightlifting. In general, you want to add stress to as many attachment points as possible. Resistance exercises are not only the best way to achieve this, but most people, including the elderly, can do these exercises.

Once reaching middle-age, far too many people are satisfied to just sit in a lounge chair and watch the idiot box. Combined with the mindless programming, not only could this destroy your muscles and bones, but could ruin your mind, to say nothing of your morals.

Several studies of elderly residents in nursing homes have shown that regular resistance exercises can significantly increase strength and mobility, as well as reduce the incidence of fractures. My elderly patients who exercise regularly, and who still work in their gardens, always amaze me. They are robust, sharp-minded, and are rarely stoop-shouldered or hunch-backed. We have seen that there is a direct connection between regular exercise and mental sharpness, now we find that it improves our mobility as well.

It is not necessary to do aerobics to experience the health benefits of exercise. All that you have heard about heart rate and cardiovascular effectiveness of the exercise is only partially true, because much of the information is age-related. In fact, the elderly could be significantly harmed by the physical demands of aerobic exercise.

A Program to Prevent Osteoporosis

The most important lifestyle modification you can make that will help to prevent or reduce osteoporosis is to change your diet. You should eat at least seven to ten servings of high-nutrient dense fruits and vegetables every day. As we have seen, the potassium and magnesium in plants protects the bones, and many high-density vegetables also contain a fair amount of calcium, which balances their high magnesium content.

Minimize meat intake. If you are not a vegetarian, eat no more than six ounces of meat twice a day. To gauge the amount of meat more conveniently, it should fit in the palm of *your* hand—not a gorilla's hand, your hand. Avoid pork and red meat altogether.

Avoid soft drinks. One study of 460 young, very active girls found that those who drank colas were five times more likely to suffer fractures than girls of equal activity who avoided soft drinks. It is suspected that because phosphorus draws calcium from bone, it is the culprit in such cases. Cow's milk is also high in phosphorus, as well as protein.

Do not substitute rice milk or soymilk, since the former is high in sugar and the latter is high in glutamate. While studies have indicated that various extracts from soybeans, such as ipriflavone, can reduce osteoporosis, I recommend that everyone (especially small children) avoid all forms of soy. Soy is also high on the list of foods that cause allergies.

For those with demonstrable osteoporosis, or with a strong family history of osteoporosis, I suggest supplementation. A single supplement which contains calcium, magnesium, zinc, vitamin K, vitamin D3, and boron should suffice. It may also contain ipriflavone.

By eating a balanced diet, heavy in fruits and vegetables, you will also get all the trace elements you need, such as manganese, molybdenum, and boron. In addition, you will need extra vitamin C to strengthen the bone matrix. This should include 500 mg vitamin C as either calcium or magnesium ascorbate three times a day. Long-term use of buffered vitamin C has been shown to increase bone mineral density.[434] Collagen forms the matrix upon which calcium is laid and this collagen in dependent on adequate amounts of ascorbate in the diet. The best buffered form is magnesium ascorbate. You can also use a combination of calcium and magnesium ascorbate.

Since omega-3 fatty acids have been shown to reduce osteoporosis, I suggest supplementing with DHA, the vital component of omega-3 fatty acid, 100 mg three times a day. To prevent DHA from oxidizing, you will also need vitamin E succinate 400 IU a day.

The amount of vitamin K needed to increase bone mineral density is much higher than the RDA provides. The recommended dose is 100 ug three times a day. However, do not take vitamin K if you are on prescription drugs for anticoagulation, since vitamin K reverses their effects. Leafy green vegetables, broccoli, green lettuce, spinach, and green tea are all rich in vitamin K. One study found that chromium picolinate reduced bone loss by inhibiting bone calcium loss.[435]

In addition, you will need to establish a regular exercise program, geared to your physical conditioning and age. It is important to exercise all of the muscles with resistance exercises or light weights. Your program should include at least three sessions a week. You can alternate more vigorous exercise days with lighter days.

Digestion, Bowel Movements, and Other Pleasant Topics

It will come as no surprise to my older readers to learn that improper digestion is one of the most frequent health complaints in those of us who have reached the "golden years." Such difficulties can include dyspepsia, chronic nausea, bloating, weight loss, and chronic constipation.

The digestive system is a series of hollow organs joined in a long tube that extends from the mouth to the anus. These organs are responsible for breaking down food into components our bodies can use for energy and for building and repairing tissues and cells.

From the mouth and esophagus, ingested substances travel into the stomach, then (partially digested) through a short tube (the duodenum) that is actually the first part of the small intestine. The liver, pancreas, and gall bladder all produce enzymes that reach the small intestine through small tubes and aid in further digestion as food moves to the large intestine, which is the last section of the digestive tract. The large intestine includes the cecum, colon, and rectum.

Distribution of bacteria in the colon is remarkably stable throughout life, unless something upsets the balance, such as chemotherapy or the use of antibiotics.[436] During early infancy, the colon's immune system takes stock of the normal bacterial flora and allows it to remain unharmed. It also neutralizes toxins secreted by certain of the bacteria. However, if this delicate system of tolerance and protection is impaired later in life, disease can result. As we age, a number of disorders can affect digestive health.

Many doctors are lost when it comes to testing and treatment. My experience has been that testing is inadequate and rarely includes functional studies of digestion. A usual work-up for GI problems includes a gallbladder series, upper and lower GI radiological examination (barium swallow and enema), and possibly an endoscopic examination both fore and aft. Basic lab work, including complete blood count (CBC), urinalysis, and a comprehensive metabolic analysis are also included. The last test includes a measure of liver enzymes.

While these surveys are certainly useful, and help to rule out a number of pre-existing diseases, they do little to evaluate risk to, or metabolic function of, the digestive tract. For example, liver enzymes indicate significant abnormalities of liver-cell function, but will not tell anything about subtle damage or abnormal liver cell detoxification that could lead to later disease, such as an inability of the liver to detoxify various chemicals, both of internal and external origin.

I frequently ordered the comprehensive digestive analysis from the Great Smokies Diagnostic Laboratory for a complete analysis of a patient's gastrointestinal function. Unfortunately, I rarely saw an analysis that was even close to normal. Most had significant risk factors for colon disease. Common abnormalities, especially in older patents, include abnormal protein digestion, low stomach acid, deficient N-butyrate, and dysbiosis—all of which can increase the risk of colon disease.

In medical school we were taught that as we age it is normal for us to have fewer bowel movements. In fact, one bowel movement a week for the elderly has long been considered adequate. This is sheer nonsense. Everyone, no matter their age, should have at least one bowel movement every day for proper elimination of toxins and prevention of pathogenic bacterial overgrowth.

A major reason for constipation is simple dehydration. Most studies have shown that the elderly are frequently dehydrated, a main cause of which is their desire to reduce the number of trips to the bathroom—especially at night. As a result, fluid intake in this group is severely inadequate, which causes increased dehydration of the bowel, leading to constipation. A main function of the large bowel is reabsorption of water. Normally, we absorb about one liter of fluid from the bowel a day. When dehydrated, we absorb even more water from the bowel and excrete less in the urine.

Inadequate intake of both soluble and insoluble fiber, both of which come from vegetables and grains, frequently accompanies dehydration. Insoluble fiber adds to the bulk of the stool making it easier to expel, while soluble fiber provides a fermentation medium, and is a source of vital nutrients for cells lining the GI tract, such as N-butyrate. In addition, these fermentation products provide beneficial bacteria with a medium for growth.

Gut Ecology

Another frequent GI disorder is called dysbiosis, an abnormality of gut ecology character-ized by an imbalance in the number of good and bad bacteria in the colon. Yes, there are little critters living in your colon! In fact, there are more bacteria and viruses living in your colon than there are cells in your entire body. Overall there may be between 400 and 500 different species of organisms living in your colon. When the balance between good and bad bacteria becomes disrupted, the entire digestive process can malfunction, leading to B_{12} deficiency, steatorrhea (fatty bowel movements), irritable bowel disease, inflammatory bowel disease, autoimmune arthritis, colon and breast cancer, and chronic fatigue.

It appears that each of the many species of good bacteria performs a specific, necessary function. The good guys help keep the colon healthy by producing helpful products, such as N-butyrate and vitamin B_{12}. They also hold the bad guys at bay. There is always a certain number of bad bacteria in our colon, but they're not really harmful unless they become overgrown, usually as a result of excessive antibiotic use. The small bowel usually has very few bacteria, but with reflux from the colon into the ileum, the main site of vitamin B_{12} absorption, these bacteria can enter the small bowel. Here, the bacteria can inhibit vitamin B_{12} absorption, resulting in severe deficiencies.

Good bacteria include *Lactobacillus* and *Bifidobacillus* species and *E. Coli*. These organ-isms must exist in sufficient numbers for the colon to be healthy. Several studies have shown that improving the good coloform bacteria can significantly improve symptoms in patients with Crohn's disease and inflammatory bowel diseases, such as ulcerative colitis. One study found that *Lactobacillus casei* greatly improved the sIgA (secretory immunoglobulin A) function in the intestine of patients with Crohn's disease, which significantly improves their symptoms.[437] Many times, it will significantly improve chronic constipation as well.

Some bacteria merely pass through the bowel while others take up residence. *L. bulgaricus* and *Streptococcus thermophilus* are two species that just pass through but have been shown to be very effective in cases of traveler's diarrhea. One species that actually takes up residence, *Lactobacillus rhamnosus*, shows much promise in controlling infantile diarrhea, especially in premature babies. Of special concern to the ulcer victim, and those with colitis, is the finding that the *Lactobacillus salivarius* species can prevent and treat infections by *Helicobacter pylori*, the causative organism in both conditions. Both the *Lactobacillus* and the *Bifidobacterium* organisms have been shown to reduce colonic inflammation in the elderly as well.

Lactobacillus ramnosus species can rapidly restore normal permeability to the intestine in cases of leaky gut syndrome, a condition in which large food components enter the blood stream. The same organism also can inhibit *Candida* yeast growth. Other species of good bacteria can stimulate the immune system, making it more effective in protecting you. For example, *Lactobacillus casei* has been shown to stimulate the activity of natural killer cells in the spleen.[438]

Many pathogenic bacteria, such as *Klebsiella* and *Proteus*, cannot metabolize longer-chained polysaccharides, whereas good bacteria, such as *Lactobacillus* and *Bifidobacterium*, can. This mixture of nutrients, supplied from the diet, protects us from bowel diseases, such as irritable bowel syndrome, constipation, diarrhea, colon cancer and inflammatory bowel disease.

When more virulent bacteria, such as *Clostridium perfringens* or *difficile*, become overgrown, serious disease can result, including the highly fatal pseudomembranous colitis, a condition where the lining of the colon sloughs off.[439] Some of the good bacterial secrete antibiotic-like chemicals that inhibit the growth of the more pathogenic species. For instance, *E. Coli* secretes a chemical called colcine, which not only stops the growth of the bad bacteria but also regulates its own growth.

It should be appreciated that not all bacteria and viruses have the same ability to cause disease, a characteristic called virulence. Organisms of high virulence cause acute, severe infections. Those of low virulence may either cause no disease or produce chronic low-grade infections. This last type usually escapes your doctor's detection.

One of the more notorious of these low-virulence organisms is the *Candida* species. While the colon may contain a small amount of yeast, large overgrowths are harmful. We know that under such conditions, the yeast can form mycelia that can penetrate the bowel wall and enter the blood stream, where it can be carried to any organ or tissue in the body.

Yeast can also enter the small bowel, resulting in numerous microscopic perforations of the wall of the bowel. This can lead to food allergies, since large molecules of food products will be able to enter the blood stream. Interestingly, food allergies may subside when the yeast invasion is cured.

I have seen three patients with ALS, and one with *Giardia* infection, all of whom had serious yeast overgrowth, and all undiagnosed by their treating physicians. Each patient experienced significant improvement of bowel function following treatment, and some improved their neurological picture as well. It is also known that patients with this neurological disorder frequently have pancreatic insufficiency.

There is some evidence that low-virulence bacteria and yeast can cause diseases remote from the digestive tract, including asthma, autoimmune diseases, and eczema.[440] Surgeons have been aware for many years that occasionally these bacteria and viruses can leak out of the colon into the blood stream, where they can produce infections at other sites.

Mobilization of colon bacteria into the blood stream also can occur during surgery, resulting in infections elsewhere. Colonic bacteria labeled with radioactive tracers have been followed traveling through the wall of the colon into blood vessels supplying the colon, where the bacteria then travel to distant locations. Any area of damage, such as that resulting from an operative wound, will act as a collecting point for these organisms. This is because serum, blood products, and dead tissue act as a perfect culture medium for the bacteria.

For years, hospitals and doctors have battled postoperative wound infections by meticulous hand washing with powerful antibacterial soaps, and even the use of expensive laminar flow devices and UV light; however, little headway has been made in preventing these infections. The best protection is good nutrition for the patient and correction of bladder infections and colon overgrowth before the patient arrives in the operating room.

Fermentation Excess and Putrefaction

When bad bacteria overgrow in the colon and enter the small bowel, malabsorption and maldigestion of foods can take place.[441] Under such circumstances, the undigested carbohydrate ferment in the colon, leading to bloating, flatulence, diarrhea or constipation, and fatigue.

Under these circumstances, the affected person will become intolerant to soluble fiber supplements, since they will increase the short-chained fatty acids that can increase fermentation. Antibiotic treatment may be required to correct the problem. Long term correction requires a low carbohydrate diet and enzyme supplementation when indicated. Garlic can suppress the overgrown bacteria and yeast.

The typical Western diet, high in fats and meats, and low in fiber, promotes the growth of a particular species of bad bacteria called *Bacteroides*. This organism secretes an enzyme called beta-glucuronidase, which can metabolize bile acids to form tumor promoters and prevent the proper metabolism of estrogens by deconjugating them. This raises blood estrogen levels, thereby increasing the risk of breast cancer. This enzyme can be reduced by taking calcium D-glucarate, which has been shown to lower breast cancer risk.

Acidity

Proper acidity is critical to proper digestion and for absorption of zinc and ferrous iron. In addition, when the stomach's acid level is low, bacteria and viruses can colonize the GI tract. Many enzymes exist in the stomach and small intestine as inactive enzymes, or pro-enzymes, that lie dormant until needed. In the stomach, pepsinogen is activated by hydrochloric acid (HCL) secreted from parietal cells, and is converted to active pepsin for protein digestion. In the small intestine, the pancreatic pro-enzymes, trypsinogen, chymotrypsin and carboxypeptidase are converted to their active enzymes as well.

As we age, our ability to maintain stomach acidity decreases. In fact, after age sixty, over 50 percent of people suffer from low stomach acidity (hypochlorhydria),[442] associated with a number of conditions such as asthma, celiac disease, chronic autoimmune disorders (rheumatoid arthritis and lupus), diabetes, food allergies, gastritis, Graves disease, hepatitis, pernicious anemia, osteoporosis, and psoriasis.

Normally, the pancreas secretes about 2.5 liters of juices a day—a rather large volume. Meanwhile, the liver and gallbladder each secrete about 700 ml of bile a day. Pancreatic secretion is controlled by the hypothalamus via the vagus nerve and special locally secreted hormones such as secretin and choleocystokinin. These hormones are activated by the presence of fats, protein, and chyme in the duodenum. Several of these hormones may be deficient in the aged. This can lead to maldigestion.

Even small decreases in pancreatic enzyme activation can produce serious digestion problems, which can lead to abdominal bloating, upset stomach, cramping pains, and diarrhea. It also leads to malnutrition, since absorption of vital nutrients, including vitamins and minerals, is impaired.

Numerous glutamate receptors also exist in the pancreas, and insulin control is strongly regulated by glutamate in the blood. As yet, we do not know the function of these receptors on digestive enzyme function. If glutamate can affect their secretion as well, then diets high in MSG could cause significant digestive problems. Intestinal muscle also contains glutamate receptors which, when overstimulated, can result in increased spasm of the intestine. This would explain the diarrhea and cramping seen in many people following a meal high in MSG.

Once food enters the small intestine, it undergoes further churning and mixing with digestive enzymes and is mixed with bile produced in the liver. Bile helps emulsify the fats in your food so that they can be digested and absorbed properly. The pancreas secretes most of the digestive enzymes in the duodenum, including proteases to break down proteins, amylase for carbohydrate digestion and lipases to break down diglycerides and triglycerides into long-chained fatty acids. Fat-soluble vitamins, such as vitamins A, E, and D, are absorbed through dissolution in the emulsified fats.

Several enzymes inside the wall of the intestine further digest oligosaccharides and proteins. These special cells also control absorption of nutrients to prevent large molecules of undigested foods from entering the blood stream. If this occurs, food allergies may result. Drugs, food additives, and inflammatory bowel diseases all can damage these delicate cells. Frequent use of nonsteroidal anti-inflammatory medications, such as ibuprofen, is a common culprit when these cells are damaged.

Diseases such as sprue, Whipple's disease, Crohn's disease, Giardiasis, cryptosporidiosis, lactose intolerance, and eosinophilic gastroenteritis all impair proper digestion and absorption of nutrients. But it should be appreciated that nutrient absorption utilizes different pathways in the intestine, so that isolated nutritional deficiencies can occur. For example, one may see fat malabsorption alone, or impaired absorption of vitamin B_{12}, iron, or zinc, while other nutrients are absorbed normally.

Leaky Gut

Many think of the GI tract as the inside of the body, but in actuality it is still *outside* us. The lining of the gastrointestinal tract protects the inside of our body from the outside: in addition to providing a place for digestion and absorption of nutrients, the GI tract is also responsible for making sure that what finally makes it into our bodies is safe. Protecting our interior is very important, since many substances in the environment, including foods, are quite toxic to us if they enter the blood stream intact.

The GI tract is also a major component of the immune system. Within the wall of the intestine are numerous lymphoid patches. Cells lining the intestine also contain antibody-producing cells, which secrete immunoglobulin A (secretory IgA). This substance protects the intestine by forming a complex with bacteria, preventing them from binding with the intestinal lining. Otherwise, bacteria could pass through the wall of the intestine and enter the lymphatics or blood stream, a process called translocation. People with poor secretory IgA experience numerous infections and food intolerance, a common finding in disorders such as autism.

Particles—both good and bad—enter the body from the GI tract by two basic mechanisms: through cells themselves (transcellular) and between cellular junctions (paracellular). Over 85 percent of passive entry is paracellular. At the site of these tight cellular junctions are channels (pores) which allow small molecules to pass. Like pores in other parts of the body, these channels can open and close as needed. Much of this traffic is controlled by electrical charges from cells.

When these junctions are altered by disease, drugs, or trauma, larger molecules can enter the blood stream, many of which can induce immune reactions. Examples of these diseases include rheumatoid arthritis, asthma, ankylosing spondylitis, food allergies, eczema, pancreatic dysfunction, acute gastritis, celiac disease, HIV infection, burn injury, cystic fibrosis, alcoholism, post-surgical infection, and endotoxemia. Drugs known to alter gut permeability include virtually all nonsteroidal noninflammatory medications (NASIDS), many chemotherapy agents, amphetamine, and cocaine. Cow's milk is also known to induce leaky gut syndrome.

When gut ecology is severely altered, we see increased translocation of bacteria and yeast into the circulatory system. Antibiotics, especially broad-spectrum varieties, can kill beneficial organisms, resulting in an overgrowth of the pathogenic, disease-causing ones. Bacterial translocation is greatly accelerated when antibiotics are combined with cortisone, a common practice.

Once microorganisms enter the blood stream they can seed into numerous organs and tissues, resulting in systemic illness. They can also result in immune suppression, and the formation of autoimmune complexes, which can present as arthritis, muscle weakness or neurological problems. Overgrowths of *Candida albicans* and *Pseudomonas aeroginosa* have also been shown to produce immune suppression.[443] This would be especially important in those with cancer and chronic infections.

In all cases of increased permeability, the problem is that large polypeptides and proteins are allowed to enter the blood stream where they elicit immune reactions, some of which, by molecular mimicry, can fool the immune system into attacking cells within one's own body.

Chemotherapy also increases gut permeability. Many anticancer agents are very toxic to the rapidly dividing cells lining the GI tract, resulting in chronic diarrhea, blood loss, and increased gut permeability. Two good bacteria, *Lactobacillus plantarum* and *L. reuteri*, have been shown to reduce significantly the severity of GI reactions to the chemotherapy agent methotrexate. Radiation of the GI tract, common with cancer treatment, can also cause increased permeability. If uncorrected, it can lead to a prolonged problem lasting years.[444]

Increased permeability is also common with Crohn's disease and inflammatory bowel diseases. In fact, measures of intestinal permeability are a good way to predict recurrences of Crohn's disease. When permeability is normal during periods of remission, the likelihood of recurrence is smaller.

Food allergies are also associated with increased permeability. Early exposure during infancy to common food allergens such as eggs, milk, and soy can precipitate long term sensitivities to these food products. A similar process can occur when the gut becomes excessively permeable during adulthood, for whatever reason. In fact, food allergies can change as permeability improves. This is not uncommon in autistic children, and in those suffering from yeast overgrowth of the bowel.

Increased gut permeability is common in rheumatoid arthritis, but we cannot tell if it is part of the disease or the result of years of taking NSAIDs. We do know that such patients frequently have antibodies to an organism called *Proteus mirabilis*. Antibody reactions against this organism are much greater in active disease than quiescent disease. It is also interesting to note that rheumatoid patients who improved after a period of fasting followed by a strict vegetarian diet experienced a fall in *Proteus* antibodies as well.

While this is not to say that this organism causes rheumatoid arthritis, is has been shown to increase significantly symptoms and accelerate the course of the disease. The same can be said of other autoimmune diseases such as lupus.

What You Can Do to Plug the Leaks!

Stop taking drugs that are known to produce leaking, primarily antibiotics and NSAIDs. If you have a condition, such as rheumatoid arthritis, that will not allow you to stop NSAIDs, you should take phosphotidylcholine with your medication. There is some evidence that when the two are combined, NASIDs bind to the phsophotidylcholine, preventing them from causing problems. While this has not been proven as yet, there is strong suggestive evidence and little to lose.

You should always take a probiotic supplement before, during and for three weeks after taking antibiotics.

Glutamine

Glutamine is an amino acid that acts as a major fuel for the small intestine. Biochemically, it is converted to glutamic acid and then to alpha-ketogluterate, which goes on to form ATP for energy. Normally, I do not advise supplementing with glutamine because in the brain it is also converted to glutamic acid, where it can contribute to excitotoxicity, but because of the severity of the leaky gut problem, a short-term course of glutamine is less dangerous than the problems associated with this disorder.

Glutamine also has been shown to lengthen intestinal villi, thicken mucosa, and increase IgA secretion. In cases of radiation and chemotherapy injury, glutamine has produced significant improvement in gut healing.

Dietary Fiber

While glutamine is the main fuel for the small bowel, the short-chained fatty acids N-butyrate, proprionate, and acetate are the colon's main fuel. Combining N-butyrate and vitamin E succinate has been shown to reduce colon cancer rates dramatically, as well as to improve colon function.

A good source of N-butyrate is oat bran and as a pure supplement called ButyrAid (www.advantagenutrition.com). Oats are also good sources of beta-glucans, the immune stimulants, as well as glutamine.

DHA

This omega-3-fatty-acid component protects the gut by reducing inflammation. Recent studies have shown that fish-oil supplements can significantly reduce the recurrence of Crohn's disease. It also may reduce colon cancer, but you have to be careful. DHA is also polyunsaturated, and therefore subject to extensive oxidation. When oxidated, it may potentially increase colon cancer rates. *It is very important always to take vitamin E with DHA and to keep the DHA in the refrigerator, to prevent oxidation.*

Flavonoids

Most flavonoids, as we have seen, are powerful and versatile antioxidants and inhibitors of lipid peroxidation. They also bind excess iron and reduce inflammation. This makes them very important for treatment of inflammatory bowel disease.

Quercetin (found in onions, tea, cranberries, and apples) is a powerful histamine inhibitor, not only making it a great supplement for hayfever and sinusitis, but also for leaky gut. Mast cells in the gut, which secrete histamine, promote the development of the leaky gut syndrome.

Flavonoids from green tea extract, primarily catechins, not only reduce inflammation and protect against free radicals, but also inhibit the growth of *Clostridium*, a very bad bacteria, and promote the growth of *Lactobacillus* and *Bifidobacterium*, both good bacteria.[445]

Probiotic Supplements
A good replacement supplement should contain all of the species of good bacteria, including *Bifidobacterium* and *Lactobacillus*. Each organism has a different function, and they also inhibit the growth of pathogenic bacteria. Both directly and indirectly, they reduce the leaky gut problem, improve secretory IgA production, and suppress yeast growth.

Saccharomyces Boulardii
Similar to baker's yeast, *Saccharomyces boulardii* prevents *Candida albicans* from translocating from the gut to lymph nodes in the abdomen, preventing the yeast from invading the rest of the body.

Food for the Good Guys
FOS, or fructo-oligosacchrides (a union of one molecule of sucrose and three of fructose), is a complex molecule found in many foods, such as Jerusalem artichokes, onions, honey, beer, oats, and bananas. Normally, only the good guys can use these sugars for growth, but the nasty organism, *Klebsiella*, can also utilize it. This organism is associated with the leaky gut syndrome and ankylosing spondylitis. It is best to culture the stool before taking this supplement, just to make sure that no *Klebsiella* is present.

Finally, it is important to avoid excess simple sugars in your diet since they promote dysbiosis, especially yeast overgrowth.

Testing Colon Function

The Great Smokies Diagnostic Laboratory does one of the most comprehensive tests for gastrointestinal function I have found. It analyzes digestive enzyme function, nutrient absorption, short-chain fatty acid content, bacterial analysis, and yeast culture, and estimates dysbiosis risk. In addition, it provides an analysis of sensitivity of the pathogenic organisms to various natural and prescription drugs; in other words, it tells you what products will kill the bad guys.

12
Protecting Your Brain

Most of us don't worry about brain health until we near our fifties. That situation changed when Michael J. Fox—who is still quite young—made the startling announcement that he has Parkinson's disease. Recent research indicates that years of accumulated free-radical damage eventually leads to aging and degeneration of the brain. Most neurological diseases do not become obvious until about 75 percent of brain cells in the affected area have died; the surviving 25 percent are extremely sick and cannot function normally, which is why treating neurodegenerative diseases such as Alzheimer's disease, Parkinson's disease, and Lou Gehrig's disease (ALS) is so difficult. By the time such a disease becomes clinically evident, there just isn't much left for doctors to work with.

Numerous toxins—including pesticides, herbicides, industrial chemicals, and heavy metals such as mercury—are stored throughout our lives in our body's fatty cells. Our bones may also contain high concentrations of aluminum, lead, and fluoride that have accumulated for decades due to chronic environmental exposure. Unfortunately, many people lose fatty tissues as they age, releasing fat-soluble toxins from cells and bones for redistribution to other fatty parts of the body. What this means is that very high concentrations of these toxins are suddenly released into the blood stream, which is akin to being poisoned all over again—only much more rapidly. Because the brain is composed of approximately 60 percent fat, it acts as a natural sink for many of these dangerous chemicals.

In addition, cells weaken and energy production dwindles as we age. Cell membranes lose much of their fluidity, enzymes are damaged, DNA undergoes multiple injuries, and reparative enzymes are less effective; as a result, we become much more vulnerable to additional toxic insults, even those originating within our own bodies.

Not only do organs sustain injury, our blood vessels—which deliver vital nutrients and oxygen to these organs and tissues—also suffer damage. The blood-brain barrier begins to fail, allowing blood-borne toxic substances to enter the brain. Furthermore, the brain's glucose-transport system begins to fail, leaving our brain starving for fuel. As free radicals and lipid-peroxidation products accumulate, synaptic connections, stem cells, and dendrites begin to dwindle—which is common in patients with Alzheimer's disease.

This may sound very frightening—and it should—but such damage is by no means inevitable. People one hundred years old can have perfectly functioning brains with robust plasticity—the capacity of the brain to develop new connections and expand dendrites into areas that have been damaged.

It even has been proposed that the millions of undifferentiated stem cells in the brain can become active at any age. Normally, stem cells can change into neurons, replacing those that have been destroyed. However, the same processes that kill neurons also destroy stem cells. In fact, stem cells may be more sensitive to these destructive processes than fully mature neurons and glial cells. High concentrations of stem cells can be found in the hippocampus of the temporal lobe, the area most affected in Alzheimer's disease.

Nutrition, Aging and the Brain

The brain has one of the highest metabolic rates of any organ in the body. Like the heart, it is never completely at rest. Even in states of deep coma, the brain has a fairly high rate of metabolic function, which means it needs a constant supply of sufficient nutrients, especially vitamins and minerals—all of which must be obtained from food. Unfortunately, too many people approach eating as nothing more than another form of instant gratification, rather than our body's way of getting the vital nutrition it needs to function properly. For too many of us, it is no longer enough for food simply to taste good—it must be *delicious* to be worth eating. Of course, what makes so many modern foods "delicious" are harmful food additives (combined with virtually nonexistent nutritional value), meaning that a lifetime of eating processed foods can lead to severe nutritional deficiencies.

Numerous studies have shown that the elderly are usually deficient in several important nutrients, especially vitamins B_6 and B_{12}, folate, and numerous minerals and trace elements.[446] Oftentimes, these deficiencies are subclinical, meaning that, while they do not produce obvious signs such as bleeding gums (vitamin C deficiency) or bowed legs (vitamin D deficiency), the body is still unable to function optimally.

Because these subtle changes in cognitive function, memory, and social behavior can be so difficult to measure, researchers in the past have assumed that these deficiencies were of no consequence. But, newer, more sophisticated and sensitive studies have shown this not to be true. One report in the early 1980s, when such theories were first being proposed, showed an association between age-related brain function and nutrition. This study looked at 260 seemingly healthy people age sixty and above.[447] Using a concept learning test, which is highly sensitive for brain malfunction, and the Wechler Memory Scale, researchers found that test subjects with even low normal values for vitamin C, riboflavin, B_{12}, and folate were cognitively impaired.

Another study used an EEG analysis to detect subtle brain dysfunction in a group of elderly subjects.[448] It is known that with aging there is an increase in slow wave activity of the brain and other changes that indicate reduced brain function. Researchers discovered a high incidence of marginal riboflavin and thiamine deficiency in these subjects, which was associated with changes in the EEG pattern in specific locations of the brain.

Riboflavin deficiency was associated with poorer memory in those with lower riboflavin intakes. Low thiamine (vitamin B_1) intake was associated with lower values for alpha-power on the EEG in both hemispheres of the frontal, temporal, and parietal lobes of the brain. Alpha-power is a measure of the brain's functional activity. The best correlation was

Evaluating Risk of Neurodegeneration

- oxidative stress status
    presence of chronic diseases such as diabetes, lupus, etc.
    toxic metal exposure: lead, mercury, aluminum
    fluoride exposure
    excitotoxin exposure
- age
    immature brain four times more sensitive to glutamate
- nutritional status
    dietary antioxidant intake
- strength of DNA repair systems
- status of cellular glutathione synthesis
- mitochondrial function
    energy status
- functional status of antioxidant enzymes
- heredity
    presence of two apoE4 genes

TABLE 12.1

between the levels of beta-carotene in the plasma and cognitive function, which, when low, also caused changes in the EEG in the frontal region of the brain.

Iron and zinc deficiencies appeared to play no part in cognitive function, but low levels of zinc did reduce right temporal lobe EEG power. This indicates that even mild nutritional deficiencies were indeed affecting brain function, but cognitive tests were not sensitive enough to measure it.

Other vitamins also appear to play a role in preserving brain function as we age. Dr. Asenath LaRue and co-workers from the Department of Psychiatry, Pathology, and Neurology at the University of New Mexico School of Medicine found that vitamin E intake early in life could predict future cognitive performance.[449] Those who had taken vitamin E for a long time were more likely to have a well-preserved ability to think and reason later in life. A more recent review devised a more accurate measure of vitamin E status by correlating it to blood cholesterol levels, and found that those with the highest serum vitamin E levels had the best memory.[450]

While many previous studies have shown a correlation between folic acid intake and preservation of memory and cognitive function, a more recent study also showed a strong correlation between poor memory and even a normal level of homocysteine if it was in the higher range.[451] Homocysteine has been found to be an independent risk factor for atherosclerosis; increased levels are found in association with deficiencies of vitamins B_6 and B_{12} and folate.

It is also metabolized into two very powerful excitotoxins, homocysteine sulphenic acid and homocysteic acid. This study of over three thousand individuals found that those who had folate levels in the upper half of values had significantly better memory than those in the lower half.

Low folate levels have also been associated with depression. Several studies have found that supplementation improved the depression in those with low values.[452] Recently, it has been demonstrated that supplementing depressed patients with S-adenosyl methionine (SAMe), often significantly improves their depression.[453] SAMe plays a vital role in brain function by acting as a methyl donor in the brain. In this capacity, it is responsible for synthesis of several neurotransmitters (norepinephrine and serotonin), DNA repair and phospholipid synthesis.

So how is folic acid connected to all this? Three vitamins act as coenzymes in the synthesis of SAMe: vitamin B_6, folic acid and vitamin B_{12}. Deficiencies in one or more of these vitamins can severely disrupt the metabolic formation of SAMe. Recent studies have found very low levels of SAMe in Alzheimer's patients, which is not surprising given that numerous studies have shown that these same three vitamins are also low in this disease as well. Remember from an earlier discussion that B_{12} deficiencies were found in 83 percent of hospitalized, and 68 percent of healthy, elderly.[454]

Fats and the Brain

While vitamins and minerals are critical for proper brain function, of equal importance is a group of fats called omega-3 fatty acids. These polyunsaturated fats are composed of two very important components, EPA (eicosapentaenoic acid) and DHA (docosahexaenoic acid), which play a particularly important part in brain function and health.

The brain is composed of approximately 60 percent fats, the majority of which are polyunsaturated. These fats make up the cell membranes that cover neurons and all the internal components of the cell such as mitochondria, endoplasmic reticulum, and golgi apparatus. DHA-type fat also makes up most synapses and dendrites—the connections between neurons.

DHA is not only very critical in brain development but also in maintenance of the brain later in life.[455] Don't forget, the brain is constantly restructured throughout life, even into the extremes of age. Unfortunately, because of food-processing methods and industrial raising of animals as meat sources, most omega-3 fatty acids have been removed from our foods.

It has been determined that the proper ratio of omega-6 fats to omega-3 fats is about 4:1. Presently, the ratio is more like 2:1. When the fatty-acid ratio of neuron membranes is abnormal, cell membranes also function abnormally. This includes the mitochondrial membrane, which is vital to cellular energy supply.[456]

Several studies have found that low intakes of DHA-type fats increase the likelihood of depression and that restoring DHA can actually relieve it.[457] Because of DHA's importance in maintaining synapses, diets containing more of this essential fat can also improve connectivity of brain circuits.[458]

In addition, mitochondrial membranes, the major energy-generating components of the cell, are heavily dependent on DHA. Any change in the membrane's fluidity can alter its ability to produce energy. Low energy equals high excitotoxicity and free-radical generation.

A high intake of N-6 fats (corn, safflower, sunflower, peanut, canola, and soybean oils) also has been shown to impair brain function and to increase the risk of neurodegenerative diseases. Most diets are filled with the bad fats. You will recall that these are the same fats that increase the risk of atherosclerosis and inflammation, and impair immune function. By maintaining a low intake of N-6 fats and a higher intake of N-3 fats, you can significantly improve the function of your brain and reduce the risk of developing a neurodegenerative disease such as Alzheimer's and Parkinson's.

Iron, a Double-Edged Sword

Iron is essential not only for proper hemoglobin function but also for the production of cellular energy, immune function, and brain function. It is especially important for learning and memory in growing children. Iron supplementation may also be necessary in endurance athletes, pregnant women, those taking arthritis medication regularly, and for those taking an aspirin a day. Later in life, it becomes less essential. Low iron levels are known to increase the likelihood of infection and can increase the generation of free radicals in tissues. Low levels are also responsible for poor wound healing.

Because of the problem of anemia, especially in premenopausal women, the government, in all its wisdom, decided to force by law, beginning in the late 1970s, the fortification of certain foods with iron. These include all grains and pasta products. Unfortunately, they seemed to have ignored the expanding medical literature demonstrating the harmful effects of too much iron, especially in the elderly and those with cancer and neurodegenerative diseases. Even Sweden, which was one of the first countries to require iron fortification of certain foods, repealed their rule in 1995 when studies indicated that iron was responsible for a significant increase in liver cancer in women.

We know for instance, that even high normal levels of iron increase tumor growth.[459] Also, during bacterial and viral infections, iron supplementation can promote the growth of these organisms, making treatment difficult. I know of many doctors who give iron supplements to patients who have severe infections.

We also know that iron plays a major role in degenerative diseases of the nervous system, as well as aging of all tissues.[460] At one time it was thought that only free iron was the culprit in these disorders, but new evidence indicates that even iron bound to ferritin can be harmful. Ferritin is a special protein that binds iron in the tissues in an attempt to prevent harm caused by free iron. It works very efficiently at lower iron levels, but is impaired when iron levels in the body are too high.

Recent studies have found that elevated iron levels are associated with all neurodegenerative diseases. This is especially true of Parkinson's disease, where iron accumulates in the substantia nigra nucleus as an early event.[461] In the presence of the pigments neuromelanin (found in the substantia nigra) and 6-hydroxydopamine (a metabolite of dopamine), iron is especially harmful.[462] This mixture produces a large amount of the free-radical precursor, hydrogen peroxide, which eventually destroys neurons, producing the same pattern of destruction seen in Parkinson's disease. There is even some evidence that people destined to develop Parkinson's disease have a defect in iron metabolism.

As we age, we accumulate more iron. The importance of this observation is demonstrated by the fact that men are four times more likely to suffer a coronary heart attack than premenopausal women at age forty-five years. At this age, men have iron stores four times higher than women. Further, men with higher iron levels have heart attack rates two times higher than men with lower levels. In both men and women, iron stores peak between age forty and sixty years.

For this reason, iron intake after a certain age should be substantially reduced. For men, that should be around twenty-five years of age, and for women, after menopause. It has even been hypothesized that women have lower incidences of heart attacks and strokes before menopause because of regular iron loss resulting from menstruation.[463] After menopause, women accumulate iron at a rate that exceeds men's—and develop heart attacks and strokes at a rate equal to men. This does not mean you should never take iron. There are actually conditions for which iron supplements are recommended, but anyone on such a program should be carefully tested and monitored.

I have seen numerous women treated by doctors who assume that all anemia in women is due to iron deficiency. As a result, and as is often the case, iron supplements were hastily given—with no tests for iron levels beforehand, and no monitoring during treatment whatsoever. I have even seen women who took iron for years before coming to me, whose doctors had never ordered follow-up studies to test their iron levels. This is a very dangerous practice, especially in the elderly, who are already accumulating too much free iron.

In addition to neurodegenerative disorders and cancer, several other diseases put people at an especially high risk of iron injury. Anyone with an autoimmune disease, such as lupus or rheumatoid arthritis, should not take iron supplements unless their levels are extremely low. It is important to emphasize that rapid correction of iron levels can actually exacerbate these disorders.

Diabetics, those with degenerative eye diseases (such as macular degeneration), or severe liver or kidney diseases, should also be very careful with iron supplementation. We know that diabetics develop a 40 percent increase in retinal glutamate levels and as a result, free-radical generation and lipid peroxidation increase by 100 percent. Iron greatly increases damage associated with glutamate-induced excitotoxicity. It is also known that high iron levels are associated with a dramatic increase in cataract formation.

Testing

First, you should be tested for iron levels, iron-binding capacity, ferritin levels and trans-ferrin saturation. If your iron level is well below normal values, you should begin taking supplements with an iron preparation. After two weeks of supplementation, the studies should be repeated. Further supplementation depends on levels at that point. I advise anyone to avoid letting iron levels reach values above the midpoint of the reference range. Once acceptable levels of iron have been achieved, supplementation should be stopped, and iron levels monitored every three to six months until they remain stable. If they will not stabilize, a through examination is called for.

Treatment

Flavonoids in vegetables—and especially tea—bind to iron in tissues, protecting them from iron-induced free-radical damage. In fact, heavy tea consumption can cause iron deficiency, especially in premenopausal women. This may explain, in part, how flavonoids protect against cancer and other degenerative diseases, especially heart attack and strokes. Quercetin, rutin, hesperidin, and curcumin are especially powerful iron-chelating flavonoids, and all can be purchased from health food stores and suppliers.

It is important to note that Vitamin C can actually overcome the blocking effect of flavonoids by dramatically increasing iron absorption, and the amount that will increase absorption is quite small. For this reason, I advise taking vitamin C on an empty stomach. Usually, cells lining the intestinal wall regulate iron absorption. Large doses of iron are less well absorbed than smaller doses, especially under conditions of iron depletion. Also, animal proteins enhance the absorption of iron. This is why iron from meat, especially red meats, is much better absorbed than from vegetables.

Hemochromatosis

Approximately 10 percent of the Caucasian population has a condition called hemochromatosis that causes a dramatic overload of iron in the body.[464] It is five to ten times more prevalent in men than women, with an overall incidence of one in three hundred people.

While hemochromatosis is a genetically inherited disorder, not everyone with the gene has the full-blown clinical expression of the disease. About 18-20 percent escape the disease. When it is expressed, we see iron levels between fifty and one hundred times higher than normal in the liver and pancreas, 25 times higher in the thyroid and 10-15 times higher in the heart and adrenal glands.

Testing

Diagnosis is usually made by iron-blood studies. Normally, less than 5 percent of iron is unbound to ferritin, but in hemochromatosis, up to 35 percent can be unbound. In those with the disorder, transferrin saturation is normally greater than 55 percent and ferritin levels are greater than 200 ug. Transferrin is a transport protein for iron when it is traveling in the blood. Generally 25 percent or less is saturated with iron. Several other conditions can also be associated with iron overload, including alcoholism, heavy smoking, African siderosis, sideroblastic anemia and thalassemia. Due to persistently high concentrations of iron, liver disease eventually appears. The constant free-radical generation caused by high free iron levels in the liver leads to liver cell destruction and fibrosis.

Treatment

We also see a dramatic increase in heart attacks and strokes in these same individuals. Most cases are treated by repeated transfusions, which is quite effective in ridding the body of excess iron. The success of this practice even lends credence to the ancient treatment of bloodletting. Maybe they weren't so ignorant after all! An easier way to remove excess iron is with a chemical known as IP-6, which tightly binds iron, preventing it from harming you. It can be taken as a capsule with meals to remove the iron from your food. When absorbed, it chelates iron from your tissues.

Stress and Brain Aging

Studies have shown that stress increases the death of specific brain cells, especially those concerned with memory and orientation, the very ones affected by Alzheimer's disease.[465] To a large degree this is due to the fact that prolonged stress of any kind dramatically increases free-radical generation and lipid peroxidation in the brain.

Two hormones, adrenaline and cortisol, appear to be responsible for most of the destructive effects. When we experience stress, both hormones are released in large concentrations and as we age, cortisol release is more prolonged. The physiological events that occur with stress are called allostasis; unrelieved stress is known as an allostatic load.

Dr. Bruce McEwen, director of the Laboratory of Neuroendocrinology at Rockefeller University, has demonstrated through a series of experiments conducted on animals the importance of the brain's response to the allostatic load. He found that unrelieved stress could destroy stem cells in a portion of the hippocampus of the brain, which is vital to memory storage and which contains more cortisol receptors than any other part of the brain.[466] In addition, stress destroyed synaptic connections and dendrites as well.

Further, he found the process was reversible if stress was eventually stopped. With his experimental animals, the limit was twenty-eight days. After that, permanent changes took place. In fact, Dr. Robert Sapolsky of Stanford University found that stress beyond this period actually killed brain cells. The mechanism of brain-cell destruction involves oxidation of these hormones, as well as interaction with the excitotoxin glutamate.

How to Protect Your Brain

Let's put it all together. The brain contains neurons that never divide, and astrocytes and microglia, which can. Those that cannot divide are vulnerable to accumulated lifetime damage from free radicals and lipid peroxidation. The DNA damage that is not repaired prevents cells from performing normal functions and the neuron suffers from impaired energy production, decreased membrane repair, and damaged neurotransmitter production.

Numerous conditions can activate the brain's special immune system, including excess iron, glutamate, certain cytokines, lipid-peroxidation products, mercury, oxidized LDL and HDL, and beta amyloid.[467] This means that as we grow older, our immune systems begin to attack our own brains.

Protecting the brain requires that we address all of these factors. For example, we know that the brain contains its own LDL- and HDL-type lipoproteins, just like those found in the blood. They become harmful only when oxidized, and can then promote excitotoxicity, free-radical production, and microglial activation.[468] Flavonoids, especially epicatechin, have been found to prevent oxidation of LDL and HDL in the brain. Epicatechin is found in grape seed extract as well as green and white tea, which may explain in part why their consumption improves cognitive ability.[469]

Hormones also play a vital role in preserving our brains. As we age, DHEA—an adrenal hormone precursor for production of the reproductive hormones estrogen and testosterone—levels begin to fall. Interestingly, the brain contains receptors for DHEA, and several studies have shown that these receptors are capable of protecting the brain against damage.[470]

Depression is a major problem in the elderly and DHEA may be able to help. One recent study found that when DHEA was given to elderly patients with major depression, all but one improved significantly.[471] The big surprise was that memory also improved significantly. The one patient that did not respond continued on the DHEA, and after six months her depression rating improved 48-72 percent and her semantic memory improved 63 percent.

The brain also contains receptors for pregnenolone. This adrenal hormone, which is a precursor of DHEA and other steroid hormones, also protects brain cells.[472] Pregnenolone also declines with aging, showing a 60 percent reduction by age seventy-five. It has many interesting properties, several of which may make it useful in protecting the brain and improving brain function. For example, it has powerful anti-inflammatory properties, which may protect against Alzheimer's disease.[473]

One advantage of pregnenolone supplementation may be its ability to restore glutamate receptors in the brain, which are commonly lost with aging. While excess glutamate acts as an excitotoxin, the receptors are necessary for memory storage.

Several ongoing studies are investigating pregnenolone's efficacy, and early results are conflicting. In one, significant behavioral complications were seen. In a more recent study using larger doses of pregnenolone, improvement was seen.[474] The reason I generally do not recommend pregnenolone supplementation, except in special situations, is that it can induce seizures in seizure-prone individuals, cause damage to the retina in cases of eye diseases and increases excitotoxicity. Because it reduces activation of the AMPA type glutamate receptor, one thought to cause the damage in MS, it may be of use in this condition. More research is needed before it can be recommended for general use. More research is needed before it can be recommended for general use.

Oxidative Stress & Aging

- Oxidation of nuclear DNA in aged brains is four times higher than younger brains.
- Mitochondrial DNA oxidizes ten times faster than nuclear DNA.
- Mitochondrial DNA has fewer repair enzymes than nuclear DNA.
- Brain DNA oxidizes fifteen times faster after age seventy.
- Aged brain is more susceptible to oxidation, even with normal antioxidant levels.

TABLE 12.2

Other hormones, such as estrogen and testosterone, also have demonstrated protective properties. We know that patients on hormone replacement therapy have a significantly lower incidence of Alzheimer's disease and Parkinson's disease.[475] Several studies also have shown that estrogens and testosterone both protect brain cells from age-related damage.[476] That there are receptors for these hormones in the brain may also help to explain behavioral changes associated with menopause.

Ginkgo Biloba, the Oldest Tree in the World

As I already mentioned, this herb has gotten a lot of attention because of its reputed ability to improve memory in the aged. We have already covered the ability of Ginkgo biloba to thin the blood slightly so as to prevent heart attack and strokes. In addition, we have seen that its flavonoids powerfully protect the walls of blood vessels and prevent oxidation of LDL cholesterol. This effect is very important in protecting the brain since oxidized LDL attached to brain cells can severely damage and even kill neurons.[477]

First, let's look at studies that have been done on less severe memory problems, such as age-related memory loss. In one study, using thirty-one people over age fifty with mild to moderate memory problems, those taking Ginkgo extract showed a significant improvement in several standardized tests of brain function.[478] In another study, eighteen elderly men and women with a slight age-related memory problem[479] were given the Ginkgo one hour before the test, and then tested repeatedly on both visual and word identification to examine information-processing by their brains. Those who took the Ginkgo extract (320 or 600 mg) demonstrated a significant improvement in brain information processing.

A French study, using significantly more patients (166 geriatric patients) than the previous two studies, found those taking the Ginkgo extract demonstrated a significant improvement in memory after three months, and that the effect continued to increase the longer they took the extract.[480] The double-blind, placebo-controlled study used strict methodological conditions to prevent error.

Dr. Pierre LeBars and his co-workers, in a fifty-two-week study of 309 patients with mild to severe dementia, also found that a significant number of the patients improved while taking the extract.[481]

It has been shown that Ginkgo biloba not only protects brain cell membranes from damage, it also restores their youthful fluidity;[482] much of this protection is linked to antioxidant flavonoids found in the herb.[483]

We know that with diseases such as Alzheimer's, connections between neurons—synapses—are most affected, and that millions of these synapses are lost long before there is a significant loss of brain cells. This is important, since synapses can be regenerated as long as neurons survive. Ginkgo biloba has been shown to be very protective of the brain's synapses.[484] Interestingly, the flavonoid, quercetin, is also very protective.

As we age a certain enzyme, called MAO-B, increases in our brain, and this enzyme can increase brain damage by producing harmful compounds. In Parkinson's disease, one of the more effective drugs works by inhibiting this enzyme. Ginkgo biloba extract also inhibits MAO-B, as do several other flavonoids.[485] It has been proposed that by inhibiting this enzyme, Ginkgo acts to relieve stress and promote a sense of calm.

Ginkgo, even in low concentrations, also directly blocks excitotoxicity, and protects brain cells in the hippocampus from injury by beta-amyloid, which is a microscopic collection of toxic crud seen in the brains of Alzheimer's patients. This crud kills surrounding brain cells by an excitotoxic process.

Finally, another way this herb may inhibit the development of dementia is by relieving brain stress. Older animals given the extract are better able to adapt to stressful situations.[486]

With all we know about Ginkgo's effectiveness in protecting the brain and in preventing strokes, it's a shame that the medical community is struggling so hard to frighten the public into avoiding it. Especially when you consider that numerous studies have demonstrated its safety—while physicians continue to prescribe drugs that are not only less effective, but have frighteningly high rates of life-threatening side effects and complications.

Increasing the Brain's Energy Supply

Mitochondria produce about 95 percent of energy within cells: a lifetime of damage to delicate membranes and DNA within these structures leads to significantly impaired energy production throughout the body and the brain. Fortunately, improving lipids in the membrane, especially DHA, goes a long way in repairing this damage. This is done by improving diet and with special supplementation. In addition, increasing your antioxidant protection (mainly vitamins, minerals, and flavonoids) can reduce further damage to this energy-generating system.

Several special supplements that stimulate mitochondria are available without prescription, and can dramatically improve energy production, thereby improving brain function. I have discussed CoQ10 throughout this book: this substance is the first in a line of five compounds that constitute mitochondria's energy-supplying cycle—called the electron transport system. CoQ10 is severely deficient in Parkinson's disease and Alzheimer's.[487] In addition to increasing brain-cell energy production, it also acts as an antioxidant, protects the brain against excitotoxicity, increases cellular glutathione levels, and has been shown to improve memory as well as other brain functions. When combined with niacinamide, CoQ10 strongly protects against the damage seen in Parkinson's disease.[488]

A recent study found that CoQ10 taken by mouth did enter the brain in useful concentrations and that it protected brain cells against excitotoxic damage. In addition, CoQ10 protected neurons from viral damage, including mumps.[489] CoQ10's protective properties stem not only from its ability to increase brain-cell energy production, but also its capacity to protect the mitochondrial membrane.[490]

Alpha-lipoic acid protects cells by acting as a powerful antioxidant, by chelating dangerous metals (arsenic, cadmium, and mercury), by increasing glucose transport into brain cells, by blocking excitotoxicity, and by altering gene expression. A recent study found that supplementing old mice with alpha-lipoic acid could significantly improve mitochondrial function, reduce lipid-peroxidation damage, and not only stop the age-related decline in overall energy production, but reverse the aging of the cell's mitochondria.[491] Another study also found that alpha-lipoic acid could reverse aging of the mitochondria, and improve memory function.[492]

L-carnitine's major function is to guide fatty acids into the cell so they can be metabolized. Another form of this nutrient, called acetyl-L-carnitine is more suited for the brain because it enters the brain more easily than L-carnitine. In addition acetyl-L-carnitine can aid in the formation of the neurotransmitter acetylcholine, which we know plays a vital role in memory.

Acetyl-L-carnitine is unique in its ability to provide a number of important protective functions. For example, it is an antioxidant, increases mitochondrial energy formation, chelates iron, increases brain glutathione levels, and increases brain levels of CoQ10.[493] It has also been shown to reduce the amount of an age pigment in the brain called lipofuscin.[494] It stabilizes membranes and reduces the loss of receptors in the brain.[495] The latter is especially important, since the loss of brain neurotransmitter receptors is one of the hallmarks of brain aging, and is especially severe in Alzheimer's disease.[496]

Both experimental and clinical studies using acetyl-L-carnitine have demonstrated a significant capacity to slow, and even reverse, the affects of aging on the brain.[497] Several studies have shown that acetyl-L-carnitine may be effective in slowing the course of Alzheimer's disease, and in improving behavior and attention span in people with the disease.[498]

By increasing brain-cell energy production and brain-cell repair, as well as providing antioxidant protection, vitamins and minerals also play an important part in protecting the brain from degeneration due to disease and aging. Most B vitamins, particularly thiamine and riboflavin, are involved in energy production. Folic acid, B_{12}, B_6, and niacinamide all contribute to DNA repair and synthesis. Vitamins C and E protect brain cells from oxidative damage and protect microvessels that feed the brain. Several studies have shown that vitamin C supplementation seems to protect the brain against Alzheimer's disease and age-related memory loss.[599]

Because it is both a powerful antioxidant and is capable of blocking excitotoxicity, magnesium is one of the most important minerals involved in protecting the brain. It is also vital for reactions that produce cellular energy. Magnesium depletion of the hippocampus also occurs in Alzheimer's disease.[500]

It is important to maintain proper levels of the antioxidant enzymes, manganese, selenium, zinc, and copper. While deficiencies can result in a significant increase in free-radical damage to the brain (thought to be a mechanism of injury in all degenerative diseases), there is also evidence that high brain concentrations can produce neurological injury. For example, excess zinc has been associated with Alzheimer's disease and excess manganese produces a neurological disorder resembling parkinsonism.

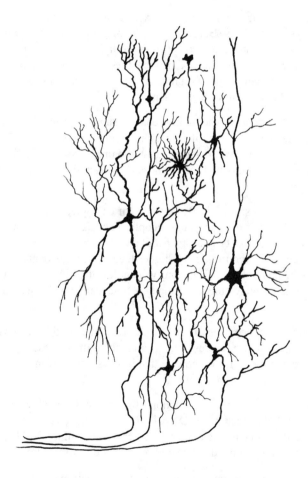

FIGURE 12.1 Drawing demonstrating the complexity of the brain's wiring.

Repairing the Damage

Nutritional abuse, toxic metal accumulations, pesticides and herbicides, industrial chemicals, viral invasions, immune disorders and other chronic diseases all add up to produce serious long-term damage to the nervous system. These factors are interrelated in that they all spur the formation of free radicals and lipid peroxidation. Virtually all mechanics of aging lead back to cellular damage caused by free radicals and lipid peroxidation.

We produce huge numbers of free radicals throughout our lives, but the reason we are totally unaware of it while we are young is that the human body has an incredible repair system that involves hundreds of highly efficient enzymes, RNA, and DNA. Only a very small amount of the injury goes unrepaired in youth.

It is instructive to examine a condition called xeroderma pigmentosum to get an idea of how important this system really is. Because the cells of people afflicted with this disease lack certain DNA repair enzymes, any exposure to sunlight causes severe, chronic damage to skin leading to multiple skin cancers. In fact, these peoples' risk of skin cancer is two thousand times higher than people with normal repair mechanisms. Even the risk of internal cancers is increased twelve times higher than normal.[501]

For those of us with normally functioning repair systems, we may be unaware that damage is occurring, but the small amount of damage that goes unrepaired begins to mount slowly. By the time we reach fifty-five, this accumulated damage begins to affect cellular function and energy production in mitochondria—whose DNA lack the numerous repair mechanisms that protect nuclear DNA.

As we age, these injuries snowball. By seventy, for example, DNA damage occurs at a rate fifteen times faster than it does in young people. Especially frightening is that the risk of increased DNA damage exists even in people with normal antioxidant levels: adequate protection for older folks requires much higher levels of antioxidants. While young people do well at ten servings a day of fruits and vegetables, the elderly need twelve servings to gain health benefits. (Interestingly, younger people gain no further advantage after ten servings.)

It has been shown that people suffering from Alzheimer's disease have impaired DNA repair. Whether this is inborn or develops as a result of the disease itself, we do not know for sure, but the evidence seems to indicate that it plays a significant role in development of the disease.[502]

Melatonin and curcumin enhance production of repair enzymes,[503] which then aid in repair of pre-existing DNA damage. When DNA is functioning properly, it can give the cell the information it needs to make repairs as well. Acetyl-L-carnitine, CoQ10, alpha-lipoic acid, and DHA can repair membrane damage and return fluidity to this vital cellular component.

Special lipid nutrients are also needed for membrane repair and are vital for maintaining a healthy nervous system: phosphotidylcholine, phosphotidylserine, phosphotidylethanolamine, and phosphotidylinositol. These special fatty acid molecules are found in rather high concentrations in egg yolks, or may be taken as supplements. Lecithin contains the major phospholipids and could significantly improve recovery from brain trauma and stroke. In addition, studies showed it improved recall in age-related memory loss and Alzheimer's dementia. Not only will lecithin aid in the repair of membranes, but it will also supply the brain with additional acetylcholine.

Phosphotidylserine has been getting a lot of attention lately because experimental studies have shown that it can restore receptors on brain cells, which permit neurotransmitters to communicate with neurons, most frequently lost in Alzheimer's disease.[504] Clinical studies using phosphotidylserine have been promising, especially for mild memory loss associated with aging. One double-blind, placebo-controlled study of 494 people between the ages of sixty-five and ninety-three found that those supplemented with 300 mg a day demonstrated a statistically significant improvement in behavioral and cognitive testing.[505] In a separate study, Dr. T. H. Crook and colleagues found that the best effects were in elderly people who had the greatest difficulty to begin with.[506] In addition to its affects on memory and cognitive brain function, phosphotidylserine also significantly relieves depression in the elderly.[507]

The big question is: what will it do for the person with Alzheimer's disease? Studies have shown a significant improvement in behavior and some improvement in memory.[508] The best results were found in people with early disease.

Basic Supplementation

Whether or not you should consider special supplementation designed to protect the brain will depend on a number of factors. If you have lived a hard life, eaten poorly, exercised too little or too much, experienced prolonged, intense stress, or suffered from a chronic disease (such as diabetes, lupus, or hypertension), you will most certainly need intensive nutritional therapy.

On the other hand, if you have always eaten nutritious foods, exercised regularly and in moderation, controlled stress, and suffered no chronic diseases, you can take minimal supplements to ensure adequate protection. For you, diet should be your main concern: a recent study found that blueberries, spinach, and strawberries provide the greatest protection against, and even reversal of, brain aging.[509]

Recommendations

Vitamin C 500 mg (buffered)
Take one three times a day on an empty stomach.

Vitamin E 400 IU
Succinate or mixed tocopherols. Take two a day.

Special Coverage for High-Risk Individuals

All of the above plus:

DHA 100 mg
Take two capsules twice a day. Keep refrigerated.

CoQ10 100 mg
Take one twice to three times a day. Take with DHA.

N-acetyl L-cysteine (NAC) 500 mg-750 mg
Take one twice a day.

Alpha-lipoic acid 50 mg
Take one two to three times a day with meals.

Niacinamide 500 mg
Take one twice a day.

Pyridoxal-5 phosphate 34 mg
Take one three times a day with meals.

Phosphotidylcholine 750 mg
Take two capsules twice a day. Keep refrigerated.

Phosphotidylserine 100 mg
Take one three times a day.

Acetyl-L-carnitine 500 mg
Take one two to three times a day.

Curcumin 500 mg
Take one twice a day. Mix with one tablespoon extra virgin olive oil or Omega-3 oil.

Quercetin 250 mg
Dissolve in oil or take a water-soluble form, twice a day

Milk Thistle 200 mg
Take two capsules twice a day.

DHEA
25-50 mg a day under medical supervision only.

Vinpocetine 10 mg
Take one twice a day.

B-100 multivitamin with minerals and no iron
Take one a day.

13
The Aging Immune System

The human immune system is a highly complex, bodywide network of specialized cells, organs, and even a separate circulatory system, which work in concert to clear infection from the body. The organs of the immune system are called lymphoid organs. Lymphatic vessels and lymph nodes comprise the special circulatory system that transports white blood cells to sites of infection throughout the body.

Lymph (after the Greek meaning "clear stream") is a clear-to-white fluid made of chyle (fluid from the intestines after digestion which contains proteins and fats), some red blood cells, and many white blood cells, especially lymphocytes. Lymphocytes are cells that attack bacteria in the blood. Operating in close partnership with blood circulation, lymph bathes the tissues of the body, and lymphatic vessels collect and move it back into the blood.

In addition to lymph nodes (scattered in the neck, armpits, and groin areas), the tonsils, adenoids, thymus, and spleen all perform specialized immune functions. Also, bone marrow of certain long, flat bones (such as the bones of the pelvis) produces cells that grow into the more specialized cells that circulate throughout the immune system. The appendix is also a lymphoid organ and helps protect the cecal part of the colon.

While immune-system processes are far too complicated for a lengthy discussion here, it is necessary to know that there are two major classes of lymphocytes: B cells, which mature within bone marrow, and T cells, which mature in the thymus (located behind the breastbone). B cells are part of the body's antibody-mediated, or humoral (after the Greek "humor," for the body's blood and lymph systems), immune system. B cells produce antibodies that circulate in blood and lymph and attach to antigens (foreign substances), marking them for destruction by other cells.

T cells also patrol for foreign invaders, but in addition to marking them, certain T cells also can attack and destroy cells. T lymphocytes are responsible for cell-mediated immunity (also called cellular immunity). They also coordinate overall immune-system response.

While the immune system ages right along with the rest of our body, it may actually do so at an increased rate because of the speed at which immune cells proliferate. During viral invasions or bacterial infections, the immune system mobilizes billions of white blood cells. Cells that divide rapidly run a higher risk of frequent genetic mutations, especially when free-radial generation is high. Antioxidant defenses naturally fall and DNA damage by free radicals may increase by as much as fifteen times as we age, making us even more susceptible to damage that accompanies infections.

This means that we run a higher risk of cancer of blood-forming tissues, such as leukemia, myeloma, and lymphoma, as well as immune incompetence. Such a situation leaves the body unable to protect itself from even common infections and increases risk for autoimmune diseases. As with so many other health-related disorders, the incidence of immune-related diseases in the population appears to be increasing—and many can be correlated directly to poor nutritional practices in all age groups.

Poor nutrition does not affect all parts of the immune system equally. Most sensitive is the cellular arm of the immune system, consisting of macrophages (specialized scavenger cells), lymphocytes (T-cells), natural killer cells, and other specialized immune cells.[510] Antibodies are less affected. This is exactly what we see with aging—cellular immunity that is depressed out of proportion to humoral antibodies.[511]

Because immune overreaction is common with aging, autoimmunity due to other factors, such as viral infections and environmental toxins, can be worse in the aged. Interestingly, autoimmunity to brain proteins is much higher in cases of Alzheimer's, Parkinson's, and Lou Gehrig's diseases (ALS).[512]

Nutrition and Immunity

Immune suppression can occur even with single nutrient deficiencies: for example, you can have excellent general nutrition, but an isolated deficiency in say, pyridoxine, will trigger immune suppression. The same is true for most of the B vitamins, vitamins C, E, and D, and magnesium, zinc, boron, iron, and selenium. Supplying these people with a balance of high-quality protein and adequate calories can quickly restore immune function to normal.

While isolated vitamin and mineral deficiencies are far more likely to occur in Western nations (more profound deficiencies are found in developing countries), there is a subgroup of elderly in this nation who do suffer from profound protein-calorie and vitamin-mineral deficiencies. These are shut-ins who live alone and have no surviving family, or at least no one to care for them on a regular basis. Only organizations such as Meals on Wheels provide such people with even semi-nutritious foods. I say semi-nutritious because, despite improved protein-calorie nutrition, the meals often contain a number excitotoxins, bad fats, and excess sugars. Still, their hearts are in the right place and they provide care that no one else seems willing to provide.

Vaccines

Because depression of immunity accompanies aging (especially cell-mediated immunity responsible for protection from viruses, bacteria and other nasties), the elderly also are more likely to experience reactivation of quiescent tuberculosis and herpes zoster, and have a reduced response to vaccination.[513]

The latter is especially important in light of the medical profession's obsession with vaccinating the elderly against influenza each year. Because many older folks are already immune-suppressed due to poor nutrition, especially vitamin A deficiency, they simply will not respond to vaccination by proper immunity. This means they have been exposed to the risk of complications from the vaccine without gaining any benefit. Few are aware that the success rate for flu vaccinations in the elderly is less than 50 percent, and that each vaccine contains the dubious bonus of mercury and aluminum doses that persist in the nervous system for decades.

Protein and calorie deficiencies have been shown to increase risk of infection significantly and to reduce the success rate of immunizations.[514] Several studies have demonstrated impaired antibody production as well as decreased levels of serum immunoglobulins, secretory IgA, thymic function, splenic lymphocytes, complement formation, and interferon production, all of which are vital to competent immune function.

Our evidence-based doctors, who seem to know little of the relationship between vaccination safety, immunity, and nutrition, never suggest nutritional supplementation. In fact, an elderly person's best protection is improved nutrition—not vaccination—as we shall see.

Vitamin A

We've known for years that successful vaccination depends on adequate vitamin A intake.[515] Attempts to vaccinate African children who suffered from vitamin A deficiencies resulted in a very high mortality rate. The same tragedy occurred when vaccinations were forced on aboriginal populations in Australia.

Deficiencies in this vitamin cause a decrease in thymus gland size, natural killer (NK) cell activity, production of interferon, and delayed hypersensitivity reactions. We also see impairment of macrophage function, an immune cell that plays a vital role in controlling viral, yeast, mycoplasma, and cancer growth.

One more devastating side effect of vaccination is the potential for encephalitis (called postvaccinal encephalomyelitis), a condition in which the immune system mistakenly attacks the coverings of neural pathways in the brain and spinal cord. Studies have shown that when vitamin A is given to an animal, either before or after vaccination, the severity of the disorder is greatly reduced.[516] There is also compelling evidence that the incidence of autism may be reduced by adequately supplementing children with vitamin A.

Carotenoids

Close to five hundred types of carotenoids exist in the plant world, thirty-four of which occur in fruits and vegetables found in the human diet. The best known of these is beta-carotene, which recently received a bad name due to a poorly conducted experiment. Rest assured that no *well-conducted* scientific study has ever demonstrated that beta-carotene causes lung cancer in nonsmokers!

A recent study in human volunteers aged fifty-six years and older found that a dose of 30 mg of beta-carotene significantly increased T-helper lymphocytes and lowered the number of T-suppressor cells. T-helper cells enhance the immune attack on bacteria, viruses, and fungi, while T-suppressor cells stop the attack, limiting peripheral damage to surrounding normal tissues.[517] A proper balance between T-helper and T-suppressor cells is vital to immune health. NK cell function also increased with beta-carotene supplementation, as well as interleukin-2. This pattern of immune alteration corrects the immune suppression abnormalities seen with aging.[518]

With aging we also see a decrease in an important immune chemical called interleukin-2, which affords protection by enhancing T-lymphocyte production and function. Carotenoids improve age-related declines in interleukin-2 production. Another cytokine, interleukin-6, increases with aging[519] and is associated with autoimmune diseases, Alzheimer's disease, and cancer.[520]

Because beta-carotene is converted, in part, into vitamin A, some have questioned if the immune stimulation seen in tests was an affect of the beta-carotene itself or of vitamin A. Recent studies, however, have shown that the carotenoids, astaxanthin, and lutein—neither of which are converted to vitamin A—can also restore lost immune function in the elderly.[521]

When taking carotenoids it is best to take a mixture that includes a number of varieties, such as beta-carotene, alpha-carotene, canthoxanthin, astaxanthin, lutein, zeaxanthin, lycopene and cryptoxanthin. Taking beta-carotene alone, especially the synthetic form, can actually reduce absorption of other carotenoids, such as lutein. Of all the carotenoids, the best source is a pair of species of unicellular organisms from the ocean called *Dunaliella salina* and *Dunaliella bardawil*. These tiny algae absorb a very high concentration of multiple forms of carotenoids. The dose is 25,000 IU daily.

Obtaining carotenoids from fruits and vegetables is preferable. Most forms are fairly heat-resistant; in fact, steaming or cooking at low temperature actually releases the carotenoids normally bound in vegetables. If you choose to rely on fresh, raw vegetables, I suggest juicing or blending to break down the cell wall and release the nutrients.

B Vitamins and Immunity

Vitamin B$_6$ (Pyridoxine)

Pyridoxine plays a major role in numerous biochemical reactions, especially those involving amino acids—which play a major role in immunity. Of these, arginine is perhaps the most important for proper immune function. A B$_6$ deficiency will promote loss of cell-mediated immunity and a slight reduction in antibody formation in response to tetanus toxoid. A combined deficiency of B$_6$ and pantothenic acid (a vitamin) can result in profound suppression of immune function.

Good sources of pyridoxine are wheat, corn, egg yolks, and meat. There are several chemical forms of vitamin B$_6$ such as pyridoxine, pyridoxal, and pyridoxamine. All three must be converted to pyridoxal-5 phosphate to be utilized. In some instances, a person may lack the enzyme needed to convert pyridoxine to its active form. This is common in those with chronic diseases, in the elderly, and in the very young. The maintenance dose for pyridoxine is 25 mg a day. Higher doses may be needed in the elderly, especially in those with atherosclerosis. While the only confirmed reports of nervous-system toxicity are for doses over two grams a day, for safety's sake I recommend a maximum dose of 500 mg per day.

Pantothenic acid is a component of coenzyme A, a primary component of energy production known as the Kreb's cycle. Eggs and yeast are the most important sources. As a supplement, 25 mg is sufficient for maintenance.

Folic Acid and Vitamin B_{12}

Folic acid and B_{12} are considered together because they play a connected role in DNA synthesis and single-carbon transfer reactions. Since immune cells multiply at a rate equal to the most malignant tumor, they require an endless supply of these two vitamins. People deficient in these vitamins demonstrate impaired antibody formation, reduced reproduction of stimulated lymphocytes, thymic atrophy, and decreased cell-mediated immunity. As with vitamin A, deficiencies of folic acid and vitamin B_{12} increase the likelihood of postvaccinal encephalomyelitis.

Folic acid should be taken in a dose of 400-800 ug a day. Vitamin B_{12} as a supplement most often comes in a form called cyanocobalamin. Cobalamin is the actual B_{12} component. Cyanide is added to make it stable for packaging. Unfortunately, activation requires that the cyanide be removed by an enzyme. If it cannot be removed, you will get no benefit from your supplement. In fact, you will be worse off, because it will act as an antivitamin, blocking the effect of the existing B_{12}.

The natural form of vitamin B_{12} is called methylcobalamin. This form does not require conversion and can be taken sublingually. Having measured levels myself, both before and after taking this form of B_{12}, I can attest to its absorptive properties. The dose for methylcobalamin is 1,000 ug a day for maintenance. Those with poor nutrition or who suffer from a chronic disease will need 5,000 ug a day.

Biotin

Only severe deficiencies of biotin will produce obvious signs of immune system injury. Under such conditions, reactions to vaccine boosters are blunted, indicating decreased antibody formation. The usual dose is 1-3 mg a day.

Other B vitamins, such as thiamine and riboflavin, play a smaller role in immune competence, and only in cases of severe deficiencies are there any observable negative effects.

Vitamin C

Vitamin C, which is water-soluble, plays a major role in the body's defense against foreign invasions. By strengthening the integrity of tissue barriers, such as connective tissue of the skin and mucous membranes, it helps to prevent harmful organisms from entering the body. And it prevents infections from becoming established by stimulating wound healing. Ascorbic acid in high concentrations can also directly kill some viruses and bacteria. In addition, it plays a major role in white blood cell function by promoting phagocytosis and cell migration.

Deficiencies in ascorbic acid (ascorbate) can result in impaired hypersensitivity reactions and complement formation, but have not been associated with cell-mediated or humoral immunity.

It is best to use buffered vitamin C since ascorbic acid is, obviously, acidic. Acidosis induced by this form can result in mouth ulcers in some people. I prefer the magnesium or calcium ascorbate form. The dose varies from 500 mg to 2 g three times a day, depending on your needs.

Several nutritionists have promoted the use of very high concentrations of this vitamin, which seems to have some merit in individual cases. The real question is whether such large doses can be absorbed. Several studies have indicated that absorption from the gut is regulated, preventing uptake of extremely high doses. It may be that with certain disorders larger concentrations are allowed to pass through the intestinal barriers. As far as I am aware, no one has tested ascorbate absorption in persons with lupus, rheumatoid arthritis, and other similar disorders. Most absorption studies have been conducted using healthy volunteers. Intravenous ascorbate can attain very high levels and appears to be helpful with serious infections such as Lyme disease.

Vitamin D

Vitamin D acts as an immunoregulatory hormone by suppressing overreactions of the immune system, which is especially important for those with autoimmune disorders. It also plays a major role in lymphocyte differentiation, that is the maturation of lymphocytes into their various types.

While much press has been given to the possible toxicity of vitamin D, it is important to realize that the skin can manufacture up to *25,000* IU of vitamin D_3 per day. While most supplement doses are limited to 400 IU, more recent studies indicate a safe and effective dose is 1,500 to 2,000 IU a day of vitamin D_3.

Vitamin E

Vitamin E is actually made of eight different components, four tocopherols and four tocotrioneols, each with a different function. While little is known about the functions of the other tocopherols, we have learned a lot about d-alpha tocopherol in particular.

Besides its role as a major membrane antioxidant, d-alpha tocopherol also plays a significant role in immunity. Supplementation with vitamin E in old mice and elderly humans has been shown to increase lymphocyte proliferation, increase delayed type hypersensitivity, lower immune-suppressing PGE_2-type eicosanoids, and prevent age-related loss of NK-cell activity.[522]

NK cells protect us against viruses, bacteria, mycoplasma, and cancer, and in the instance of cancer, vitamin E may induce antigenic changes in cancer cells that make them more susceptible to immune destruction.[523]

One very important observation related to the vaccine issue is that combined with low vitamin E intake, attenuated viruses can become pathogenic. Doses several times the RDA levels enhance antibody activity against antigens and improve clearance of particulate matter by a special lymph cleaning system (reticuloendothelial system).

Vitamin E requirements are linked to polyunsaturated fat intake, such as corn, safflower, sunflower, and the omega-3 oils. Because these oils are easily oxidized, they can be very destructive to cells and tissues. Vitamin E occurs naturally in such oils and keeps them from oxidizing in the body; unfortunately, most vitamin E is removed during processing, and few companies add it back. Extra virgin olive oil is a monounsaturated oil and so is very resistant to oxidation, not only because it is mostly saturated, but because it contains numerous powerful antioxidant flavonoids.

Some studies have found that excess vitamin E can actually suppress immune function but most of these used doses of 2,000 IU or greater. Immune suppression has also been reported, but not confirmed, with doses as low as 800 IU. It is important to note that most of these studies used a form of vitamin E with very little antioxidant function, and poor absorption and tissue distribution, which may have deleterious effects on the immune system that wouldn't be associated with natural (mixed tocopherols) or succinate forms (dry vitamin E).

I recommend for maintenance 400 IU of mixed tocopherols, not to contain either dl-tocopherol or d-alpha tocopherol acetate. For those at high risk of neurological disease, cancer, or atherosclerosis I recommend 1,000 IU of d-alpha tocopherol succinate once a day.

Minerals, Supplements, and Immunity

Several studies have shown that supplementation with vitamins and minerals in combination can correct age-related immune suppression.[524] For example, one double-blind, placebo-controlled study using eighty-one elderly hospitalized people (over sixty-five years old) found that in those given a supplement mixture containing zinc, selenium, vitamins C and E, and beta-carotene showed a significant improvement in antioxidant defense, including antioxidant enzymes, as well as a significant reduction in infections over the two-year period of observation. This study also found that over two-thirds of these elderly patients had deficiencies in vitamin C, folate, selenium, and zinc when the study began.

Another double-blind, placebo-controlled study, also among the elderly, found that the trace elements zinc and selenium, but not the vitamins, reduced the incidence of infections over the two-year observation period.[525] This does not mean that vitamins do not play a significant role in preventing infections, just that they cannot work alone. We have already known for some time that minerals, especially zinc and selenium, play a critical role in immune function.

Iron

Iron is a very precarious mineral: levels that are either too low or too high increase free-radical generation. The immune system seems to function well within a rather broad range of iron levels, but significantly low levels can interfere with immune function. For example, low iron levels are associated with decreased killing power by phagocytes (scavenger cells), reduced ability to stimulate lymphocyte mobilization, fewer NK cells, and decreased interferon production. Iron has no affect on antibody production.

Studies on people in poorer countries demonstrate that iron supplements, when given to those deficient in the mineral before infection develops, significantly reduce morbidity and mortality from infectious diseases. Iron deficiency also impairs wound healing.

Iron supplementation should only be given with great caution to a person who has an active infection. Many virulent organisms—especially viruses, bacteria, and mycoplasmic organisms—utilize iron just as we do. Iron supplementation in individuals with infections and cancer has produced some disastrous results.[526] During infections, supplementing your diet with iron, or eating high iron-containing foods, such as red meats, greatly increases the growth of the viruses and bacteria and will prolong your illness by making it more difficult for your immune system to clear the infection.[527] Cancer cells are also highly iron-dependent, growing rapidly and metastasizing in the presence of iron.[528] Even high normal levels of iron can spur cancer growth.

Before beginning iron supplementation, have an entire iron panel done, including iron levels, total iron-binding capacity, transferritin saturation, and ferritin levels. How will you know if you are iron-deficient? If your iron panel shows that your ferritin level is less than 12 ug/l and your transferrin is less than 16 percent saturated, you will need supplementation. If your iron levels are drastically low, take lower doses of iron over a longer period of time rather than very high doses all at once. After three weeks of supplementation, iron levels should be checked. If you are in the mid-range or slightly lower, stop supplementation.

For those having difficulty absorbing iron, I suggest taking vitamin C with the iron since this vitamin is known to enhance iron absorption. Also avoid vegetables and other flavonoids, including tea, when you take your iron supplement. Plant flavonoids bind the iron and reduce absorption. For this reason, iron from meat sources is much better absorbed than iron from vegetables.

Phytic acid (inositol hexaphosphate or IP-6) also binds iron and prevents its absorption. In addition, it is a powerful antioxidant. Phytic acid is found in very high concentrations in colostrum, the first milk to arrive from the breast. It is also found in many fruits, grains, and vegetables. A specially formulated form of phytic acid, called Cellular Forte with IP-6 ™ is used to treat cancers of many types. One of its major effects is to prevent iron from reaching cancer cells. Its iron binding power is so great that it is also used to treat the iron-overload disease hemochromatosis.

Composed of 98 percent iron, carbonyl is the best form of iron to take. Because it is highly concentrated, 18 mg of carbonyl is equal to 54.4 mg of ferrous fumerate, and 150 mg of ferrous gluconate, two commonly prescribed forms of iron. The advantage of the carbonyl form is that it is well-tolerated and has a wide margin of safety. For more information about iron and health I strongly recommend *The Iron Time Bomb* by Bill Sardi.

The body has a remarkable system to prevent excessive iron absorption. If you are deficient, iron absorption increases. If you have an excess of iron in your tissues, iron absorption is reduced by 50 percent. For this reason, I recommend taking iron supplements every other day, if you need supplementation at all.

Zinc

Zinc deficiency is fairly common among the elderly. This very important mineral plays a vital role in hundreds of metabolic reactions as part of metalloenzymes (metal-containing enzymes). Severe deficiency can cause widespread atrophy of the lymph nodes and decrease lymphocyte counts. Other studies have reported depressed NK-cell activity, reduced antibody production, and impaired delayed hypersensitivity reactions. Zinc also plays a major role in the thymic hormone, thymulin, which is very important for cellular immunity.

Excessive zinc can impair immunity by inhibiting bactericidal and macrophage function and neutrophils. As with all minerals, oversupplementation should be avoided. The usual dose for maintenance is 15 mg a day.

Selenium

This element has gotten a lot of attention over the last several years. Early experiments demonstrated that selenium—like vitamins A and E, and the carotenoids—could enhance antibody titers following vaccination in experimental animals.

Much of the scientific literature on selenium concerns its ability to enhance the killing of tumor cells. For example, one study demonstrated that supplementing with selenium produced a significantly greater capacity of the immune system to kill tumor cells and produce tumor necrosis factor-alpha (a tumor killing cytokine) than in animals with normal levels of selenium. The mineral appeared to be able to increase the ability of the body to generate cytotoxic (tumor-cell-killing) macrophages.[529]

Several human studies have shown a strong correlation between selenium intake and lowered cancer risk. One such study done in China found that a mixture of beta-carotene, selenium and alpha-tocopherol significantly lowered total cancer mortality. A similar study found the same relationship in Americans. A recent, impressive study measured the level of selenium proteins in the blood of 12,500 middle-aged men and 400 cancer cases, and found that those with the lowest selenium proteins (selenoprotein P) had cancer rates five times higher than those with the highest levels.

Selenium also plays a major role in glutathione peroxidase function, an enzyme vital for neutralizing hydrogen peroxide. It is thought that enhanced immunity is imparted by selenium's effects on this enzyme.

Selenium normally exists in the plasma in two forms, selenocysteine (selenoprotein P) and seleniomethionine. Both appear to work equally well in immune-system enhancement and in preventing cancer. An excellent source is a garlic-extract-enhanced selenium supplement, which supplies the extra benefits of garlic's powerful cancer-inhibiting, antibacterial and antiviral phytochemicals.

The usual dose is 100-200 ug a day. Doses above 400 ug a day are potentially toxic.

Omega-3 Fatty Acids

A study reported in the journal, *Nutrition*, in 1990 described the significant immune-enhancing effects of omega-3 fatty acids.[530] Subsequent studies have proposed a mechanism for this effect, including suppression of special enzymes (COX-II) known to produce substances (the eicosanoid PGE_2) that suppress immunity and promote inflammation.

We now know that omega-6 oils profoundly suppress immunity and promote inflammation by stimulating the production of these inflammatory chemicals.[531] As a result, they also promote infections and the growth and spread of cancers.

Unfortunately, most oils used in developed countries are of the omega-6 type and few processed foods contain omega-3 fatty acids. As a result, the vast majority of Americans are severely deficient in omega-3 fatty acids, an imbalance that promotes disease and immune suppression. In my nutritional practice, I frequently order the Essential Fatty Acid Analysis though the Great Smokies Diagnostic Laboratory. This test breaks down the various metabolic products and the results are displayed on a helpful diagram, one side of which is a breakdown of omega-6 fatty acids and the other the omega-3 fatty acids.

I rarely find a person whose test results indicate normal omega-3 fatty acid components. Most are severely deficient in EPA and DHA, the main components of omega-3 fatty acids. The DHA is primarily responsible for protecting the immune system and inhibiting cancer growth. Many people's tests are also very high in the omega-6 product arachidonic acid, which promotes inflammation and cell degeneration.

To benefit from DHA supplementation, it is necessary to *decrease* omega-6 fatty-acid intake. This means giving up virtually all processed foods—which is just about the only thing most Americans eat. It is interesting to note that the USDA is currently conducting experiments in feeding fishmeal to cattle to increase the amount of omega-3 fatty acids in the meat. Cattle that graze on plants and grasses have naturally higher omega-3 levels in their meat than those fed grain.

The safest way to benefit from omega-3 fatty acids is to take DHA, which is derived from an algae, directly. It is usually steam-distilled and contains no mercury. Recent studies have shown that DHA reduces immune overactivity, which has been shown to be beneficial in autoimmune diseases, neurodegenerative diseases, and autism.

I recommend that your fish oil supplement contain at least 500 mg of DHA and that you remember to keep it in the refrigerator.

Special Immune Stimulants

Most of us have heard that the herb echinacea boosts the immune system, and a lot of people take it during cold season. Several studies have shown that indeed echinacea does boost immune function of mononuclear cells, especially NK cells. Panax ginseng has the same properties. Both herbs boost immunity in both normal individuals and those with depressed immune systems.[532] Unfortunately, if use is continued for more than two weeks, there is a significant reduction in immune stimulation.

A recent study found that NAC (N-acetyl L-cysteine) could reduce the effects of common viral infections such as influenza. In this study of 262, mostly elderly, people, those given NAC (600 mg twice daily for six months) experienced a significant decrease in influenza-like episodes, severity of symptoms, and length of time in the bed as compared to matched controls.

The study also demonstrated that those taking the NAC had a better immune response than the controls. While they still were infected by the virus, their symptoms were mild compared to those who did not take the supplement. NAC, as you will recall, increases cellular glutathione levels, preventing free-radical damage triggered by the virus. This is another way the elderly can avoid taking the influenza vaccine every year. In all studies involving NAC, it was well-tolerated and produced no significant side effects.

Cellular Forte with IP-6™ is another popular immune stimulant, which works in diverse ways. Normally, it is used to treat cancer, but it is excellent for treating viral infections as well. One of the interesting ways it kills viruses, bacteria, mycoplasma, and cancer cells is by robbing them of iron. All of these dangerous characters require large amounts of iron to grow and reproduce.

Because of its powerful iron-binding capacity, this product should be used only for short durations. Long-term use could result in severe iron-deficiency anemia. In general, one to two weeks is a safe length of time to use Cellular Forte with IP-6™.

A similar supplement called MGN-3 also binds iron and may have slightly better immune-enhancing effects than Cellular Forte with IP-6™.

Another immune-enhancing supplement getting a lot of attention these days is beta 1,3/1,6 D-glucan, extracted from baker's yeast and mushrooms.[533] Basically, it is a polysaccharide molecule that activates macrophages, the primary initiator of the immune system. In fact, the macrophage has beta 1,3 D-glucan receptors on its surface that play a major role in this activation process. Studies have shown that beta 1,3 D-glucan not only enhances cellular immunity, it is also a powerful radioprotectant, capable of protecting cells from damage, even with very high doses of radiation. Beta 1,6 D-glucan alone is a poor immune stimulant. Only combined with the 1,3 form is it effective.

By stimulating the cells most involved in immunity against cancer and infections, beta 1,3 glucan has been shown to be effective against a variety of cancers including melanoma, breast cancer and leukemia, and infections, including yeast, bacteria, and viruses. When combined with traditional medications, such as chemotherapy agents and antibacterial drugs, it significantly enhances their effectiveness.

There is some evidence that beta 1,3 glucan extracted from baker's yeast is superior to that extracted from mushrooms. If you have a yeast infection, you do not have to worry about the product being extracted from yeast as long as you buy a highly purified brand, such as the ImmuDyne brand called Macroforce™ or Imucell™ by Biopolymer Engineering, Inc.

For maintenance of immunity, you should take a lower dose, such as 2.5 mg once or twice a day. Higher doses are reserved for cancer treatments and for those with active infections. Because of the heavy demand for vitamin C by macrophages, extra vitamin C is also recommended. The higher dose Macroforce product even includes extra vitamin C.

Another concern is the risk of aggravating autoimmune diseases by excessive immune stimulation. Autoimmune diseases such as lupus, rheumatoid arthritis and thyroiditis are all caused by an over-stimulation of humoral immunity (antibodies). Another benefit of beta 1,3 D-glucan is that it stimulates only cellular immunity and not humoral immunity. ImmuDyne recently released a new product that combines beta 1,3 D-glucan with IP-6. It is recommended for cancer patients or patients with severe immune deficiencies.

Lyme Disease and Rickettsia

Rickettsia are bacterial intracellular parasites, considered a separate group of bacteria because they have the common feature of being spread by ticks, fleas, mites, and lice.

Perhaps the most familiar rickettsial disease is Lyme disease, a bacterial infection spread by ticks. The causative bacteria, *Borrelia burgdorferi*, is a corkscrew shaped microorganism (called a spriochete) that resembles the syphilis organism. More than 100,000 cases of Lyme disease have been reported to the CDC since 1982, and it is spreading rapidly across the United States, going from fourteen states at the time it was discovered in 1972 to forty-eight states by 1992.[534]

Lyme disease manifests as an inflammatory disease that affects the skin in the early stage, and spreads to the joints, nervous system, and other organ systems in its later stages. If diagnosed within a few weeks, most cases can be cured easily with antibiotics. Yet, even a short delay can lead to a life of misery and possibly to death.

The disease is notoriously difficult to diagnose. The least accurate test, the ELISA, is known to return an unusually high number of false negative results. The Western Blot Test is more accurate, but can produce false negatives in the 30 to 40 percent range. The PCR (polymerase chain reaction), which measures the bacteria's DNA, is by far the most accurate, but if the organisms are hiding in body tissues, the PCR test also may be negative. Once antibiotic treated is begun, the PCR test becomes a more accurate measure as dead organisms are released into the blood, exposing their DNA.

Once the organism enters the body, it quickly leaves the blood stream and burrows deep into tissues throughout the body. Chronic infections can lead to severe arthritis, cardiac injury, and neurological injury. In addition, infected individuals often suffer from headaches, muscle pains, weakness, and fatigue.

It is much more difficult to cure the disease once it has burrowed into tissues and organs. One reason is the phenomenon of stealth bacterial conversion (L-form bacteria), where the bacteria becomes invisible to the body's immune system, as well as to antibiotics. When this occurs, the only way to combat the organism is to give antibiotics over a long period of time, usually more than three months. Even then, some cases remain uncured.

Neuroborreliosis

In the nervous system, the organism can cause a condition called neuroborreliosis, which appears to involve the glutamate neurotransmitter system. In fact, viral infection acts through the same mechanism. It has been shown that the bacteria or virus activates microglia in the nervous system, which move around within the brain and spinal cord seeking out the spirochetes. When it encounters them, the microglia are activated and begin to pour out large amounts of free radicals and immune chemicals (cytokines). Together, these two block the uptake mechanism for the glutamate neurotransmitter.[535]

As we have seen, elevated glutamate levels in the nervous system can result in widespread damage to neurons and other normal cells. The more intense the immune response, the greater the damage. Yet something worse can occur if the immune system is impaired. While a normal response will end an infection quickly, a prolonged response—which is the result of an impaired or unbalanced immune system—can produce long-term damage, leading eventually to neurodegeneration.[536] This happens because glutamate levels that remain elevated for long periods of time will cause the death of large numbers of neurons.

We also know that, when activated, microglial cells themselves secrete two excitotoxins, glutamate and quinolinic acid, in large quantities.[537] This may be why neurologic disorders are sometimes associated with Lyme disease. In essence, our own immune systems, especially if they are impaired by disease, can cause damage over and above the infection the system is attempting to cure.

In fact, quinolinic acid and glutamate account for most damage associated with nervous system infections. In addition, certain cytokines secreted by these immune cells block the glutamate transport proteins that normally prevent glutamate accumulation. Viral encephalitis has been linked with this particular mechanism. It also emphasizes the importance of avoiding dietary MSG and aspartame.

Babesiosis

Another disease caused by ticks (especially the deer tick) is known as babesiosis, a parasitic infection caused by a protozoa living in the red blood cells, much like malaria, which is more likely to occur in the spring and summer months: tick season.

Until recently, babesiosis was thought to affect only animals, but now is recognized as one of the most widespread blood parasites in the world, second only to trypanosomes;[538] however, more infections probably occur than are reported. The biggest problem is that many doctors still have never heard of the disease, and therefore do not know to test for it.

The infection can be either asymptomatic or produce rapid death, especially in those who already have weakened immune systems. Some people may have the disease and never know it because their immune system clears the infection before symptoms manifest. In others, the disease may cause mild symptoms such as muscle aches and joint pains or headaches, while others suffer severe weakness, headaches, migratory muscle pains, joint arthritis, nausea, and vomiting.

Because the organisms frequently invade the heart muscle, heart failure is a major risk in severely affected individuals.[539] This is especially likely in someone whose spleen has been removed, or in those suffering from extreme immune suppression. In such cases, the blood and organs are filled with babesia organisms. Blood transfusion and high doses of anti-malarial medications are necessary.

The babesia organism can also invade the brain, and pediatricians have been warned to suspect babesia infection in children showing sudden behavioral changes. The infection is very similar to cerebral malaria. As with Lyme disease, neurological damage is most likely produced by an immune-triggered excitotoxic reaction.

Ehrlichosis

A third tick-borne disease, Ehrlichosis, is caused by the *Ehrlica chaffeenis* organism, a bacteria that lives within cells. While some people will experience no symptoms, others will experience chills, fever, flu-like symptoms, weakness, muscle pains, chronic fatigue, and headaches.

Dual Infection

Until recently, it was not recognized that two or more rickettsial infections could co-exist in the same person, however it is now estimated that 10 percent of people diagnosed with Lyme disease are also infected with another rickettsial organism. This would be especially true for those who have been treated for Lyme disease, yet never recover. These unfortunate people may be suffering from Lyme disease along with babesia or Ehrlichia. Most unfortunate is that the strategy for curing these diseases differ, so diagnosing and treating only one does not solve the problem.

It follows that someone suffering from a dual infection will experience symptoms much worse than those infected with only one organism, including severe muscle pains, arthritis, heart damage, intense weakness, night sweats, and neurological disorders. Babesia can result in severe shortness of breath as well. Both babesia and Lyme organisms can damage the heart.

Because at least two of these diseases can infect the nervous systems, special precautions must be taken when treating them. It has been known for some time that when people are treated with antibiotics or antiprotozoal medications, they may suffer from acute worsening during the course of the treatment, called the Herxheimer reaction. This is because tissues and blood are suddenly flooded with dead and dying organisms. Once the dead organisms are cleared, symptoms begin to improve.

This brings us to a special concern of mine: killing organisms too rapidly without sufficient protection. When microorganisms invade tissues, the immune system sends in billions of white blood cells (mostly lymphocytes, phagocytes, and NK cells) to kill the organism. As part of this process, the white blood cells generate a storm of free radicals and release powerful cytokine immune chemicals that result in inflammation of surrounding tissues.

It is possible that the microorganism massacre releases such a large antigenic load that the ensuing immune response is greatly magnified, producing exaggerated damage to the surrounding normal tissues. In the case of the heart and nervous system, this could have devastating consequences leading to heart failure or neurological deterioration.

To help prevent this, it would be wise to increase antioxidant and anti-inflammatory vitamin, mineral, and flavonoid intake significantly before beginning the antibiotic/antiprotozoal course.[540] This is especially true if you will also be taking immune stimulants in conjunction with those medications. Doing so will greatly improve your chances of a good recovery free of severe complications.

I recommend beginning the following supplements at least several days to several weeks before starting the medications.

Alpha-lipoic acid 200 mg
Take one twice a day with meals.

Vitamin E succinate 400 IU
Take one twice a day.

Vitamin C (as ascorbate) 1,000 mg
Take three times daily on an empty stomach. Do not eat for one hour afterward to prevent iron absorption.

N-acetyl L-cysteine (NAC) 750 mg
Take one twice a day. This will increase cellular glutathione, which reduces cellular damage.

Quercetin 500 mg
Take two capsules twice a day with food.

Curcumin 500 mg
Take one three times a day with food.

Multivitamin/mineral (without iron or copper)
Start one of the following immune stimulants two days after the Herxheimer reaction subsides.

CoQ10 150 mg (oil based)
Take one three times a day with meals. This will increase your energy level, improve immune function, strengthen the heart muscle, and protect the brain.

Beta-1,3/1,6 D-glucan (Macroforce™) 7.5 mg
Take two capsules three times a day on an empty stomach and do not eat for one hour afterwards. After two weeks stop the supplement.

Other immune stimulants are also useful. Of particular interest is Lactoferrin, which also chelates iron. I would avoid IP-6 because of the danger of excessive iron removal. Chronic infections naturally cause a severe loss of iron and this can increase fatigue, free radical generation, and risk of heart failure.

It is also vital to take probiotic organisms during antibiotic treatment and for at least one month afterward. This should include prebiotic (bacteria food) such as FOS.

The high-dose antioxidants and anti-inflammatory supplements should be continued throughout the treatment period. Afterwards, switch to your regular maintenance supplements that I discussed earlier.

One of the greatest dangers during prolonged antibiotic treatment is a secondary yeast infection and overgrowth in the colon, which could lead to a rapid infiltration of yeast organisms throughout the body causing your symptoms to return. In addition, the yeast will depress immunity and can trigger the same excitotoxic reactions as the rickettsial organisms. Stool test for dysbiosis should be done following completion of antibiotic treatment.

What About All Those Stories Concerning Dangerous Supplements?

Virtually every day another headline appears exposing the dangers of nutritional supplements. Vitamin C causes cancer! Vitamin C causes heart attacks! Herbs destroy the liver! Vitamin E causes hemorrhages! Ginkgo biloba can result in hemorrhaging! What is going on? Are supplements really that dangerous?

Make no mistake: behind all of these scare stories is money, the love of which is the root of all evil. The alternative medicine sector of health care has grown into a multi-billion dollar business and people are abandoning traditional medical care for these alternatives. They are sick and tired of the way they are being treated by their doctors, and tired of taking bags full of pills that often make them sicker than the condition for which they are taking them. Pharmaceutical companies, feeling the pinch in their pocketbooks, are fighting back any way they can. What they have chosen to do is attempt to discredit natural health treatments and portray them as both dangerous and ineffective.

Wait, you say, it isn't pharmaceutical companies from whom we're hearing scare stories. It's *universities and doctors* who are pointing out the dangers of alternative medicine. True. So let's follow the money.

Major funding of medical schools often comes from pharmaceutical company grants and gifts. One pharmaceutical giant recently donated $20 million to one of our most prestigious medical centers. It would be disingenuous to pretend that amount of money doesn't carry serious influence.

Pharmaceutical companies also fund many of the research projects conducted in our major medical centers. Doctors in private practice receive mountains of free samples, and often are sent on luxurious vacations in exotic places. Many carry out drug trials for the pharmaceutical giants, for which they receive compensation.

When I was in medical school, pharmaceutical reps would take us to lunch at some of the best restaurants, give us leather medical bags, expensive medical textbooks, stethoscopes, and other "toys" to buy our loyalty. They were always friendly, and over time, we did become close friends with them. In private practice, we joked that a drug rep couldn't see us unless he brought some toys.

The 1960s and 1970s saw an attack on such practices, and soon the federal government stepped in and outlawed much of this activity. A significant number of doctors refused to see drug reps, leaving pharmaceutical companies with few avenues to the prime source of their sales. After all, only doctors could prescribe medications.

At first, pharmaceutical companies stepped up advertising, some of which ran for four pages, in the medical journals and weekly magazines sent to doctors' offices. Soon, such ads constituted the medical journals' major source of funding, and while they continue to deny it, publishers are influenced by the pharmaceutical industry in choosing which articles to print. Articles concerning alternative treatments, such as the use of nutritional supplements, are few in number in clinically oriented journals, and usually are routinely rejected in favor of articles extolling the virtues of a prescription drug or surgical procedures.

Editors of these journals dispute such contentions, puff up their chests, and portray themselves as standard bearers of virtue and truth. This is pure hubris: they favor their friends, and the pharmaceutical companies who pay their bills. You must realize that most editorial staff members of these scientific journals, as well as editors-in-chief, also receive research funding from pharmaceutical companies, and even hold stock in the companies from which they take money! Their prejudice is towards paradigms that support their funded research. Competing ideas, especially those that endanger their funding, are quickly rejected and buried in some lesser-known journal or never published.

Ulcers: A Case Study In Money Medicine

Take the case of Dr. B. J. Marshall, an Australian physician who, in 1984, noticed that his patients with gastric ulcer disease often had a particular bacterial organism growing in their stomachs. This organism, *Helicobacter pylori*, had been cultured in the past but was considered to be an opportunistic invader and not the cause of the disease.

At the time, pharmaceutical companies were selling billions of dollars of medications to control stomach acid. In fact, an early one called Tagamet saved its maker from major financial difficulty. Soon, other companies were manufacturing similar drugs and spending huge amounts of money to capture the loyalty of doctors, including gastroenterologists, treating ulcers.

Meanwhile, Dr. Marshall continued to amass evidence that ulcer disease was an infectious disorder, not due to excess acid secretion. He attempted to have his work published in several gastroenterology journals, all to no avail. It just wasn't "interesting" enough, or there wasn't enough "evidence," was the refrain. All the time, the stock for the manufacturers of acid-inhibiting drugs continued to rise. Marshall even tried to address gastroenterologists at their annual meeting. No way, he was told. Finally, he was able to meet with one of the higher-ups in the world of gastroenterology and present his case. Much to his credit, this man did listen and realized that Dr. Marshall was onto something very important.

Now, the high priests of medicine will deny that their ties to the pharmaceutical companies had anything to do with these events, but common sense says otherwise. Money is a very powerful influence, even subconsciously.

Had it not been for the valiant efforts of two people working against an entire industry, people would still be spending millions of dollars every year on ulcer medication that is virtually useless and without a treatment that addresses the *cause* of the condition. The truth, unfortunately, has not been so lucky in many other cases of modern medical cover-ups, as the examples of Drs. Phyllis Mullenix and John Yiamouyiannis vividly attest.

It is interesting to note that treatment today for the *H. pylori* infection is still based on pharmaceutical drugs: Biaxin and the acid-lowering Prilosec. It seems that *H. pylori* is easier to kill when stomach acid is low. However, acid-controlling medications now are only given during the course of treatment for the microorganism. Still ignored is the fact that the *H. pylori* organism is also very sensitive to garlic extract and vitamin C, both of which can be taken for extended periods of time with much greater safety.

Treating the infection with Biaxin, or any other antibiotic, also increases the likelihood of yeast overgrowth in the colon and dysbiosis. Evidence-based doctors are not routinely giving their patients probiotics when they give antibiotics, despite abundant scientific evidence that they should.

How It Works Today

Getting back to our story, the pharmaceutical companies soon realized they didn't need to influence the doctors; they could go directly to the patients. Proof? We are now inundated with TV, radio, and magazine ads extolling the virtues of any number of prescription drugs, the big moneymakers. In one ad, a beautiful woman walks though a field of lilies, silk scarf flowing in the breeze, as a soothing voice tells us how Nasal Blow can free you from all your allergies and give you a full life. As the commercial ends, a subdued voice, speaking a mile-a-minute, informs you that users may experience seizures, heart palpitations, explosive diarrhea, bone-marrow failure, and transient psychotic episodes of suicidal tendencies while taking the medicine.

Despite the commercial success of these campaigns, manufacturers must still contend with the problem of massive customer dissatisfaction with their products and the side effects. As more and more people gravitate to natural remedies, the panic among the pharmaceutical executives is reaching a crescendo. You are now witnessing the results of their latest brain storm: discredit natural remedies and scare the public to death.

Unfortunately, it's working. People think beta-carotene will give them lung cancer and that vitamin C causes cancer, kidney stones, and even heart attacks and strokes. Now we're being told that St. John's Wort is ineffective and Ginkgo biloba induces brain hemorrhages.

The vast majority of stories emanating from the media arise from single case reports, letters-to-the-editor, and poorly conducted research that would never be accepted by the guardians of knowledge occupying the seats of power in our medical universities, and who control the scientific journals. When those working in the area of nutraceuticals attempt to have a paper published in a traditional medical journal, they meet stiff resistance. Yet, those same journals will accept virtually anything from anyone as long as it criticizes non-traditional medicine.

One modern ploy of the medical hierarchy is to release an article summary before the issue in which it is slated to appear is distributed to subscribing doctors. This assures that the media will dutifully inform the general public of the latest danger from non-traditional medicine without giving anyone a chance to critically examine and respond to the article. By the time doctors do read, analyze, and respond to the whole article, it is considered old news by the media—who are already on to next month's big medical news.

Upon its release by the media, the public is told that the story comes from one of the most prestigious medical journals in the known universe, so who could possibly criticize it? This is what we are up against. But, you should understand that to the pharmaceutical companies and the evidence-based medical hierarchy this is a "take-no-prisoners" war.

Are Vitamins Dangerous?

Some clinicians have objected to the use of vitamin supplements on the basis of real or imagined dangers transposed from completely different vitamins than the ones being advocated. For example, we frequently hear that vitamins in general can be dangerous.

When asked for scientific documentation, you'll usually receive stories of toxicity related to megadoses of vitamin A (especially in children), vitamin D excess (which is difficult to document except in serious extremes), liver failure with time-release niacin, or reports on the neurotoxicity of large doses of vitamin B_6. While these toxicities do exist, they are quite rare and never occur when nutritional supplementation is designed by competent physicians versed in their appropriate use. Rather than a call to avoid the use of supplements, it should be a call for physicians to be trained in the proper and scientific use of supplements.

Vitamin A Toxicity

Most acute cases of vitamin A toxicity have occurred in infants given massive doses of the vitamin, usually from 50,000-4,000,000 IU over a short period of time.[541] Most adult cases involved doses greater than 100,000 IU a day over prolonged periods of time. Risk below this level is most often seen with associated medical disorders, such as low body weight, protein malnutrition, alcohol consumption, and ascorbic acid deficiency. Between 1976 and 1987, fewer than ten cases per year were reported in the United States. Obviously, vitamin A toxicity is not a big problem in this country. Doses between 5,000-10,000 IU are, without question, safe.

Beta-Carotene Toxicity

Extensive reviews of the safety of beta-carotene have shown no evidence of toxicity at any concentration, even in pregnant women and small children. In doses of 30-150 mg per day for over fifteen years, no adverse effects have been seen.[542] It should be noted that synthetic beta-carotene acts differently than the natural form. Fruits and vegetables contain principally what is called the all-trans form and only small quantities of the less functional forms (isomers 9-cis and 13-cis). Rats fed synthetic beta-carotene are seen to have a drastic reduction in liver carotenoid stores,[543] a condition that has not been observed with natural beta-carotene. Upon absorption, beta-carotene is metabolized into numerous other types of carotenoid compounds, none of which appear to be toxic to normal cells, but which are *significantly* toxic to tumor cells.

Concern has been raised recently by the ATBC and CARET clinical trials involving beta-carotene supplementation and a link to increased cancer rates of the lungs and prostate in those exposed to asbestos or engaged in heavy smoking and/or heavy alcohol consumption. It should be noted that those who only smoked occasionally did not show an increased cancer rate with supplement use. In the Physicians' Health Study, no increase in cancer was seen with prolonged supplementation.

These studies have been criticized on several grounds. For example, early malignant lesions could have existed in the study subjects at the time of the study, thereby negatively affecting the results. Also, the subjects, because of their poor health practices, were more likely to suffer from multiple nutritional deficiencies having had poor immune status to begin with.

It is well known that antioxidants work together. Single antioxidant supplementation in subjects deficient in other antioxidant vitamins would increase the likelihood of the production of oxidized forms of beta-carotene—that is, the beta-carotene itself becomes a free radical. The lungs, a high-oxygen atmosphere, would increase the likelihood of pro-oxidant conversion as well.

Another explanation for the possible procarcinogenic effect seen in these studies is that using a synthetic form of beta-carotene may reduce the tissue concentration of more important antioxidant and anticarcinogenic carotenoids, such as canthaxanthin and lutein. In the ATBC trial, supplementation with synthetic beta-carotene lowered lutein levels. Animal studies have shown that mixed carotenoids, such as *Spirulina* and *Dunaliella* species of algae, have significantly greater tumor-killing ability than beta-carotene alone. No antioxidant vitamin or flavonoid should be taken alone.

Vitamin E Safety

Today we hear a lot about "evidence-based medicine," by which is really implied "scientifically" based medicine. But just how scientific is the purported danger of vitamin E quoted by medical authorities? A review of the claims of complications is to be found in letters-to-the-editor, individual reports (anecdotal cases), and uncontrolled studies.

After an extensive review of available animal research and human data, Bendich and Machlin concluded that even in doses as high as 3,200 mg a day, few adverse effects were seen.[544] Most of the adverse reports claimed in individual case reports have not been seen in larger controlled studies, the kind purists always demand. Still, many will quote anecdotal cases when it suits their argument.

All reports of vasopathic hepatotoxicity, a condition that causes liver destruction following vitamin E intake, have occurred only in premature infants receiving intravenous alpha tocopherol acetate.[545] It was even suggested that a polysorbate carrier was the true culprit, and not vitamin E. No cases have been reported following oral vitamin E usage, and never in adults.

Necrotizing enterocolitis and sepsis have also been reported, but again only in very low birth weight, premature babies given high doses of vitamin E. Neither sepsis nor necrotizing enterocolitis have been reported in mature neonates, children, or adults taking vitamin E supplementation. At doses of 1,000 mg or less a day, vitamin E enhances immune function, especially in the elderly and in those with nutritionally related immune suppression.[546]

Thrombophlebitis has been reported in an uncontrolled series but larger, controlled studies have not reported such a complication. While reduced thromboxane production by vitamin E has been proposed, carefully conducted studies have found no affect of megadose vitamin E on bleeding-time, prostacyclin production, platelet aggregation or other coagulation parameters in human test subjects.[547] A more recent study found that vitamin E can inhibit platelet adhesion, a major factor in the clotting mechanism, but only to a modest degree, and no more than taking a single aspirin would.[548]

In the ATBC study of Finnish men, smokers supplemented with 50 mg of vitamin E experienced a 50 percent increase of hemorrhagic strokes as compared to the control group. It is known that smokers have very low ascorbate levels, something that would have increased their likelihood of cerebral hemorrhage because of blood vessel weakness in the brain. Such vessel damage has been repeatedly shown in smokers.

While most controlled studies have found no significant effects of high vitamin E intake on blood coagulation and bleeding times, it can produce problems in vitamin-K-deficient individuals, a condition common in advanced-cancer patients. This problem can be prevented easily simply by supplementing with vitamin K. In patients taking anticoagulants, such as warfarin, there is no evidence that vitamin E has a deleterious effect on clotting factors or bruising, which was determined in an extensive review of cardiac patients on warfarin who received either 100 mg or 400 mg a day of vitamin E.[549]

Ascorbic Acid/Ascorbate Safety

One frequently cited complication associated with large-dose vitamin C supplementation is an increased risk of oxalate renal stones. There is not a *single* proven case of oxalate stone ever reported due to ascorbate consumption. This fear is based on the idea that oxalate is a major metabolite of ascorbic acid metabolism.[550] Hyperoxaluria does not occur with high intakes of vitamin C because the metabolic conversion to oxalate is saturated before such levels are reached. Ingestion of doses as high as four grams acutely, or long term at three grams a day, does not increase oxalate production.[551] The confusion concerning vitamin C and oxalate stones has arisen due to the fact that, in tests, ascorbic acid in urine exposed to air is rapidly oxidized to oxalate—which does *not* happen in the body.[552]

Vitamin C is associated with one major potential complication: the promotion of iron absorption and concomitant triggering of hydroxyl radical production. Excess iron has been associated with increased cancer induction, accelerated tumor growth, and metastasis. Of particular concern is the patient with hemochromatosis, since excess vitamin C can precipitate fatal reactions. Such patients should be tested for ferritin, iron content, and transferritin saturation before supplementation. There is no evidence that in normal people ascorbate promotes excess iron absorption to pathological levels.[553] Despite this, I recommend that ascorbate should be taken only between meals and always should be combined with flavonoids to inhibit possible excess iron absorption.

In addition, magnesium and calcium ascorbate are preferable to ascorbic acid because of the potential of increasing the acid load of the plasma.

Vitamin B₆ (Pyridoxine) Toxicity

Over a decade ago, reports began to surface concerning a neuritis following the use of vitamin B_6 in very large doses. The dose used in the report was massive: 2,000 mg! Most of the affected people recovered once they stopped taking the vitamin, but a few did experience persistent neurological deficits. Doses below 500 mg a day rarely cause nerve problems and, except in very special instances, there are very few indications for such a huge dose. For example, doses up to 500 mg a day, when given to autistic children, improve about 50 percent of the children without significant side effects. Doses this high are used to stop seizures in a rare childhood disorder called pyridoxine sensitive seizures. In fact, it is the only thing that will stop the seizures and prevent deterioration to the point of dementia. Higher doses are also used to lower elevated homocysteine levels. Considering that a standard dose is 25-50 mg a day, the possibility of side effects is practically non-existent.

Vitamin B$_{12}$ and Folate

There is no known toxicity associated with even very large doses of vitamin B$_{12}$. Folate or folic acid is composed particularly of glutamic acid, which has raised the question of safety in terms of brain excitotoxicity. Dr. John Olney has shown that very high doses of folic acid can be brain-toxic through an excitotoxic mechanism. This may be due to the release of glutamate from the molecule. Doses should be limited to no more than 1,500 ug per day.

Niacin, B$_3$

Niacin occurs in several forms, including niacinamide (nicotinamide). Taking very large doses (2-4 grams) of the form niacin (or nicotinic acid) can cause flushing and intensive itching. This form is used mainly for its effects on fat mobilization and lipid-lowering effects.

Over a decade ago, a time-release form was created to overcome this flushing effect. Unfortunately, it also resulted in several cases of massive liver failure resulting in liver transplant. More than anything, this should serve as a potent reminder that altering natural compounds may result in dangerous—even fatal—pharmaceutical side effects.

Nicotinamide is not toxic and has never been shown to produce liver toxicity, even in very large doses. Unfortunately, it has no affect on cholesterol or other plasma lipids. A new form called inositol hexaniacinate also prevents the flushing, and lowers cholesterol without observed liver toxicity. This is not to say that liver toxicity cannot occur, but it is extremely rare.

Herbs

Each of the thousands of herbs of which we know contains numerous phytochemicals—including flavonoids, sterols, and special chemicals peculiar to each plant. It is important to remember that many of these complex compounds have not been adequately studied, and some can be quite toxic, possibly even resulting in death. Herbs should only be used with caution and in most cases for limited periods of time.

One of the first herbs to make the news for its toxicity was chaparral, which causes severe liver damage. Several people who took the herb ended up needing liver transplants. Another plant extract that has gotten a bad name is the weight-loss product, ephedria. Virtually all reports of severe reactions have been related to obvious abuse. Further, problems always will accompany any weight-loss product, especially when used by teenage girls, who often take doses far exceeding those recommended when they become desperate to lose weight. Many herbs with hypoglycemic properties also can cause problems. Many are brain stimulants and can, under certain circumstances cause mania, panic attacks, insomnia, and even seizures.

On the other hand, many herbs have safely been used for thousands of years by millions of people, and some have been studied in the laboratory for their medicinal properties. Ginkgo biloba is a wonderful example: it contains numerous powerful antioxidants, as well as special compounds that increase blood flow through numerous arteries, including those in the brain. It also improves glucose uptake by brain cells and has shown impressive results in Alzheimer's disease patients.

Reports of hemorrhages associated with Ginkgo should be taken with a healthy portion of salt. Most are single anecdotal reports that in no way make a scientific link to Ginkgo biloba. Hemorrhages that have been reported occurred in elderly patients due to atrophied brains with thinned and fragile blood vessels. Certain blood vessels pass through the skull and enter the surface of the brain, virtually suspended in space: it doesn't take much to rupture one of these vessels in a damaged brain.

I find it strange that, despite the much larger number of reports of brain hemorrhages in elderly people who take aspirin every day, evidence-based doctors do not hesitate to put their patients on such a ridiculous treatment. No matter how many come in with brain hemorrhages, the connection is simply ignored. Ginkgo biloba does not reduce platelet adhesiveness any more than one aspirin a day.

I would much rather have my elderly patients take Ginkgo biloba every day than aspirin. Unlike aspirin, Ginkgo biloba will not erode holes in the stomach or result in GI bleeding. Also, it improves memory in the elderly, protects the brain against the effects of aging, and may play a major role in preventing degenerative brain disorders.

14
Preparing for a Trip to the Hospital

A Ton of X-rays, A Lifetime of Damage

When I was a neurosurgery resident, we used to laugh about getting a hernia from lifting some patient's x-ray folders. They were four inches thick and weighed a ton. Perusing these folders would usually disclose: a complete GI x-ray with a gallbladder series, upper and lower GI with barium swallow and barium enema, a scout film of the abdomen, numerous chest x-rays, pelvic films, arteriograms, cystograms, and every other type of gram but a Billy Graham.

During my tenure as a medical student, the big rage was a yearly chest x-ray for early detection of lung disease, especially cancer. I, for one, never liked the idea of being radiated, but medical students at the time were required to have yearly chest x-rays. I invented some clever ways to avoid it, but as far as I know, all my classmates dutifully allowed their bodies to be radiated annually for some absurd policy. I also avoided all dental x-rays. I just didn't trust the medical profession.

This is what surprises me about my colleagues: they all remember the way medicine was practiced in a medical center. Fortunately for most professors, the public is unaware of what really goes on in the medical industry and how incompetent some medical professors really are—which is not to indict everyone in the profession. There are indeed some excellent professors in our medical centers, but there are also a frighteningly large number of turkeys. Yet, my colleagues still wait for the next shining beacon to come from medical meccas, telling us what faddish new treatment we should all follow next and what we should believe. I find that frightening.

We've known for decades that when x-rays pass through cells, they damage numerous cell components, including cell membranes, enzymes and most importantly, DNA—both in the nucleus and in the mitochondria. While the vast majority of injury is repaired, some persists and with each exposure, the new damage compounds pre-existing damage. Added to this is normal damage that results from free radicals constantly generated during metabolism and by other toxic exposures.

In our youth, we are able to tolerate and repair most of this damage. But, as we age, our repair mechanisms are faulty. Unfortunately, we receive most of our diagnostic x-ray exposure when we are the least likely to tolerate it, in our advanced years. In addition, people are quite frequently x-rayed when they are at their weakest and have the lowest levels of antioxidants: when they are sick.

An Average Hospital Experience

Take, for example, a person who has had chronic diarrhea and abdominal pains, and has been unable to eat a full meal for over a month. He is weak, disoriented from hunger, and has lost twenty pounds during his illness. Evidence-based doctors rush him to the hospital, start an IV consisting of dextrose and water, and start x-raying everything in sight. Despite the fact that the patient has had little or nothing to eat, except for some MSG-laden soup, for the past month, the evidence-based doctors make no attempt to supply even basic nutrition.

After a full set of x-rays, CT scans, and blood work, our hapless patient is taken to a room and plopped in a bed. For the rest of his stay—no matter how long it may be—he will not receive any vitamins, minerals or trace elements, and only the worst forms of proteins, fats and calories imaginable. He'll be reduced to subsisting on mostly water and sugar.

It never seems to occur to our evidence-based doctor that when someone is suffering from a severe vitamin B deficiency, especially thiamine, giving copious quantities of carbohydrates can precipitate an explosive onset of Wernicke's syndrome, which destroys vital brain pathways in the brain stem and hypothalamus. A magnesium deficiency, which this patient certainly will have, will magnify the destruction. Of course, our evidence-based doctor doesn't know this because it's nutrition, and he was asleep in class when they briefly mentioned these facts, or else he was out to lunch with the drug detail rep.

Because of severe nutritional depletion, the patient's glutathione levels also are very low, significantly increasing the likelihood of free-radical damage. Since he also has very few diet-supplied antioxidants and low levels of intrinsic antioxidant enzymes for protection, when combined with even normal generation of numerous free radicals and lipid peroxidation products, this can produce a considerable amount of cellular and organ damage. Because these processes are all biochemical, our evidence-based doctor is lost—since there are no drugs to prescribe as antioxidants.

Finally, the good doctor decides that it's time for some nutrients, but his only source is prepackaged canned liquid feedings. It's probably not too far off the mark to assume that most doctors who order this stuff have never read the label; they just trust that the folks at the pharmaceutical company put all the right stuff in it. Besides, it's just nutrition—not the sacred cow of real science.

In case you're interested, a quick check of the ingredient list for most liquid feedings reveals a bevy of pro-inflammatory oils that are known to suppress immunity and promote lipid peroxidation, as well as hydrolyzed proteins very high in glutamate and aspartate. To top off our delectable concoction, a bunch of sugar is thrown into the mix, which increases free-radical damage and worsens neurological damage.

Okay, this is a worst case scenario. What about someone who sees her doctor as an outpatient and is sent for a few tests. Let say that these tests include a chest x-ray series and a mammogram. The mammogram is done every six months because of fibrocystic disease.

Our patient is thirty years old, an otherwise healthy woman, eating the usual American diet of processed foods, few vegetables, and plenty of high-sugar goodies. She runs ten miles a week, and to top it all off, she works long hours at a very stressful job.

This combination of a poor diet, running, and stress greatly increases free-radical generation and depletes her body's store of antioxidant nutrients. As a result, long before she even arrives for her x-ray series, she has accumulated a significant amount of free-radical and lipid-peroxidation damage. In her condition, the cumulative x-ray exposure will be much more damaging. Because she is still relatively young, her body should be able to repair much of the damage. But because she has an inborn defect in certain DNA-repair enzymes in her breast, she will not be able to repair a fair amount of the damage in that area.

Her risk of radiation-induced cancer rises with each exposure to the x-rays. The risk has been calculated to be 3 percent per year for the normal person; however, her risk is much higher, especially since she is being x-rayed every six months. Because of accumulative injury to her DNA, eventually a particular sequence of gene damage will occur, activating oncogenes for breast cancer. The very test that was supposed to provide early detection of breast cancer actually *induced* the cancer.

If we add to this story the fact that her evidence-based doctor put her on iron supplements many years ago, her risk would be even higher—much higher. Sadly, due to the combination of poor nutrition and high iron, her prognosis is much worse than if she had practiced good nutrition and avoided iron supplements. It is important to point out that recent studies have shown that women who consume seven to ten servings of cruciferous vegetables a day and still get breast cancer are able to convert their cancers to a form that is less likely to metastasize.

Does this mean that everyone should avoid all x-rays? Not necessarily, but it is essential to understand that x-rays are harmful, and it is important to avoid any that are not absolutely necessary. If you know in advance that you will have x-rays taken, you should take supplements beforehand that are known to reduce cellular damage. I recommend:

Vitamin C (buffered): 500 mg three times a day on an empty stomach
Quercetin: 500 mg three times a day
Vitamin E succinate or natural form vitamin E: 400 IU twice a day
Niacinamide: 500 mg daily
Folate: 800 ug a day
Methylcobalamin: 1,000 ug a day
N-acetyl-L-cysteine: 750 mg a day
Alpha-lipoic acid: 200 mg twice a day
Selenium: 200 ug a day

Start these supplements at least three weeks before x-rays are taken.

The best protection is to take a full spectrum of vitamins and minerals daily, which could be especially important since you never know when you will have an emergency that will require you to have a number of x-rays and scans done immediately.

Cancer is not the only danger presented by excessive x-rays. It has also been shown that the DNA of Alzheimer's patients' brains are especially sensitive to x-ray-induced radiation damage. Likewise, repeated x-rays and brain scans can produce additive DNA damage, leading to an increased risk of neurodegenerative diseases. I believe our society takes x-ray radiation far too lightly. I know quite a few people who have dental x-rays routinely without so much as a thought as to the radiation damage to sensitive tissues, including the brain, from scatter radiation. This is especially a concern when combined with fluoride treatments and dental amalgam, since both are carcinogenic.

Preparing for Surgery

Most surgery is elective; that is, you have time to prepare yourself nutritionally for the inevitable trauma that accompanies any sort of invasive procedure. If you have not followed a good program of nutrition or taken supplements, then you will need a minimum of three weeks to a month to prepare.

Most important—and no matter what kind of surgery you are having—is to build up your magnesium stores. Magnesium is one of the most important protective factors for the brain and heart. It also improves blood flow through every organ and tissue, improves pulmonary and kidney functions, and prevents postoperative blood clots from forming in the legs.

You may say: if I am having a hernia repaired, why do I need to worry about my brain or heart? The answer in all cases is anesthesia. While complications due to anesthetization are much less frequent than they were forty years ago, they do still happen. If your heart stops, one major complication is brain damage secondary to a loss of oxygen to the brain. Magnesium will protect your brain significantly during such events. It will also protect your heart against irregular rhythms.

One of the most frightening complications following surgery is pulmonary embolism, usually from blood clots originating in veins in the pelvis or legs. Physicians have devised all sorts of ways to prevent this deadly complication, from small doses of heparin after surgery to special self-inflating leg wraps. Several studies have shown that magnesium alone can reduce the risk of such problems significantly. I have never had a patient develop a pulmonary embolism after surgery since I began using magnesium supplementation in my patients.

If your surgeon is a reasonable person, and will agree to add one or two grams of magnesium to your IV fluids during surgery, you will have maximum protection. You might also suggest he or she add a healthy dose of vitamins to your IV fluids as well!

Anesthesia Precautions

Several recent reports have noted that nitrous oxide gas can precipitate a severe fall in vitamin B_{12} levels, producing disorientation and acute-onset B_{12}-deficiency symptoms, including a loss of sensation in the limbs. For this reason, it is vital to take 2,000 ug of methylcobalamin supplements daily for at least a month before surgery.

Many anesthetic gases are fluorine-based. Studies have shown that the fluoride may produce significant injury to neurons: in fact, the potential for danger is even greater because you are under the stress of surgery, your immune system is suppressed, and the gas easily penetrates the brain.

The main way to counteract the toxic effects of fluorine-based anesthetic gases is to increase your calcium intake. Again, if your surgeon will agree, have him or her put 500 mg of calcium chloride in your IV solution during surgery. Fluoride interferes with calcium, leading to heart irregularity. The extra calcium will counteract this effect.

It is also important to have a high level of antioxidants in your cells and plasma during anesthesia to protect your cells from hypoxia and ischemia (low oxygen and decreased blood flow). While these problems may not be the result of the anesthesia, they can result from large blood losses during surgery.

After Your Surgery

Once back in your room, you struggle to make out those clustered shapes about you through blurred, goo-filled eyes, and attempt to speak. But, all you hear is raspy crowing. The shock of waking up from deep anesthesia is definitely something you have to experience to appreciate.

Depending on the type of surgery you have had, food will appear on your tray that day, or many moons later. In the meantime, you will be fed evidence-based sugar water. (Don't go to the hospital and ask your doctor if your IV is evidence-based sugar water. It will only confuse him or her.)

The first day will be one of maximum stress. Pain will, most likely, be intense and your entire body will be struggling to return to normal. As a result of surgery and anesthesia, your immune system will be profoundly suppressed, and will remain so for more than two weeks. Your liver will be stressed from all the medications as well as the anesthesia it has had to detoxify. If your detoxification capacity was low to begin, it will be even worse after surgery.

For major surgeries, it will take anywhere from forty-eight hours to three days for your GI tract to crank up again. The pain and surgical manipulation temporarily paralyzes the intestines. Once it wakes up, and the doctor is satisfied with the music he hears through his stethoscope, he will start you off on some liquids. Unfortunately, these liquids are often broth—another name for MSG and hydrolyzed protein.

In the liquid form, MSG is rapidly absorbed, instantly raising your blood glutamate levels. From your blood it enters your brain, making you feel confused and disoriented. Your thoughts are jumbled and you may have a sense of racing thoughts that won't stop. In addition, the MSG will disrupt your GI tract, making you nauseated and possibly producing diarrhea. Some people will even experience severe intestinal cramping. Your evidence-based doctor will assume your symptoms are just the result of surgery or anesthesia.

As if that isn't bad enough, the high glutamate will stimulate the glutamate receptors in your pancreas causing a rush of insulin, which can produce a profound hypoglycemic response that will leave you trembling, intensely hungry, and profusely sweating, and may make concentration difficult. The nurse will call your evidence-based doctor, who will then pull something out of his hat to explain it away and satisfy the nurse so she will leave him alone.

The high glutamate level also will increase your pain by stimulating pain receptors in the spinal cord. This will require more pain medication, which will further suppress your immunity. (All pain medications suppress immunity.) If you receive blood, your immunity will be suppressed profoundly. This is because transfusions stimulate the generation of the eicosanoid PGE_2. Multiple transfusions can suppress immunity to the same degree seen in AIDS cases.

Because of the stress of surgery, your body has been depleted of a significant store of B vitamins, as well as several minerals. Magnesium depletion secondary to high rates of IV infusions, long-term poor dietary intake, and stress can lead to multiple complications. One problem, confirmed in several case reports, is the precipitation of severe confusion, disorientation and even coma secondary to magnesium loss following surgery. Recovery usually occurs following magnesium-replacement therapy.

Magnesium is especially important to those who undergo neurosurgical, cardiac, or vascular operations. One big problem cardiovascular surgeons face is a dramatic magnesium-level drop following use of the cardiac pump. This greatly increases the risk of fatal cardiac arrhythmia and neurological complications. Most cardiovascular surgeons are aware of this and make attempts to correct the problem during and after surgery.

Some of my cardiovascular-surgeon friends have told me that it actually is very difficult to replace magnesium once it begins its precipitous drop. This is because the magnesium in the tissues, where most magnesium resides, is extremely low long before the patient arrives for surgery: the surgeon is then forced to play catch-up. To prevent this complication, you should start magnesium replacement long before surgery.

Unfortunately, it may take as long as six months to replace magnesium by oral supplementation. The only solution is to have magnesium given in an IV before surgery. Since serum levels of magnesium are an unreliable measure, the doctor will have to check urinary levels of magnesium. When a large spillover persists, your tissues should be saturated with the mineral.

Very few neurosurgeons are aware of the need for magnesium during surgery, even though an incredible amount of research demonstrates that magnesium is one of the most powerful and important brain protectants known. Low magnesium greatly increases excitotoxicity, free-radical generation, and the risk of seizures in neurosurgical patients. And, as we have seen, low magnesium is common in the healthy population and even more common in the unhealthy population.

Steroids and diuretics—both mainstays of neurosurgeons—cause profound magnesium depletion. I have seen patients being given several grams of steroids and large doses of powerful diuretics for prolonged periods of time, in an effort to combat brain swelling. The doctors were not even aware that their treatments were making the situations much worse.

Most neurosurgeons also fail to provide their patients with nutrient supplementation, despite the fact that their own journals carry numerous articles about free radicals, lipid peroxidation, and brain protection. There is abundant evidence that a combination of flavonoids, magnesium, selenium, zinc and the antioxidant vitamins can protect the brain significantly both during and after surgery. Yet, surgeons often fail to apply this knowledge to the care of their patients.

Wound Healing

It has been known for many years that nutrition plays a major role in proper wound healing. Animals made deficient in vitamin C and the bioflavonoids heal poorly, and the strength of the healing itself is poor. Supplementation with ascorbate increases the tensile strength of the scar, speeds healing, and inhibits infections.

While profound degrees of vitamin C deficiency are rare, subclinical deficiency is common, resulting in impaired wound healing. The stress of anesthesia and surgery increase vitamin C depletion, which can occur over a matter of hours. Proper wound healing also requires zinc, which plays a major role in collagen synthesis.

Several studies have shown that curcumin (extracted from turmeric) can increase the rate of wound healing and promote the healing of injured muscle. It also is a very powerful and versatile antioxidant. Other fruit- and vegetable-based flavonoids, such as hesperidin, rutin, and quercetin, are powerful antioxidants, chelate excess iron, and have antibacterial activity. They also stimulate the immune system.

A proper balance of high-quality proteins and calories is also important. The highest quality protein is from egg whites. If you are not allergic to egg-white protein, I suggest eating the whites of two to three eggs twice a day several weeks before your surgery and for one month afterward. Chicken, turkey, and well-cooked pork also supply quality proteins. Beef should be avoided because of the real risk of Mad Cow Disease (prion disease).

What about vegetarians? The problem with the vegan diet is that vegetables do not supply all the essential amino acids needed for healing and immune function. It is important that vegetarians and vegans eat a wide variety of fruits and vegetables to get as many of the essential amino acids as possible. Many are gulping down amino acid concoctions to replace these lost amino acids, but I discourage this practice since most are high in free glutamic acid, which can produce the same damage as MSG.

Soybeans do supply some missing amino acids in the vegan diet, but it lacks other essential amino acids and has additional problems. It contains protease blockers that can interfere with enzyme function and inhibit the thyroid. The soybean has one of the highest glutamate levels of any plant, and when solubilized or hydrolyzed, the glutamate is freed to do its damage. This is particularly true of liquid soy products, such as soymilk and free amino acid products. Some liquid soy products even have extra hydrolyzed soy protein added, which increases the glutamate content considerably.

We have known for some time that the body requires an adequate calorie supply to be able to incorporate protein into muscle and tissues. Protein intake alone results in no protein deposition at all: this is why most pharmaceutical companies and makers of liquid diets initially added a lot of sugar to their products.

The problem with sugar is that it stimulates insulin release that can produce spells of hypoglycemia or, in the diabetic, hyperglycemia. It also suppresses the immune system, promotes the growth of bacteria and yeast, and eventually increases free-radical injury. To combat these problems, manufacturers have switched to maltodextrin, which is absorbed more slowly.

If you are on an unrestricted diet while in the hospital, you should avoid sugars and eat complex carbohydrates, such as whole-grain rice and breads, and sweet potatoes. Good luck trying to find these in your hospital! I find it humorous that hospitals today, in an effort to pretend to care about nutrition, have hired dietitians to monitor the food that patients are eating. In fact, these well-meaning staff members go around scribbling little notes on patient charts about protein and caloric requirements—which is good—but then they never choose foods that are nutritious.

I am always appalled when I see a patient's food tray. It usually contains a glass of tea, tap water, beef or chicken smothered in gravy, the usual green peas and a little pile of mashed potatoes with a trough filled with brown gravy. The peas taste like wax, the potatoes like wallpaper paste, and the gravy like greasy wallpaper paste. To the side is a dessert topped with ice cream or whipped cream.

For breakfast, there's sugar-coated cereal, milk, several slices of burned, grease-soaked bacon, toast, eggs, and several packets of margarine. The bacon is full of saturated fat and replete with carcinogenic heterocyclic amines, as well as nitrates and nitrites. The toast is usually made from white bread, and the eggs have been cooked in corn oil or some other immune-suppressing oil. The margarine is full of trans fatty acids and the milk is full of antigenic proteins.

None of these meals is conducive to good health, healing, and recovery from surgery. Unfortunately, many dietitians know little or nothing about types of fats, quality proteins, food additives, fluoride, carbohydrate metabolism, or immune function. Our evidence-based doctors are not much better. All they care about is that the patient is eating. To them, food is food. After all, patients in hospitals eat exactly what doctors and dieticians eat.

I once asked a hospital dietician to exclude MSG-containing foods for my patients. She returned days later to tell me that all the food delivered to the hospital came in huge crates and ingredients were not listed. The only solution is to have your family prepare your meals and bring them to the hospital. That is the only way you will know what you are eating and that it is nutritious.

The Cancer Patient in the Hospital

Fiber

The American diet is notoriously low in fiber, a substance which plays several important roles in preventing cancer. Higher fiber intake increases stool bulk, shortens the time food and digestive products stay in the colon, and helps remove various digestive toxins. Vegetables and fruits are excellent sources of fiber. Red beet fiber in particular has been shown to lower bowel cancer risk.

In general, one should consume about 25-35 grams of fiber a day—easily accomplished if you stick with the recommended eight to ten servings of fruits and vegetables a day. (Juicing will remove the insoluble fiber.) Fruits and vegetables are better sources of fiber than bran and grain products, but they should all be included in the diet. Other high-fiber foods include: apples, bananas, oranges, prunes, raisins, raspberries, strawberries, broccoli, brussels sprouts, cabbage, carrots, parsnips, spinach, sweet potato, legumes (beans), and whole grains.

Iron and Disease

I have already noted that iron plays a vital role in the development, growth, and spread of cancer.[554] Several experiments have shown that iron also increases the development of cancer in experimental animals exposed to carcinogenic chemicals. Even slight elevations in iron intake—at levels considered to be normal—significantly increase cancer growth. In one experiment, iron-fed animals developed two to five times more tumors than animals fed a low-iron diet.

As a powerful free-radical-generating substance, excess iron can damage all components of cells, leading to cancer formation. It is also associated with risk for increased heart attacks and strokes, degenerative brain disorders, arthritis, and other degenerative diseases associated with aging. Iron absorption is increased by ascorbic acid (vitamin C), red meat, and elevated estrogen levels. Cooking in iron skillets will substantially increase the iron content of food. In the past, iron skillets were so effective at increasing iron intake that they were used to treat anemia.

Some fruits and vegetables also inhibit iron absorption and prevent iron overload.[555] The most effective are oranges, grapefruit, onions, apples, cranberries, and various berries. Tea, both green and white, is also useful. This is why it is important to eat mixed meals, that is meals containing fruits and vegetables as well as proteins, carbohydrates, and fiber.

While anemia can lower immunity, taking iron during an active infection or with a known cancer can increase the growth of both. If you are anemic due to low iron, replacement must be done slowly and should be carefully monitored by blood tests. Significantly low iron levels also can interfere with immunity.

Patients with cancer need special nutrition and, unfortunately, they rarely get it. Many of my cancer patients tell me that when they ask their oncologist what they should be eating, they are told, "Just eat anything. All that matters is that you eat." More evidence-based medicine.

The idea that even a single specialist treating cancer patients might have no idea about the impact of foods on cancer growth is appalling. Hundreds of scientific papers have been published, most in the last decade, on the affects of nutrients on cancer-cell growth. Yet, oncologists don't read them; instead, they read the articles about the latest chemotherapy agent or new combination therapy. After all, vegetable farmers are not going to take them out to lunch or invite them to exotic resorts in Hawaii.

Let's look at a typical cancer patient's visit to the hospital. Once a diagnosis is suspected, the doctor will most likely admit you for a biopsy, with the option of surgical removal if the biopsy is positive. It all depends on the type of cancer. Once again, it's sugar water in the vein. If the biopsy comes back with a diagnosis of a highly malignant cancer, the doctor may opt to proceed with surgery immediately.

A very complicated surgery may last for many hours. With prolonged anesthesia, you will be exposed to the fluorine-containing anesthetic gases in addition to the stress of the surgery, which will severely depress your immune system. If blood loss is significant during surgery, you might receive one or more units of blood. This not only exposes you to possible blood-borne diseases, such as hepatitis, HHV-6, Epstein Barr virus, cytomegalovirus, or even HIV, but the transfusions themselves will depress your immune system severely for several weeks.

Any viruses transmitted by the transfusion will be incorporated in your cells and organs and never leave. With immune suppression, the viruses will proliferate. This not only makes you feel worse, but can also depress your immune function even further. Patients are rarely told that blood transfusions may contain dozens of viruses that are never included in screening programs.

After surgery, you will have one or more IV infusions in your arm, dripping more sugar water plus antibiotics and other medication, but no nutrients. At that time, the stress of surgery and anesthesia, plus the pain, all combine to increase adrenal stress hormone release, mainly cortisol and epinephrine. These hormones will depress your immunity and increase metabolism. The trauma of surgery will greatly increase your metabolic rate, increasing free-radical generation, and putting a huge demand on your antioxidant systems. Unfortunately, it also will severely deplete your B vitamins (including B_{12}), vitamin C, and magnesium stores.

Your evidence-based doctors will not do anything to replace your lost nutrition at this critical point. They will be too busy pumping you full of more medicines. Mind you, most of these medicines are necessary in your situation; it's just that your body needs more than what it's getting and, as we have seen, detoxification depends heavily on your nutrition.

If your surgery is extensive or involves your GI tract, you will not be fed for some time. In the past, all you would receive would be sugar water intravenously, even if you could not eat for a month. Today at least, evidence-based doctors have finally learned that sick people need nourishment. It took a long time to get there, but they have finally arrived.

Depending on the type of surgery you have had, and how sick you are, you may require what is referred to as hyperalimentation. This consists of high-intensity, intravenous nutrient feeding. In an effort to get you to assimilate your proteins and amino acids, the infusion will contain 50 percent glucose, a very high concentration of sugar. As we have seen, glucose in high concentrations further depresses immunity and increases free-radical damage.

In the early days of hyperalimentation therapy, doctors eventually learned that people also needed fats in their diets, especially if the IV feeding continued over a prolonged period of time. More and more reports of patients exhibiting fatty-acid deficiency symptoms were being seen. The manufacturers of these infusions then created a fat solution called IntraLipid, composed mainly of triglycerides.

The problem with fat infusions is that they can inhibit the immune system as well, the very thing you do not want to do in the surgical patient, and especially in the cancer patient. Gradually, we have learned that the type of fats makes a lot of difference. Omega-3 fatty acids enhance tumor immunity and reduce inflammation, and omega-6 fatty acids depress immunity and promote inflammation. You need a mixture of both, because omega-6 fats are essential.

Once you are back on a regular diet, you must avoid oils containing omega-6 fats and replace them with omega-3 fats and extra virgin olive oil. This means no corn, safflower, sunflower, peanut, or canola oils. The omega-3 oils should not come from flaxseed oil; rather they should come directly from a combination of EPA and DHA oils (fish oils).

A high intake of fruits and vegetables is vitally important, especially cruciferous vegetables, such as cauliflower, broccoli, and brussels sprouts. Kale, blueberries, blackberries, raspberries, strawberries, and spinach are also all important in protecting you against free-radical damage and inhibiting the growth and spread of your cancer.

Eat at least ten servings of a variety of vegetables every day. Blenderizing would be even better since it releases phytochemicals for maximum absorption. While you're in the hospital you can have your family bring your mix to your room in a portable cooler. The fruits should be as special sugar-free blends.

While fruits contain numerous antioxidants and cancer-inhibiting compounds, they also have a lot of sugar, and cancer growth is sugar-dependent. For this reason, cancer patients should avoid fruit altogether. Furthermore, don't resume fruit consumption until your cancer is well under control.

What to Eat at Home

Once home, you can control your diet more easily. Maintain a diet of ten servings of fruits and vegetables a day, preferably blenderized, and avoid bad fats and simple sugars as much as possible. Follow the dietary guidelines outlined in the Program For Vascular Health in chapter ten.

15
A Word About Doctors

Throughout this book, I have given the medical profession a pretty hard time, especially concerning how medicine is practiced—so-called evidence-based medicine, and I contend that much of that criticism is well-deserved. Yet, doctors also deserve a lot of praise at the same time. Most doctors are extremely hard-working, dedicated, very intelligent men and women. Their level of skill in diagnosing and treating disease within the bounds of their training is exceptional.

As a neurosurgeon, I have known many surgeons, in many sub-specialties, who serve their profession with the skill of the most talented of artists. They work very long hours at a pace few others in our society could even attempt, and they do this almost every day and night of the week. They sacrifice many of their weekends, lose enormous amounts of sleep, and have little time to spend with their families.

As if they are not under enough stress, the government, litigation lawyers, and insurance companies have placed them under a burden that is close to destroying the profession. This not only includes a dramatic loss of income, but threats of stiff jail sentences for minor coding errors and other bureaucratic mistakes, no matter how innocent. Doctors are so stressed out that they are retiring early, changing professions, and turning to drugs and alcohol in alarming numbers.

As a result of all this, patients are also suffering. Because doctors' expenses have skyrocketed and operating funds dwindled, they have to see twice as many patients as they normally would. This means that each patient will be hurried through so that they can see the next one. As a result, the patient has little time to discuss anything with the doctor, and the doctor has little time to even get to know patients.

To save on expenses, doctors form huge groups, which means you may see a different doctor on each visit. The doctor you see knows nothing about you, other than the few notes scribbled by the last doctor. This crazy system was largely created because of the insurance companies and the Medicare/Medicaid system. Medicare pays about forty cents on the dollar and Medicaid about twenty cents. The paperwork necessary for these payer systems costs the doctor a large share of his income.

I have dug ditches, tarred roofs, laid concrete, worked digging holes to plant telephone poles in the scorching Louisiana summer heat, and worked as a carpenter's helper in a sweltering attic, but nothing is as stressful, physically demanding, and exhausting as performing surgery.

To get some idea of just how difficult it is, go over to your kitchen table and stand there for three hours. No, you can't just stand there. Lean over the table about thirty degrees for the entire time. After three hours, you can walk around the block, and then come back to your table lean over again for another three hours. Do this from 7:30 a.m. until 7:00 p.m.

After you finish your last standing episode, walk around the block one more time. (Walking around the block is like making rounds, which you have to do between surgeries.) To make it realistic, you would have to get in your car, drive through the traffic, park, and then walk around the block somewhere else. You see, doctors often make rounds in several hospitals. By then it is eight or nine o'clock at night. Then you can go home and eat some cold supper. Your family has already eaten and the kids are fast asleep in their beds, so you sit by yourself and eat alone.

This gives you a little time to read the paper, sift through the mail and maybe watch a little television before bedtime. After all, you will have to get up at 6:30 a.m. so you can do it all over again. Finally, you lie down in your soft bed, totally exhausted, adjust your pillow, and quickly sink into a deep sleep. Just as you enter the wonderful world of dreams you're jolted awake by the phone. After all, you are on emergency call. Groggily, you answer the phone, only to realize that you have to get out of your nice warm bed, get dressed, and drive to the emergency room.

So, get out of your bed. Sure it's 3:00 a.m., but you have an emergency to see. Continuing our exercise, go get in your car, drive around for twenty or thirty minutes, and then come back to your house and once again, stand by the kitchen table for another four hours. You can't leave to go to the bathroom, eat, or get a cup of coffee. Just stand there—leaning over, of course. Isn't it nice to see the sun coming up, shining through your window?

Feeling a little achy? Eyes rather heavy? Go ahead, stretch that aching back and quickly grab something to eat. After all, you still have a long day of surgery and seeing emergencies ahead of you. Your first surgery case is at 7:30 a.m. Sharp. Let's see, you stood up all day in surgery the day before, walked an equivalent of two miles on rounds, slept for three hours, and then performed surgery from 3:00 a.m. to 6:00 a.m. Feeling a little tired? Muscles aching? Joints screaming at you? Too bad, you have work to do. This is just a sample of the life of a surgeon. Many times, the stress, workload, and all-nighters are much worse than this.

The problem with the medical profession is not necessarily a lack of dedication or laziness or arrogance, even though, admittedly, there are doctors with some real personality problems. The problem is with the educational institutions which train doctors, and the AMA which influences them. Medical education underwent a significant change with the discovery of various pharmaceutical drugs used to treat disease. Closely connected with this is an overwhelming faith in science and technology as a means to solve all of our problems.

With the growth of pharmaceutical giants and the development of newer drugs for a variety of previously untreatable diseases, medical education began to incorporate this new knowledge into its educational curriculum. Pharmacology courses became a mainstay and biochemistry and nutrition took a back seat. Biochemistry was looked upon as nothing more than an obstacle when I was in medical school. In fact, some instructors viewed it as nothing more than a way to weed out academically weak students, almost an initiation.

I single out biochemistry because it is intimately connected with nutrition. Nutrition is a scientific discipline concerned with the ways food consumption fulfills the biochemical needs of the body. I remember that most of my fellow classmates just wanted to get through what they called "the nonsense" and move on to the clinical material. After all, they wanted to be practicing doctors, not scientists.

Once the basic sciences requirements were fulfilled, all of the material to which we had been exposed—the biochemistry, physiology, and biophysics—went out the window, forgotten to make room for the really "useful" stuff. During the clinical years of study, we were taught diagnosis and the treatment of disease. Not surprisingly, all of the treatment was directed towards pharmaceutical medicine and no attention was given to nutritional support or treatments. Everything we had learned in biochemistry was ignored—unless it was useful to explain the mode of action of a pharmaceutical drug.

The pharmaceutical giants saw this as a tremendous opportunity. Using their financial power, they could influence what was being taught to budding doctors. First, they made enormous grants to the medical schools. With federal funding cuts, their money became the life-blood of the schools as well as a source of grants to professors for basic research. Who pays the piper chooses the song.

Ever looking for a way to enhance their influence, pharmaceutical manufacturers began to entice doctors to participate in expensive paid vacations, either to visit the factory or give lectures and attend meetings in exotic places. In addition, they started paying doctors to conduct clinical tests of their products.

Recently, pharmaceutical companies have launched an even more clever plan. Whereas, in the past they depended on frequent visits to the doctors' offices by drug reps to convince doctors to use their drugs, now they've bypassed doctors altogether and advertise directly on television and the radio, urging people to *tell* their doctors they want to try the advertised drug. Obviously, the plan has worked beautifully.

The problem is that doctors, both academic and those in private practice, are exposed constantly to propaganda from the major pharmaceutical companies. Doctors' entire educations have been based on a belief in pharmaceutical agents to treat disease, with no consideration given to the role of nutrition. This is not to say that the pharmaceutical companies haven't tried to get in on the nutrition business, because they did. The problem was that their product cost infinitely more than a similar product that could be purchased from a local health food store at a fraction of the cost.

As a result, many abandoned their natural-products lines. But, a problem arose. While the pharmaceutical industries grew, so did the nutrition industry. Nutritional science has undergone a virtual explosion in the last two decades, and in the process we have discovered numerous ways to prevent and treat nutritionally diseases that in the past were considered incurable. This terrified the pharmaceutical industry.

Not only was this information appearing in numerous scientific journals and books, it was flowing to the general public through numerous sources: newsletters, popular books and especially the Internet. The truth is that the Internet has revolutionized medical care in this country. Patients with a variety of diseases are now searching the internet and finding enormous amounts of information, and have access to renowned experts and basic research that before remained obscure.

The problem that has arisen from this trend is that patients are often better informed than their doctors about their particular illness. Most doctors, either consciously or unconsciously, assume they represent the best that medical knowledge has to offer. They firmly believe that medical centers, bastions of research and scientific breakthroughs, are the repository of this knowledge and that since their source of training and continuing education arises from these elitist centers, they should be listened to, and patients should mind the business of being good, unquestioning patients.

As a result of this belief, there is often a clash of wills when knowledgeable patients intervene on the turf of the doctors. The doctor may be thinking, "Who is this person to dare challenge me? I have had the best medical training in the world." It also is embarrassing when a patient presents the doctor with information with which he or she is unfamiliar. Instead of saying, "I don't know," which would challenge their preeminence in the field, doctors will frequently mumble something about such information either being unproven, or that studies have disproved it, or there is no evidence of a benefit. In truth, they often know absolutely nothing about the topic. Again, this is a result of years of indoctrination by the medical elite, who, in turn, are under the influence of pharmaceutical companies.

You must also appreciate that doctors have very little time for outside study, especially in fields unfamiliar to them. In order to become knowledgeable in the field of nutrition, they would have to relearn a lot of biochemistry and pour through a tremendous amount of nutritional literature. In their busy lives, they simply don't have time for it. Most practice medicine based on what they learned in their residency. The only education they receive afterwards is usually sponsored by pharmaceutical companies or medical supply companies.

If you scan most clinical journals, you will see that they are filled from cover to cover with ads from pharmaceutical companies and medical supply dealers. These are very expensive ads. In addition, many of these companies give grants to the journals in which they advertise. Unfortunately, this is also true of many nutrition journals as well. Doctors tend to read the articles that deal with new drugs being developed, new surgical techniques, and advances in diagnosis. The scattered nutritional or biochemical articles are rarely read.

The number of articles about nutrition now published in these journals is growing so fast that pharmaceutical companies are getting worried. As a result, they and their medical-center cohorts have launched a drive to scare the public into abandoning nutraceutical treatments. I have discussed this issue throughout the book: most of these scare stories are bogus and should be ignored.

Now that you understand better why doctors think the way they do, you can understand better their reluctance to comply with your wishes to include nutrition in your care. The information is foreign to them, and most have no idea what the scientific and clinical literature has to say supporting their use. I just ask that you appreciate how hard doctors work and that most are extremely sincere in their desire to get you well.

There is no doubt that advances in medicine and surgery have saved millions of lives and relieved a tremendous amount of suffering. But, we can do much better if we combine nutritional treatments with conventional medicine and surgery. In many instances, nutrition can cure diseases that do not respond to conventional medical treatment.

16
The Role of Fats in Health

Most of us think of fat as something that we should get rid of, diet off, or have removed by surgery. Likewise, dieticians and the media have convinced us that we should reduce the amounts of fats we eat to 30 percent of calories ingested or below, often making little distinction as to which types of fats are harmful and which are good. With the advent of Dr. Atkins's "new" diet, all this was turned on its head and suddenly we were told we can eat all the fats we want; that it is sugar that is the real enemy. So, what are we to believe?

Well, Dr. Atkins was half right. Sugar is the biggest enemy we face in the world of nutrition and health. Yet, the answer is not to engorge ourselves on fats of every type. Over the past thirty years, scientists have learned a great deal about fat metabolism and how different fats affect our health. It turns out that fats play a major role in most of the cell's metabolism and when certain fats are eaten in excess, they can act like powerful drugs.

One of the things you have learned by reading this book is that the human body is one of the most complex systems in the entire universe. Even a single cell's complexity is so enormous that despite some of the most sophisticated instruments and gifted scientific minds in the world, the cell's function remains shrouded in mystery. Tens of thousands of reactions, special molecules, and DNA mechanisms interact in a way that baffles even the most brilliant of our cell biologists.

What we do know is that fats play a major role in our cells' functions. Most of us are familiar with saturated, monounsaturated, and polyunsaturated fats, but cells also contain very specialized fats such as ceramide, sphingomyelin, phosphotidylcholine, phsophotidylethinolamine, phosphotidylserine, phosphotidylinositol, gangliosides, cerebrosides, triglycerides, arachidonic acid, docosahexaeonic acid, ecosapentaenoic acid, and dozens more.

These fats control cell membrane function, regulate immunity, control ion channels and receptors, regulate inflammation mechanisms, regulate transcription factors, control blood pressure, regulate DNA gene expression, and are precursors of steroid hormones. In addition, they are intimately connected to and help regulate every other system in the body. In essence, our dietary fats can play a major role in how well our bodies function.

A Short Course on Lipid Chemistry

Those of you not interested in how things work may want to skip this section. I find that a growing number of people are interested in how things work the way they do. In addition, it helps us understand better why we need to follow certain dietary programs and take certain supplements.

Lipids include fats, oils, and waxes. We will be concerned with fats and oils. All lipids are insoluble in water because water is polar and lipids are non-polar. This is why oil floats on the surface of water and if you shake it up, it forms thousands of tiny lipid bubbles. Most fats and oils exist in foods as triglycerides. These are molecules made up of three (tri) chains of fat linked to a glycerol molecule (glyceride). Glycerol is a three-carbon molecule.

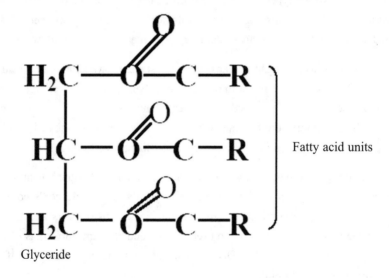

Glyceride

Figure 1: Triacylglycerol (triglyceride) composed of a glycerol side chain and three attached fatty acid units.

Fats are, in fact, fatty acids. What makes them acids is that on one end of the long chain of carbon and hydrogen atoms they have a carboxyl acid structure (COOH). Common fatty acids include palmitic, stearic, oleic, linoleic, and linolenic acids. It is these fatty acids that are chemically joined by their acidic tails to the glycerol molecule. The lengths of these fatty acids vary—some are short like the three carbon butyric acid, others are medium length such as the seven carbon caprylic acid, and still others are long chained such as docosahexaenoic acid at twenty-two carbons in length.

Bonded to each of the carbon atoms are varying numbers of hydrogen atoms. If all the carbon atoms have a full complement of hydrogen atoms the fat is called saturated. If one or more of the pairs of carbon atoms is missing a hydrogen atom, it is considered unsatu-rated. When hydrogen atoms are missing from two adjacent carbon atoms a double bond forms. This causes the fat molecule to bend, something like a boomerang. Saturated fats are straight. Fats with a single double bond are called monounsaturated fats. This is seen with oleic acid found in olive oil. Fats having more than one unsaturated bond are called polyun-saturated fats. Examples include fish oils, arachidonic acid, and linoleic acid.

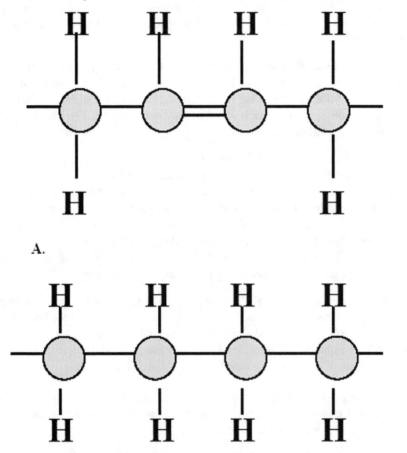

Figure 2:   A. Unsaturated fat with two double bonds between the carbon atoms.
            B. Saturated fat with no double bonds between carbons.

The shape of the fat molecule plays a major role in how these fats function in the body. The saturated fats are solid like lard and butter, whereas the unsaturated fats tend to be liquid, as we see with the vegetable oils. Within cells this can determine how well the membrane works. Saturated fats interfere with the movement of special molecules that normally travel along the membrane. We call this property fluidity. Polyunsaturated fats increase fluidity and saturated fats reduce fluidity.

Normally, fats in nature are fully hydrogenated; that is, all the carbon atoms have a full complement of hydrogen atoms. In order to make liquid fats, such as corn oil, into hard fats that can be used in margarine, food chemists add hydrogen atoms to the oil. This requires heat, pressurized hydrogen, and a metal catalyst. Because the fully saturated fats are too hard, the chemists partially hydrogenate the oil, leaving some of the double bonds, hence the name partially hydrogenated oil.

In nature, both of the hydrogen atoms attached to the carbon atoms making up the double bond are located on the same side. We call this a cis configuration. For example, oleic acid is referred to as cis-9-octadecenoic acid in the language of organic chemistry. When the hydrogen atoms are on opposite sides it is referred to as a trans fat. The cis form is bent while the trans form is straight as an arrow.

Because the trans fats have a straight configuration, they no longer fit into the cell membranes properly, making the cell function abnormally. In addition, the trans form interferes with certain enzymes, leading to things like atherosclerosis, heart attacks, strokes, and degenerative brain disorders. For decades, the USDA and their scientists denied that trans fats were harmful. It was the untiring efforts and scientific work of lipid scientist Dr. Mary G. Enig that eventually exposed the health disaster related to these fats. Millions of unsuspecting and trusting Americans were harmed and many died because of this collusion between industry and government, something previously called fascism.

Fatty acids are named in several ways. First, they are classified according to the number of carbon atoms they possess, usually from one to twenty-four. At one end of the long chain of carbon atoms is an acid group (called a carboxyl group and designated COOH). This acid group can react with a number of molecules, including cholesterol and glycerol. At the other end is a methyl group (CH_3). This is called the omega end of the molecule.

The designation for unsaturated fats is the delta symbol, Δ, which tells where the double bond is located. For example, Δ-9 means the double bond is located at the ninth carbon counting from the acidic end of the fatty acid.

Most people have heard of omega-3 fatty acids. The use of the term omega (or with the Greek symbol Ω) comes from the older chemical nomenclature. It simply means that the first double bond is to be found on the third carbon atom counting from the methyl end of the molecule, the omega end.

When scientists get bored, they like to rename everything, which can keep laymen confused. The new chemical term for omega-3 oils is N-3 oils. Corn, safflower, sunflower, peanut, and soybean oils are referred to as N-6 oils, as is alpha-linoleic acid. Olive oil contains the N-9 oil called oleic acid.

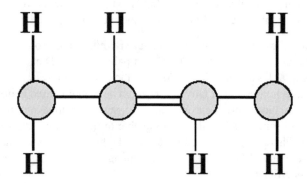

Trans-form of unsaturated fatty acid. The hydrogens are on opposite sides of the carbon.

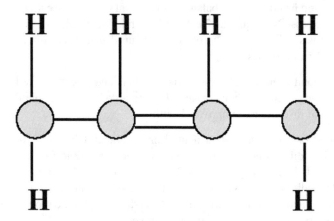

Cis-form of unsaturated fatty acid. Both hydrogens are on the same side of the carbon.

Figure 3: Forms of unsaturated fatty acid configuration

When you see a fatty acid referred to in most scientific articles, you will see something like 18:3 N-3. This means the oil is eighteen carbons long, has three double bonds, and is in the family of omega-3 oils. DHA is designated 22:6 N-3 and EPA 20:5 N-3.

Essential and Non-essential Fats

These two terms cause a lot of confusion among laymen and doctors alike. Basically, an essential oil is one that cannot be manufactured by the body and must be supplied in the diet.

Alpha-linolenic acid (18:3 N-3) is an essential oil; it must be supplied by the diet. Diets deficient in this oil will eventually result in death. Alpha-linoleic acid (18:2 N-6) is also an essential oil. It cannot be manufactured by the cells and must be supplied in the diet as well.

Non-essential oils are those that can be manufactured within cells from other molecules, such as sugars, some amino acids, and mainly from palmitic acid. Diets deficient in these oils cause no problem, at least theoretically. As with the case of non-essential amino acids, under certain conditions non-essential fatty acids cannot be manufactured in quantities sufficient for health. This includes during chronic illnesses, severe trauma, and toxic poisoning. In addition, infants and some small children are unable to manufacture these fatty acids in sufficient quantities. There is some question as to whether older people have sufficient ability to create these required fats. We know that with aging these desaturase and elongase enzymes become less efficient.

Good Fats and Bad Fats

In this chapter, I will refer to fats frequently as being either "good" or "bad." In truth, they are all required for good health. It is the balance and amount of these essential fats to which I am referring. In excess, N-6 fats can be very harmful, increasing the risk of cancer, diabetes, atherosclerosis, heart attacks, strokes, and neurodegenerative diseases, and can worsen a great number of diseases.

The good fats (N-3) tend to be in short supply in our diets and in excess are less harmful than the N-6 fats. In fact, significantly increasing the amount of N-3 fats in our diets reduces the risk of a number of diseases and improves health.

The monounsaturated fats (N-9) are either neutral or beneficial. Oleic acid, found in high concentrations in olive oil, has been shown to have powerful anticancer effects, especially against breast cancer. It inhibits a gene (HER-2/neu) known to make some breast cancers very aggressive. In addition, extra virgin olive oil contains a number of flavonoids that prevent inflammation and neutralize free radicals and lipid peroxidation. One special flavonoid, called hydroxytyrosol, is especially protective.

The typical Western diet is severely deficient in N-3 oils and heavily laden with N-6 oils. The ratio of N-6 to N-3 oils varies from 10:1 to as high as 45:1. It has been estimated that we consume fifty times more N-6 fats than are necessary for good health. Most diets in my native state of Mississippi are in the latter range. Mississippi has the record in gross obesity in the United States and, as a result, extremely high rates of heart attacks, strokes, and cancer. It has been estimated that we consume fifty times more N-6 fats than are necessary for good health.

It is important that you understand that we not only have to correct the ratio of good to bad fats, we have to change the absolute amounts we eat as well. For example, a person could have a ratio of 25:1 of N-6 to N-3 and change this to a 1:1 ratio simply by eating a lot more N-3 fats or taking supplements. Yet, he or she would still be taking in too many N-6 fats. A number of studies have shown that a high intake of N-6 fats, even in the face of high N-3 intake, interferes with the good effects of the increased N-3 oil consumption.

What is needed is to reduce drastically N-6 fat consumption while increasing N-3 consumption. Virtually all processed foods, fast foods, and hospital foods are very high in N-6 fats and devoid of N-3 fats. When I go to the grocery store, I have a habit of looking at other peoples' grocery baskets. I am amazed when I see nutritionally uneducated mothers, with their fat little children tagging along, filling their baskets with processed foods as well as cakes, ice cream, candies, and pies.

If only they were informed, they would see that every one of those products is loaded with N-6 fats—corn oil, safflower oil, sunflower oil, peanut oil, canola oil, and soybean oil (a favorite of food manufacturers). At home and at school, the children are consuming fried chicken nuggets, French fries, potato chips, cookies, pastries, and donuts as if they were going out of style. If that wasn't bad enough, most of these foods are laden with excitotoxic additives that have been shown to produce gross obesity and the relatively new Metabolic Syndrome (also known as syndrome X or insulin resistance syndrome), which is a cluster of conditions that often occur together including obesity, high blood sugar, high blood pressure, and high lipids, which can lead to cardiovascular disease. We are being told that 41 million people in the United States have the Metabolic Syndrome and most don't know it. In addition, another 13 million have type-2 diabetes. The types of oils we eat play a major role in both of these related conditions. More about this later.

What Makes the Bad Fats Bad

The N-6 fats play a major role in how cells work. They do this by being converted by special enzymes into powerful chemicals called eicosanoids. (Figure 4). The basic N-6 fatty acid is called alpha-linoleic acid (18:2 N-6). This is the fatty acid present in all the vegetable oils the American Heart Association and the government previously told you to eat in unlimited amounts. The more the better, they preached.

Several enzymes react with this fatty acid, converting it to a longer chain fatty acid called arachidonic acid. This fatty acid is stored within the membranes of all our cells. What is important to remember is that the more bad fats we eat, the more of them we have in our cells. Some small amount is essential, but when present in excess amounts, they are converted into even more powerful chemicals that produce intense inflammation and generate huge numbers of free radicals and lipid peroxidation products.

When a person eats large amounts of these bad fats, it's like being sick with a virus all the time, because in both situations the body is undergoing chronic inflammation. Viruses and bacteria make us feel sick because they trigger this very same fat to produce an inflammatory reaction to the microorganism that spreads throughout the body.

When one takes an aspirin, it is the action of the aspirin blocking the enzymes needed to convert this fat into the inflammatory chemicals during the viral attack that makes one feel

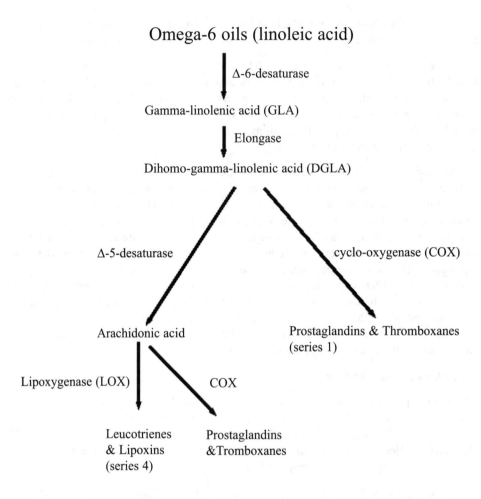

Figure 4-A: Omega-6 oils are metabolized along pathways that lead to an increase in inflammation.

better. It's not the virus that makes the body feel achy, feverish, and fatigued; rather it's the inflammatory chemicals generated by the body in response to the attack. Eating too many N-6 fats can do the very same thing; it is just not as obvious.

It is this subtle, smoldering inflammation that eventually contributes to the diseases plaguing our society, including diabetes, atherosclerosis, heart attacks, strokes, neurodegenerative diseases, autoimmune disorders, and even cancer. One study, in which a large number of cancer patients were examined, found that over 70 percent had one or more chronic diseases ten to seventeen years before they developed their cancer. The common

Omega-3 oils

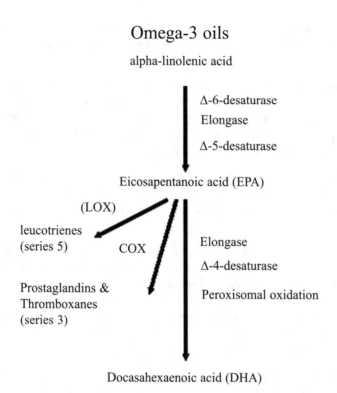

alpha-linolenic acid

Δ-6-desaturase

Elongase

Δ-5-desaturase

Eicosapentanoic acid (EPA)

(LOX)

leucotrienes
(series 5)

COX

Elongase

Δ-4-desaturase

Prostaglandins &
Thromboxanes
(series 3)

Peroxisomal oxidation

Docasahexaenoic acid (DHA)

Figure 4-B: Docosahexaenoic acid generation from alpha-linolenic acid. This mechanism is insufficient to supply adequate DHA. Many things interfere with the enzymes needed to generate DHA including age, chronic disease, alcohol, and viral infections. DHA produces powerful anti-inflammatory chemicals such as resolvin and NPD1 (10, 17s-docosatriene). EPA produces anti-inflammatory leucotrienes and prostaglandins.

link was chronic, smoldering inflammation. Most things known to increase cancer risk also cause inflammation.

Inflammation stimulates the production of enormous numbers of destructive free radicals and lipid peroxidation products, which damage cell membranes, the mitochondria, and DNA.

This also explains why cancer tends to grow faster in the face of inflammation. The common food additive carrageenan is known to trigger powerful inflammation when injected or even rubbed on the skin. It activates the same inflammatory pathways that N-6 fats activate. Even doses so dilute that they don't produce obvious inflammation will still cause cancers to grow significantly faster and spread widely. This is because, like our diets high in N-6 fats, it's not enough to make us feel really bad, but enough to activate the enzymes triggering cancer growth and spread.

A number of experiments have shown that diets high in N-6 fats stimulate cancer growth and spread. In fact, one species of lab rats never develops metastasis unless it is fed N-6 fats. Then the cancer will spread like wildfire. Adding arachidonic acid, the fat originating from alpha-linoleic acid (N-6 fat), will do the same thing. Some foods, like organ meats (spleen and liver) and egg yolks, contain very high levels of arachidonic acid.

Ironically, a baby's brain and a child's brain need a lot of arachidonic acid for normal development. As one gets older, one requires much less. All of these N-6 fats make autoimmune diseases, such as Lupus, rheumatoid arthritis, Crohn's disease, and ulcerative colitis worse—much worse.

Once the bad fats are converted into an excess of these inflammatory eicosanoids, they can interact with a number of other cell systems to cause even more problems. For example, they can stimulate harmful immune cytokines and interfere with the workings of the immune system. There are certain cytokines that make us feel bad during a viral illness. The worst of the cytokines, when in excess, are tumor necrosis factor alpha (TNF-alpha) and interleukin 1β (IL-1β°). Both of these cytokines are elevated in a number of disorders, including Lupus, rheumatoid arthritis, ulcerative colitis, and even autism.

One product generated by too much N-6 fats in the diet is called prostaglandin E2 (PGE2), which has been shown to stimulate intense inflammation and to suppress the immune system powerfully. A number of studies have shown that PGE2 stimulates the growth of cancer and promotes its spread by this very mechanism. The more N-6 fats one eats, the more harmful PGE2 is produced.

How We Got Into This Dilemma

At the turn of the twentieth century, the American diet began to change. Before this period, foods contained more N-3 oils and far fewer N-6 oils. People cooked with lard, a saturated animal fat, and cattle were fed through grazing. Both of these events changed the ratio of N-6 to N-3 fats in our diets.

When cattle graze on grasses, they are consuming some alpha-linolenic acid, an N-3 oil. This healthy oil is incorporated into their tissues, which ultimately ends up in the meats we consume. In addition, people ate more vegetables, usually freshly grown in their own gardens. With the formation of more and more corporate farms, feeding methods and growing methods changed.

Increasingly, cattle were fed grains devoid of N-3 fats and often higher in N-6 fats. Corporate farms utilized fertilizers devoid of most of the essential minerals needed by plant foods and crop rotation began to disappear. As a result, soils became more and more depleted, while at the same time they became more contaminated with herbicides and insecticides.

Many pesticides contain mercury and fluoride. With each year's application, soil contents of these contaminants increased. Crops grown in these soils were not only devoid of major nutrients, but also contained high levels of fluoride and other toxic metals.

With the growth of interstate trucking on a large scale, locally grown crops were displaced by regional crops that were then picked and shipped across country. Today, we have international shipping of crops that line our grocery shelves. To be able to have these transported crops arrive fresh, they are picked before the foods are fully mature, which translates into even lower nutrient contents.

If all this was not bad enough, dyes are added to many foods to make them appear healthier—apples and tomatoes redder, peppers more colorful, and strawberries deeper red. Newer biodegradable pesticides are now more toxic and are applied to certain vegetables with waxes that make make it impossible to wash off. Today, MSG is sprayed on crops, which makes it impossible to avoid this dangerous additive (called Auxigrow™). Ironically, MSG has been shown to stimulate hunger by lowering blood glucose, something that elates the food industry.

Fats, Government, and Industry

In the late 1880s, most meals were prepared using beef tallow, refined lard, or coconut butter. From 1880s until the early 1900s, American diets contained anywhere from 30 to 43 percent of fats.

Dr. Mary Enig, in her book *Know Your Fats*, stated that documents from General Foods Company in the 1930s recommended 40 percent fats in diets.[556] Other sources recommended even higher percentages, as high as 60 percent. It is also instructive that even then, scientists recognized that saturated fats were more stable and safer to use and that unsaturated (vegetable oils) were subject to becoming rancid (oxidizing) and were often unsafe.

In 1910, the food industry introduced the process of hydrogenation of vegetable oils to make them more solid. Unsaturated fats were liquid and were difficult to sell. The new lard-like product called Crisco entered the market in 1911, and was an immediate success. This was the cooking fat my mother used.

Corn and peanut oils entered the market place in the 1930s and margarines hit the market in the 1940s. Margarines are 90 percent vegetable oils (usually corn oil), which were hydrogenated to make them solid. By the 1950s, these "seed oils" had taken over the cooking oil market and were a big success in the rapidly expanding fast food rage.

Dr. Enig notes noted that by the late 1950s, American researcher Ancel Keys announced that the growing epidemic of coronary heart disease was due to people eating these hydrogenated vegetable fats. In an effort to head off this alarming announcement, vegetable oil manufacturers mounted a massive public relations campaign to promote the idea that it was only the saturated fat component of these new fats that was the problem, not the hydrogenated polyunsaturated vegetable oils.

As we learned earlier, in fact, these oils were not fully hydrogenated; they were only partially hydrogenated, creating high concentrations of trans fatty acids. The edible oil industry began to promote the idea that polyunsaturated oil (mainly corn oil) was healthy and saturated fats were unhealthy.

By 1965, the American Heart Association (AHA) changed its recommendations by removing any negative references to trans fats and removing the suggestion that people decrease their intake of hydrogenated oils. This new statement was then promoted by government health agencies. After all, it came from the prestigious American Heart Association, the leader in heart health recommendations.

Magazines, radio and TV ads, and other media outlets were flooded with propaganda (backed by the AHA) stating that polyunsaturated oils were much healthier than saturated fats.

The government entered the arena in a big way when its scientists, working under the auspices of the National Heart Lung and Blood Institute, endorsed the view that saturated fats were the main culprit in heart disease. Unfortunately, these studies did not take into account the high trans fatty acid contents of the diets studied.

By 1984, the government put together the National Institutes of Health Cholesterol Consensus Conference to promote the use of the new oils and discourage the use of saturated fats. The National Cholesterol Education Program arose from this meeting with the specific purpose of promoting the consumption of margarine and partially hydrogenated vegetable fats. The government scientists removed any references to the harmful effects of trans fatty acids from their printed material and brochures used for public education.

To convince the public that the major danger to their health was saturated fats, the edible oil industry (primarily the soybean oil producers) and the Center for Science in the Public Interest (CSPI) led a campaign to attack the use of saturated fats and the tropical oils, such as palm oil (which is a very healthy oil).

This campaign resulted in a dramatic increase in the use of partially hydrogenated oils containing high levels of trans fatty acids. Soon, virtually every product using oils now contained these harmful trans fats. The increase in trans fatty acids in foods is illustrated by the finding that in 1982 a sample food contained 2.4 grams of trans fatty acid. By 1992, this identical food contained 19.2 grams.

According to the Department of Agriculture, a typical serving of chicken nuggets contains 33 to 43 grams of fat, of which 35 percent to 40 percent are trans fats. That's 12 to 18 grams of health-destroying trans fats. I still see unknowing parents feeding their children this terrible junk.

The question is: how many people suffered a heart attack, stroke, cancer, neurodegenerative disease, or worsening of their particular disease because of the CSPI and federal government/industry collusion? How many people died as a result of this secretly, profit driven campaign? Those who scream for more power to the government and more regulation by the government should remember that it was only by the power of the government that these terrible changes in our foods took place. Certainly, the media played a major role, but then the media always runs to the government scientists for the final word on health recommendations. This includes the medical centers, which usually are state institutions or heavily dependent on government/industry funding, or both.

The Health Benefits of N-3 (omega-3) Fatty Acids

All cells in the body contain N-3 fatty acids. In fact, the eye's retina and brain's neuron cell membranes contain 50 percent N-3 fats and preferentially extract them from the blood over other fats. N-3 fatty acids are important to the normal functioning of all cells, including the internal workings (organelles) within the cell, such as mitochondria, golgi apparatus, endoplasmic reticulum, and the nuclear membrane. Recent studies have shown that these special fatty acids do a lot more than just make up the structure of cell membranes. They also regulate a large number of genes, interact with cell membrane proteins, control cellular messenger molecules, regulate signal transduction, control hormone receptors, regulate a number of enzymes, and are precursors of the eicosanoids.

Because they play such an important role in cell function, especially brain cells, our dietary intake of these special oils is critical to our health. Our youth are consuming a steady diet of junk foods high in harmful N-6 fats. Ironically, parents are the ones feeding their children these health-destroying diets. The schools are doing their share as well.

Now let us look at the health impact of such diets and what we can do to change things.

N-3 Oils and The Brain

In 1998, scientists observed, upon examining a variety of people living in France, New Zealand, and Japan, that there was a strong correlation between the incidence of heart attacks and major depression. How these two seemingly unrelated conditions could be linked was not to be discovered until subsequent studies were done. These studies found that both conditions were significantly lower in populations eating fish as the main staple.

Despite Japan's problems with overcrowding and high stress levels, they still had the lowest level of major depression. A number of studies have confirmed this early finding. New studies have shown that consumption of diets high in N-6 fats increased rates of major depression, and diets high in N-3 oils lowered depression rates. Trans fats played a major role as well.

Dr. Andrew Stoll, Director of the Psychopharmacology Research Laboratory in McLean Hospital in Boston, relates a case history of a researcher suffering from bipolar disorder of such severity that she was unable to work or relate to her friends.[557] Between her episodes of depression, she experienced explosive anger that was unresponsive to powerful psychotropic medications. In fact, she said the side effects of the medications were as bad as the bipolar symptoms.

In desperation, she entered one of Dr. Stoll's research protocols in which N-3 oils were being used as a primary treatment. Within two weeks, all of her symptoms disappeared. Dr. Stoll found that supplying large doses of N-3 oils could dramatically reduce or even cure patients suffering from major depression, bipolar disorder, and violent behavior.

The N-3 oils have a number of beneficial effects on the brain. One of the most researched is its effect on synaptic function, the microscopic connections between neurons. N-3 oils improve synaptic function by improving membrane fluidity, enhancing neurotransmitter control, preventing excitotoxicity, improving glutamate (NMDA) receptor function, and reducing microglial activation. It is the DHA component of omega-3 oils that has the greatest benefit.

Depression

Depression has become a major problem in Western societies, with rates increasing at younger ages than ever before, even in pre-teens. For example, people born before 1945 are 100 times less likely to suffer from major depression than those born later. The incidence of depression continues to climb, along with anxiety disorders, insomnia, violent suicides, and teen violence. What could possibly explain these horrifying statistics? A growing amount of data indicates it might be our diet.

A number of studies have been done using people with major depression or by looking at large populations to see if risks are decreased or increased with varying amounts of the oils in the diets. The majority of these studies, especially the better conducted ones, show a positive effect. That is, supplying N-3 oils, either by supplementation or by diet, reduces depression and reduces the risk of developing depression.[558]

Even animal studies found a reduction in depression in rats, using special tests to determine depression. In one such study, in which researchers compared coconut oil and fish oil enhanced diets in pregnant rats and their offspring, it was found that lifelong intakes of fish oils produced a significant reduction in depression.[559] Careful measurements of EPA and DHA by the scientists, the major components of fish oils, found high levels in the cerebral cortex and hippocampus.

As I pointed out, chronic inflammation has been linked to depression. This is because the inflammatory cytokines and chemokines (inflammatory chemicals of the immune system) activate inflammation within the brain as well, causing the release of toxic chemicals and altering neurotransmitters. Depression is a major side effect of people receiving interferon (an immune cytokine) for the treatment of chronic hepatitis, viral infections, and cancer.[560]

A number of studies have shown that depression during infections, such as the flu, is the direct result of these inflammatory chemicals in the brain.

Interestingly, N-3 fats have been shown to reduce depression caused by inflammation in an animal model.[561] This is because N-3 fats, both the EPA and DHA component, reduce inflammation.

In another study from Washington University School of Medicine Department of Psychiatry, thirty-seven patients with bipolar disorder were either given supplements containing a low dose of N-3 fats (1 to 2 grams a day) or diets devoid of additional N-3 oils.[562] All patients were experiencing persistent irritability despite ongoing psychotherapy and psychotropic drugs before the supplementation. Those taking the N-3 supplements demonstrated a significant reduction in irritability.

The authors of the study suggested using N-3 oils to reduce irritability in other psychiatric conditions such as schizophrenia and borderline personality disorder. A recent review found that five out of six double-blind, placebo controlled studies found discovered a significant benefit of using DHA in schizophrenia.

One recent study suggested a link between overactivation of an enzyme that causes inflammation called 5-LOX (lipoxygenase) enzyme, and anxiety and depression. N-6 oils are known to enhance the activity of this enzyme significantly, while N-3 oils suppress it, thus reducing inflammation and depression.[563] Most of the pharmaceutical anti-inflammatory drugs, such as aspirin, ibuprofen, and naproxen, do not suppress this enzyme.

One of the more impressive human studies was done in northern Finland, in which 2,721 males and 2,968 females were followed from birth until age 31.[564] After controlling for all relevant interfering factors, they found that women who rarely ate fish had a 260 percent increased risk of developing major depression. No reason was discovered for the lack of correlation in men.

Another large study, done in Rotterdam, in which 3,884 people over age fifty-five were examined, found that the ratio of N-6 to N-3 oils was higher in depressed patients (that is, they had an excess of bad N-6 oils), but only in those with a normal C-reactive protein (CRP).[565]

Ironically, those with elevated CRP levels (indicative of active inflammation) had a normal ratio, even in depressed patients. Of course, they are considering a 4:1 ratio as being normal, yet studies show that the optimal ratio for brain health is 1:1 and no more than 2:1. In essence, both the people with normal CRP and those with elevated CRPs had too much N-6 oils on board.

Another explanation for the lack of different ratios in those with elevated CRP is that they were most likely sicker, and we know that free radicals and lipid peroxidation products can also cause depression, especially when diets are antioxidant poor. Importantly, low levels of N-3 fatty acids in the plasma increased the risk of depression in most elderly people.

It is known that N-3 oils enhance the sensitivity of the serotonin receptor in the brain, and low serotonin is associated with depression, anxiety, violence, and suicide. When the receptor is more sensitive, even low levels of serotonin can become sufficient for brain function, that is, in reducing depression, suicide, and aggressive behavior.

Another neurotransmitter affected by N-3 oils is dopamine. Dopamine is known to enhance motivation and drive. It is a feel-good neurotransmitter. Depressed patients are frequently deficient in this neurotransmitter. Several studies have shown that N-3 oils enhance dopamine levels in the frontal lobes and limbic system (mesolimbic and nucleus accumbens), areas controlling behavior and mood. Diets low in N-3 oils lower frontal lobe dopamine levels and thereby affect behavior and even memory (via mesocortical pathways).[566]

Because the amount of N-3 fatty acid in the mother (during pregnancy) and in the breast milk (during lactation), plays such a critical role in the baby's brain level of serotonin and dopamine, it is vital that pregnant women get a sufficient amount of N-3 oils, especially the DHA component.[567] This may, in fact, prevent the depression and high suicide rate we are seeing in our youth.

One particularly frightening aspect of depression is the finding that depressed people experience a loss of neurons in their hippocampus, the memory area of the brain. This loss of brain, called atrophy, usually occurs with severe, chronic depression.[568] Follow-up studies found that even younger patients with less prolonged depression also had smaller hippocampi. Worse still, even those without brain loss frequently suffered from an impairment of memory and learning ability.

The omega-3 oils (N-3 oils) can significantly reduce this damage and prevent memory loss. This is because the membranes of brain cells are composed of 25 percent N-3 fats, mostly the DHA component. DHA has also been shown to stimulate the growth of brain cell filaments (dendrites) and synapses, essential to brain function.

Finally, one factor being totally ignored by everyone is the finding that the process of vaccination induces prolonged immune activation, not only in the body proper, but also in the brain. A number of studies have shown that such immune stimulation can induce severe depression. I have often wondered how many of the suicides in high school and college students could be linked to recent vaccinations against pneumonia, pneumococcal meningitis, or other vaccine boosters. No one has looked at this.

A new study has found that a diet high in N-3 fatty acids significantly reduces depression caused by vaccination in experimental animals.[569] With our children subsisting on a diet high in depression-causing N-6 fats and low in depression-reducing N-3 fats in the face of an expanded vaccine schedule, it is no wonder that we are seeing a rise in violence, rage, and aggressive behavior, and an increase in suicides in our youth.

Stress and Good Fats

Most would agree that we live in a stressful world, and it is getting more stressful all the time. A considerable amount of research demonstrates that chronic, unrelieved stress can cause damage to the brain. The mechanism seems to be through a combined effect of two stress hormones—glucocorticoids (steroids) and norepinephrine.

These studies have shown that both hormones can kill brain cells, especially in the memory areas of the brain (hippocampus). It appears that both hormones trigger excitotoxicity, the same process caused by MSG. A recent study found that N-3 oils, even in low doses, could suppress the release of norepinephrine.[570] This is also important in hypoglycemia, since the worst symptoms—shakiness, irritability, weakness, and aggression—are all caused by the release of norepinephrine as the blood sugar falls.

Suppression of norepinephrine may be one of the ways DHA prevents brain loss associated with depression as previously discussed. Norepinephrine in excess damages brain cells by forming neurotoxic compounds, free radicals, and lipid peroxidation products.

New Mothers Who Kill: Postpartum Depression

It has been observed that some women, soon after giving birth, suffer from such overpowering oppressive depression that it can lead to suicide or even murder. There is an old saying, "If mama ain't happy, ain't nobody happy." New research throws light on this widespread problem of deep depression following the birth of a child.

Extensive research has shown a clear connection between brain levels of the neurotransmitter serotonin and violence, depression, and suicide. As we have seen, there is also a clear connection between a low intake of N-3 oils and low brain serotonin levels. In addition, low dopamine, also seen in N-3 oil deficiency, is associated with a loss of excitement about life, making the world seem dull, uninteresting, and dark. Under such conditions, every day is filled with drudgery and soon overwhelming fatigue sets in.

Extremes of this deficiency may result in situations in which the mother may kill herself or murder her children and even her spouse.

So, what is behind such a deficiency that is peculiar to pregnant women? Careful studies have shown that the N-3 fatty acids, especially DHA, are so critical to the baby's brain formation and growth that the baby will take large amounts from the mother's blood and tissues. It does this by a special placental mechanism that selectively removes the DHA from the mother's blood as it circulates through the placenta.

When the mother's diet is devoid of N-3 oils, even greater amounts of the mother's N-3 fatty acids are removed by the baby. Studies have shown that the amounts of N-3 fatty acids available for the baby are directly proportional to the mother's intake. The same is true of her breast milk. For example, mothers living in areas where fish is a staple had about 2.78 percent of their breast milk composed of DHA, whereas mothers not eating a fish diet had only 0.82 percent as DHA. American women, on average, have between 0.05 percent and 0.59 percent DHA, an extremely low level.

Another study looked at a number of countries and found that as fish consumption increased, rates of postpartum depression decreased and vice versa. A Belgian study measured the level of N-3 fatty acids in ten women who developed postpartum depression compared to thirty-eight normal women and found significantly lower levels of N-3 fatty acids in their serum.[571] The evidence is pretty strong, but few obstetricians are telling their patients to supplement with DHA.

It has been shown that the mother loses the greatest about of N-3 fatty acids during the last trimester of her pregnancy. This is because the baby's brain is undergoing a tremendous spurt in growth and internal development, making it a very critical period.

With each succeeding pregnancy, the mother's N-3 levels continue to fall, eventually making the mother's N-3 fatty acid so low that dramatic reductions in frontal lobe dopamine and serotonin can lead to major depression and possibly violence. In addition, norepinephrine levels also fall in the frontal lobe, which can contribute to depression.[572]

To prevent this devastating disorder, I recommend that all pregnant or lactating mothers take 500 mg to 1000mg of DHA a day. This will build up their body stores and protect both them and their babies. I would recommend either take marine oils with a low EPA content (no more than 30 percent) or just pure DHA. This is because the EPA component of N-3 oils can thin the blood and you do not want to lower your blood coagulation too low, so as to prevent excessive bleeding during delivery. DHA has little effect on blood coagulation.

Because of this effect of EPA, it is a good idea for young women on birth control pills to take fish oils with a higher content of EPA (50 to 60 percent) to prevent blood clots, a major complication of this form of contraception. Birth control pills can produce blood clots in the calves, pelvis, and even the brain. The latter produces a very crippling stroke and even death. As a neurosurgeon, I have seen these birth control pill-induced strokes far too often. In addition, clots in the legs can migrate to the lungs, producing fatal pulmonary embolisms.

Protecting Your Baby

As we have seen, these N-3 fatty acids are so critical to the baby's brain development that it will take DHA from the mother's body to assure adequate levels. Having multiple births and having a number of babies over all has have been shown to reduce the DHA level in the babies significantly. It is also important to appreciate that with each pregnancy, the mother's store of N-3 fatty acids continues to fall, so that the last child gets the lowest amount of essential DHA.[573] If she has four or more children, the problem becomes of major concern. We commonly see behavioral, learning, and language problems in the last child. Unfortunately, if the mother's levels are drastically low to start with, there is not even enough for the baby to steal.

Even women who have multiple births (multigravidae) at the same time will have babies with lower DHA levels.

The good news is that enhancing her diet with N-3-containing oils or taking DHA supplements can repair the deficit in the baby's brain within as little as two weeks.[574] Unfortunately, if she delays taking the supplemental DHA too long, possible irreversible damage can occur because critical brain developmental milestones will have passed. During this period of brain development, things are moving very fast.

In addition, major stresses such as excessive vaccination, mercury, lead, and aluminum exposure, are much more damaging in a child with low N-3 fatty acid levels.[575] It has been shown that N-3 fatty acids are major protectors of the brain, both by affecting membrane function and by reducing excitotoxicity.[576]

Interestingly, a recent study found that DHA levels in the blood, and hence brains, of autistic kids were significantly lower than normal, while N-6 fatty acid levels were normal.[577]

Because N-3 fatty acids play such a vital role in brain cell membranes, especially dendrites and synapses, and regulate a number of genes, control ion channels, control neurotransmitter release and receptor sensitivity, regulate enzymes, and regulate eicosanoid synthesis, they play a major role in brain development as well as its ongoing physiology.

Experiments using rats found that if they were fed a diet low in N-3 fatty acids, they developed dry, scaly skin, lost hair and weight, and eventually died of kidney failure. Similar findings were seen in children living off intravenous feeding devoid of N-3 fats.

It is established that the brain has one of the highest contents of DHA and arachidonic acid of any tissue in the body. In fact, the brain will preferentially remove DHA from the blood over other types of fats. Neurons cannot make DHA or arachidonic acid (another essential fat used by the brain). As we have seen, this need for DHA is so tremendous the baby will take DHA from the mother's tissues. Likewise, after birth, especially during the first four months, the baby's need for high levels of DHA continues. Breast milk contains both arachidonic acid and DHA.

Until recently, commercial formulas did not contain either of these essential nutrients, despite the fact this was known decades before. In one human study, it was shown that breast fed babies had IQ levels 8.3 points higher than bottle fed-babies.[578] It is important to note that this study was done in preterm infants. Most studies have shown that the greatest effect of supplemental DHA and arachidonic acid occurs in preterm infants and not full term infants. This is because the brain is more immature and therefore growing more rapidly in preterm infants.

In the studies that followed the children to at least four years of age, it was found that those supplemented with DHA had better problem-solving abilities, alertness, and overall intelligence than bottle-fed babies. The studies that found little or no difference usually stopped at age one year, far too young to assess higher cognitive function. In addition, they compared the DHA-supplemented babies to breast-fed babies, not formula-fed babies.

A number of studies have shown better visual development in babies fed DHA, even using objective tests such as the visual evoked potential test.[579] This may be because the retina contains greater than 50 percent DHA in its cellular membrane fatty acid content. Neurons contain about 25 percent. We also know that DHA plays a major role in photoreceptor function and rhodopsin regeneration for color vision.

Because arachidonic acid is also critical to a baby's brain growth and development, a few other facts need to be reviewed. It is known that N-3 fatty acids reduce arachidonic acid levels in the brain, not something we want to do. Arachidonic acid increases the ability of a brain growth chemical (Nerve Growth factor or NGF) to enhance the sprouting of dendrites, important connecting elements in the brain. In fact, deficiencies in arachidonic acid are less reversible than DHA deficiencies. It is now known that it is the EPA that actually causes the problem, not the DHA component.

During pregnancy, mom will supply all the arachidonic acid the baby needs. After delivery, breast milk is the major source. Since arachidonic acid is derived from N-6 fats and we are consuming fifty times more of these fats than necessary for health, there is no shortage in mother's milk. But, as we have seen, a severe shortage in DHA commonly occurs. In some studies ratios of N-6 to N-3 fats were as bad as 25:1 to 45:1 in American women's breast milk.

Women should exclusively breast feed their babies, if at all possible, for a minimum of six months, optimally for one year. Breast milk supplies essential immune protection, essential fatty acids, and psychological closeness to the baby. It is known that breast-feeding reduces the risk of diabetes, hypertension, asthma, and atopic dermatitis. I also point out that flaxseed oil is not to be given to babies or small children. The enzymes necessary for conversion of the alpha-linolenic acid in flaxseed into DHA and EPA work poorly at this age, not allowing sufficient production of these essential fatty acids.

After breast-feeding, either at six months or one year, when the child begins to eat table foods, it is a good idea to feed your child an egg three times a week. Egg yolk not only contains high levels of arachidonic acid and phospholipids, but some also contain high concentrations of DHA (Christopher Eggs, Eggland's Best, etc.). Brands of these N-3 enhanced eggs are given in the appendix.

What About Brain Protection for Adults?

N-3 oils protect the adult brain for the same reasons they protect the child's brain. Most people assume that after birth the brain is fully formed and no further development takes place. Nothing could be further from the truth. The brain is always remolding itself and developing new circuits, a process we call plasticity. The more we learn and use our minds, the more active this process becomes. Optimal plasticity depends on an adequate supply of DHA in the diet.

It is known that the frontal lobes have the most DHA and that it is very sensitive to dietary deficiencies. It is the frontal lobes that allow us to direct our attention, control social urges, establish memories, and understand certain aspects of language (theory of mind).

With aging, DHA levels in the brain begin to decline, as do arachidonic acid levels. People with Alzheimer's disease have very low levels of both fatty acids, and they have an abundance of oxidative products of DHA, called neuroprostanes. This indicates that extensive lipid peroxidation is occurring in the Alzheimer's diseased brain, which again indicates chronic inflammation of the brain. This is something controlled by flavonoids, vitamin E and N-3 oils.

Likewise, a high intake of alpha-linoleic acid, an N-6 fatty acid, has been shown to increase cognitive decline in the elderly when compared to control patients, in one study.[580] Patients on higher N-3 fatty acid diets showed reduced cognitive decline.

Of particular importance is the finding that DHA plays a major role in synaptic function and synaptic protection against excitotoxicity. The greatest and earliest damage in Alzheimer's disease involves the synapse. In one study it was found that DHA in particular protected cholinergic neurons from excitotoxic damage, even when high levels of excitotoxins were used.[581] Some independent studies have shown improvement, even in those with moderate to severe Alzheimer's disease.

In addition, all of the neurodegenerative diseases are thought to be caused by chronic inflammation of the brain, or certain parts of the brain, via microglial activation (the brain's immune cell). Since the production of eicosanoids, especially the inflammatory types, are regulated by N-6 and N-3 fatty acids, they play a major role in these diseases, with opposite effects. Too much N-6 fatty acids combined with too little N-3 oils promotes brain inflammation. High intakes of N-3 oils, both EPA and DHA, reduce inflammation. DHA reduces inflammation by a different mechanism than does EPA.

It is known that as we age we become progressively more allergic to our own brains. Researchers measuring antibodies to brain proteins have demonstrated this in a number of studies. Some have proposed this to be an explanation for why our immune system begins to be less effective as we age. N-3 fatty acids are immune modulators, as they reduce the immune overactivity seen with brain autoimmunity.

You may recall that those who live on diets high in fish, such as the Inuit of Greenland, rarely develop autoimmune diseases. This is because the N-3 fats reduce immune injury to the brain and other tissues.

In addition, by thinning the blood slightly and improving endothelial cell function (cells lining the blood vessels), N-3 oils improve blood flow through the brain. Impaired blood flow is common in all types of dementia, including Alzheimer's disease.

It is also known that brain levels of the special fat arachidonic acid are lower in Alzheimer brains. Studies conflict as to whether enhancing the arachidonic acid in the diets of the elderly is harmful or helpful. If helpful, an easy way to increase brain ararchidonic acid is to eat eggs three to four times a week. By using the N-3 enhanced eggs, you can increase DHA at the same time. A small amount of GLA (gamma-linolenic acid, an N-6 fatty acid) has been shown to reduce inflammation and to increase brain arachidonic acid to normal levels as well.

A number of studies indicate that high levels of arachidonic acid worsen neurological damage during a stroke as with other cases of excitotoxic damage. This bad effect can be eliminated simply by taking 700 mg of N-acetyl-L-cysteine (NAC) a day. NAC greatly increases cellular glutathione levels. Glutathione is one of the most important cell protection molecules against free radical attack and lipid peroxidation products. By decreasing the amount of N-6 fats you ingest, you can add even more protection.

Excessive alcohol drinking also has been shown to lower brain DHA and arachidonic acid levels significantly.[582] Alcohol is a powerful glutamate receptor blocker, but once one sobers up, sensitivity to glutamate excitotoxicity increases significantly. When combined with low DHA levels, the degree of damage is greatly magnified. This may explain the brain atrophy, confusion, and memory loss seen in alcoholics.

Taken together, these studies indicate that low levels of DHA in the brain interfere with the dynamic plasticity of the brain, which allows us to learn, remember, and expand our minds. My son, Damien, made the observation that the more we learn and expand our minds intellectually, the more conscious we become. I think this is true.

In addition, with aging our brain's blood vessels become atherosclerotic, thereby reducing blood flow to the brain. The brain is so dependent on glucose and oxygen that, at about 1 to 2 percent of body weight, it consumes approximately 25 percent of both from the general circulation. N-3 fats can reduce atherosclerosis, increase blood flow to the brain and make the brain more efficient at extracting glucose from the blood.

Violence and Aggression in Our Society

The news media is filled with stories of violent teenage assaults and even incredible acts of aggression by small children; road rage, airplane rage, and every other kind of rage, plagues our society. In large part, I believe this is because of the destruction of religiosity in the

West, which undermines teaching people how to love one another and behave in a civil manner. Yet, there is growing evidence that nutritional deficiency may play a major role in extremes of violence and in violent suicide.

In one interesting study, scientists had forty-one medical students and pharmacology students take either 1.5 to 1.8 grams of DHA oil or soybean oil during a transition between low stress and high stress periods to see the affect on aggression scores.[583] The low stress was measured during summer vacation and high stress during final exams. The control students eating a typical American diet containing soybean oil increased their aggression scores significantly, but the students taking the DHA supplement showed no increased aggression.

With drugs saturating our youth culture, increased aggression associated with such drugs as cocaine has become more common. The idea that diet may make the difference between aggressive, violent cocaine users and non-violent users was recently tested.[584] What they found was that on admission and testing at the controlled testing unit, the violent cocaine users had significantly lower N-3 fatty acid levels, especially DHA, than the non-violent drug users. Unfortunately, they did not test to see if supplementation with DHA would reduce aggression in these individuals.

Because frequent drug users, especially cocaine addicts, have such poor diets, one would expect a high degree of N-3 deficiency in some. Other studies have shown that deficiencies in a multitude of vitamins, especially B vitamins, also increased violence, suicide, and aggression.

We can quickly see how a number of toxicities and nutritional deficiencies interact to increase aggression, suicide, and violence. It is known that elevated lead levels are strongly associated with violence, aggression, and suicide. It also has been shown that water lead levels are significantly higher in fluoridated communities and, likewise, crimes of violence and aggression are also higher. Accumulating evidence indicates that fluoride itself may initiate excitotoxicity and cause brain damage.[585] A person who is deficient in N-3 oils and multivitamins would be at much greater risk than one having better nutrition. This has been shown in the case of lead and violence.

Another study looked at aggression in the elderly. FBI statistics indicate that violence between elderly couples is on the increase. In this double blind, placebo controlled study, they found that aggression did not change in the placebo group but decreased significantly in the group taking the DHA (1.5 gram a day).[586] Lower doses were found to have little beneficial effect. Of interest was the finding that in villagers who had low stress there was little difference in aggression between the placebo group and the DHA supplemented group. It was only the high-stress university employees that showed the greatest benefit; that is, the people most likely to express aggression under tension.

Likewise, diets high in N-6 fats have been shown to increase aggression and violent suicides significantly. In fact, diets with low intakes of N-3 oils and high N-6 intakes have been shown to increase violent and angry behavior in boys aged six to twelve years.

The average American diet is loaded with N-6 fats, such as corn, soybean, safflower, sunflower, peanut, and canola oils. The leading source is pastries and breads. Virtually all processed breads and pastries are made with N-6 oils. Most fast foods, especially French fries, are soaked in N-6 fats. Our children are being stuffed with these harmful, aggression- and suicide-inducing fats every day of their lives, almost from birth. School lunch programs are filled to the brim with these oils. At the same time, our youth are being denied N-3 oils that reduce aggression, violence, and suicide.

When you combine overvaccination, mercury and lead exposure, fluoridation, pesticides and fungicide exposure, and a dozen other toxic encounters with poor nutrition, you create a social time bomb. Only parents can reverse this. Stop supplying your children with brain-damaging foods and give them healthy foods that have been proven to protect the brain as well as the rest of the body. You owe it to your children. To do less is to destroy the lives of your own children.

N-3 Fats and the Cardiovascular System

A growing number of studies have shown that N-3 oils significantly reduce the incidence of cardiovascular disease by a number of mechanisms. What led to the interest in N-3 oils as a protector against vascular disease, especially heart attacks and strokes, was the observation that Greenland Eskimos rarely developed cardiovascular diseases as compared to people eating Western diets.[587] When these Eskimos began to eat Western diets, they developed heart attack and stroke rates equal to most Americans, demonstrating that it wasn't genetic.

Subsequent studies of other populations with fish as a dietary staple showed the same thing. In fact, even eating fish once or twice a week significantly lowered disease rates. In one such study, it was found that men who ate as little as 1.2 ounces of fish daily, as compared to men who ate no fish, reduced their risk of coronary heart disease (heart attacks) by 38 percent and death from heart attacks by 67 percent.[588] This is especially true for sudden cardiac deaths.

The reason for the greater reduction in death from heart attacks (myocardial infarction or MI) is that N-3 fatty acids dramatically reduce the risk of arrhythmias, a leading cause of death following an MI. It does this by reducing the irritability of the heart, which increases dramatically following an MI. In one study, it was found that intravenous N-3 oils could control even some of the most difficult, drug-resistant arrhythmias.[589]

Extensive studies on the mechanisms involved in reducing arrhythmias indicate that N-3 oils work by altering sodium and calcium channels in the membranes of heart muscle fibers, which are responsible for cardiac irritability following an MI.[590] The DHA component of N-3 oils, not the EPA component, appears to play the major role in protecting the heart.[591]

Importantly, the N-3 oils have no deleterious effects on the normal heart's rhythm.[592] Likewise, GLA also has been found to reduce the risk of arrhythmias.[593]

It has also been shown that it makes a lot of difference how a fish is cooked. Researchers at the Cardiovascular Health Research Unit at the University of Washington demonstrated that cardiovascular protection occurs only by eating fish that was baked or broiled and not fried.[594] Most people, at least in the South, eat their fish fried.

Farm raised fish contain very little N-3 oils and offer little other than significant amounts of dioxin, mercury, pesticides, and fungicides. The vast majority of salmon, even if labeled wild, has have been shown to be farm raised and therefore low in these healthy oils.

One question I am frequently asked is whether flaxseed oil can replace fish oils when trying to prevent cardiovascular disease. Actually, the results are rather mixed, as would be expected. You will recall that I said babies, small children, those with chronic illnesses, and the elderly often have difficulty converting the alpha-linolenic acid into EPA and DHA. The older we get the more difficulty we have.

For those who can convert the alpha-linolenic acid, results have shown a reduction in cardio-vascular disease and arrhythmia.[595] Unless one has been specifically tested to see if he or she can convert this oil, one would not depend on flaxseed oil for protection.

The Science: How N-3 Oils Protect the Cardiovascular System

N-3 oils reduce the risk of cardiovascular disease, both directly and indirectly. They do so directly by correcting lipid profiles, improving blood flow (especially through microscopic vessels), reducing autoimmunity to oxidized lipoproteins, reducing harmful eicosanoid production and increasing beneficial eicosanoids, correcting endothelial cell function, and reducing smooth muscle proliferation.

Indirectly, they improve insulin function at the cell surface, reduce the risk of the Metabolic Syndrome, lower blood pressure, reduce chronic inflammation, and modulate the immune system. All of these things help prevent cardiovascular disease.

In chapter 9, I explained that atherosclerosis occurs because of chronic inflammation within the walls of the blood vessels, and that a variety of things could trigger this inflammation. While viruses and bacteria have been known to act as triggers, recent evidence indicates that MSG (and other excitotoxins), mercury, lead, and possibly fluoride (as fluoroaluminum) can also act as triggers. In fact, they often act either additively or synergistically.

Since food based excitotoxin taste enhancers (MSG, hydrolyzed protein, soy protein extract, etc.) are added to virtually all processed foods in enormous amounts, our blood vessels are constantly exposed to a high level of free radicals, which they produce. This has been shown experimentally. One way free radicals do their damage is by activating the inflammatory eicosanoids, such as PGE2. This eicosanoid is generated by N-6 fatty acids.

It is ironic that the self-appointed, orthodox medical elite declared vegetable oils, most of which are N-6 oils, to be the answer to cardiovascular health and a way to prevent atherosclerosis. Newer studies indicate that in fact N-6 oils may be the culprit. Even more intriguing, during the original studies on atherosclerosis it was observed that the oxidized fatty acids in the walls of blood vessels were made mainly of polyunsaturated N-6 oils—the very same as those promoted by the medical elite. This was over seventy years ago.

The question to be asked is: how many people became crippled or died over the past seventy years, a period during which this bad advice was being followed religiously by millions of people who trusted the food manufacturers and government? The numbers reach into the millions, with over 700,000 dying of heart disease each year and several million suffering from atherosclerotic diseases over the same period. This doesn't even consider the trans fatty acid debacle, which only recently has been addressed by food manufacturers and the government. Kept from the public was the fact that both groups fought viciously against scientists such as Dr. Mary Enig, who had proven the harm decades before. This seems to be an ongoing theme.

Atherosclerosis and Hypertension

Hypertension is an aggravating factor in the production of atherosclerosis. Likewise, atherosclerosis can lead to hypertension as well, since a normal blood pressure depends on elastic blood vessels.

In one study sixty-three obese, hypertensive men were placed in one of three treatment groups: 1. Weight loss alone; 2. Diet including 3.65 grams of fish N-3 oils, and; 3. Both combined. Interestingly, they found that both weight loss alone and fish oil diet alone produced significant reductions of both systolic and diastolic blood pressure, but combining fish oil with weight reduction produced even more dramatic reductions in blood pressure. For example, weight loss alone caused a drop in systolic BP of 5.5mm Hg and fish oil alone caused a fall in systolic BP of 6.0 mm Hg, whereas combining the two caused a drop of 13 mm Hg in systolic and 9.3 mm Hg diastolic pressures.

Subsequent studies have shown that the effect is due solely to the DHA component of the fish oils. In one such study, reported in the 2000 issue of the journal *Circulation*, researchers found that in a double-blind, placebo controlled study of fifty-six obese, mildly hyperlipidemic men, that those fed DHA (4 grams/day), but not EPA or control oil (olive oil), showed improved blood flow under conditions of acetylcholine, norepinephrine, and L-NMMA infusion (an NO blocker).[596] These are all tests used to aggravate hypertension.

It was concluded that DHA caused the vessel to dilate, and therefore lower blood pressure, mainly by increasing the production of prostanoids and a special protein released from the endothelial cells called hyperpolarizating factor. It may also increase nitric oxide production, a major vasodilator of blood vessels generated within the endothelial cells lining all blood vessels. In addition, DHA has been shown to reduce epinephrine release and is a more effective suppressor of thromboxane-like vasoconstrictor responses than EPA.

A more recent study demonstrated for the first time that DHA alone had little effect on vascular smooth muscle cell production of nitric oxide (NO), but in the presence of low concentrations of IL-1β, it produced a dramatic elevation in nitric oxide production, and acted through the p44/42 MAPK system.[597]

IL-1β is an immune cytokine that increases in the face of inflammation, and especially during chronic inflammation. This means that under such conditions, DHA improves blood flow, endothelial cell function, and lowers blood pressure if it is too high. In addition, N-3 oils lower triglycerides, elevate healthy HDL-cholesterol and convert the dangerous small density LDL-cholesterol into the protective large buoyant LDL type. Some cardiologists and internists become alarmed when they see an elevation of LDL-cholesterol in their patients taking N-3 oils, not knowing that it has increased their protective form of the lipid.

It is known that proliferation or overgrowth of smooth muscle cells, cells found in all arterial blood vessels, plays a major role in atherosclerosis and restenosis following coronary vessel surgery, a major cause of heart attack in people having had coronary by-pass surgery.

Research indicates that this overgrowth of smooth muscle cells is triggered by chemical factors released from aggregating platelets that are known to accumulate at the site of atherosclerosis and sites of vessel injury, such as we see with surgery. These platelets release growth factors, such as platelet-derived growth factor, epidermal growth factor and transforming growth factor-ß, as well as others such as serotonin, thromboxane A2, norepinephrine, histamine, and platelet activating factor.

Both EPA and DHA inhibit 5HT (serotonin) receptor mRNA rather powerfully. That is, these N-3 fatty acids reduce the number of receptors found on smooth muscle cells and thus prevent them from overgrowing. Since this overgrowth is the major mechanism by which atherosclerosis develops, this makes these two N-3 fatty acid components major weapons against atherosclerosis. Yet, by the response of traditional medicine, you would never know it. They still rely on dangerous drugs such as the statin cholesterol-lowering drugs.

While EPA is slightly more potent in suppressing overgrowth of the smooth muscle cells, when in combination, even in small doses, DHA plus EPA have powerful effects. This allows one to use N-3 oils with high levels of DHA and low levels of EPA.

Finally, we also know that most of the trouble in atherosclerosis begins in the thin layer of cells lining all blood vessels, called the endothelial cells. These cells act as regulators of the rest of the arterial wall. By generating nitric oxide, they regulate the dilation of arteries, both protecting them and preventing abnormal elevations in blood pressure. They also send a number of chemical messengers to the other layers of the blood vessel.

Studies have shown that an adequate supply of magnesium is especially important to the proper functioning of these endothelial cells, which explains the connection between low magnesium and high rates of heart attacks and strokes. In addition, N-3 fatty acids, especially DHA, plays a major role in the health of these cells. By inhibiting platelet-activating factors, N-3 fatty acids prevent the platelets from attaching to the surface of the arterial wall, which prevent the initiation of the atherosclerosis process from even starting.

As you can see, all of this is very complicated, much more so than I have outlined in this brief review.

Why Greenland Eskimos Rarely Get Autoimmune Diseases

A number of scientific studies have shown that Greenland Eskimos rarely, if ever get autoimmune diseases, such as Lupus, rheumatoid arthritis, and thyroiditis. Yet, if they adopt the typical Western diet, they have the same high incidence as others eating this diet. The tremendous rise in autoimmune diseases of all types has alarmed health officials, those enigmatic individuals who always seem to dwell in the dark.

The connection to N-3 fatty acid consumption fits the pattern well. When Westerners switch to a diet low in N-6 fats and higher in N-3 oils, their autoimmune diseases either improve or, on occasion, disappear altogether. Studies that showed little or no effect are ones that did not reduce the N-6 fat intake or add known powerful antioxidants to the diet, such as cruciferous vegetables.

Experimental studies using animal models genetically prone to autoimmune disease (resembling human cases) have consistently shown a tremendous benefit from a diet high in N-3 oils. We know that humans develop autoimmune diseases only if they are genetically prone to do so. Upon being exposed to certain environmental triggers, they may develop the full blown disease. These triggers can include certain viruses, pesticides, mercury, and various industrial chemicals.

Human experiments also indicate that a diet high in N-3 oils and low in N-6 oils may benefit people with a variety of autoimmune diseases. The greatest evidence is for diseases such as Lupus, autoimmune glomerulonephritis, multiple sclerosis, and rheumatoid arthritis. Some evidence also exists for psoriasis, Sjogrens syndrome, ulcerative colitis, and Crohn's disease. Benefits also have been shown for neurodegenerative diseases, diabetes, and atherosclerosis, all of which have immune components involved in their pathology.

The mechanism by which N-3 oils benefit these conditions involves their powerful anti-inflammatory effects as well as their ability to affect intercellular signaling, cytokine levels, transcription factor activity, and even gene expression.[598]

A number of studies using experimental models of human autoimmune diseases demonstrate that the animals fed increased amounts of N-3 oils have significantly longer lifespans than those fed N-6 oils (corn oil).[599] Likewise, several studies have shown that when caloric restriction is combined with N-3 oils, (eating fewer sugars and high glycemic carbohydrates), results are even better.[600]

It appears that eating too many calories worsens these diseases by increasing the generation of damaging immune complexes and immune factors and increasing free radical generation.

The dramatic improvement in combining N-3 oil supplementation with restricted calories is critical to all those having one of these terrible diseases. This can mean being free of harmful drugs used in most of these diseases and living a longer, healthier life.

Most of the drugs used to treat autoimmune diseases are powerful immune suppressing drugs and cytokine blocking drugs (such as Enbrel® that blocks TNF-α), both of which can produce dramatic increases in risk of cancer development and even fatal infections. Treatments using dietary changes (reducing calories and increasing flavonoid intake) and supplemental N-3 oils represent a safe alternative.

For the person with an autoimmune disease, I would recommend the following:

Get tested for food allergies and avoid all foods that produce even modest reactions.

Take N-3 oil supplements (preferably liquid forms, not those in gelatin capsules) that contain both N-3 oils and GLA in a balanced mixture.

Avoid N-6 oils, such as corn, safflower, sunflower, peanut, canola, and soybean oils.

Eat at least five servings of fresh, washed vegetables a day (avoid fruits because of high caloric content).

Drink 8 ounces of blenderized vegetables a day.

Avoid vegetables of the nightshade family (tomatoes, bell peppers, potatoes, etc.) unless well cooked.

Eat only complex carbohydrates that contain high fiber, such as beans, peas, and lentils.

Drink only filtered water, free of pesticides, industrial chemicals, and fluoride.

Exercise regularly, but only at moderate levels. No aerobics. Resistance exercises are best.

Have mercury amalgam fillings removed by a dentist trained in the IAOMT technique.

Avoid vaccinations (when possible), especially the mercury-containing flu vaccine.

Take magnesium citrate or citrate/malate, two capsules twice a day for for two weeks, then increase to two capsules three times a day between meals.

The Effect of N-3 Oils on Immunity

It is known that N-6 oils are powerful suppressors of immunity, especially cellular immunity. This is why N-6 oils such as corn and safflower consistently have been shown to promote the growth and spread of cancers and worsen inflammatory diseases, such as Lupus and rheumatoid arthritis.

While N-3 oils also can suppress immune reactions, they have opposite effects on cancer growth and spread, that is, they strongly suppress their growth and spread. In fact, DHA has been shown to cause cancer cells to commit suicide (apoptosis), while protecting and strengthening normal cells.

There are many diseases in which one would want to calm down the immune system; for example, the autoimmune diseases such as Lupus, rheumatoid arthritis, Crohn's disease, ulcerative colitis, immune thyroiditis, multiple sclerosis, Alzheimer's disease, Parkinson's disease, and psoriasis. In fact, clinical studies have shown a positive benefit for all of these diseases. Again, better results would be seen with these diseases if researchers had reduced the intake of N-6 fats and increased the intake of antioxidants at the same time.

Recent studies indicate that N-3 oils may be useful in treating multiple sclerosis by suppressing lymphocyte overactivity. It is the lymphocytes that play a role in destroying the covering insulation of the nerves (myelin). Even more important is that the N-3 oils, especially DHA, suppress the microglial cells near the damaged area, and it is these cells that cause most of the damage. To a large degree these microglial cells do their damage by an excitotoxic mechanism. DHA has been shown to protect against excitotoxicity directly.

As you may recall, omega-3 oils are composed of two major components: EPA and DHA. Recent studies have shown that EPA powerfully suppresses interleukin-10, a cytokine that plays a major role in preventing autoimmunity and that powerfully suppresses immune overreaction and inflammation—a good thing.[601] This is why I prefer either pure DHA or an oil that has low amounts of EPA.

A number of plant extracts and antioxidants have been shown to reduce microglial activation and therefore reduce autoimmune damage. For example, DHA, EPA, vitamin D3, vitamin E, silymarin, curcumin, and quercetin have all been shown to suppress these inflammatory cells in the brain and other tissues.

As stated previously, the anti-inflammatory and immune modulating effects of N-3 oils may explain why such inflammatory diseases as Alzheimer's dementia and Parkinson's disease are much less common in people with a high intake of N-3 oils.

N-3 Oils and Cancer Treatment and Prevention

An abundance of new evidence indicates that a higher intake of N-3 oils protects against a number of cancers, especially breast cancer, prostate cancer, leukemia, melanoma, colon cancer, and malignant histocytic cancers. Even more exciting is the finding that these same oils, especially the DHA component, suppress the growth and spread of these same cancers and enhance the effectiveness of certain chemotherapy drugs against the cancers.

Prostate Cancer

A Swedish study reported in the journal *Lancet* found that among 6,272 Swedish men followed for thirty years, those who ate no fish had two to three times the incidence of prostate cancer as those who ate either moderate or large amounts of fish.[602]

A new study also found that the growth of prostate cancer cells is suppressed by a cell signal molecule called peroxisome proliferators-activated receptor-γ (PPAR-γ) and that DHA is a powerful stimulator of PPAR-γ. In addition, prostate cancers utilize a special enzyme called COX-2 to stimulate their growth, the same enzyme suppressed by anti-inflammatory medications such as ibuprofen and Celebrex™.[603]

In this study it was found that both DHA and Celebrex™ suppressed prostate cancer growth, but that they both worked even better when combined. While Celebrex™ has been removed from the market because of cardiovascular deaths, a number of natural substances also suppress COX-2 enzymes. These include quercetin, luteolin, apigenin, vitamin E, and curcumin—all of which are available as supplements. Together, DHA, vitamins E and D3, and flavonoids are powerful ways to prevent and even treat prostate cancer.

Breast Cancer

A recent study reported in the journal *Cancer Science* found that there was no relationship between saturated or total fat consumption and breast cancer in Japanese women but, that those who ate the greatest amount of fish per week had a dramatically lower risk of getting the disease—a whopping 50 percent lower.[604]

While most think that breast cancer rates in Japanese women are are low because of soy consumption, in fact it has little or nothing to do with soy. The Japanese eat some of the highest amounts of omega-3 oils and have the highest vegetable (flavonoids) intakes in the world, both of which powerfully prevent breast cancer as well as other cancers.

Herceptin™, one of the newer breast cancer chemotherapy drugs touted by the pharmaceutical industry, depends on the presence of a special cancer cell receptor in certain types of highly aggressive breast cancers called the HER-2/neu receptor. A new study found that N-3 fatty acids also suppress this receptor.[605] Animal tests found that N-3 oils powerfully suppressed breast cancer growth and the spread of the cancers. Herceptin™ has a lot of bad side effects, whereas DHA has none.

What if you could change your diet while you were pregnant and prevent breast cancer, not only in yourself, but in your new baby daughter as well? A new study indicates that you may be able to do just that. Most of the most highly aggressive breast cancers occur in young women who have a strong family history of breast cancer.

Scientists used a special animal model utilizing mice that are genetically prone to very high rates of breast cancer as adults, just as we see in these women. When these mice were fed a diet high in N-6 fats (as we have in most Americans' diets) 100 percent of the babies grew up to develop breast cancer.

Yet, when the mothers were fed N-3 oils either during pregnancy or when the newborns were fed an N-3-containing formula after weaning, there was a greater than 40 percent reduction in the incidence of breast cancer when the babies grew up. Incredibly, when given the N-3 oils throughout the pregnancy and after birth, there was an 87 percent reduction in breast cancer as adults.

If this holds up in people, it means that merely adding N-3 oils to your diet during pregnancy and the diet of your baby daughter after birth can virtually eliminate your daughter's risk of developing breast cancer. It is known that DHA can alter the genes in cells, preventing cancer-genes (oncogenes) from becoming active.

Two of the big guns used by oncologists against breast cancer are Taxol and Taxomere, both highly toxic and not always effective. A recent study appearing in the *European Journal of Cancer Prevention* found that DHA significantly enhanced the effectiveness of both drugs against even previously drug-resistant breast cancers.[606]

Leukemia

Growing evidence indicates that N-3 fats may be a powerful weapon against leukemia. For example, it is known that both EPA and DHA components suppress leukemia cell growth and induce these cells to commit suicide (apoptosis).

In one animal model of myeloid leukemia, which normally kills 100 percent of mice, it was found that DHA added to their diet significantly prolonged life.[607] Subsequent studies confirmed this and showed the mechanism, which involved gene activation and activation of apoptosis mechanisms. In addition, DHA increased the effectiveness of the anti-leukemia drug AraC.

Another study found that both GLA and EPA suppressed the growth of leukemia cells and killed leukemic cells.[608] Combining the two oils increased the effectiveness. What this means is that a combination of EPA, DHA, and GLA provides us with a powerful weapon against leukemia. Other studies have shown that quercetin, especially when combined with resveratrol and ellagic acid, powerfully suppress leukemia.

One recent weapon used by oncologists in fighting the battle against leukemia is a compound called arsenic trioxide, which has been shown to kill leukemic cells, but not in all forms of leukemia. One recently released study found that adding DHA to the diet greatly increased the effectiveness of this drug against previously resistant forms of the disease.[609]

Colon Cancer

For some time it was known that the oil conjugated linolenic acid (CLA) significantly reduced the risk of developing colon cancer. The same can be said for GLA. But new evidence indicates that another oil may be equally, if not more, effective against this terrifying disease, and that is N-3 oils—especially the DHA component.

Prevention is one thing, but treatment of existing colon cancer can be much tougher. It is now evident that DHA also kills colon cancer cells selectively. The mechanism is by increasing free radicals and lipid peroxidation products in the cancer cells. Vitamin E can partially erase this benefit by suppressing lipid peroxidation.

This would mean that colon cancer patients under active treatment should avoid vitamin E until the cancer is eradicated. Like many nutrients, DHA been also shown to enhance the effectiveness of chemotherapy and to make it less toxic to normal cells. This was dramatically shown in a recent study in which the response to the highly toxic AraC drug on normal colon cells and colon cancer cells were compared.[610]

The researchers found that DHA, even in small doses, increased the toxicity of the drug to colon cancer cells some thirty times as compared to a minimal toxicity to normal cells. In essence, the DHA made the drug more effective in treating the cancer and in protecting the normal colon cells.

Curcumin, which has been shown to have a strong ability to prevent and even treat colon cancer, is soluble in N-3 oils. As a preventative, you can mix 1,000 mg of GLA and 1,000 mg of CLA in 1 tbsp of omega-3 oil. Once mixed, add ¼ tsp of Unique-E (a pure form of vitamin E) liquid to the oils and 250 mg of curcumin powder. Take this mixture twice to three times a day.

A unique form of DHA, called conjugated DHA, similar to the CLA, has been shown to be even more powerful in killing cancer cells.[611]

Other Cancers

Tests using DHA against melanoma cells in culture have shown promising results against this nasty cancer. One study found that there were two types of melanoma cells, one that was sensitive to destruction and growth suppression by DHA and another that was resistant.[612]

Earlier studies have demonstrated that the flavonoid quercetin (found in high concentrations in teas, onions, shallots, apples, and cranberries) inhibits the growth and spread of melanomas and can induce apoptosis as well. You can mix quercetin powder from a capsule into the oil mix I discussed before, since quercetin is oil soluble. This combination is active against both types of melanoma cells.

It is known that some cervical cancers are quite resistant to chemotherapy (vincristine). A new study found that EPA, DHA, and GLA all increased the ability of this chemotherapy agent to kill cervical cancer cells and that they also suppressed growth and spread of the cancer by themselves.[614]

One of the most deadly cancers is that of the pancreas. Using human pancreatic cancer cells, researchers have recently shown that DHA is unique in that it induces the cancer cells to kill themselves by an apoptosis mechanism.[61] It causes the cancer cells, but not normal cells, to lose their glutathione, and this causes them to burn up (by free radicals and lipid peroxidation). Ironically, DHA has an opposite effect on normal cells—that is, it increases their protective glutathione.

Another way DHA combats cancer is by preventing cholesterol from entering the cancer cell membrane. It does this by replacing it. This makes the cancer cell very vulnerable to immune attack and even chemotherapy. In addition, DHA powerfully inhibits the ability of cancers to grow new blood vessels (called angiogenesis), something essential to their growth and spread.

DHA and EPA combat cancer in a number of ways, utilizing cell mechanisms that are beyond the scope of what can be explained in this book. For more information on how to combat cancer nutritionally you can refer to my book *Natural Strategies for Cancer Patients*.

N-3 Fats, Diabetes, the Metabolic Syndrome, and Hypertension

There is growing evidence that N-3 oils can have a profoundly protective effect in preventing a number of deadly diseases, including diabetes, hypertension, atherosclerosis, heart attacks, strokes, cancer, autoimmune disorders, neurodegenerative diseases, and recently, the Metabolic Syndrome.

A new study, soon to be released in the journal *Endocrinology*, found that N-3 oils, when added to the diet early in life, seems to turn off the genes responsible for hyperlipidemia (high bad fats in the blood) and hypertension. Using a rat model of human hypertension, researchers found that if pregnant rats are exposed to dexamethasone (a powerful steroid), their offspring will develop high blood pressure as adults. But, if the mothers are fed increasing amounts of N-3 oils, they do not develop hypertension.

Another interesting study was done using children born with dangerously high blood lipids (familial hypercholesterolemia and familial combined hyperlipidemia), who are known to have a high risk of atherosclerosis early in life. In a double blind, crossover, placebo-controlled study it was found that adding DHA to their diets (1.2 grams a day) significantly improved their blood vessel function, which translates into less hypertension and atherosclerosis.[615]

Increasingly, we are seeing that altering our nutrition can spare us serious diseases later in life, even hereditary diseases. N-3 oils have been shown to reduce significantly the incidence of diabetes in children born to high-risk mothers.

The ability of N-3 oils to do this is based on their capacity to alter a number of genes and their ability to reduce inflammation. DHA is known to reduce atherosclerosis risk by a group of its byproducts called resolvins. These reduce inflammation in the walls of arteries and this blocks the process that causes the crud to build up within arteries. Likewise, DHA reduces inflammation in other tissues and this reduces the risk of the Metabolic Syndrome.

The Metabolic Syndrome is an alteration of metabolism causing abnormal blood lipids (high triglycerides, low HDL-cholesterol, and high bad form LDL-cholesterol), hypertension, and type-2 diabetes. We are now seeing an explosion of this syndrome that is affecting millions of our youth. Overall, some 41 million Americans are affected by this disorder, making it a major killer.

We know that a diet high in sugar, certain saturated fats, and N-6 fats can cause this syndrome. It is less well known that MSG and similar food additives also can cause the syndrome. As you saw in chapter 7, excitotoxins can cause gross obesity in newborn animals either exposed to MSG during pregnancy or soon after birth. There is a strong correlation between obesity and the Metabolic Syndrome—especially abdominal obesity. This is the fat within the abdomen and not that under the skin.

One of the newer innovations in preventing and treating diabetes is the use of drugs that stimulate a particular receptor on the genes of cells called peroxisome proliferator-activated receptors (PPARs). Ironically, DHA is a very powerful activator of PPARs and has been shown to prevent diabetes by reversing insulin resistance.

Newer studies have also shown that the PPARs protect the stomach and intestines from ulceration. In fact, this may be how glutamine aids in intestinal healing.[616] This provides us with an alternative to glutamine for gut healing, since glutamine increases glutamate levels in tissues and can worsen excitotoxicity. In addition, PPARs prevent hypertension and reduce inflammation, the mechanism of the Metabolic Syndrome.

What this means is that DHA is a powerful and extremely safe way to enhance PPARs and so reduce the risk of the Metabolic Syndrome and its complications. In addition, DHA has been shown to reduce the number of fat cells, especially stomach fat, the very same fat that causes Metabolic Syndrome.

We also know that abdominal fat releases a special set of inflammatory cytokines (called adipokines) that result in hypertension, diabetes, and abnormal lipids in the blood (the Metabolic Syndrome). While CLA will reduce the excess fat from the fat cells, DHA actually reduces the number of fat cells, which is much better.[617] Combined, CLA and DHA offer a powerful weapon against excess abdominal fat and so the Metabolic Syndrome.

The abnormal blood lipids are also corrected by increasing dietary DHA intake. A number of studies have shown that DHA and N-3 oils substantially lower triglyceride levels, raise HDL-cholesterol levels, and increase the healthy LDL levels (large, buoyant type). Some doctors would be shocked to hear that you might want a higher LDL level, but there are two forms of LDL—a large, buoyant form that actually reduces the risk of atherosclerosis (like HDH) and a small, dense form that increases risk. Even though these tests are now available, most doctors still do not order them. It is the good large, buoyant form that is increased by DHA.

Conclusion

As we have seen, N-3 (omega-3) oils offer a cornucopia of healthy benefits well beyond any known pharmaceutical drug in terms of efficacy and safety. Because they modulate immune inflammatory reactions in the body, the N-3 oils, especially DHA, can play a major role in preventing and treating a wide array of diseases, such as diabetes, Metabolic Syndrome, hypertension, autoimmune diseases, vaccine reactions, atherosclerosis (heart attacks and strokes), cancer, stomach ulcers, and neurodegenerative diseases (Alzheimer's dementia, Parkinson's disease, and ALS). In addition, they aid in weight loss and improve brain function.

There are many brands of N-3 oils. Most are either derived from fish or algae. Fish get the oils from eating algae. The most important consideration in choosing an oil is the purity and the balance of the EPA and DHA. Most fish oils have far too much EPA and too little DHA. It is the DHA component that is responsible for most of the beneficial effects.

At this writing, I am designing an N-3 oil supplement that will improve the benefits of the taking omega-3 oils. All oils should be kept in the refrigerator to prevent oxidation of the oil, which would make it unhealthy. In fact, I recommend that all supplements should be kept in the refrigerator to maintain freshness and extend their shelf life.

In general, I do not advocate taking supplements in gel-cap or gelatin capsules. The gelatin, if derived from cattle, is a very high-risk product for bovine spongioform encephalopathy (BSE or mad cow disease). It is also high in the excitotoxins glutamate and fluoride. Instead, I prefer a liquid form.

There is some debate as to which is better, the triglyceride form or the ester form of N-3 oils. After reviewing the scientific literature, I feel the ester form is superior since it has excellent distribution in the brain, is of higher purity than the triglyceride form, and has extremely good bioavailability. It is also important to remember that you must not only increase your intake of N-3 oils, but at the same time decrease your intake of N-6 oils. Studies indicate that the average person is consuming fifty times more N-6 oils than is required by the body. The N-6 oils interfere with the normal metabolism of the good oil components and dramatically increase inflammation.

In my opinion, the government's promotion of eating more vegetable oil-containing foods has resulted in the deaths and disabilities of millions of people worldwide. Likewise, I believe their denial of the danger of trans fatty acids (partially hydrogenated oils) for over thirty years may have killed millions.

Afterword

Although I have discussed many ways you can protect yourself against disease and injury by utilizing modern scientific knowledge, this book necessarily has been unable to cover the entire field of health and disease-prevention through good nutrition and supplementation. New information is continually being added to our body of knowledge, and will have to be included in subsequent books. My primary purpose has been to emphasize that your best protection while navigating the health care system is to become involved in your own treatment. You must learn about your disease, how to prevent future disease, and the best ways to treat your particular problem. This takes a great deal of work!

As we have seen, doctors are in the midst of a very difficult period. Insurance companies, government agencies, liability lawyers, and an ever-constraining healthcare system have battered them beyond endurance. Managed care and HMOs have destroyed the best of American medical care and have produced a nation of dispirited doctors. This affects you directly, since many doctors' primary aims are to retire early. They are terribly overworked, financially strapped, and afraid of their patients—and as a result want only to get through each day and go home.

Even when doctors want to provide the best care that medical science can offer, insurance companies and government payers (Medicare/Medicaid) often will not let them. What little decision-making is left to them entails jumping through seemingly endless, infuriating bureaucratic hoops. As a result, many find it's a lot easier to avoid even *attempting* to treat you.

Due to this abysmal state of affairs, your health is dependent on your own determination, ingenuity, and hard work. You must learn as much as you can about how the body functions in both health and sickness. In addition, you must study all your treatment choices, including nutritional options. With the Internet, you have a tremendous resource that was not available to patients twenty years ago. While it can be cluttered with confusing, often contradictory, information, if you persevere you will eventually develop a better idea of your health needs. This is especially true if you have the good fortune to find a health care professional who is knowledgeable about nutritional science. While this is rare in many parts of the country (including my own), fortunately, the demand for such practitioners is growing by leaps and bounds.

If you have learned anything from this book, I hope that you now understand that the body is a whole organism encompassing many *inter*dependent systems. Modern science likes to divide things and examine systems in isolation. Little work has been done on how all the body's systems work together, and more importantly, how disease arising from one part of the body can affect numerous other systems, often at great distances from the source of the disease.

In addition, modern medicine has all but ignored the affects of various additives used in processed foods, especially the problems associated with accumulated, synergistic effects. The same is true of environmental toxins. As we have seen, the most neglected area of all is the affect of these toxins on the nervous system. Tens of thousands of such chemicals have never been tested to determine their combined, long-term effects.

Another serious problem is widespread use of vaccines. The medical hierarchy has assumed that vaccinations are much safer than actual experience has shown, and the connection to learning disorders, such as ADD/ADHD and autism, has been virtually ignored by these elitists. There is overwhelming evidence that over-vaccination and vaccination under conditions of immune impairment can have substantial deleterious affects on the developing nervous system. As with so many problems, medical elitists simply have refused to objectively examine the issue.

I also hope that you now realize that nutritional medicine is not outside the scope of science and that so-called "orthodox" medicine is not the only true and scientifically based medical model. The nutritional basis of disease is just as scientific as orthodox medicine, which I have attempted to demonstrate throughout this book. What makes orthodox medicine "orthodox" is that its leaders have wrested control from nutritional scientists, who actually have more complete and scientifically based methods of treating disease and maintaining health. Despite the fact they frequently stand on very shaky scientific ground, the orthodox medical industry has also wooed the favor of the main media outlets in this country so they always get the last word in any argument.

I tell my patients that every major medical journal and surgical specialty journal contains at least one nutrition-based article in virtually every issue. The problem is that doctors do not read them. Instead, they focus on articles concerning the newest surgical techniques, diagnostic tests, or expensive drug treatments. My theory is that the nutrition articles are ignored because doctors simply don't understand them, especially if there is a lot of biochemistry involved. In addition, nutritional treatments will not increase a doctor's sagging income the way an exorbitant new procedure can.

The big secret among doctors is that when they arrived at medical school, they were told that first-year biochemistry flunked out most medical students, and they learned to hate and dread it. In fact, among all subjects, this is the one that continues to wash out the greatest number of students. At our twentieth reunion, my fellow alumni were still vehement in their hatred for our old biochemistry teacher—who was really a great guy—even two decades after graduating from medical school!

As a biochemistry major in undergraduate school, and having taken postgraduate biochemistry courses, I actually found the medical school course to be fairly easy. In truth, I enjoyed biochemistry more than any other subject. Unfortunately, it was also the last and only course or instruction I encountered anywhere that dealt with the subject of nutrition. Throughout my ten years of medical and neurosurgical training I never heard a single word about nutrition.

The only time doctors ever learn anything about biochemistry or nutrition is in connection with a pharmaceutical drug's mode of action or a very focused review of a disease process. Actually applying biochemical/nutritional knowledge to patient care was and is as rare as hen's teeth. Nutrition is essentially biochemistry, and medical care devoid of nutritional considerations is like a car without wheels. It goes nowhere.

Take something as simple as a common infection. When most doctors see a patient with an infection (e.g., pneumonia), their first thought is to culture the organism, identify it, and specify an antibiotic appropriate to effectively treat it. This is basic medicine, something all doctors are taught from day one. But simply giving the antibiotic leaves a huge gap in properly treating the patient. It is rare, in my experience, that doctors will place such a patient on probiotic organisms and prebiotic support nutrients to assure the growth of friendly organisms.

We all learned in medical school that broad-spectrum antibiotics kill both pathogenic disease-causing organisms, as well as beneficial colon bacteria, and that an overgrowth of pathogenic bacteria caused by the antibiotic can lead to the often fatal condition called pseudomembraneous colitis. But, we were never taught what to do about it. We were also not told that one of the most common secondary problems with frequent or prolonged antibiotic usage is yeast overgrowth (Candidia albicans) and that it can lead to numerous and severe long-term complications.

We were *not* taught about the importance of nutrition in immune function, and that antibiotics work better when we utilize nutritional non-specific immune stimulation. In addition, most doctors do not seem to understand that certain foods, particularly fats, can severely impair the immune system, causing antibiotics to fail and an infection to spiral out of control. Few doctors know that iron supplements can cause existing infections to become deadly and uncontrollable—all of this despite the numerous studies that have appeared in peer-reviewed medical journals emphasizing the importance of nutrition in controlling infections. These are the articles that they skip over to read about the latest prescription drug.

Throughout this book I have provided examples of the importance of utilizing what we know about the biochemistry of disease and the enormous importance of nutritional treatment in conjunction with conventional treatment modalities. Until doctors acknowledge these truths, it will be your responsibility to learn and practice good nutrition so that you can prevent disease and protect your own life if you do become ill. This will require discipline. It has been said that the undisciplined life is not worth living. We now know that the undisciplined life will also be short and full of misery.

Endnotes

Chapter 3
Mercury: The Silent Killer

[1] Weiss B, Clarkson TW. Toxic chemical disasters and the implications of Bhopal for technology transfer. *Milbank Quarterly* 64(1986): 216-240.

[2] Kanluen S, Gottlieb CA. A clinical pathological study of four adult cases of mercury inhalation toxicity. *Arch Path Lab Med* 115(1991): 56-60.

[3] Teueg C, Sanfilippo DJ, et al. Acute and chronic poisoning from residential exposures to elemental mercury: Michigan 1989-1990. *Clin Toxicol* 30(1982): 63-67.

[4] Stock A. Die gefahrlichkeit des quecksilberdampfes. Z Angew. *Chem* 39(1926): 461-488.

[5] Gay DD, Cox RD, Reinhardt JW. Chewing releases mercury from fillings. *Corresp Lancet* 1(1985): 985-986.

[6] Svare CW, et al. The effects of dental amalgams on mercury levels of expired air. *J Dental Research* 60(1981): 1668-1671.

[7] Vimy MJ, Lorscheider FL. Intra-oral air mercury released from dental amalgam. *J Dental Res* 64(1985): 1069-1071. Patterson JE, et al. Mercury in human breath from dental amalgams. *Bull Environ Contam Toxicol* 34(1985): 459-468.

[8] Fredin B. Studies on the mercury release from dental amalgam fillings. *Swed J Biol Med* 3(1988), 8-15.

[9] Zander D, Ewers U, et al. Studies on human exposure to mercury II. Mercury concentrations in urine in relation to the number of amalgam fillings. *Zbl Hyg* 190(1990): 325-334.

[10] Vimy MJ, Lorscheider FL. Intra-oral mercury released from dental amalgams. *J Dent Res* 64(1985): 1069-1071. Bjorkman L, Lind B. Factors influencing mercury evaporation rates from dental amalgam fillings. *Scand J Dental Res* 100(1992): 354-360.

[11] Barregard L, Sallsten G, Jarvholm B. People with high mercury uptake from their own dental amalgam fillings. *Occup Environ Med* 52(1995): 124-128.

[12] Begerow J, Zander D, et al. Long-term mercury excretion in urine after removal of amalgam fillings. *In Arch Occup Health* 66(1994): 209-212.

[13] Kraub P, Deyhle M, et al. Field study of Mercury Content in Saliva. *Universitat Tubingen* 8/29/00.

[14] Uzzell B, Oler J. Chronic low-level mercury exposure and neuropsychological functioning. *J Clin Exp Neuropsychol* 8(1986): 581-593.

[15] Stonehouse CA, Newman AP. Mercury vapour release from a dental aspirator. *British Dental Journal* 190(2001): 558-560.

[16] Ngim CH, Foo SC, et al. Chronic neurobehavioral effects of elemental mercury in dentists. *British Journal of Internal Medicine* 49(1992): 782-790.

[17] Ritchie KA, MacDonald EB, et al. Psychomotor testing of dentist with chronic low level mercury exposure. *J Dent Res* 74(1995): 420.

[18] Echeverria D, Heyer NJ, et al. Behavioral effects of low-level exposure to elemental Hg among dentists. *Neurotoxicol Teratol* 17(1995): 161-168.

[19] Bucio L, Gareia C, et al. Uptake, cellular distribution and DNA damage produced by mercuric chloride. *Mutation Research* 423(1999): 65-72.

[20] One study showed that strand breaks within the DNA occurred at low doses of mercury, below that causing obvious toxic cell damage, and the damaging effect on DNA increased with increasing concentrations of mercury exposure. [Ariza ME, Holliday J, Williams MV. Mutagenic effect of mercury (II) in eukaryotic cells. *In Vivo* 8(1994): 559-563.] This may explain the association between mercury exposure and brain tumors, as well as other degenerative brain disorders.

[21] Bulat P, Dujic I, et al. Activity of glutathione peroxidase and superoxide dismutase from workers occupationally exposed to mercury. *Int Arch Occup Environ Health Supp* 71(1998): S37-39. This included a significant fall in glutathione peroxidase and superoxide dismutase (SOD) enzyme levels.

[22] Yoshino Y, Mozai T, Nakao K. Biochemical changes in the brain in rats poisoned with an alkyl mercuric compound with special reference to the inhibition of protein synthesis in brain cortex slices. *Neurochem* 13(1996): 1223-1230.

[23] Recent studies have shown that mercury interferes with a special membrane enzyme called sodium-potassium ATPase (Na$^+$/K$^+$ ATPase), which is necessary for energy production.

[24] It also can cause swelling of the astrocytes in the nervous system, which is important since the astrocyte plays a major role in regulating glutamate levels in the nervous system, among many other vital functions. [Aschner M, Vitarella D, et al. Methylmercury-induced astrocytic swelling is associated with activation of the Na$^+$/K$^+$ antiporter, and is fully reversible by amiloride. *Brain Res* 799(1998): 207-214.] This effect of methylmercury is similar to what we see with aging of neurons and with neurodegenerative diseases.

[25] Lorsheider FL, Vimy MJ, et al. Mercury vapor exposure inhibits tubulin binding to GTP in rat brain: a molecular lesion also present in human Alzheimer's brain. *FASEB J* 9(1995): A-3845.

[26] Rajanna B, Hobson M, et al. Effects of cadmium and mercury on Na+/K+ ATPases and the uptake of 3H-dopamine in rat brain synaptosomes. *Archives of Inter Physiology and Biochemistry* 98(1990): 291-296. Oudar P, Caillard L, Fillon G. In vitro effects of organic mercury on the sertonergic system. *Pharmacology and Toxicology* 65(1989):245-248. Rajanna B, Hobson M. Influence of mercury on uptake of dopamine and norepinephrine by rat brain synaptosomes. *Toxicol Lett* 27(1985): 7-14.

[27] Part of the reason is that the antioxidant enzyme catalase converts metallic mercury to Hg^{+2}, which passes through the blood-brain barrier with great difficulty, thus trapping the ionic mercury in the brain.

[28] Swensson A, Ulifvarson U. Distribution and excretion of mercury compounds in rats over a long period after a single injection. *Acta Pharmacol* 26(1968): 273-283.

[29] Sorensen FW, Larsen JO, et al. Neuron loss in cerebellar cortex of rats exposed to mercury vapor: a stereological study. *Acta Neuropathol (Berl)* 100(2000): 95-100.

[30] Highest in the Purkinje cells and Bergman glial cells, with considerable amounts also found in the astrocytes of the medullary layer of the cerebellum. [Warfvinge K. Mercury distribution in the neonatal and adult cerebellum after mercury vapor exposure of pregnant squirrel monkeys. *Environ Res* 83(2000): 93-101.]

[31] Szasz A, Barna B, et al. Chronic low-dose maternal exposure to methylmercury enhances epileptogenecity in developing rats. *J Dev Neurosci* 17(1999): 733-742.

[32] Nadorfy-Lopez E, Torres SH, et al. Skeletal muscle abnormalities associated with occupational exposure to mercury vapours. *Histology and Histopathology* 15(2000): 673-682. They found atrophy of the type IIB muscle fibers, thickening of the basement membrane and capillary alterations indicative of mercury damage.

[33] Aschner M, Rising L, Mullansy KJ. Differential sensitivity of neonatal rat astrocyte cultures to mercuric chloride (MC) and methylmercury (MeHg): studies on K+ and amino acid transport and metallothionein (MT) induction. *Neurotoxicol* 17(1996): 107-116.

[34] Audesirk G, Audsirk T. Neurite Development. In *Developmental Neurotoxicology*. Harry GJ (ed). Boca Raton: CRC Press, 1994, p 75.

[35] This can include effects on adhesion molecules, cytoskeletal element formation, regulation and formation of ion channels, effects on intracellular transduction pathways that normally regulate transcription, translocation and modification of proteins, alteration of hormones and effects on the development and regulation of neurotransmitters, all very complicated processes.

[36] Jenson KF, Catalano SM. Brain morphogenesis and developmental neurotoxicology. In *Handbook of Developmental Neurotoxicology*. Slikker W, Chang LW (eds). San Diego: Academic Press, 1998, p 15.

[37] Ben-Ozer EY, Rosenspire AJ, et al. Mercury chloride damages cellular DNA by a non-apoptotic mechanism. *Mutant Res* 470(2000): 19-27.

[38] It does this by altering the integrity of the inner layer of the mitochondrion, where all of the energy-producing enzymes rest. [Weinberg JM, Harding PG, Humes HD. Mitochondrial bioenergetics during the initiation of mercuric chloride-induced renal injury. *J Biol Chem* 257(1982): 60-67.]

[39] Soderstrom S, Fredriksson A, et al. The effects of mercury vapor on cholinergic neurons in the fetal brain: studies in the expression of nerve growth factor and its low-and high-affinity receptors. *Develop Brain Res* 85(1995): 96-108. Several of the neurotransmitters, such as glutamate, glycine, acetylcholine, and serotonin, in too high a concentration, can damage or even kill neurons. Both mercury vapor and methylmercury can alter the development of cholinergic neurons (that secrete the neurotransmitter, acetylcholine).

[40] Chang LW, Guo GL. Fetal Minamata disease. Congenital methylmercury poisoning. In *Handbook of Developmental Neurotoxicology*. Slikker W and Chang LW (eds). San Diego: Academic Press, 1998, pp 507-515.

[41] Suzuki K, Martin PM. Neurotoxicants and Developing Brain. In *Developmental Neurotoxicology*. Harry GJ (ed). Boca Raton: CRC Press, 1994, pp 18-19.

[42] Gilbert SG, Grant-Webster KS. Neurobehavioral effects of developmental methylmercury exposure. *Environ Health Perspect* 103(1995): 135-142.

[43] Watanabe C, Yin K, et al. In utero exposure to methylmercury and SE deficiency converge on the neurobehavioral outcome in mice. *Neurotoxicol Teratol* 21(1999): 83-88.

[44] Seppananen K, Kantola M, et al. Effect of supplementation with organic selenium on mercury status as measured by mercury in pubic hair. *J Trace Elem Med Biol* 14(2000): 84-87.

[45] Lee JH, Kang HS, Roh J. Protective effects of garlic juice against embryotoxicity of methylmercury chloride administered to 344 pregnant Fischer rats. *Yonsei Med J* 40(1999): 483-489.

[46] Vimy MJ, Takahashi Y, Lorscheider FL. Maternal-fetal distribution of mercury (203Hg) released from dental amalgam fillings. *Am J. Physiol* 258(1990): R939-945.

[47] Polifka JE. Drug and Chemical Contaminants in Breast Milk. Effects on Neurodevelopment of the Nursing Infant. In *Developmental Neurotoxicology*, Harry GJ (ed). Boca Raton: CRC Press, 1994, p 393.

[48] Letz R, Gerr F, et al. Residual neurological deficits 30 years after occupational exposure to elemental mercury. *Neurotoxicol* 21(2000): 459-474.

[49] Sundberg J, Jonsson S, et al. Lactational exposure and neonatal kinetics of methylmercury and inorganic mercury in mice. *Toxicol Apply Pharmacol* 154(1999): 160-169.

[50] Oskarsson A, Schutz A, et al. Total and inorganic mercury in breast milk and blood in relationship to fish consumption and amalgam fillings in lactating women. *Arch Environ Health* 51(1996): 234-241.

[51] WHO/FAO. Toxicological evaluation of certain foods additives and contaminants. WHO Food Additive Series: 24. Cambridge: Cambridge University Press, 1989, pp 295-328.

[52] Razagui IB, Haswell SJ. Mercury and selenium concentrations in maternal and neonatal scalp hair: relationship to amalgam-based dental treatment received during pregnancy. *Bio Trace Elem Res*. 81(2001): 1-19.

[53] Sandborgh-Englund G, Ask K, Belfrage E, Ekstrand J. Mercury exposure in utero and during infancy. *Journal of Toxicology and Environmental Health* 63(2001): 317-320.

[54] Suzuki K. Martin PM. Neutrotoxicants and Developing Brain. In *Developmental Neurotoxicology*, Harry GJ (ed). Boca Raton: CRC Press, 1994.

[55] Letz R, Geer F, et al. Residual neurological deficits 30 years after occupational exposure to elemental mercury. *Neurotoxicol* 21(2000): 459-474.

[56] Murata K, Weihe P, et al. Delayed evoked potentials in children exposed to methylmercury from seafood. *Neurotoxicology Teratology* 21(1999): 343-348.

[57] Yeates KO, Mortensen ME. Acute and Chronic Neuropsychological consequences of mercury vapor poisoning in two early adolescents. *J Clin Exp Neuropsychol* 16(1994): 209-222.

[58] Windebank AJ, McCall JT, Dyck PJ. Metal neuropathy. In *Peripheral Neuropathy*. Dyck PJ, Thomas EH, et al. (eds). Philadelphia: Saunders, 1984, pp 2133-2161.

[59] Fredriksson A, Dencker L, et al. Prenatal coexposure to metallic mercury vapor and methylmercury produce interactive behavioral changes in adult rats. *Neurotoxicol Teratol* 19(1996): 129-134.

[60] Hartman DE. Neuropsychological Toxicology. *Identification and Assessment of Human Neurotoxic Syndromes*. New York: Olenum Press, 1995, p 131.

[61] Grandjean P, Budtz-Jorgensen E, et al. Methylmercury exposure biomarkers as indicators of neurotoxicity in children aged seven years. *Am J Epidemiol* 150(1999): 301-305.

[62] Gerhard I, Waibel S, et al. Impact of heavy metals on hormonal and immunological factors in women with repeated miscarriages. *Human Reproduction Update* 4(1998): 301-309.

[63] Gerhard I. Amalgam aus gynakologischer sicht. *Der Frauenarzt* 36(1995): 627-628.

[64] Koller L. Immunotoxicology of heavy metals. *Immunopharmacol* 2(1980): 269-279.

[65] Moszezynski P, Sowinski S, et al. Lymphocyte, T and NK cells in men occupationally exposed to mercury vapors. *J Occup Med Environ Health* 8(1995): 49-56.

[66] Queiroz MLS, Perlingeiro RCR, et al. Immunoglobulin levels in workers exposed to inorganic mercury. *Pharmcol Toxicol* 74(1994): 72-75.

[67] Warfringe K, Hansson H, Hultman P. Systemic autoimmunity due to mercury vapor exposure in genetically susceptible mice: dose-response studies. *Toxicol Appl Pharmacol* 132(1995): 299-309.

[68] Hultman P, Johamsson U, et al. Adverse immunological effects and immunity induced by dental amalgam and silver alloy in mice. *FASEB J* 8(1994): 1183-1190.

[69] Ekstrand J, Bjorkman I, et al. Toxicological aspects on the release and systemic uptake of mercury from dental amalgams. *Eur J Oral Sci* 106(1998): 678-686.

[70] Ellermann-Eriksen S, Christensen MN, Mogeusen SC. Effect of mercury chloride on macrophage-mediated resistance against infection with herpes simplex virus type 2. *Toxicol* 93(1994): 269-287.

[71] Perlingeiro RC, Queiroz ML. Polymorphonuclear phagocytosis and killing in workers exposed to inorganic mercury. *J Immunopharmacol* 16(1994): 1011-1017.

[72] Zdolsek JM, Soder O, Hultman P. Mercury induces in vivo and in vitro secretion of interleukin-1 in mice. *Immunopharmacol* 28(1994): 201-208, 1994.

[73] Nadarajah V, Neiders ME, et al. Localized cellular inflammatory responses to subcutaneous implanted dental mercury. *J Toxicol Environ Health* 49(1996): 113-125.

[74] Siblerud RL. A comparison of mental health of multiple sclerosis patients with silver/mercury metal fillings and those with fillings removed. *Psycol Rep* 70(1992): 1139-1151.

[75] Ben-Ozer EY, Rosenpire AJ, et al. Mercury chloride damages cellular DNA by a non-apoptotic mechanism. *Mutation Research* 470(2000): 19-27. The binding of mercury to DNA is so intense that it occurs at concentrations below that necessary to cause damage to other cellular proteins, such as glutathione and SOD. [For more information see, Ariza ME, Holliday J, Williams MV. Mutagenic effect of mercury (II) in eukaryotic cells. *In Vivo* 8(1994): 559-563.]

[76] Boffetta P, Merler E, Vainio H. Carcinogenicity of mercury and mercury compounds. *Scand J Work Environ Health* 19(1993): 1-7.

[77] Al Saleh I, Shiwari N. Levels of cadmium, lead, and mercury in human brain tumors. *Biology Trace Elements Research* 79(2001): 197-203.

[78] Oliveiva RR, Malm O, Guimaraes JR. Distribution of methylmercury and inorganic mercury in neonate hamsters dosed with methylmercury during fetal life. *Environmental Research* 86(2001): 73-79.

[79] Schionning JD, Eide R, et al. Detection of mercury in rat spinal cord and dorsal root ganglion after exposure to mercury vapor. *Ex Mol Pathol* 58(1993): 215-228.

[80] The mercury has accumulated in the lysosomes of the neurons. Lysosomes are small packets of enzymes located within all cells, which are activated to dissolve a cell when it is fatally injured.

[81] Louwerse ES, Buchet J-P, et al. Urinary excretion of lead and mercury after oral administration of meso-2,3-dimercaptosuccinic acid in patients with motor neuron disease. *Int Arch Occup Environ Health* 67(1995): 135-138.

[82] Tandon L, Kasarskis EJ, Ehmann WD. Elemental imbalance studies by IAA on extraneuroal tissues from amyotrophic lateral sclerosis patients. *J Radio Anal Nuclear Chem* 195(1995): 13-19.

[83] Pamphlett R, Waley P. Motor neuron uptake of low-dose inorganic mercury. *J Neurol Sci* 135(1996): 63-67.

[84] Brookes N. Specificity and reversibility of the inhibition by HgCl2 of glutamate transport in astrocyte cultures. *J Neurochem* 50(1988): 1117-1122.

[85] Ehmann WD, Markesbery WR, et al. Brain trace elements in Alzheimer's disease. *Neurotoxicol* 7(1986):197-206.

[86] Eggleston DW, Nylander M. Correlation of dental amalgam with mercury in brain tissue. *J Prosthet Dent* 58(1987): 704-707. Nylander M, Freiberg L, Lind B. Mercury concentrations in the human brain and kidneys in relation to exposure from dental amalgam fillings. *Swed Dent J* 11(1987): 179-187.

[87] It may be that all of the various causes proposed for this disease are either connected to a central or final mechanism, such as free-radical injury or excitotoxicity. For example, we know that mercury promotes free-radical generation in the brain as well as acceleration of excitotoxicity. When neurons are exposed to glutamate, neurofibrillary tangles, exactly like those seen with Alzheimer's disease, will form. In fact, three relatively specific immune

complexes seen with Alzheimer's disease (ALZ-50, E52 and ubiquitin) will form as well, when high concentration of glutamate are added to brain cell cultures.

[88] Wenstrup D, Ehmann WD, Markesbery WR. Trace element imbalances in isolated subcellular fractions of Alzheimer's disease brains. *Brain Res* 533(1990): 125-131.

[89] Thompson CM, Markesbery WR, et al. Regional brain trace element studies in Alzheimer's disease. *Neurotoxicol* 9(1988): 1-7.

[90] Hock C, Drasch G, et al. Increased blood mercury levels in patients with Alzheimer's disease. *J Neural Transm* 105(1998): 59-68.

[91] Mercury has been shown to interfere with this polymerization process by interfering with the binding of GTP to tubulin dimers in the brain.

[92] Pendregrass JC, Haley BE, Vimy MJ, et al. Mercury vapor inhibits binding of GTP to tubulin in rat brain: similarity to a molecular lesion in Alzheimer's diseased brain. *Neurotoxicol* 18(1997): 315-324.

[93] Yuan Y, Atchison WD. Comparative effects of inorganic divalent mercury, methylmercury and phenylmercury on membrane excitability and synaptic transmission of CA1 neurons in hippocampal slices of the rat. *Neurotoxicol* 15(1994): 403-412.

[94] In one study, development of antibodies to glial fibrillary acid protein (GFAP), a protein associated with neurofilaments, was so typical of mercury exposure that it was proposed as a sensitive test for such exposure. Elevated antibodies were seen in the cortex, hippocampus and cerebellum in this study.

[95] Charleston JS, Body RL, et al. Changes in the number of astrocytes and microglia in the thalamus of the monkey Macaca fascicularis following long-term subclinical methylmercury exposure. *Neurotoxicol* 17(1996): 127-138.

[96] Peraza MA, Ayala-Fierro F, et al. Effects of micronutrients on metal toxicity. *Environ Health Perspectives* 106, suppl 1(1998): 203-216.

[97] Sorg O, Schilter B, et al. Increased vulnerability of neurons and glial cells to low concentrations of methylmercury in a prooxidant situation. *Acta Neuropathol* 96(1998): 621-627.

[98] DePalma G, Mutti A, et al. Case-control study of polymorphic xenobiotic-metabolizing enzymes in Parkinson's disease. Abstract of 7th Annual Meeting of International Neurotoxicological Association. July 4-9, 1999, Leicester, UK. *Neurotoxicol* 21(2000): 615-640, p 632.

[99] Finkelstein Y, Vardi J, et al. The enigma of Parkinsonism in chronic borderline mercury intoxication, resolved by challenge with penicillamine. *Neurotoxicol* 17(1996): 291-295.

[100] Seidler A, Hellenbrand W, et al. Possible environmental, occupational, and other etiological factors for Parkinson's diseases—a case-control study in Germany. *Neurology* 46(1996): 1275-1284.

[101] Goldfrank LR, Flomenbaum NE. *Goldfrank's Toxicologic Emergencies*. Norwalk, Connecticut: Apple & Lange, 1994.

[102] Quig D. Cysteine metabolism and metal toxicity. *Alter Med Rev* 3(1998): 262-270.

[103] Adachi T, Ischido M, Kunimoto M. Studies on protective factors for cell death of cerebellar neurons induced by methylmercury. Abstract of 7th Annual Meeting of International Neurotoxicological Association. July 4-9, 1999, Leicester, UK. *Neurotoxicol* 21(2000): 615-640, p 627.

[104] Aschner M, Yao CP, Allen JW. Transfection and overexpression of metallothionein-I (MT-1) in MT1/MT II knockout (MT-KO) mice increases their resistance to methylmercury (MeHg)-induced cytotoxicity. Abstract of 7th Annual Meeting of International Neurotoxicological Association. July 4-9, 1999, Leicester, UK. *Neurotoxicol* 21(2000): 615-640, p 626.

[105] Duhr EF, Pendergrass JC, et al. Hg EDTA complex inhibits GTP interaction with the E-site of brain beta-tubulin. *Toxicol Appl Pharmacol* 122(1993): 273-280.

[106] Skare I, Engqvist A. Amalgam restorations—an important source of human exposure of mercury and silver. *Lakartidningen* 15(1992): 1299-1301.

[107] Dunn J, Clarkson TW, Magus L. Ethanol-increased exhalation of mercury in mice. *Br J Ind Med* 35(1978): 241-244.

[108] Tamashiro H, Arakaki M, et al. Effect of ethanol on methyl mercury toxicity in rats. *J Toxicol Environ Health* 18(1986): 595-606.

[109] Hursh JB, Greenwood MR, et al. The effect of ethanol on the fate of mercury vapor inhaled by man. *J Pharmacol Ex Ther* 214(1980): 520-522.

[110] Desi I, Papp A, Nagymajteni L. Investigation of combined subchronic lead, mercury and ethanol exposure on neurophysiological process in rats. Abstract of 7th Annual Meeting of International Neurotoxicological Association. July 4-9, 1999, Leicester, UK. *Neurotoxicol* 21(2000): 615-640, pp 627-628.

Chapter 4
Fluoride: What Have They Done to Us Now?

[111] Lovejoy HB, Bell ZG, Vizena TR. Mercury exposure evaluation and their correlation with urine mercury excretion. 4: Elimination of mercury by sweating. *J Occup Med* 15(1973): 590-591.

[112] Ziegelbecker D. *Fluoride* 14(1981): 123-128.

[113] Diesendorf M. *Nature* (Jul 10, 1990): 322.

[114] Tsutsui T, et al. Sodium fluoride-induced morphological and neoplastic transformation, chromosome aberrations, sister chromatid exchanges, and unscheduled DNA synthesis in cultured Syrian hamster embryo cells. *Cancer Research* 44(1984): 938-941.

[115] Jones CA, et al. Sodium fluoride promotes morphological transformation of Syrian hamster embryo cells. *Carcinogenesis* 9(1988): 2279-2284.

[116] Duffy P, et al. Giant cells in the bone marrow of patients on high-dose fluoride treatment. *Ann Intern Med* 75(1971): 745-747.

[117] Taylor A, Taylor NC. Effect of fluoride on tumor growth. Proceeding *Soc Experm Biol Med* 65(1965): 252-255.

[118] Decision of Paul W. Aitkenhead vs Borough of West View in the Court of Common Pleas of Allegheny County, Pennsylvania, No. DG 4585-78 (1978) and Decision of Illinois Pure Water vs Director of the Department of Public Health of the State of Illinois, in the Third judicial Circuit, Madison County, No. 56315 (1982).

[119] Yiamouyiannis JA, Burke D. Fluoridation of public water systems and cancer death rates in humans. Presented at the 67th Annual Meeting Society Biological Chemist. *Fed Mer Soc Exp Biol*, June 1976.

[120] Yiamouyiannis, John. *Fluoride the Aging Factor: How to Recognize and Avoid the Devastating Effects of Fluoride.* Delaware, Ohio: Health Action Press, 1993 (3rd ed), pp 82-84 and 167.

[121] Hoover RN, et al. Time trends for bone and joint cancers and osteosarcomas in the Surveillance, Epidemiology and End Results (SEER) Program. *Review of Fluoride: Benefits and Risk, DHHS* (Feb 1991): F1-F7.

[122] Cohn PD. A Brief Report on the Association of Drinking Water Fluoridation and the Incidence of Osteosarcoma among Young Males. New Jersey Department of Health, Trenton, NJ, Nov 1992.

[123] Yiamouyiannis JA. Fluoridation and cancer: the biology and epidemiology of bone and oral cancer related to fluoridation. *Fluoride* 26(1993): 83-96.

[124] Grandjean P, et al. Cancer incidence and mortality in workers exposed to fluoride. *Journal of National Cancer Institute* 84(1992): 1903-1909.

[125] Klein W, et al. DNA repair and environmental substances. Report of the Austrian Society of Atomic Energy, Seiberdorf Research Center, 2613(1976), pp 1-9.

[126] Aardema MJ, et al. Sodium fluoride-induced chromosomal aberrations in different stages of the cell cycle: a proposed mechanism. *Mutation Research* 223(1989): 191-203.

[127] Anuradha CD, Kanno S and Hirano S. Fluoride induces apoptosis by caspase-3 activation in human leukemia HL-60 cells. *Arch Toxicol* 74(2000): 226-230.

[128] Meng ZQ, Zhang B. Chromosomal aberrations and microneuclei in lymphocytes of workers at a phosphate fertilizer factory. *Mutation Research-Genetic Toxicology and Environmental Mutagenesis.* 393(1997): 283-288.

[129] Takahashi K. Fluoride-linked Down syndrome births and their estimated occurrence due to water fluoridation. *Fluoride* 31(1998): 61-73, 1998.

[130] Danielson C, et al. Hip fractures in Utah's elderly population. *JAMA* 268(1992): 746-748. This study is important because the Mormon group avoided practices that might influence the results of other studies, such as smoking and drinking alcohol.

[131] Sowers MR, Clark MK, et al. A prospective study of bone mineral content and fracture in communities with differential fluoride exposure. *A J Epidem* 133(1991): 649-660.

[132] Rueqserrer P, Rueqserrer E, et al. Natural causes of osteoporosis and fluoride therapy: a longitudinal study using quantitative computed tomography. (Abstract) *J Comput Assist Tomogr* 9(1985): 626-627.

[133] Dure-Smith BA, et al. Calcium deficiency in fluoride-treated osteoporotic patients despite calcium supplementation. *J Endocrinol Metab* 81(1996): 269-275.

[134] Spittle B. Psychopharmacology of fluoride: a review. *Inter Nat Clin Psychopharmacol* 9(1994): 79-82.

[135] Rotton J, Tikofsky RS, Feldman HT. Behavioral effects of chemicals in the drinking water. *J Appl Psycho* 67(1982): 230-238.

[136] Li XS, Zhi JL, Gao RO. Effect of fluoride exposure on intelligence in children. *Fluoride* 28(1995): 189-192.

[137] Mullenix PJ, Denbesten PK, Schunior A, Kernan WJ. Neurotoxicity of sodium fluoride in rats. *Neurotoxicology and Teratology* 17(1995): 169-177.

[138] Ekstrand J. Pharmacokinetic aspect of topical fluoride. *J Dental Research* 66(1987): 1061-1065.

[139] Whitford GM, Pashley DH, Reynolds KE. Fluoride tissue distribution: Short-term kinetics. *Am J Physiol* 236(1979): F141-F148.

[140] Varner JA, Jenson KF, et al. Chronic administration of aluminum-fluoride or sodium-fluoride to rats in drinking water: Alterations in neuronal and cerebrovascular integrity. *Brain Research* 784(1998): 284-298.

[141] Wang Y, Guan Z, Xiao K. Changes of coenzyme Q content in the brain tissues of rats with fluorosis. *Chang Hua Yu Fang Tsa Chih* 31(1997): 330-333.

[142] van der Voet GB, Schijns O, de Wolf FA. Fluoride enhances the effect of aluminum chloride on interconnections between aggregates of hippocampal neurons. *Arch Physiol Biochem* 107(1999): 15-21.

[143] Guan ZZ, Wang YN, et al. Influence of chronic fluorosis on membrane lipids in rat brain. *Neurotoxicol Teratol* 20(1998): 537-542. The most drastically affected were phosphotidylethanolamine, phosphotidylserine and phosphotidylcholine.

[144] Yiamouyiannis, John. *Fluoride the Aging Factor: How to Recognize and Avoid the Devastating Effects of Fluoride.*. Delaware, OH: Health Action Press, 1993 (3rd ed), p 92.

[145] Hodge H. The safety of fluoride tablets or drops, continuing evaluation of the use of fluorides. AAAS Symposium, Boulder, Co: Westview Press, 1979, p 253.

[146] Bobek S, Kahl S, Ewy Z. Effect of long-term fluoride administration on thyroid hormone levels in rats. *Endocrinol Exp* 10(1976): 289-295.

[147] Zhao W, Zhu H, et al. Long-term effects of various iodine and fluorine doses on the thyroid and fluorosis in mice. *Endoc Regu* 32(1998): 63-70.

[148] Matthesis P. Thyroid disease in Down's syndrome: Clinical perspectives, and directions of research. Originally presented at the 2nd International Symposium on Biomedical and Psychoeducational Aspects of Down's Syndome, Mexico City, April 24, 1997.

[149] Chinoy NJ, Sharma A. Amelioration of fluoride toxicity by vitamins E and D in reproductive functions of male mice. *Fluoride* 31(1998): 203-216.

[150] Chinoy NJ , Sequeira E. Effects of fluoride on the histoarchitecture of reproductive organs of the male mouse. *Reproductive Toxicology* 3(1989): 261-267.

[151] Messer HH, Armstrong WD, Singer L. Fertility impairment in mice on a low fluoride intake. *Science* 177(1972): 893-894.

[152] Bastiat F. *Selected Essays on Political Economy*. Irvington-on-Hudson: Foundation for Economic Education, 1964.

[153] Heller KE, Eklund SA, Burt BA. Dental caries and dental fluorosis at varying water fluoride concentrations. *J Pub Health Dent* 57(1997): 136-143.

Chapter 5
Other Toxic Metals to Avoid

[154] Sherlin DMG, Verma RJ. Vitamin D ameliorates fluoride-induced embryotoxicity in pregnant rats. *Neurotoxicology and Teratology* 23(2001): 197-201.

[155] Phil RD, Parkes M. Hair element content in learning disabled children. *Science* 198(1977): 205-206.

[156] Marlowe M, Errera J, Jacobs J. Increased lead and cadmium burdens among mentally retarded children and children with borderline intelligence. *Am J Men Def* 87(1983): 477-483.

[157] Thatcher RW, Lester ML, et al. Effects of low levels of cadmium and lead on cognitive functioning in children. *Arch Environ Health* 37(1982): 159-166.

[158] Mederiros DM, Pellum LK. Elevation of cadmium, lead, and zinc in the hair of adult black female hypertensives. *Bull Environ Contam Toxicol* 32(1984): 525-532. Borgman RF, Lightsey SF, Roberts WR. Hair element concentrations and hypertension in South Carolina. *Roy Soc Health J* 101(1982): 1-2.

[159] Dally S, Maury P, et al. Blood cadmium level and hypertension in humans. *Clin Toxicol* 13(1978): 403-409.

[160] Waalkes MP, Rehm S, et al. Cadmium exposure in rats and tumors of the prostate. *IARC Scientific* 118(1992): 391-400.

[161] Frery N, Nessmann C, et al. Environmental exposure to cadmium and human birthweight. *Toxicology* 79(1993): 109-118.

[162] Such as inhibiting basal adenylate cyclase activity in the cerebellum, cerebrum and brainstem, and by altering cell membrane formation, especially in the synapses.

[163] Goldstein GW. Neurologic concepts of lead poisoning in children. *Ped Ann* 21(1992): 384-388.

[164] Rice D. Developmental Lead exposure. Neurobehavioral Consequences. In *Handbook of Developmental Neurotoxicology*. Slikker W, Chang LW (eds). San Diego: Academic Press, 1998, pp 539-557.

[165] Mushak P, Davis JM, et al. Prenatal and postnatal effects of low level lead exposure: integrated summery of a report to the US Congress on childhood lead poisoning. *Env Res* 50(1989): 11-36. Winneke G, Altmann L, et al. Neurobehavioral and neuropsychological observations in six-year-old children with low lead levels in East and West Germany. *Neurotoxicology* 15(1994): 705-714.

[166] Kuhn W, Winkel R, et al. High prevalence of parkinsonim after occupational exposure to lead-sulfate batteries. *Neurology* 50(1998): 1885-1886.

[167] Altmann L, Weinberg F, et al. Impairment of long-term potentiation and learning following chronic lead exposure. *Toxicology Letters* 66(1993): 105-112.

[168] Bradbury MWB, Deane R. Permeability of the blood-brain barrier to lead. *Neurotoxicology* 14(1993): 131-136. Fluoride and chorine enhance the absorption of lead into the brain, and calcium, EDTA and N-acetyl-L-cysteine inhibit its uptake by the brain. Simons, TJB. The role of anion transport in the passive movement of lead across the human red cell membrane. *J Physiology* 378(1986): 287-312.

[169] Markovac J, Goldstein GW. Picomolar concentrations of lead stimulate brain protein kinase C. *Nature* 334(1988): 71-73. Protein Kinase C activation occurs at a concentraton as low as 10^{-5} M.

[170] Naarla JT, Loikkanen JJ, et al. Lead amplifies glutamate-induced oxidative stress. *Free Radical Biology and Medicine* 19(1995): 689-693.

[171] Nevin R. How lead exposure relates to temporal changes in IQ, violent crime, and unwed pregnancy. *Environ Res* 83(2000): 1-22.

[172] Tang HW, Huel G, et al. Neurodevelopmental evaluation of 9-month-old infants exposed to low levels of lead in utero: involvement of monoamine neurotransmitters. *J Appl Toxicol* 19(1999): 167-172.

[173] Bellinger D, Needleman HL, et al. A follow-up study of academic attainment and classroom behavior of children with elevated dentine lead levels. *Biol Trace Element Res* 6(1984): 207-223.

[174] Bellinger D, Leviton A, et al. Pre and Postnatal lead exposure and behavioral problems in school aged children. *Environ Res* 66(1994): 12-30.

[175] Sciarillo W, Alexander A, and Farrell K. Lead exposure and child behavior. *Am J Public Health* 82(1992): 1356-1360.

[176] Yiin LM, Rhoads GG, Lioy PJ. Seasonal influences on childhood lead exposure. *Environ Health Perspect* 108(2000): 177-182.

[177] Cremin JD Jr, Luck ML, Laughlin NK, Smith DR. Efficacy of succimer for reducing brain lead in a primate model of human lead exposure. *Toxicology Applied Pharmacology* 161(1999): 283-293.

[178] Soldatovic D, Vujanovic D, Matovic V, Plamenac Z. Compared effects of high oral magnesium and of EDTA chelating agent on chronic lead intoxication in rabbits. *Magnesium Research* 10(1997): 127-133.

[179] Markesbery WR, Ehmann WD. Brain Trace Elements in Alzheimer's Disease. In *Alzheimer's Disease*. Terry RD, Katzman R, Bick KL (eds). New York: Raven Press, Ltd, 1994, pp 353-367.

[180] Bondy SC, Guo-Ross SX, Pien J. Mechanisms underlying the aluminum-induced potentiation of the pro-oxidant properties of transition metals. *Neurotoxicology* 19(1998): 65-71.

[181] Ibid

[182] Verstraeten SV, Golub MS, et al. Myelin is a preferential target of aluminum-mediated oxidative damage. *Arch Biochem Biophys* 15(1997): 289-294.

[183] Jones DL, Kochian LV, et al. Aluminum interaction with plasma membrane lipids and enzyme metal binding sites and its potential role in Al cytotoxicity. *FEBS Lett* 400(1997): 51-57. This is true for the enzymes enolase, pyruvate kinase, ATPase, myosin, calpain, proteinase K, phospholipase A$_2$ and arginase.

[184] Coburn JW, Mischel MG, et al. Calcium citrate markedly enhances aluminum absorption from aluminum hydroxide. *Am J Kidney Dis* 17(1991): 708-711.

[185] Allain P, Gauchard F, et al. Enhancement of aluminum digestive absorption by fluoride in rats. *Res Commun Mol Pathol Pharmacol* 91(1996): 225-231.

[186] Deng Z, Coudray C, et al. Effect of acute and chronic coingestion of ALCl3 with citrate or polyphenolic acids on tissue retention and distribution of aluminum in rats. *Biol Trace Elem Res* 76(2000): 245-256.

[187] Crapper DR, Krishman SS, et al. Brain aluminum distribution in Alzheimer's disease and experimental neurofibrillary degeneration. *Science* 180(1973): 511-513.

[188] Xu N, Majidi V, et al. Determination of aluminum in human brain tissue by GF-AAS. *J Anal Atomic Spec* (1992): 749-751. This study found aluminum levels of 3.83 ug/g in the inferior parietal lobule of the Alzheimer's patients' brains compared to a level of 1.70ug/g in normal brains matched for age. Similar differences were found in the other areas of the brain normally damaged by Alzheimer's disease.

[189] Markesbery WR, Ehmann WD. Brain Trace Elements in Alzheimer's Disease. In *Alzheimer's Disease.* Terry RD, Katzman R, Bick KL (eds). New York: Raven Press, Ltd, 1994, pp 353-386.

[190] Yumoto S, Kakimi S, et al. Demonstration of Aluminum in the Brain of Patients with Alzheimer's Disease. In *Progress in Alzheimer's and Parkinson's Diseases.* Fisher, et al, (eds). New York: Plenum Press, 1998, pp 293-300.

[191] Jones KR, Black MJ, Oorschot DE. Do aluminum and/or glutamate induce Alzheimer's PHF-like formation? An electron microscopic study. *J Neurocytol* 27(1998): 59-68.

[192] Savory J, Huang Y, et al. Reversal by desferrioxamine of tau protein aggregates following two days of treatment in aluminum-induced neurofibrillary degeneration in rabbit: implications for clinical trials in Alzheimer's disease. *Neurotoxicology* 19(1998): 209-214.

[193] Bouras C, Giannakopoulos P, et al. A laser microprobe mass analysis of brain aluminum and iron in dementia pugilistica: comparison with Alzheimer's disease. *Eur Neurol* 38(1997): 53-58.

[194] Cambell A, Hamai D, Bondy SC. Differential toxicity of aluminum salts in human cells lines of neural origin: implications for neurodegeneration. *Neurotoxicology* 22(2001): 63-71.

[195] Yoshida S, Mitani K, et al. Bunina body formation in amyotrophic lateral sclerosis: a morphological-statistical and trace element study featuring aluminum. *J Neurol Sci* 130(1995):88-94. The aluminum accumulated near the intracellular inclusion body for the disease called a Bunina body, as well as the endoplasmic reticulum. It was proposed that the aluminum, in the face of low magnesium levels, caused the DNA to malfunction near the endoplasmic reticulum.

[196] Kasarskis EJ, Tandon L, et al. Aluminum, calcium, and iron in the spinal cord of patients with sporadic amyotrophic lateral sclerosis using laser microprobe mass spectrometer: a preliminary study. *J Neurol Sci* 130(1995): 203-208.

[197] Wakayama I, Nerurkar VR, et al. Comparative study of chronic aluminum-induced neurofilamentous aggregates with intracytoplasmic inclusions of amyotrophic lateral sclerosis. *Acta Neuropathol (Berl)* 92(1996): 545-554.

[198] Tanridag T, Coskun T, et al. Motor neuron degeneration due to aluminum deposition in the spinal cord: a light microscopical study. *Acta Histochem* 101(1999): 193-201.

[199] Yasui M, Ota K. Aluminum decreases the magnesium concentration of spinal and trabecular bone in rats fed a low calcium, high aluminum diet. *J Neurolog Sci* 15(1998): 37-41.

[200] Sarin S, Gupta V, Gill KD. Alterations in lipid composition and neuronal injury in primates following chronic aluminum exposure. *Biol Trace Elem Res* 59(1997): 133-143. These enzymes include Na+ K+ ATPase, acetyl-cholinesterase and 2',3'-cyclic nucleotide phosphohydrolase.

[201] Szutowicz A, Bielarczyk H, et al. Effects of aluminum and calcium on acetyl-CoA metabolism in rat brain mitochondria. *J Neurochem* 71(1998): 2447-2453.

[202] Kumar S. Biphasic effect of aluminum on cholinergic enzymes of rat brain. *Neurosci Lett* 248(1998): 121-123.

[203] Francis PT, Cross AJ, Bowen DM. Neurotransmitters and neuropeptides. In *Alzheimer's Disease*. Terry RD, Katzman R, Bick KL (eds). New York: Raven Press, Ltd, 1994, pp 247-261.

[204] Deloncle R, Huguet F, et al. Chronic administration of aluminum L-glutamate in young mature rats: effects on iron levels and lipid peroxidation. *Toxicol Lett* 104(1999): 65-73.

[205] Meglio L, Oteiza PI. Aluminum enhances melanin-induced lipid peroxidation. *Neurochem Res* 24(1999):1001-1008.

[206] Julka D, Gill KD. Effect of aluminum on regional brain antioxidant defense status in Wister rats. *Res Exp Med (Berl)* 196(1996): 187-194.

Chapter 6
The Vaccine Controversy

[207] Miller, Neil Z. *Vaccinations: Are They Really Safe and Effective? A Parent's Guide to Childhood Shots.* Santa Fe, NM: New Atlantean Press, 1999.

[208] Orenstein WA, Heseltine PN, et al. Rubella vaccine and susceptible hospital employees: poor physician participation. *JAMA* 245(1981): 711-713.

[209] Dye, Michael. *Vaccinations: Deceptions and Tragedy.* NC: Hallelujah Acres, 1999.

[210] Beck MA. The influence of antioxidant nutrients on viral infection. *Nutr Rev* 56(1998): S140-S146.

Chapter 7
Food Additives That Can Kill: The Taste That Kills

[211] Lucas DR, Newhouse JP. The toxic effect of sodium L-glutamate on the inner layers of the retina. *Archives of Ophthalmology* 58(1957): 193-201.

[212] Olney JW. Brain lesions, obesity and other disturbances in mice treated with monosodium glutamate. *Science* 165(1969): 719-721.

[213] Seal RP, Amara SG. Excitatory amino acid transporters: a family in flux. *Annual Review of Pharmacology and Toxicology* 39(1999): 431-456.

[214] Thurston JH, Warren SK. Permeability of the blood-brain barrier to monosodium glutamate and effects on the components of the energy reserve in newborn mouse brains. *Journal of Neurochemistry* 18(1971): 2241-2244.

[215] Zuccarello M, Anderson DK. Interaction between free-radicals and excitatory amino acids in the blood-brain barrier disruption after iron injury in the rat. *Journal of Neurotrauma* 10(1993): 397-403. Elovaara I, Palo J, et al. Serum and cerebrospinal fluid proteins and the blood-brain barrier in Alzheimer's disease and multi-infarct dementia. *European Neurology* 26(1987): 229-234. Gupta A, Agarwal R, Shukla GS. Functional impairment of blood-brain barrier following pesticide exposure during early development in rats. *Human and Experimental Toxicology* 18(1999): 174-179. Mooradian AD. Effect of aging on the blood-brain barrier. *Neurobiology of Aging* 9(1988): 31-39.

[216] Isokawa M, Levesque MF. Increased NMDA responses and dendritic degeneration in human epileptic neurons in slices. *Neuroscience Letters* 132(1991): 212-216.

[217] Pellegrini-Giampietro DE, Cherici G, Alesiani M, et al. Excitatory amino acid release and free-radical formation may cooperate in the genesis of ischemia-induced neuronal damage. *The Journal of Neuroscience* 10(1990): 1035-1041.

[218] Choudhary P, Malik VP, Puri S, Ahluwalia P. Studies on the effects of monosodium glutamate on hepatic microsomal lipid peroxidation, calcium, ascorbic acid and glutathione and its dependent enzymes in adult male mice. *Toxicology Letters* 89(1996): 71-76.

[219] Halliwell B, Gutteridge JMC. *Free Radicals in Biology and Medicine.* (3rd ed.) Oxford University Press, 1999, pp 156-158.

[220] Olanow CW. A radical hypothesis for neurodegeneration. *Trends in Neurosciences* 16(1993): 439-444. Han D, Sen CK, Roy S, et al. Protection against glutamate-induced cytotoxicity in C6 glial cells by thiol antioxidants. *American Journal Physiology* 273(1997): R1771-R1778.

[221] Alante A, Calissano P, Bobba A, et al. Glutamate neurotoxicity, oxidative stress and mitochondria. *FEBS Letters* 497(2001): 1-5.

[222] Montal M. Mitochondria, glutamate neurotoxicity and the death cascade. *Biochemistry, Biophysics Acta* 1366(1998): 113-126. Henneberry RC, Novelli A, Cox JA, Lysco PG. Neurotoxicity at the N-methyl-D-Aspartate receptor in energy-compromised neurons. *Annals of the New York Academy of Science* 568(1989): 225-233.

[223] Perros P, Deary IJ, et al. Brain abnormalities demonstrated by magnetic resonsance imaging in adult IDDM patients with and without a history of recurrent severe hypoglycemia. *Diabetes Care* 20(1997): 1013-1018.

[224] Matthews RT, Yang L, et al. Coenzyme Q10 administration increases brain mitochondrial concentrations and exerts neuroprotective effects. *Proc Natl Acad Sci* 95(1998): 8892-8897.

[225] Michaelis EK. Two different families of NMDA receptors in mammalian brain: physiological function and role in neuronal development and degeneration. *Advances in Medicine and Biology* 341(1993): 119-128.

[226] Bar-Peled O, Ben-Hur H, et al. Distribution of glutamate transporter subtypes during human brain development. *Journal of Neurochemistry* 69(1997): 2571-2580.

[227] Frieder B, Grimm VE. Prenatal glutamate causes long-lasting cholinergic and adrenergic changes in various brain regions. *J Neurochemistry* 48(1987): 1359-1365.

[228] Olney JW. Excitatory neurotoxins as food additives: an evaluation of risk. *Neurotoxicology* 2(1980): 163-192.

[229] Klingberg H, et al. Long-term effects on behavior after postnatal treatment with monosodium L-glutamate. *Biomed Biochem Acta* 46(1987): 705-711.

[230] Yu T, Zhao Y, Shi W, et al. Effects of maternal oral administration of monosodium glutamate at a late stage of pregnancy on developing mouse fetal brain. *Brain Research* 747(1997): 195-206.

[231] FASEB Report on Safety of Monosodium Glutamate. 1995.

[232] Carter LT, Levesque L. Monosodium glutamate-induced changes of aggression and open-field activity in rats. *Neurobehavioral Toxicology* 1(1979): 247-251.

[233] Blaylock RL. Neuropharmacology as a long-range strategic war policy. *Medical Sentinel* 7(2001): 10-15.

[234] Karler R, Calder LD. Excitatory amino acids and the actions of cocaine. *Brain Research* 582(1992): 143-146. Cador M, Bjijou Y, Cailhol S, Stinus L. D-amphetamine-induced behavioral sensitization: implication of a glutamatergic medial prefrontal cortex-ventral tegmental area innervation. *Neuroscience* 94(1999): 705-721. Wolf ME, Xue CJ.Amphetamine-induced glutamate efflux in the rat ventral tegmental area is prevented by MK-801, SCH 23390, and ibotenic acid lesions of the prefrontal cortex. *J Neurochemistry* 73(1999): 1529-1538.

[235] Bunyan J, Elspeth A, Murrell A, Shah PP. The induction of obesity in rodents by means of monosodium glutamate. *British Journal of Nutrition* 35(1976): 25-39.

[236] Kanarek RB, Marks-Kaufman R. Increased carbohydrate consumption induced by neonatal administration of monosodium glutamate to rats. *Neurobehavioral Toxicology Teratology* 3(1981): 343-350.

[237] Nikoletseas MM. Obesity in exercising, hypophagic rats treated with monosodium glutamate. *Physiology & Behavior* 19(1977): 767-773.

[238] Iwase M, Yamamoto M, et al. Obesity induced by neonatal monosodium glutamate treatment in spontaneous hypertensive rats. An animal model of multiple risk factors. *Hypertensive Research* 21(1998): 1-6.

[239] Vaarala O, Knip M, Paronen J, et al. Cow's milk formula feeding induces primary immunization to insulin in infants at genetic risk for type 1 diabetes. *Diabetes* 48(1999): 1389-1394.

[240] A good review is to be found in *Nutrition Reviews*. Vol 58 No. 3, March 2000.

[241] Blaylock, RL. *Excitotoxins: The Taste That Kills*. Health Press, 1997.

[242] Fuster JM. The prefrontal cortex-an update: Time is of the essence. *Neuron* 30(2001): 319-333.

[243] Gill SS, Pulido OM. Glutamate receptors in peripheral tissues: current knowledge, future research, and implications for toxicology. *Toxicol Pathology* 29(2001): 208-223.

[244] Natelson BH, Chang Q. Sudden Death. A neurocardiac phenomenon. In *Neurology Clinics*. Brillman J (ed). Philadelphia, May 1993, WB Saunders Company. Pp 293-308.

[245] Oida K, Nakai T, Hayashi T, et al. Plasma lipoproteins of monosodium glutamate-induced obese rats. *International J Obstetrics* 8(1984): 385-391.

[246] Kim YW, Kim JY, Lee SK. Surgical removal of visceral fat decreases plasma free fatty acid and increases insulin sensitivity on liver and peripheral tissues in monosodium glutamate (MSG)-obese rats. *Journal Korean Medical Science* 14(1999): 539-545.

[247] Smith JD, Terpening CM, Schmidt SO, Gums JJG. Relief of fibromyalgia symptoms following discontinuation of dietary excitotoxins. *Annals Pharmacotherapy* 35(2001): 702-706.

[248] Ren K, Williams GM, Hylden JLK, et al. The intrathecal administration of excitatory amino acid receptor antagonist selectively attenuated carrageenan-induced behavioral hyperalgesia in rats. *Journal of Pharmacology* 219(1992): 234-243.

[249] Gill SS, Pulido OM. Glutamate receptors in peripheral tissues: current knowledge, future research, and implications for toxicology. *Toxicol Pathol* 29(2001): 208-223.

[250] Lin JY, Pan JT. Single-unit activity of dorsomedial arcuate neurons and diurnal changes of tuberoinfundibular dopaminergic neuron activity in female rats with neonatal monosodium glutamate treatment. *Brain Research Bulletin* 48(1999): 103-108. Maiter D, Underwood LE, et al. Neonatal treatment with monosodium glutamate:

effects of prolonged growth hormone (GH)-releasing hormone deficiency on pulsatile GH secretion and growth in female rats. *Endocrinology* 128(1991): 1100-1106.

[251] Van Den Pol AN, Wuarin J-P, Dudek FE. Glutamate, the dominant excitatory transmitter in neuroendocrine regulation. *Science* 250(1990): 1276-1278.

[252] Nemeroff CB, Lamartiniere CA, Mason GA, et al. Marked reduction in gonadal steroid hormone levels in rats treated neonatally with monosodium L-glutamate: further evidence for disruption of hypothalamic-pituitary-gonadal axis regulation. *Neuroendocrinology* 33(1981): 265-267. Miskowlak B, Limanowski A, Partyka M. Effect of perinatal administration of monosodium glutamate (MSG) on the reproductive system of the male rat. *Endokrynol Pol* 44(1993): 497-505.

[253] Miskowiak B, Kesa B, Limanowski A, et al. Long-term effect of neonatal monosodium glutamate (MSG) treatment on reproductive system of the female rat. *Folia Morphol (Warz)* 58(1999): 105-113.

Macho L, Jezova D, et al. Postnatal monosodium glutamate treatment results in attenuation of corticosterone metabolic rate in adults rats. *Endocrine Regulation* 33(1999): 61-67. Miskowiak B, Partyka M. Effect of neonatal treatment with MSG (monosodium glutamate) on thyroid of the adult male rats. *Histology and Histopathology* 14(1999): 63-67.

[254] Hsieh Y-L, Hsu C, Lue S-I, et al. The neonatal neurotoxicity of monosodium L-glutamate on the sexually dimorphic nucleus of the preoptic area of rats. *Neuroscience* 19(1997): 342-347.

[255] Skuletyova I, Kiss A, Jezova D. Neurotoxic lesions induced by monosodium glutamate result in increased adrenopituitary proopiomelanocortin gene expression and decreased corticosterone clearance in rats. *Neuroendocrinology* 67(1998): 412-420.

[256] Didier M, et al. Chronic glutamate toxicity causes DNA damage. *Neurol* 44(1994): A236.

[257] Raz A, Levine G, Khomiak Y. Acute local inflammation potentiates tumor growth in mice. *Cancer Letters* 148(2000): 115-120.

[258] Neurotransmitter may promote brain tumor growth. *Cancer Watch* 10(Sept. 2001): 140-141.

[259] Kato K, Hamada N, et al. Depression of delayed-type hypersensitivity in mice with hypothalamic lesion induced by monosodium glutamate: involvement of neuroendocrine system in immunomodulation. *Immunology* 58(1986): 389-395.

[260] Vowerk CK, Gorla MS, Dreyer EB. An experimental basis for implicating excitotoxicity in glaucomatous optic neuropathy. *Survey Ophthalmology* 43(1999): S142-S150.

[261] Kowluru RA, Engerman RL, Case GL, Kern TS. Retinal glutamate in diabetes and effect of antioxidants. *Neurochemistry International* 38(2001): 385-390.

[262] Olney JW. The toxic effects of glutamate and related compounds in the retina and the brain. *Retina* 2(1982): 341-359.

[263] Blaylock RL. Food additive excitotoxins and degenerative brain disorders. *Medical Sentinel 4* 6(1999): 212-215.

[264] Blaylock RL. Phytonutrients and metabolic stimulants as protection against neurodegeneration and excitotoxicity. *Journal of the American Nutraceutical Association* 2(2000): 30-39.

[265] Saito K, Markey SP, Heyes MP. Effects of immune activation on quinolinic acid and neuroactive kynurenines in the mouse. *Neuroscience* 51(1992): 25-39.

[266] Beal MF, Bradley T, Koroschetz HW. Do defects in mitochondrial energy metabolism underlie the pathology of neurodegenerative disease? *Trends in Neurosciences* 16(1993): 125-131.

[267] Blaylock RL. Neurodegeneration and aging of the central nervous system: Prevention and treatment by phyto-chemicals and metabolic nutrients. *Integrative Medicine* 1(1998): 117-133.

[268] Jagust WJ, Seab JP, Huesman RH, et al. Diminished glucose transport in Alzheimer's disease: Dynamic PET studies. *Journal of Cerebral Blood Flow and Metabolism* 11(1991): 323-330.

[269] Hoyer S. Abnormalities of glucose metabolism in Alzheimer's disease. *Annals New York Academy of Science* 640(1991): 53-58.

[270] Breitner JCS. Inflammatory processes and anti-inflammatory drugs in Alzheimer's disease: A current appraisal. *Neurobiology of Aging* 17(1996): 789-794.

[271] Zaman Z, Roche S, Frost PG, et al. Plasma concentrations of vitamins A and E and Carotenoids in Alzheimer's disease. *Age and Aging* 21(1992): 91-94.

[272] Wei JY. Age and the cardiovascular system. *New England Journal of Medicine* 327(1992): 1735-1739.

[273] Kashii KM, Honda Y, Tamura Y, et al. Protective effects of methylcobalamin, a vitamin B12 analog, against glutamate-induced neurotoxicity in retinal cell culture. *Invest Opthalmol Visual Science* 38(1997): 848-854.

[274] Ruiz F, Alvarez G, Pereira R, et al. Protection by pyruvate and malate against glutamate-mediated neurotoxici-ty. *Neuroreport* 9(1998): 1277-1282.

[275] Muller U, Krieglstein J. Prolonged pretreatment with alpha-lipoic acid protects cultured neurons against hypox-ic, glutamate, or iron-induced injury. *Journal of Cerebral Blood Flow and Metabolism* 15(1995): 624-630.

[276] Beal MF, et al. Coenzyme Q10 and nicianamide are neuroprotective against mitochondrial toxins in vivo. *Neurology Suppl* 2(1994): A177.

[277] Petanceska SS, Nagy V, Frail D, Gandy S. Ovariectomy and 17ß-estradiol modulate the levels of Alzheimer's amalyoid ß peptides in brain. *Neurology* 54(2000): 2212-2217.

[278] Skaper SD, Facci L, Kee WJ, Strijbos PJ. Potentiation by histamine of synaptically mediated excitotoxicity in cultured hippocampal neurons: a possible role for mast cells. *Journal of Neurochemistry* 76(2001): 47-55.

[279] Katoh Y, Niimi M, Yamamoto Y, et al. Histamine production by cultured microglial cells in the mouse. *Neuroscience Letters* 305(2001): 181-184.

Chapter 8
Pesticides and Other Chemicals in Our World

[280] Lang L. Are pesticides a problem? *Environmental Health Perspectives* 101(1993): 578-583.

[281] Hartman DE. *Neuropsychological Toxicology, Second Edition* New York: Plenum Press, 1995, p 328.

[282] Coye MJ. The health effects of agricultural productions: The health of the agricultural workers. *Journal of Public Health Policy* 6(1985): 349-370.

[283] He F. Neurotoxic effects of insecticides—current and future research: A review. *Neurotoxicology* 21(2000): 829-836.

[284] Duffy FH and Burchfiel JL. Long term effects of the organophosphate sarin on EEGs in monkeys and humans. *Neurotoxicology* 1(1980): 667-689.

[285] Thrasher JD, Madison R, Broughton A. Immunological abnormalities in humans exposed to chlorpyifod: prelim-inary observations. *Archives of Environmental Health* 48(1993): 89-93.

[286] Livingston JM, Jones CR. Living area contamination by chlordane used for termite treatment. *Bulletin of Environmental Contamination Toxicology* 27(1981): 406-411.

[287] Ahlboom J, Fredricksson A, Ericksson P. Exposure to an organophosphate (DFP) during a definite period in neonatal life induces permanent changes in brain muscarinic receptors and behavior in mice. *Brain Research* 677(1995): 13-19.

[288] Koopman-Esseboom C, Weisglas-Kuperus N, de Ridder MAJ, et al. Effects of polychlorinated biohenyl/dioxin exposure and feeding type on infants' mental and psychomotor development. *Pediatrics* 97(1996): 700-706.

[289] Murray, Michael T. *The Healing Power of Foods*. Rocklin Prima Publishing 1993 p 24.

[290] Bagga D, Anders KH, et al. Organochlorine pesticide content of breast adipose tissue from women with breast cancer and control subjets. *J. National Cancer Institute* 92(2000): 750-753.

[291] He F. Neurotoxic effects of insecticides—current and future research: a review. *Neurotoxicology* 21(2000): 829-836.

[292] Engel LS, Checkoway H, et al. Parkinsonism and occupational exposure to pesticides. *Occup Environ Med* 58(2001): 582-589.

[293] Bhatt MH, Elias MA, Mankodi AK. Acute and reversible parkinsonism due to organophosphate pesticide intoxication: five cases. *Neurology* 52(1999): 1467-1471.

[294] Thacker P. Ecology. A new wind sweeps the plains. *Science* 292(Jul 2001): 2427.

[295] Crinnion WJ. Environmental medicine, Part 4: Pesticides—biologically persistant and ubiquitous toxins. *Alternative Medicine Review* 5(2000): 432-447.

[296] Polifka JE. Drug and Chemical Contaminants in Breast Milk. Effects on Neurodevelopment of the Nursing Infant. In *Handbook of Developmental Neurotoxicology*. Slikker W, Chang LW (eds). San Diego: Academic Press, 1998, pp 383-402.

[297] Eriksson P, Talts V. Neonatal exposure to neurotoxic pesticides increases adult susceptibility: a review of current findings. *Neurotoxicology* 21(2000): 37-47.

Chapter 9
Atherosclerosis: Hardening of the Arteries

[298] Purdey M. High-dose exposure to systemic phosmet insecticide modifies the phosphatidylinositol anchor on the prion protein: the origins of new varient transmissible spongioform encephalopathies? *Medical Hyposthesis* 50(1998): 91-111.

[299] Newman TB, Tulley SB. Carcinogenicity of lipid-lowering drugs. *JAMA* 275(1996): 55-60.

[300] Gold LS, Slone TH, Stern BR, et al. Rodent carcinogens: setting priorities. *Science* 258(1992): 261-265.

[301] Hearn JA, DeMaio SJ, Roubin GS, et al. Predictive value of lipoprotein(a) and other serum lipoproteins in the angiographic diagnosis of coronary artery disease. *American Journal of Cardiology* 66(1990): 1176-1180.

[302] Muhlenstein JB. Chronic infection and coronary artery disease. *Science and Medicine* November/December 1998, 16-25.

[303] Fong IW. Emerging relations between infectious diseases and coronary artery disease and atherosclerosis. *CMAJ* 163(2000): 49-56.

[304] Joshipura KJ, Ascherio A, et al. Fruit and vegetable intake in relation to risk of ischemic stroke. *JAMA* 282(1999): 1233-1239.

[305] Albert CM, Hennenkens CH, et al. Fish consumption and risk of sudden cardiac death. *JAMA* 279(1998): 23-28.

[306] Charnock JS. Omega-3 polyunsaturated fatty acids and ventricular fibrillation: the possible involvement of eicosanoids. *Prostaglandins, Leukotrienes and Essential Fatty Acids* 61 (1999): 243-247.

[307] Daviglus ML, Stampler J, et al. Fish consumption and the 30-year risk of fatal myocardial infarction. *N Eng J Med* 336(1997): 1046-1053.

[308] Green P, Fuchs J, et al. Effects of fish-oil ingestion on cardiovascular risk factors in hyperlipidemic subjects in Israel: a randomized double-blind crossover study. *Am J Clin Nutr* 52(1990): 1118-11124.

[309] Mori TA, Burke V, et al. Purified eicosapentaenoic and docosahexaenoic acid have differential effects on serum lipids and lipoproteins, LDL particle size, glucose and insulin in mildly hyperlipidemic men. *Am J Clin Nutr* 71(2000): 1085-1094.

[310] Bierenbaum ML, Reichstein R, Watkins TR. Reducing atherogenic risk in hyperlipemic humans with flax seed supplementation: a preliminary report. *Journal of the American College of Nutrition* 12(1993): 501-504.

[311] Blair SN, Kohl HW, Barlow MS. Physical activity, physical fitness, and all causes of mortality in women: Do women need to be active? *J Am Coll Nutr* 12(1993): 368-371.

[312] Urho M, Kujala MD, et al. Relationship of leisure-time physical activity and mortality. The Finnish Twin Cohort. *JAMA* 279(1998): 440-444.

[313] Lind K, Tonstad S, et al. Body mass index and patterns of mortality among Seventh-Day Adventists. *Int J Obesity* 15(1991): 397-406.

[314] Lind KD, Tonstad S, Kuzma JW. Self-report of physical activity and patterns of mortality in Seventh-Day Adventist men. *J Clin Epidemiol* 44(1991): 355-364.

Chapter 10
Stroke and Heart Attack: Are They Really Inevitable?

[315] Schmid-Elsaesser R, Zausinger S, Hungerhuber E, et al. Neuroprotective effects of combination therapy with tirilazad and magnesium in rats subjected to reversible focal cerebral ischemia. *Neurosurgery* 44(1999): 163-172.

[316] Steiner M, Glantz M, Lekos A. Vitamin E plus aspirin compared with aspirin alone in patients with transient ischemic attacks. *Am J Clin Nutr* 62(1995): 1381S-1384S.

[317] Bourgain RH, Andries R, Braquet P. Effect of Ginkgolide PAF-acether antagonist on arterial thrombosis. *Advances in Prostaglandin Thromboxane and Leukotriene Research* 17B(1987): 815-817. Also see, Smith PF, Maclennan K, Darlington CL. The neuroprotective properties of the Ginkgo biloba leaf: a review of the possible relationship to platelet-activating factor (PAF). *Journal of Ethnopharmacology* 50(1996): 131-139.

[318] Noda Y, Anzai K, Mori A, et al. Hydroxyl and superoxide anion radical scavenging activities of natural source antioxidants using computerized JES-FR30 ESR spectrometer system. *Biochemistry Molecular Biology International* 42(1997): 35-44. In this study the greatest scavenging effect was in decreasing order of activity: green tea extract, pycnogenol, Ginkgo biloba extract, and a blend of fruit and vegetable extracts. For the superoxide radical, the order from greatest to least was Ginkgo biloba, pycnogenol, beta-catechin, tea, and the fruit and vegetable blend.

[319] Goldman R, Finkbeiner S. Therapeutic use of magnesium sulfate in selected cases of cerebral ischemia and seizure. *New England Journal of Medicine.* 319(1988): 1224-1225.

[320] Schuschke DA. Dietary copper in the physiology of the microcirculation. *J Nutr* 127(1997): 2274-2281.

[321] Calvani M, Arrigoni-Martelli E. Attenuation by acetyl-L-carnitine of neurological damage and biochemical derangement following brain ischemia and reperfusion. *In J Tissue React* 21(1999): 1-6.

[322] Ayoub IA, Lee EJ, et al. Nicotinamide reduces infarction up to two hours after the onset of permanent focal cerebral ischemia in Wistar rats. *Neurosci Lett* 259(1999): 21-24.

[323] Gomez MN. Magnesium and cardiovascular disease. *Anesthesiology* 89(1998): 222-240.

[324] Rimm EB, Stampfer MJ. Antioxidants for vascular disease. *Medical Clinics of North America* 84(2000): 239-249.

[325] Folkers K, Vadhanavikit S, Mortensen SA. Biochemical rationale and myocardial tissue data on the effective therapy of cardiomyopathy with coenzyme Q10. *Proceeding of the National Academy of Sciences* 82(1985): 901-904.

[326] Folkers K, Littarru GP, Ho L, et al. Evidence for a deficiency of coenzyme Q10 in human heart disease. *International Journal of Vitamin Research* 40(1970): 380-390.

[327] Soja AM, Mortensen SA. Treatment of congestive heart failure with coenzyme Q10 illuminated by meta-analysis of clinical trials. *Molecular Aspects of Medicine* 18 suppl(1997): S159-S168.

[328] Baggio E, et al. Italian multicenter study on the safety and efficacy on coenzyme Q10 as adjunctive therapy in heart failure. *Mol Aspects Med* 15 supp (1994):C287-294.

[329] Nohr D, Bowry VW, Stocker R. Dietary supplementation with coenzyme Q10 results in increased levels of circulating lipoproteins and increased resistance of human low-density lipoprotein to the initiation of lipid peroxidation. *Biochem Biophys ACTA* 1126(1992): 247.

[330] Alleva R, Tomasetti M, Battino M, Curatola G, Littarru GP, Folkers K. The roles of coenzyme Q10 and vitamin E on the peroxidation of human low density lipoprotein subfractions. *Proc Natl Acad Sci USA* 92(1995): 9388-9391.

[331] Vary TC, Neely JR. Sodium dependence of carnitine transport in isolated perfused adult rat hearts. *American Journal of Physiology* 244(1983): H247.

[332] Tripp ME, Shug AL. Plasma carnitine concentrations in cardiomyopathy patients. *Biochemistry Medicine* 32(1984): 199.

[333] Feldman AM, Waber LJ, DeMent SH, et al. Plasma carnitine levels in adults with dilated cardiomyopathy. *Heart Failure* 3(1987): 39.

[334] Pierpont MEM, Judd D, Goldberg IF, et al. Myocardial carnitine in end-stage congestive heart failure. *American Journal of Cardiology* 64(1989): 56.

[335] Gottlieb SS, et al. Prognostic importance of serum magnesium concentration in patients with congestive heart failure. *J Am Coll Cardiol Failure* 16(1990): 827-831.

[336] Gueux E, Mazur A, et al. Magnesium deficiency affects plasma lipoprotein composition in rats. *Minerals Trace Elem* 514(1991): 222-228.

[337] Chang C, Varghese J, et al. Magnesium deficiency and myocardial infarct size in the dog. *J Am Coll Cardiol* 5(1985): 280-289.

[338] Teo K, Yusuf S, et al. Effects of intravenous magnesium in suspected acute myocardial infarction. Overview of randomized trials. *MJ* 303(1991): 1499-1503.

[339] Altura BM, Carella A, Turlapaty PD. Hypomagnesmia and vasoconstriction: possible relationship to etiology of sudden death, ischemic heart disease and hypertensive vascular diseases. *Artery* 9(1981): 212-231.

[340] Kafka H, Langevin R, Armstrong PW. Serum magnesium and potassium in acute myocardial infarction. *Arch Internal Medicine* 147(1987): 465-469.

[341] Gertz S, Wajnberg R, Kurgan A, et al. Effect of magnesium sulfate on thrombus formation following partial arterial constriction: Implications for coronary vasospasm. *Magnesium* 6(1987): 225-235.

[342] Dickens BF, et al. Magnesium deficiency in vitro enhances free-radical-induced intracellular oxidation and cytotoxicity in endothelial cells. *Federation of the European Biochemical Society* 311(1992): 187-191.

[343] Kamikawa T, Kobayashi A, Yamashita T, Hayashi H, Yamazaki N. Effects of coenzyme Q10 on exercise tolerance in chronic stable angina pectoris. *Am J Cardiol* 56(1985): 247-251.

[344] Ibid

[345] Koltringer P, Langsteger W, Klima G, et al. Hemorheologic effects of Ginkgo biloba extract Egb 761. Dose-dependent effect of Egb 761 on microcirculation and viscoelasticity of blood. *Forsch Med* 111(1993): 170-172.

[346] Kanowski S, Herrmann WM, Stephan K, et al. Proof of efficacy of the Ginkgo biloba special extract Egb 761 in outpatients suffering from mild to moderate primary degenerative dementia of the Alzheimer type or multi-infarct dementia. *Pharmacopsychiatry* 29(1996): 47-56.

[347] He J, Whelton PK, et al. Aspirin and the risk of hemorrhagic stroke: a meta-analysis of randomized control trials. *JAMA* 280(1998): 1930-1935.

[348] Lianda L, et al. Studies in Hawthorn and its active principle. I Effect on myocardial ischemia and hemodynamics in dogs. *Journal of Traditional Chinese Medicine* 4(1984): 283-288.

[349] Schmidt U, et al. Efficacy of the Hawthorn (Crataegus) preperation LI 132 in 78 patients with chronic congestive heart failure defined as NYHA functional class II. *Phytomedicine* 1(1994): 17-24.

[350] Menotti A, Keys A, et al. Seven Countries Study. First 20-year mortality data in 12 cohorts of six countries. *Ann Med* 21(1989): 175-179.

[351] Ascherio A, Rimm EB, et al. Intake of potassium, magnesium, calcium and fiber and risk of stroke among US men. *Circulation* 98(1998): 1198-1204.

[352] Moran JP, Cohen L, et al. Plasma ascorbic acid concentration relate inversely to blood pressure in human subjects. *Am J Cin Nutr* 57(1993): 213-217.

[353] Grant WB. Milk and other dietary influences on coronary heart disease. *Alter Med Rev* 3(1998): 281-294.

[354] Burr ML, Butland BK. Heart disease in British vegetarians. *A J Clin Nutr* 48(1988): 830-832.

[355] Matthew W, Gillman MD, et al. Protective effects of fruits and vegetables on development of stroke in men. *JAMA* 273(1995): 113-1117.

[356] Yochum L, Kushi LH, et al. Dietary flavonoid intake and risk of cardiovascular disease in postmenopausal women. *Am J Epidemiology* 149(1999): 943-949.

[357] Knekt P, Jarvinen R, et al. Flavonoid intake and coronary mortality in Finland: a cohort study. *BMJ* 312(1996): 478-481.

[358] Arai Y, Watanabe S, et al. Dietary intakes of flavonols, flavones and isoflavones by Japanese women and the inverse correlation between quercetin intake and plasma LDL cholesterol concentration. *J Nutr* 130(2000): 2243-2250. Also see, Kimira M, Arai Y, et al. Japanese intake of flavonoids and isoflavonoids from foods. *J Epidemiology* 8(1998): 168-175.

[359] Singh RB, Niaz MA, et al. Effect on mortality and re-infarction of adding fruits and vegetables to a prudent diet in the Indian Experiment of Infarct Survival (IEIS). *J Am Coll Nutr* 12(1993): 255-261.

[360] Stoll AL. *The Omega-3 Connection.* New York: Simon & Schuster, 2001.

[361] Mozar HN, Bal DG, Farag SA. Human Cancer and the food chain: an alternative etiologic perspective. *Nutrition and Cancer* 12(1989): 29-42.

[362] Cerhan JR, Cantor KP, Williamson K, et al. Cancer mortality among Iowa farmers: recent results, time trends, and lifestyle factors (United States). *Cancer Causes Control* 9(1998): 311-319.

[363] Vaarala O, Knip M, Paronen J, et al. Cow's milk formula feeding induces primary immunization to insulin in infants at genetic risk for type 1 diabetes. *Diabetes* 48(1999): 1389-1394.

[364] Grant WB. Milk and other dietary influences on coronary heart disease. *Alternative Medicine Review* 3(1998): 281-294.

[365] Ferrer JF, Kenyon SJ, Gupta P. Milk of dairy cows frequently contains a leukemogenic virus. *Science* 213(1981): 1014-1016.

[366] Hodgson JM, Puddey IB, et al. Acute effects of ingestion of black and green tea on lipoprotein oxidation. *Am J Clin Nutr* 71(2000): 1103-1107.

[367] Geleijnse JM, Launer LJ, et al. Tea flavonoids may protect against atherosclerosis: The Rotterdam Study. *Arch Intern Med* 159(1999): 2170-2174.

[368] Frankel EN, Kanner J, et al. Inhibition of oxidation of human low-density lipoproteins by phenolic substances in red wine. *Lancet* 341(1993): 454-457.

[369] Fuhrman B, Lavy A, et al. Consumption of red wine with meals reduces the susceptability of human plasma and low density lipoproteins to lipid peroxidation. *Am J Clin Nutr* 61(1995): 549-554.

[370] deRijke YB, Demacker PNM, et al. Red wine consumption does not affect oxidizability of low-density lipoproteins in volunteers. *Am J Clin Nutr* 63(1996): 329-334.

[371] Cook JD, Reddy MB, Hurrell RF. The effect of red and white wine on nonheme-iron absorption in humans. *Am J Clin Nutr* 61(1995): 800-804.

[372] Fitzpatrick DF, Hirschfield SL,et al. Endothelium-dependent vasorelaxing activity of wine and other grape products. *Am J Physiol* 265(1993): H774-H778.

[373] Miksicek RJ. Estrogenic flavonoids: structural requirements for biological activity. *Proc Soc Exp Biol Med* 208(1995): 44-50.

[374] Parodi PW. The French paradox unmasked: the role of folate. *Med Hypothesis* 49(1997): 313-318.

[375] Zierath JR, Wallberg-Henriksson H. Exercise training in obese diabetic patients. Special consideration. *Sports Med* 14(1992): 171-189.

[376] Siow RC, Richards JP, et al. Vitamin C protects vascular smooth muscle cells against apoptosis induced by moderately oxidized LDL containing high levels of lipid hydroperoxides. *Atherosclerosis Thrombosis and Vascular Biology* 19(1999): 2387-2394. Also see, Chambers DJ, Astras G, et al. Free radicals and cardioplegi: organic antioxidants as additives to the St Thomas Hospital Cardioplegic solution. *Cardiovascular Research* 23(1989): 351-358. In this study they found that by adding vitamin C to the postop cardioplegic solution, the recovery of aortic flow increased 70.2 percent and 72.1 percent. Also see, Riemerssma RA, Wood DA, et al. Low plasma vitamin E and C increased risk of angina in Scottish men. *Annals of the New York Academy of Science* 570(1989): 291-295. And finally, Wilkerson IB, Megson IL, et al. Oral vitamin C reduces arterial stiffness and platelet aggregation in humans. *Journal of Cardiovascular Pharmacology* 34(1999): 690-693. Volunteers given vitamin C experienced a significant reduction in augmentation index, a measure of arterial stiffness, and the ADP-induced platelet aggregation, a measure of platelet adhesiveness.

[377] Salonen JT, Nyyssonen K, et al. Antioxidant supplementation in atherosclerosis prevention (ASAP) study: a randomized trial of the effect of vitamins E and C on 3-year progression of carotid atherosclerosis. *Journal of Internal Medicine* 248(2000): 377-386.

[378] May JM. How does ascorbic acid prevent endothelial dysfunction. *Free Radical Biolology and Medicine* 28(2000): 1421-1425.

[379] Losonczy KG, Harris TB, Havlik RJ. Vitamin E and vitamin C supplement use and risk of coronary heart disease mortality in older persons: the Established Populations for Epidemiologic Studies of the Elderly. *American Journal of Clinical Nutrition* 64(1996): 190-196.

[380] Avena R, Arora S, et al. Thiamine (vitamin B_1) protects against glucose- and insulin-mediated proliferation of human infragenicular arterial smooth muscle cells. *Annals of Vascular Surgery* 14(2000): 37-43.

[381] Harjai KJ. Potential new cardiovascular risk factors: left ventricular hypertrophy, homocysteine, lipoprotein (a), triglycerides, oxidative stress, and fibrinogen. *Annals of Internal Medicine* 131(1999): 376-386. Also see Kark JD, Selhub J, Adler B, et al. Nonfasting plasma total homocysteine level and mortality on middle-aged and elderly men and women in Jerusalem. *Annals of Internal Medicine* 131(1999): 321-330.

[382] Josten E, van de Berg A, et al. Metabolic evidence that deficiencies of vitamin B-12 (cobalamin), folate, and vitamin B6 occur commonly in elderly people. *Am J Clin Nutr* 58(1993): 468-476.

[383] Levene CI. The Effect of Maternal Pyridoxine Deficiency on the Development of Atherosclerosis in the Child. In *Life Stress. Volume III of A Companion to The Life Sciences.* Day SB (ed). New York: Van Nostrand Reinhold Company, 1982, pp 238-245.

[384] Ide N, Lau BH. Garlic compounds protect vascular endothelial cells from oxidized low density lipoprotein-induced injury. *Journal of Pharmacology* 49(1997): 908-911.

[385] Steiner M, Lin RS. Changes in platelet function and susceptibility of lipoproteins to oxidation associated with administration of aged garlic extract. *J Cardiovasc Pharmacol* 31(1998): 904-908.

[386] Bordia A, Verma SK, Srivastava KC. Effect of garlic (Allium sativum) on blood lipids, blood sugar, fibrinogen and fribrinolytic activity in patients with coronary artery disease. *Prostaglandins Leukotrienes and Essential Fatty Acids* 58(1998): 257-263.

[387] Koscielny J, Klussendorf D, et al. The antiatherosclerotic effect of Allium sativum. *Atherosclerosis* 144(1999): 237-249.

[388] Das I, Khan NS, Sooranna SR. Potent activation of nitric oxide synthase by garlic: a basis for its therapeutic applications. *Current Research Opinion* 13(1995): 257-263.

[389] Waterhouse AL, Walzem RL. Nutrition of Grape Phenolics. In *Flavonoids in Health and Disease.* Rice-Evans CA, Packer L, Marcel Dekker (eds). New York, 1998, pp 359-385.

[390] Gendre PMJ, Laparra J, et al. Procyanidolic oligomer preventive action on experimental lathyrism in the rat. *Ann Pharmaceutiques Franciases* 43(1985): 61-71.

[391] Heneit JP. Veno-lymphatic insufficiency. 4,729 patients undergoing hormonal and procyanidol oligomer therapy. *Phlebologie* 46(1993): 313-325.

[392] Corbe C, Boissin JP, Siou A. Light vision and choriretinal circulation. Study of the effect of procyanidolic oligomers. *J French Opthamol* 11(1988): 453-460.

[393] Ayoub IA, Lee EJ, Ogilvy CS, et al. Nicotinamide reduces infarction up to two hours after the onset of permanent focal cerebral ischemia in Wister rats. *Neurosci Letts* 259(1999): 21-24.

Chapter 11
Other Disorders of Aging

[394] Yamaguchi Y, Tanaka S, et al. Reduced serum dehydroepiandrosterone levels in diabetic patients with hyperinsulinemia. *Clin Endocrinol* 49(1998): 377-383.

[395] Abbasi F, McLaughlin T, Lammendola C, et al. High carbohydrate diets, triglyceride-rich lipoproteins, and coronary heart disease risk. *American Journal Cardiology* 85(2000): 45-48.

[396] Anderson JW, Gowri MS, Turner J, et al. Antioxidant supplementation effects on low-density lipoprotein oxidation for individuals with type 2 diabetes mellitus. *Journal of the American College of Nutrition* 18(1999): 451-461.

[397] Gisinger C, Jeremy J, Speiser P, et al. Effect of vitamin E supplementation on platelet thromboxane A2 production in type I diabetic patients. *Diabetes* 37(1988): 1260-1264.

[398] Tzeng SH, Ko WC, Ko FN, Teng CM. Inhibition of platelet aggregation by some flavonoids. *Thrombosis Research* 64(1991): 91-100.

[399] Paolisso G, Balbi V, Volpe C, et al. Metabolic benefits deriving from chronic vitamin C supplementation in aged non-insulin dependent diabetics. *Journal of the American College of Nutrition* 14(1995): 387-392.

[400] Anderson JW, Gowri MS, Turner J, et al. Antioxidant supplementation effects on low-density lipoprotein oxidation for individuals with type 2 diabetes mellitus. *Journal of the American College of Nutrition* 18(1999): 451-461.

[401] Rohdewald P. Pycnogenol. In *Flavonoids in Health and Disease*. Rice-Evans CA, Packer L (eds). New York: Marcel Dekker, Inc., 1998, pp 405-419.

[402] Hertzog MGL, Feskens EJM, Hollman PCH, et al. Dietary antioxidant flavonoids and risk of coronary heart disease, The Zutphen Elderly Study. Lancet 342: 1007-1011, 1993.

[403] Samman S, Philippa M, Wall L, Cook N. Flavonoids and coronary heart disease: Dietary perspectives. I, Rice-Evans CA, Packer L (eds). New York: Marcel Dekker, Inc., 1998, pp 469-481.

[404] Hultberg B, Agardh CD, Agardh E, et al. Poor metabolic control, early age at onset, and marginal folate deficiency are associated with increasing levels of plasma homocysteine in insulin-dependent diabetes mellitus. A five-year follow-up study. *Scandanavian Journal of Clinical Laboratory Investigation* 57(1997): 595-600.

[405] Sidhu GS, Singh AK, et al. Enhancement of wound healing by curcumin in animals. *Wound Repair Regeneration* 6(1998): 167-177.

[406] Bloomgarden ZT. Antioxidants and Diabetes. *Diabetes Care* 20(1997): 670-673.

[407] Mayer JH, Tomlinson DR. Prevention of defects of axonal transport and nerve conduction velocity by oral administration of myo-inositol or an aldose reductase inhibitor in streptozotocin-diabetic rats. *Diabetologia* 25(1983): 433-438.

[408] Tutuncu NB, Bayraktar M, Varli K. Reversal of defective nerve conduction with vitamin E supplementation in type 2 diabetes: a preliminary study. *Diabetes Care* 21(1998): 1915-1918.

[409] Sagaram M, Satoh J, Wada R, et al. *Diabetologia* 39(1996): 263-269.

[410] Ziegler D, Gries FA. Alpha lipoic acid in the treatment of diabetic peripheral and cardiac autonomic neuropathy. *Diabetes* 46 suppl 2(1997):62:-66.

[411] Ziegler D, Schatz H, Conrad F, et al. Effects of treatment with the antioxidant alpha-lipoic acid on cardiac autonomic neuropathy in NIDDM patients. A 4-month randomized controlled multicenter trial (DEKAN Study). *Diabetes Care* 20(1997): 369-373.

[412] Van Baak MA, Borghouts LB. Relationships with physical activity. *Nutrition Reviews* 58(2000): S16- S21.

[413] Hotamisligil GD, Spiegelman BM. Tumor necrosis factor-alpha: a key component of the obesity-diabetes link. *Diabetes* 43(1994): 1271-1278. Also see Arner P, Caro JF, et al. Increased adipose tissue expression of tumor necrosis factor-alpha in human obesity and insulin resistance. *Journal of Clinical Investigation* 95(1995): 2409-2415.

[414] Hu Q, Ishii E, Nakagawa Y. Differential changes in relative levels of arachidonic acid in major phospholipids from rat tissues during the progression of diabetes. *Journal of Biochemistry* 115(1994): 405-408. And, Dang AQ, Faas FH, Lee JA, Carter W. Altered fatty acid composition in the plasma, platelets and aorta of the streptozotocin-induced diabetic rat. *Metabolism* 37(1988): 1065-1072.

[415] Anderson RA, Cheng N, Bryden NA, et al. Elevated intakes of supplemental chromium improve glucose and insulin variables of people with type II diabetes. *Diabetes* 46(1997): 1786-1791.

[416] Anderson RA. Chromium, glucose intolerance and diabetes. *J Am Coll Nutr* 17(1998): 548-555.

[417] Fields M, Lewis CG. Impaired endocrine and exocrine pancreatic functions in copper-deficient rats: the effect of gender. *Journal of the American College of Nutrition* 16(1997): 346-351.

[418] Verma S, Carn MC, NcNeill JH. Nutritional factors that can favorably influence the glucose/insulin system: vanadium. *Journal of the American College of Nutrition* 17(1998): 11-18. It was shown to increase glucose transport, oxidation and glycogen synthesis.

[419] Faure P, Benhamou PY, Perard A, et al. Lipid peroxidation in insulin-dependent diabetic patients with early retinal degenerative lesions: effects of an oral zinc supplementation. *European Journal Clinical Nutrition* 49(1995): 282-288.

[420] Barskaran K, Ahmath BK, et al. Antidiabetic effect of a leaf extract from Gymnema sylvestre in non-insulin-dependent diabetes mellitus patients. *Journal of Ethnopharmacology* 30(1990): 295-305.

[421] Sotaniemi EA, Haapakoski E, Rautio A. Ginseng therapy in non-insulin-dependent diabetic patients. *Diabetes Care* 18(1995): 1373-1375.

[422] Cunnane SC, Ganguli S, Menard C, et al. High alpha-linoleic flaxseed (linum usitaissimum): some nutritional properties. *British Journal of Nutrition* 69(1993): 443-453.

[423] Sharma RD, Raghuram TC, Rao NS. Effect of fenugreek seeds on blood glucose and serum lipids in type I diabetes. *European Journal of Clincial Nutrition* 44(1990): 301-306.

[424] Broadhurst CL. Nutrition and non-insulin dependent diabetes mellitus from an anthropological perspective. *Alternative Medicine Review* 2(1997): 378-399.

[425] Cumming R, Cummings SR, Nevitt MC, et al. Calcium intake and fracture risk: results from a study of osteoporotic fractures. *Amer J Epidemiol* 145(1997): 926-934.

[426] New SA, Robins SP, Campbell MK, et al. Dietary influences on bone mass and bone metabolism: further evidence of a positive link between fruit and vegetable consumption and bone health. *American Journal of Clinical Nutrition* 71(2000):142-151.

[427] Brandi MI. Flavonoids: biochemical effects and therapeutic applications. *Bone and Mineral* 19(1992): S3-C14.

[428] Marsh AG, Sanchez TV, Michelsen O, et al. Vegetarian lifestyle and bone mineral density. *American Journal of Clinical Nutrition* 48(1988):837-841.

[429] Vermeer C, et al. Role of vitamin K in bone metabolism. *Annual Review of Nutrition* 15(1995): 1-22.

[430] Bourgoin BP, et al. Lead content of 70 brands of dietary calcium supplements. *American Journal of Public Health* 83(1993): 1155-1160.

[431] Parfitt AM. Bone remodeling and bone loss: understanding the pathophysiology of osteoporosis. *Clinical Obstretics and Gynecology* 30(1987): 789-811.

[432] Halpner AD, Kellermann G, Ahlgrimm MJ, et al. The effect of an ipriflavone-containing supplement on urinary N-linked telopeptide levels in postmenopausal women. *Women's Health Gender Based Medicine* 9(2000): 995-998.

[433] Khachaturian ZS. The role of calcium regulation in brain aging: re-examination of a hypothesis. *Aging* 1(1989): 17-34. Also see, Orrenius S, Burkitt MJ, Kass GEN, et al. Calcium ions and oxidative cell injury. *Annals of Neurology* 32(1992): S33-S42. And Hubschmann OR, Nathanson MA. The role of calcium and cellular membrane dysfunction in experimental trauma and subarachnoid hemorrhage. *Journal of Neurosurgery* 62(1985): 698-793.

[434] Leveille SG, LaCroix AZ, Koepsell TD, et al. Dietary vitamin C and bone mineral density in postmenopausal women in Washington State, USA. *Journal of Epidemiology and Community Health* 51(1997): 479-485.

[435] McCarthy MF. Anabolic effects of insulin on bone suggest a role for chromium picolinate in preservation of bone density. *Medical Hypothesis* 45(1995): 241-246.

[436] Simon GL, Gorbach SL. The human intestinal flora. *Digestive Diseases Science* 31 Suppl 9(1986): 147S-162S.

[437] Malin M, Suomalainen H, Saxelin M, et al. Promotion of IgA immune response in patients with Crohn's disease by oral bacetriotherapy with Lactobacillus GG. *Ann Nutr Metabol* 40(1996): 137-145.

[438] Ginsberg DI, Drapeau C, Jensen GS. Probiotic bacteria and the immune system. *JAMA* 3(2000): 44-50.

[439] Nord CE, Edlund C. Impact of antimicrobial agents on human intestinal microflora. *Journal of Chemotherapy* 2(1990): 218-237.

[440] Ionescu G, Kiehl R, Ona L, Schuler R. Abnormal fecal microflora and malabsorption phenomena in atopic eczema patients. *Advances in Medicine* 3(1990): 71-89.

[441] Royall D, Wolever TMS, Jeejeebhoy KN, Clinical significance of colonic fermentation. *American Journal of Gastroenterology* 85(1990):1307-1312.

[442] Vellas B, Belas D, Albarede JL. Effects of aging process on digestive functions. *Comprehensive Therapy* 17(1991): 46-52.

[443] Marshall JC, Christou NV, Meakins JL. Immunomodulation by altered gastrointestinal tract flora. *Arch Surg* 123(1988): 1465-1469.

[444] Yeoh E, Hortowitz M, Russo A, et al. A retrospective study of the effects of pelvic irradiation for carcinoma of the cervix on gastrointestinal function. *J Radiat Oncol Bio Phys* 26(1993): 229-237.

[445] Yamamoto T, Juneja LR, Chu D, Kim M. *Chemistry and Applications of Green Tea*. Boca Raton: CRC Press, 1997.

Chapter 12
Protecting Your Brain

[446] Lowenstein FW. Nutritional status of the elderly in the United States of America. *Journal of the American College of Nutrition* 1(1982): 165-177. Also see, Carmel R, Green R, Jacobsen DW, et al. Serum cobalamin, homocysteine, and methylmalonic acid concentrations in a multiethnic elderly population: ethnic and sex differences in cobalamin and metabolite abnormalities. *American Journal of Clinical Nutrition* 70(1999): 904-910. Manore and co-workers found that 32 percent of healthy elderly, with low incomes, were deficient in vitamin B6. Manore MM, Vaughan LA, Carroll SS, Leklem JE. Plasma pyridoxal-5 phosphate concentration and dietary vitamin B6 intake in free living, low-income elderly people. *American Journal of Clinical Nutrition* 50(1989): 339-345.

[447] Goodwin JS, Goodwin JM, Garry PJ. Association between nutritional status and cognitive functioning in a healthy elderly population. *JAMA* 249(1983): 2917-2921.

[448] Tucker DM, Penland JG, Sandstead HH, et al. Nutrition status and brain function in aging. *Am J Clin Nutr* 52(1990): 93-102. This included a slowing of the mean alpha-wave frequency, as well as an increase in beta wave activity.

[449] La Rue A, Koehler KM, Wayne SJ, et al. Nutritional status and cognitive functioning in a normally aging sample: a 6-year reassessment. *American Journal of Clinical Nutrition* 65(1997): 20-29.

[450] Perkins AJ, Hendrie HC, Callahan CM, et al. Association of antioxidants with memory in a multicenter elderly sample using the Third National Health and Nutrition Examination Survey. *Am J Epidemiol* 150(1999): 37-44.

[451] Morris MS, Jaques P, Rosenberg IH, Selhub J. Hyperhomocystenemia associated with poor recall in the third National Health and Nutrition Examination Survey. *American Journal of Clinical Nutrition* 73(2001): 927-933. Also see Selhub J, Bagley LC, Miller J, Rosenberg IH. B vitamins, homocysteine, and neurocognitive function in the elderly. *American Journal of Clinical Nutrition* 71 suppl(2000): 614S-620S.

[452] Shorvon SD, Carney MW, Chanarin I, Reynolds EH. Neuropsychiatry of megaloblastic anemia. *British Medical Journal* 281(1980): 1036-1038.

[453] Bell KM, Plon L, Bunney WEJ, Potkin SG. S-adenosylmethionine treatment of depression: a controlled clinical trial. *American Journal of Psychiatry* 145(1988): 1110-1114.

[454] Joosten E, van den Berg A, Riezler R, et al. Metabolic evidence that deficiencies of vitamin B-12 (cobalamin), folate, and vitamin B-6 occur commonly in elderly people. *American Journal Clinical Nutrition* 58(1993): 478-476.

[455] Horrocks LA, Yeo YK. Health benefits of docosahaexaenoic acid (DHA). *Pharmacological Research* 40(1999): 211-225.

[456] Stillwell W, Jenski LJ, Crump FT, Ehringer W. Effect of docosahexaenoic acid on mouse mitochondrial membrane properties. *Lipids* 32(1997): 497-506. And Suzuki H, Manabe S, Wada O, Crawford MA. Rapid incorporation of docosahexaenoic acid from dietary sources into brain microsomal, synaptosomal and mitochrondrial membranes in adult mice. *International Journal of Vitamin Research* 67(1997): 272-278.

[457] Weidner G, Conner SL, Hollis JF, Conner WE. Improvements in hostility and depression in relation to dietary change and cholesterol lowering. *Annals Internal Medicine* 117(1992): 820-823.

[458] Ikemoto A, Kobayashi T, Watanabe S, Okuyama H. Membrane fatty acid modifications of PC12 cells by arachidonate or docohexaenoate affect neurite outgrowth but not norepinephrine release. *Neurochemical Research* 22(1997): 671-678.

[459] Stevens RG, Jones DY, Micozzi MS, Taylor PR. Body iron stores and the risk of cancer. *New England Journal of Medicine* 319(1988): 1047. This was based on an analysis of the NHANES study of 14,407 individuals. It was found that those with the highest transferrin saturation had the highest incidence of cancer, especially of the lung, colon, bladder and esophagus.

[460] Connor JR. Proteins of iron regulation in the brain in Alzheimer's disease. In *Iron and Human Disease*. Lauffer RB (ed). Boca Raton: CRC Press, 1992, pp 366-390.

[461] Hirsh EC, Brandel JP, et al. Iron and aluminum increase in the substantia nigra of patients with Parkinson's disease: an x-ray microanalysis. *Journal of Neurochemistry* 56(1991): 446-451.

[462] Good PF, Olanow CW, Perl DP. Neuromelanin-containing neurons of the substantia nigra accumulate iron and aluminum in Parkinson's disease: A LAMMA study. *Brain Research* 593(1992): 343-346.

[463] Sullivan JL. Stored Iron as a Risk Factor for Ischemic Heart Disease. In *Iron in Human Disease.* Lauffer RB (ed). Boca Raton: CRC Press, 1992, pp 295-309.

[464] For more information on this disorder see, *The Iron Disorder's Institute Guide to Hemochromatosis.* Garrison C (ed). Nashville, Tenn.: Cumberland House Press, 2001. For more information on the best method of treating the disorder, see Bill Sardi's *The Iron Time Bomb.*

[465] McEwen B, Sapolshy R. Stress and cognitive function. *Current Opinion in Neurobiology* 5(1995): 205.

[466] Magrinos A, McEwen B, Flugge C, Fuch E. Chronic psychosocial stress causes apical dendritic atrophy of hippocampal neurons in subordinate tree shrews. *Journal of Neuroscience* 16(1996): 3534. Also, Bhargava HK, Latitha T, Telang SD. Corticosterone administration and lipid metabolism in brain regions during development. *Indian Journal of Biochemistry and Biophysics* 28(1991): 214-218.

[467] Sugawa M, Ikeda S, Kushima Y, et al. Oxidized low density lipoprotein caused CNS neuron death. *Brain Research* 76(1997): 165-172. Hull M, Strauss S, Berger M, et al. The participation of interleukin-6, a stress-inducible cytokine, in the pathogenesis of Alzheimer's disease. *Behavioral Brain Research* 78(1996): 37-41. Once activated, the microglia launch an immune attack that includes the release of excitotoxins and inflammatory cytokines, such as interleukin 1ß, 12, and 6. These dramatically increase inflammation, free radical production and lipid peroxidation all of which damage the brain. The cytokines increase the autoimmune attack on the brain as well.

[468] Draczynska-Lusiak B, Doung A, Sun AY. Oxidized lipoproteins may play a role in neuronal cell death in Alzheimer's disease. *Molecular Chemistry and Neuropathology* 33(1998): 139-148.

[469] Huindmarch PT, Quinlin PT, Moore KL, Parkin C. The effects of black tea and other beverages on aspects of cognition and psychomotor performance. *Psychopharmacology* 139(1998): 230-238.

[470] Barger SW, Chavis JA, Drew PD. Dehydroepiandrosterone inhibits microglial nitric oxide production in a stimulus-specific manner. *Journal of Neuroscience* 62(2000): 503-509.

[471] Wolkowitz OM, Reus VI, Roberts E, et al. Dehydroepiandrosterone (DHEA) treatment of depression. *Biological Psychiatry* 41(1997): 311-318.

[472] Wu F-S, Gibbs TT, Farb DH. Pregnenolone sulfate: a positive allosteric modulator at the N-methyl-D-aspartate receptor. *Molecular Pharmacology* 40(1991): 333-336.

[473] Popovic M, Caballero-Bleda M, Puelles L, Popovic N. Importance of immunological and inflammatory processes in the pathogenesis and therapy of Alzheimer's disease. *International Journal of Neuroscience* 95(1998): 203-236.

[474] Roberts E. Pregnenolone—from Seyle to Alzheimer and a model of the pregnenolone sulfate binding site on the GABA receptor. *Biochemcial Pharmacology* 49(1995): 1-16. Also see Gursoy E, Cardounel A, Kalimi M. Pregnenolone protects mouse hipocamppal (HT-22) cells against glutamate and amyloid beta protein toxicity. *Neurochemical Research* 26(2001): 15-21.

[475] Tsang KL, Ho SL, Lo SK. Estrogen improves motor disability in parkinsonian postmenopausal women with motor fluctuations. *Neurology* 54(2000): 2292-2298.

[476] Ditkoff EC, Crary WG, Cristo M, Lobo RA. Estrogen improves psychological function in asymptomatic postmenopausal women. *Obstetrics and Gynecology* 78(1991): 991-995. Also, Gouras GK, Xu H, Gross RS, et al. Testosterone reduces neuronal secretion of Alzheimer's ß-amyloid peptides. *PNAS* 97(2000): 1202-1205. Also see Hammond J, Le Q, Goodyer C, et al. Testosterone-mediated neuroprotection through the androgen receptor in human primary neurons. *Journal of Neurochemistry* 77(2001): 1319-1326.

[477] Yan LJ, Droy-Lefaix MT, Packer L. Ginkgo biloba extract (Egb 761) protects human low density lipoproteins against oxidative modification mediated by copper. *Biochemistry Biophysics Research Communication* 212(1995): 360-366.

[478] Rai GS, Shovlin C, Wesnes KA. A double-blind placebo controlled study of Ginkgo biloba extract (tanakan) in elderly outpatients with mild to moderate memory impairment. *Current Medical Research Opinion* 12(1991): 350-355. This study used the Digital Copying sub-test of the Kendrick battery and the computerized version of a classification task. The study was extended over a six-month period.

[479] Allain H, Raoul P, Lieury A, et al. Effect of two doses of Ginkgo biloba extract (Egb 761) on the dual-coding test in elderly subjects. *Clinical Therapeutics* 15(1993): 549-558.

[480] Taollandier J, Ammar A, Radourdin JP, et al. Treatment of cerebral aging disorders with Ginkgo biloba extract. A longitudinal multicenter double-blind drug vs placebo study. *Presse Med* 15(1986): 1583-1587.

[481] LeBars PL, Latz MM, Berman N, et al. A placebo-controlled, double-blind, randomized trial of an extract of Ginkgo biloba for dementia *JAMA* 278(1997): 1327-1332.

[482] Klein J, Chatterjee SS, Loffelholz K. Phospholipid breakdown and choline release under hypoxic conditions: inhibition by bilobalide, a constituent of Ginkgo biloba. *Brain Research* 755(1997): 347-350.

[483] Maitra I, Marcocci L, Droy-Lefaix MT, Packer L. Peroxyl radical scavenging activity of Ginkgo biloba extract Egb 761. *Biochemical Pharmacology* 49(1995): 1649-1655.

[484] Ramassmy C, Girbe F, Christen Y, Costenin J. Ginkgo biloba extract Egb 761 or trolox C prevent the ascorbic acid/Fe 2^+ induced decrease in synaptosomal fluidity. *Free Radical Research Communication* 19(1993): 341-350.

[485] White HL, Scates PW, Cooper BR. Extracts of Ginkgo biloba leaves inhibit monoamine oxidase. *Life Science* 58(1996): 1315-1321. Other flavonoids that inhibit MAO-B include chlorogenic acid, (+)catechin, taxifolin, (-) epigallocatechin gallate, fiscetin, curcumin, silymarin, green tea extract, and rutin.

[486] Rapin JR, Lamproglou I, Drieu K, DeFeudis FV. Demonstration of the "antistress" activity of an extract of Ginkgo biloba (Egb 761) using a discrimination task. *Gen Pharmacology* 25(1994): 1009-1016.

[487] Schapira AHV, Cooper M, Dexter JB, et al. Mitochondrial complex I deficiency in Parkinson's disease. *Journal of Neurochemistry* 54(1990): 823-827. Gibson GE, Shenu KF, Blass JP, et al. Reduced activities of thiamine-dependent enzymes in the brains and peripheral tissues of patients with Alzheimer's disease. *Archives of Neurology* 45(1988): 836-840.

[488] Beal MF, et al. Coenzyme Q10 and niacinamide are neuroprotective against mitochondrial toxins in vivo. *Neurology* suppl 2(1994): A177.

[489] Edlund C, Holmberg K, Dallner G, et al. *Journal of Neurochemistry* 63(1994): 634-639.

[490] Matthews RT, Yang L, Browne S, et al. Coenzyme Q10 administration increases brain mitochondrial concentrations and exerts neuroprotective effects. *Proceedings of the National Academy of Sciences USA* 95(1998): 8892-8897.

[491] Hagen TM, Ingersall RT, Lykkesfeldt J, et al. (R)-alpha-lipoic acid-supplemented old rats have improved mitochondrial function, decreased oxidative damage, and increased metabolic rate. *FASEB Journal* 13(1999): 411-418. Alpha-lipoic acid is found in two chemical forms: the R-form and the S-form. The most powerful is the R-form. The commercial form of the supplement is a mixture of the R and S forms.

[492] McGahon BM, Martin DSD, Horrobin DF, Lynch MA. Age-related changes in LTP and antioxidant defenses are reversed by an alpha-lipoic acid-enriched diet. *Neurobiology of Aging* 20(1999): 655-664. In this study alpha-lipoic acid restored the level of arachidonic acid in the cell membrane to that seen in young rats. This fatty acid plays a major role in cell signaling, and hence learning and memory. In addition the age-related impairment of glutamate

release at the synapse was also reversed. Of special interest was the reduction in the immune cytokine, interleukin 1ß, which is also associated with brain aging.

[493] Carta A, et al. Acetyl-L-Carnitine and Alzheimer's disease: Pharmacological considerations beyond the cholinergic sphere. *Annals New York Academy of Science* 695(1993): 324-326.

[494] Amenta F, Ferrante F, Lucreziotti R, et al. Reduced lipofuscin accumulation in senescent rat brain by long-term acetyl-L-carnitine treatment. *Archives of Gerontology and Geriatrics* 9(1989): 147-153.

[495] Castorina M, Ambrosini AM, Giuliani A, et al. A cluster analysis study of acetyl-L-carnitine effect on NMDA receptors in aging. *Experimental Gerontology* 28(1993): 537-548.

[496] Serra M, Ghiani CA, Foddi MC, et al. NMDA receptor function is enhanced in the hippocampus of aged rats. *Neurochemistry Research* 19(1994): 483-487.

[497] Ghiradi O, Milano S, Ramacci MT, Angelucci L. Long-term acetyl-L-carnitine preserves spatial learning in the senescent rat. *Progress in Neuropsychopharmacology and Biological Psychiatry* 13(1989): 237-245.

[498] Sinforiani E, et al. Neuropsychological changes in demented patients treated with acetyl-L-carnitine. *International Journal of Clinical Pharmacologic Research* 10(1990): 69-74. Also see Sano M, et al. Double-blind parallel design pilot study of acetyl levocarnitine in patients with Alzheimer's disease. *Archives Neurology* 49(1992): 1137-1141.

[499] Morris MC, Beckett LA, Scherr PA, et al. Vitamin E and Vitamin C supplement use and risk of incident Alzheimer's disease. *Alzheimer's Disease and Associated Disorders* 12(1998): 121-126. And Paleologos M, Cummings RG, Lazarus R. Cohort study of vitamin C intake and cognitive impairment. *American Journal of Epidemiology* 148(1998): 45-50.

[500] Glick JL. Dementias: the role of magnesium deficiency and an hypothesis concerning the pathogenesis of Alzheimer's disease. *Medical Hypothesis* 31(1990): 211-225.

[501] Legerski RJ. DNA repair capability and cancer risk. *The Cancer Bulletin* 46(1994): 228-232.

[502] Robison SH, Munzer S, Tandan R, et al. Alzheimer's disease cells exhibit defective repair of alkaylating agent-induced DNA damage. *Annals of Neurology* 21(1987): 250-258. Also see, Li JC, Kaminskas E. Deficient repair of DNA lesions in Alzheimer's disease. *Biochemistry and Biophysics Research Communication* 129(1985):733-738.

[503] Reiter RJ, Tan D, Osuna C, Gitto E. Actions of melatonin in the reduction of oxidative stress. A review. *Journal of Biomedical Science* 7(2000): 444-458. And Rajakrishnan V, Viswanathan P, Rajasekaran KN, Menon VP. Neuroprotective role of curcumin from curcuma longa on ethanol-induced brain damage. *Phytotherapy Research* 13(1999): 571-574.

[504] Cohen SA, Muller W. Age-related alterations of NMDA-receptor properties in the mouse forebrain: partial restoration by chronic phosphotidylserine treatment. *Brain Research* 584(1992): 174-180.

[505] Cenacchi T, Bertoldin T, Farina C, et al. Cognitive decline in the elderly: a double-blind, placebo-controlled multicenter study on efficacy of phosphotidylserine administration. *Aging* 5(1993): 123-133.

[506] Crook TH, Tinklenberg J, Yesavage J, et al. Effects of phosphotidylserine in age-associated memory impairment. *Neurology* 41(1991): 644-649.

[507] Maggioni M, Picotti GB, Bondiolotti GP, et al. Effects of phosphotidylserine therapy in geriatric patients with depressive disorders. *Acta Psychoatr Scandanavia* 81(1990): 265-270.

[508] Crook T, Petrie W, Wells C, Maddari DC. Effects of phosphotidylserine in Alzheimer's disease. *Psychopharmacology Bulletin* 28(1992): 61-66. Also see Delwaide PJ, Gyselynck-Mambourg AM, Hurlet A, Ylieff M. Double-blind randomized controlled study of phosphotidylserine in senile demented patients. *Acta Neurologica Scandanavia* 73(1986): 136-140.

[509] Joseph JA, Shukitt-Hale B, Denisova NA, et al. Reversals of age-related declines in neuronal transduction, cognitive, and motor behavioral deficits with blueberry, spinach, or strawberry dietary supplementation. *The Journal of Neuroscience* 19(1999): 8114-8121.

Chapter 13
The Aging Immune System

[510] Chandra RK. Rosette-forming T-lymphocytes and cell-mediated immunity in malnutrition. *British Medical Journal* 3(1975): 608-609.

[511] Lesourd BM, Mazari L, Ferry M. The role of nutrition in immunity on the aged. *Nutritional Reviews* 56(1998): S113-S125.

[512] Mrak RE, Griffin WS. Interleukin-1 and the immunogenetics of Alzheimer's disease. *Journal of Neuropathology* 59(2000): 471-476.

[513] Powers DC, Sears SD, Murphy BR, et al. Systemic and local antibody responses in elderly subjects given live or inactivated influenza A virus vaccines. *Journal of Clinical Microbiology* 27(1989): 2666-2671.

[514] Woodward B. Protein, calories, and immune defenses. *Nutrition Reviews* 56(1998): S84-S92.

[515] Semba RD, Muhilal, Scott AL, et al. Effect of vitamin A supplementation on IgG subclass responses to tetanus toxoid in children. *Clinical Diagnosis and Laboratory Immunology* 1(1994): 172-175.

[516] Racke MK, Burnet D, Pak SH, et al. Retinoid treatment of experimental allergic encephalomyelitis, IL-4 production correlates with improved disease control. *Journal of Immunology* 154(1995): 450-458.

[517] Santos MS, Gaziano JM, et al. ß-carotene-induced enhancement of natural killer cell activity in elderly men: an investigation of the role of cytokines. *American Journal of Clinical Nutrition* 68(1998): 164-170.

[518] Santos MS, Meydani SN, Leka L, et al. Natural killer cell activity in elderly men is enhanced by beta-carotene supplementation. *Amer J Clin Nutr* 64(1996): 772-777.

[519] Ershler WB, Sun WH, Binkley N, et al. Interleukin-6 and aging: blood levels and mononuclear cell production increase with advancing age and in vitro production modifiable by dietary restriction. *Lymphokine and Cytokine Research* 12(1993): 225-230.

[520] Mrak RE, Sheng JG, Griffin ST. Glial cytokines in Alzheimer's disease: Review and pathological implications. *Human Pathology* 26(1995): 816-823.

[521] Gradelet S, Astorg PO, et al. Effects of canthaxanthin, astaxanthan, lycopene and lutein on liver xenobiotic-metabolizing enzymes in the rat. *Xenobiotica* 26(1996): 49-58. Also see Astrog P, Gradelet S, et al. Effects of provitamin A or non-provitamin A carotenoids on liver xenobiotic-metabolizing enzymes in mice. *Nutrition and Cancer* 27(1997): 245-249.

[522] Meydani SN, Yogeeswaran G, Liu S, et al. Fish oil and tocopherol-induced changes in natural killer cell-mediated cytotoxicity and PGE synthesis in young and old mice. *J Nutr* 118(1988): 1245-1252.

[523] Gogu SR, Blumberg JB. Vitamin E enhances murine natural killer cell cytotoxicity against YAC-1 tumor cells. *J Nutritional Immunology* 1(1992): 31-38.

[524] Girodon F, Lobard M, Galan P, et al. Effect of micronutrient supplementation on infection in institutionalized elderly subjects: a controlled trial. *Ann Nutr Metab* 41(1997): 98-107.

[525] Johnson MA, Porter KH. Micronutrient supplementation and infection in institutionalized elders. *Nutrition Reviews* 55(1997): 400-404.

[526] Brock JH. Iron and Immunity. *J Nutr Immunology* 2(1993): 47-106.

[527] Sardi Bill. *The Iron Time Bomb: How Iron Adversely Affects Your Health*. San Dimas, California: Here and Now Books, 1999.

[528] Nelson RL. Iron and colorectal cancer risk: human studies. *Nutrition Reviews* 59(2001): 140-148.

[529] Kiremidjian-Schumacher L, Roy M, Wishe HI, et al. Effect of selenium supplementation on macrophage-mediated tumor cytodestruction. *J Nutr Immunology* 1(1992): 65-79.

[530] Kinsella JE, Lokesh B, Broughton S, Whelan J. Dietary polyunsaturated fatty acids and eicosanoids: Potential effects on the modulation of inflammatory and immune cells: An overview. *Nutrition* 6(1990): 24-44.

[531] Noland MR, Kennedy DG, et al. Feeding corn oil to vitamin E-deficient pigs increases lipid peroxidation and decreases tissue glutathione concentrations. *International Journal of Nutritional Research* 65(1995): 181-186.

[532] See DM, Broumand N, Sahl L, Tilles JG. In vitro effects of echinacea and ginseng pn natural killer and antibody-dependent cell cytotoxicity in healthy subjects and chronic fatigue syndrome or acquired immunodeficiency syndrome patients. *Immunopharmacology* 35(1997): 229-235.

[533] Blaylock RL. Yeast beta 1,3-glucan and its use against anthrax infection and in the treatment of cancer. *JANA* 5(2002): 5-6.

[534] Golightly M, Benach J. Tick-borne diseases. *Reviews in Med Micro*. 10(1999): 1-10.

[535] Keller JN, Mark RJ, et al. 4-hydroxynonenal, an aldhydic product of membrane lipid peroxidation, impairs glutatmate transport and mitochondrial function in synaptosomes. *Neuroscience* 80(1997): 685-696.

[536] Ensoli F, Fiorelli V, et al. Immune-derived cytokines in the nervous system: epigenic instructive signals or neuropathogenic mediators? *Crit Rev Immunol* 19(1999): 97-116.

[537] Saito K, Markey SP, Heyes MP. Effects of immune activation on quinolinic acid and neuroactive kyurenines in the mouse. *Neuroscience* 51(1992): 25-39.

[538] Homer MJ, Aguilar-Delfin I, et al. Babesiosis. *Clin Microbiol Rev* 13(2000): 451-469.

[539] Hatcher JC, Greenberg PD, et al. Severe babesiosis in Long Island: review of 34 cases and their complications. *Clin Infect Dis* 32(2001): 1117-1125.

[540] Blaylock R. New developments in the prevention and treatment of neurodegenerative diseases using nutraceutical and metabolic stimulants. *JANA* 5(2002): 15-32.

[541] Meyers DG, Maloley PA, Weeks D. Safety of antioxidant vitamins. *Archives of Internal Medicine* 156(1996): 925-935.

[542] Diplock AT. Safety of antioxidant vitamins and beta-carotene. *American Journal of Clinical Nutrition* 62 suppl: 1510s.

[543] Levin G, Yeshurun M, Mokaday S. In vitro antiperoxidative effect of 9-cis beta-carotene compared to that of the all-trans isomer. *Nutrition and Cancer* 27(1997): 293-297.

[544] Bendich A, Machlin LJ. Safety of oral intake of vitamin E. *American Journal of Clinical Nutrition* 48(1988): 612-619.

[545] Centers for Disease Control. Unusual syndrome with fatalities among premature infants: association with a new intravenous vitamin E product. *Morbidity and Mortality Weekly Report* 33(1984): 198-199.

[546] Meydani SN, Dayong W, et al. Antioxidants and immune response in aged persons: overview of present evidence. *American Journal of Clinical Nutrition* 62 suppl(1995): 1462S-1476S.

[547] Fritzgerald GA, Brash AR. Endogenous prostacyclin and thromboxane biosynthesis during chronic vitamin E therapy in men. *Annals of the New York Academy of Science* 393(1982): 209-211.

[548] Steiner M. Vitamin E, a modifier of platelet function: rational and use in cardiovascular disease. *Nutrition Reviews* 57(1999): 306-309.

[549] Corrigan JJ, Ulfers LL. Effect of vitamin E on prothrombin levels in warfarin-induced vitamin K deficiency. *American Journal of Clinical Nutrition* 34(1981): 1701-1705.

[550] Hagler L, Herman RH. Oxalate metabolism. II Urinary oxalate and the diet. *American Journal of Clinical Nutrition* 26(1973): 758-765.

[551] Sestlli MA. Possible adverse health effects of vitamin C and ascorbic acid. *Seminars in Oncology* 10(1983): 299-304.

[552] Harris AB, Vitamin C induced hyperoxaluria. *Lancet* 321(1976):366.

[553] Bendich A, Cohen M. Ascorbic acid safety: analysis of factors affecting iron absorption. *Toxicology Letters* 51(1990): 189-201.

Chapter 14
Preparing for a Trip to the Hospital

[554] Stevens RG. Iron and Cancer. In *Iron and Human Disease*. Lauffer RB (ed). Boca Raton: CRC Press, 1992, pp 333-347.

[555] Morel I, Lescoat G, Cogrel P, et al. Antioxidant and iron-chelating activities of the flavonoids catechin, quercetin, and diosmetin on iron-loaded rat hepatocyte cultures. *Biochemical Pharmacology* 45(1993): 13-19.

Chapter 16
The Role of Fats in Health

[556] Enig, Mary G. Know Your Fats. Bethesda Press,(2004).

[557] Stoll, Andrew L. The Omega-3 Connection. Simon & Schuster, New York, 2001.

[558] Colin A, Reggers J, et al. Lipids, depression and suicide. Encophale 2003; 29: 49-58.

[559] Naliwaiko K, Araujo RL, et al. Effects of fish oil on the central nervous system: potential antidepressant? Nutr Neuroscience(2004); 7:91-99.

[560] Capuron L, Ravaud A, Dantzer R. Early depressive symptoms in cancer patients receiving interleukin 2 and/or interferon alfa-2b therapy. J Clin Oncol 2000; 18: 2143-51.

[561] Watanabe S, Kanada S, et al. Dietary N-3 fatty acids selectively attenuate LPS-induced behavioral depression in mice. Physiol Behavior(2004); 81: 605-613.

[562] Sagducu K, Dokucu ME, et al. Omega-3 fatty acids decreased irritability of patients with bipolar disorder in an add-on, open label study. Nutr J(2005); 4: 6.

[563] Manev E, Manev H. 5-Lipoxygenase as a putative link between cardiovascular and psychiatric disorders. Crit Rev Neurobiol(2004); 16: 181-186.

[564] Timonen M, Horrobin D, et al. Fish consumption and depression: the Northern Finland 1966 birth cohort study. J Affect Disord(2004); 82: 447-452.

[565] Tiemeier H, van Tuijl HR, et al. Plasma fatty acid composition and depression are associated in the elderly: the Rotterdam Study. Am, J Clin Nutr(2003); 78: 40-46.

[566] Zimmer L, Vancassel S, et al. The dopamine mesocorticolimbic pathway is affected by deficiency in N-3 polyunsaturated fatty acids. Am J Clin Nutr(2002); 75: 662-667.

[567] Kodas E, Galineau L, et al. Sertononergic neurotransmission is affected by N-3 polyunsaturated fatty acids in the rat. J Neurochem(2004); 89: 695-702.

[568] Hickie I, Naismith S, et al. Reduced hippocampal volumes and memory loss in patients with early- and late-onset depression. British Journal of Psychiatry(2005); 186: 197-202.

[569] Watanabe S, Kanada S, et al. Dietary N-3 fatty acids selectively attenuate LPS-induced behavioral depression in mice. Physiol Behav.(2004); 81:605-13.

[570] Hamazaki K, Itomura M, et al. Effect of omega-3 fatty acid-containing phospholipids on blood catecholamine concentrations in healthy volunteers: a randomized, placebo-controlled, double-blind trial. Nutrition.(2005) Jun; 21(6):705-10.

[571] DeVriese SR, Christotophe AB, Maes M. Lower serum N-3 polyunsaturated fatty acids (PUFA) levels predict the occurrence of postpartum depression: further evidence that lowered n-PUFA are related to major depression. Life Sci(2003): 73: 3181-3187.

[572] Chalon S, Delion-Vancassel S, et al. Dietary fish oil affects monoaminergic neurotransmission and behavior in rats. J Nutr(1998); 128: 2512-2519.

[573] Al MD, van Houwelingen AC, Hornstra G. Relation between birth order and maternal and neonatal docosahexaenoic acid status. Eu J Clin Nutr(1997); 51: 548-553

[574] Lim S-Y and Suzuki H. Changes in maze behavior of mice occur after sufficient accumulation of docosahexaenoic acid in brain. J Nutr(2001); 131: 319-324.

[575] Robinson DR, Xu L-L, et al. Suppression of autoimmune disease by dietary N-3 fatty acids. J Lipid Research(1993);34: 1435-1444.

[576] Lauritzen I, Blondeau N, et al. Polyunsaturated fatty acids are potent neuroprotectors. The EMBO Journal(2000); 19, 1784-1793.

[577] Vancassel S, Durand G, et al. Plasma fatty acid levels in autistic children. Prostaglandins Leukot Essent Fatty Acids(2001); 65: 1-7.

[578] Lucas A, et al. Breast milk and subsequent intelligence quotient in children born preterm. Lancet(1992); 339: 261-264.

[579] Auestad N, Scott DT, et al. Visual, cognitive, and language assessments at 39 months: a follow-up study of children fed formulas containing long-chain polyunsaturated fatty acids to 1 year of age. Pediatrics.(2003); 112:e177-83.

[580] Kalmijn S, et al. Polyunsaturated fatty acids, antioxidants, and cognitive function in very old men. Amer J Epidem(1997); 145: 33-41.

[581] Hogyes E, Nyakas C, et al. Neuroprotective effect of developmental docosahexaenoic acid supplement against excitotoxic brain damage in infant rats. Neuroscience.(2003);119:999-1012.

[582] Pawlosky RJ, Bacher J, Salem N Jr. Ethanol consumption alters electroretinograms and depletes neural tissues of docosahexaenoic acid in rhesus monkeys: nutritional consequences of a low N-3 fatty acid diet. Alcohol Clin Exp Res.(2001); 25:1758-65.

[583] Hamazaki T, Sawazaki S, et al. The effect of docosahexaenoic acid on aggression in young adults. A placebo-controlled double blind study. J Clin Invest(1996); 97 1120-1134.

[584] Buydens-Branchey L, Branchey M, et al. Polyunsaturated fatty acid status and aggression in cocaine addicts. Drug Alcohol Depend(2003); 71: 319-323.

[585] Blaylock RL. Excitotoxicity: A possible central mechanism in fluoride neurotoxicity. Fluoride(2004); 37: 301-314.

[586] Hamazak T, Theinprasert A, et al. The effect of docosahexaenoic acid on aggression in elderly Thai subjects-a placebo-controlled double-blind study. Nutr Neuroscience.(2002) Feb; 5(1):37-41.

[587] Kromann N, Green A. Epidemiological studies in the Upernavik district, Greenland. Incidence of some chronic diseases 1950-1974. Acta Med Scand.(1980); 208(5):401-6.

[588] Daviglus ML, Stamler J, et al. Fish consumption and the 30-year risk of fatal myocardial infarction. N Engl J. Med(1997); 336: 1046-1053.

[589] Schrepf R, Limmert T, Claus Weber P, Theisen K, Sellmayer A. Immediate effects of N-3 fatty acid infusion on the induction of sustained ventricular tachycardia. Lancet.(2004) May 1; 363(9419):1441-1442.

[590] Xiao YF, Ke Q, Wang SY, Yang Y, Chen Y, Wang GK, Morgan JP, Cox B, Leaf A Electrophysiologic properties of lidocaine, cocaine, and N-3 fatty-acids block of cardiac Na+ channels Eur J Pharmacol.(2004) Feb 6; 485(1-3):31-41.

[591] McLennan P, Howe P, Abeywardena M, Muggli R, Raederstorff D, Mano M, Rayner T, Head R. The cardiovascular protective role of docosahexaenoic acid. Eur J Pharmacol.(1996) Apr 4; 300(1-2):83-9.

[592] Geelen A, Brouwer IA, Zock PL, Kors JA, Swenne CA, Katan MB, Schouten EG (N-3) fatty acids do not affect electrocardiographic characteristics of healthy men and women. J Nutr.(2002);132(10):3051-4.

[593] Charnock JS. Gamma-linolenic acid provides additional protection against ventricular fibrillation in aged rats fed linoleic acid rich diets. Prostaglandins Leukot Essent Fatty Acids.(2000) Feb; 62(2):129-34.

[594] Mozaffarian D, Lemaitre RN, Kuller LH, Burke GL, Tracy RP, Siscovick DS Cardiac benefits of fish consumption may depend on the type of fish meal consumed: the Cardiovascular Health Study. Circulation.(2003) Mar 18; 107(10):1372-7

[595] Djousse L, Rautaharju PM, et al. Dietary linolenic acid and adjusted QT and JT intervals in the National Heart, Lung, and Blood Institute Family Heart study. J Am Coll Cardiol.(2005); 45(10):1716-22.

[596] Mori TA, Watts GF, et al. Differential effects of eicosapentaenoic acid and docosahexaenoic acid on vascular reactivity of the forearm microcirculation in hyperlipedemic, overweight men. Circulation(2000); 102: 1264-1269.

[597] Hirafuji M, Machida T, et al. Docosahexaeonic acid potentiates interleukin-1ß induction of nitric oxide synthase through mechanism involving p44/42 MAP activation in rat vascular smooth muscle. J Pharmacol Sci.(2005); 99:113-6.

[598] Simopoulos AP. Omega-3 fatty acids in inflammation and autoimmune diseases. J Am Coll Nutr.(2002); 21:495-505.

[599] Fernandes G, Bysani C, et al. Increased TGF-beta and decreased oncogene expression by omega-3 fatty acids in the spleen delays onset of autoimmune disease in B/W mice. J Immunol.(1994) Jun 15; 152(12):5979-87.

[600] Muthukumar AR, Jolly CA, Zaman K, Fernandes G. Calorie restriction decreases proinflammatory cytokines and polymeric Ig receptor expression in the submandibular glands of autoimmune prone (NZB x NZW)F1 mice. J Clin Immunol.(2000) Sep; 20(5):354-61.

[601] Verlengia R, Gorjao R, et al. Comparative effects of eicosapentaenoic acid and docosahexaenoic acid on proliferation, cytokine production and pleiotrophic gene expression in Jurkat cells. J Nutr Biochemistry(2004); 15: 657-65.

[602] Terry P, Lichtenstein P, et al. Fatty fish consumption and risk of prostate cancer. The Lancet 357:(2001); 1764-1766.

[603] Narayanan NK, et al. A combination of docosahexaenoic acid and celecoxib prevents prostate cancer cell growth in vitro and is associated with modulation of nuclear factor-kappB, and steroid hormone receptors. In J Oncol(2005); 26: 785-92.

[604] Wakai K, Tamakoshi K, et al. Dietary intakes of fat and fatty acids and risk of breast cancer: a prospective study in Japan. Cancer Science(2005); 96: 590-9.

[605] Yee LD, Young DC, et al. Dietary (N-3) polyunsaturated fatty acids inhibit HER-2/neu-innduced breast cancer in mice independently of the PPARgamma ligand rosiglitazone. J Nutr(2005); 135: 983-8.

[606] Menendez JA, Lupu R, Cleomer R. Exogenous supplementation with omega-3 polyunsaturated docosahexaenoic acid (DHA: 22:6N-3) synergistically enhances taxane cytotoxicity and downregulates Her-2/neu (c-erbB-2) oncogene expression in human breast cancer cells. Eur J Cancer Prev(2005); 14: 263-70.

[607] Jenski LJ, Zerouga M, Stillwell W. Omega-3 fatty acid-containing liposomes in cancer therapy. Proc Soc Exp Biol Med(1995); 210: 227-33.

[608] Gillis RC, Daley BJ, et al. Eicosapentaenoic acid and gamma-linolenic acid induce apoptosis on HL-60 cells. J Surg Res(2002); 107: 145-153.

[609] Stulan S, Baumgartner M, et al. Docosahexiaenoic acid enhances arsenic trioxide-mediated apoptosis in arsenic trioxide-resistant HL-60 cells. Blood(2003); 101: 4990-7.

[610] Cha MC, Lin A, et al. Low dose docosahexaenoic acid protects normal colonic epithelial cells from araC toxicity. BMC Pharm(2005); 5: 7.

[611] Danabara N, Yuri T, et al. Conjugated docosahexaenoic acid is a potent inducer of cell cycle arrest ad apoptosis and inhibits growth of colo 201 human colon cancer c ells. Nutr Cancer(2004); 50: 71-9.

[612] Albino AP, Juan G, et al. Cell cycle arrest and apoptosis of melanoma cells by docosahexaenoic acid: association with decreased pRb phsophorylation. Cancer Res(2000); 60: 4139-45.

[613] Madhavi N, Das UN. Effect of n-6 and N-3 fatty acids on the survival of vincristine sensitive and resistant human cervical carcinoma cells in vitro. Cancer Letters(1994); 84: 31-41.

[614] Merendino N, Loppi B, et al. Docosahexaenoic acid induces apoptosis in the human PaCa-44 pancreatic cancer cell line by active reduced glutathione extrusion and lipid peroxidation. Nutr Cancer(2005); 52: 225-33.

[615] Engler MM, Engler MB, et al. Docosahexaenoic acid restores endothelial function in children with hyperlipidemia: results from the EARLY study. Int J Clin Pharmacol Ther.(2004) Dec; 42(12):672-9.

[616] Sato N, Moore FA, et al. Differential induction of PPAR(gamma) by luminal glutamine and iNOS by luminal arginine in the rodent post ischemic small bowel. Am J Physiol Gastrointest Liver Physiol(2005); 27: in press.

[617] Flachs P, Horakova O, et al. Polyunsaturated fatty acids of marine origin upregulate mitochondrial biogenesis and induce beta-oxidation in white fat. Diabetetologia(2005); (in press).

Appendix I: Recommended Sources

Nutritional Supplements

A. C. Grace Company
903-636-4368
P.O. Box 570
Big Sandy, TX 75755
www.acgraceco.com
Maker of Unique E, the purest form of natural vitamin E made. It can be purchased as a liquid, which is preferable to gelatin capsules.

Biocodex Laboratories
877-356-7787
www.biocodexUSA.com
Maker of Flurastor™ Saccharomyces boulardii.

Biopolymer Engineering, Inc.
651-675-0300
Maker of Imucell™, a highly purified form of beta-1,3/1,6-D-glucan immune stimulant.

Douglas Laboratories
800-245-4440
www.douglaslabs.com

Carlson
888-234-5656
www.carlsonlabs.com
Maker of Super Omega-3™ supplement.

Garden of Life
www.gardenoflifeusa.com
Maker of FYI™ for inflammation.

ImmuDyne, Inc.
888-246-6839
www.immudyne.com
Makers of Macroforce™, a highly purified beta-1,3/1,6-D-glucan immune stimulant.

Longevity Science
www.longevity-science.net
800-933-9440

Metagenics
800-692-9400
www.metagenics.com

OmegaBrite
800-383-2030
www.omegabrite.com
Makers of 98% pure omega-3 fish oil.

Perque LLC
800-525-7372
www.perque.com
Manufactures an excellent sublingual vitamin B_{12}.

The Pharmanex
800-800-0260
www.pharmanex.com
Makes several purified formulas.

PhytoPharmica
800-553-2370
www.PhytoPharmica.com
PhytoPharmica makes numerous high-quality supplements, including Cellular Forte with IP-6 which is used for treatment of various cancers, among its many other uses.

Pure Encapsulations
www.PureCaps.com
800-753-2277
This company makes several well-designed nutraceutical products.

Source Naturals, Inc.
800-815-2333
www.sourcenaturals.com
Carries a broad line of nutrient supplements and one of the better forms of beta 1,3/1,6-glucan in 100mg and 250 mg doses.

Specialty Pharmacy
877-866-4979
Carries a large selection of high quality nutrients, with special dosing and combinations. Tim Rigdon, compounding pharmacist and owner.

Standard Process
800-848-5061
www.standardprocess.com
Manufacturer of high-quality herbs and natural products.

Thorne Research
800-228-1966
www.thorne.com
This company makes very high-quality supplements, but does not sell directly to the public. Get their products through your pharmacist or health food store.

Vitamin Research Products, Inc.
800-877-2447
www.vrp.com
Makers of Extend Core multi-vitamin supplement, as well as an array of other dietary supplements.

Vita-Mix
800-848-2649
www.vitamix.com
Vita-Mix manufactures high-powered blenders, available in several different models.

Diet and Food

The Country Hen
508-982-5414
www.countryhen.com
Eggs contain 170 mg omega-3 per egg.

Gold Circle Farms Eggs
888-599-4DHA
Chickens are fed all-natural vegetarian diet. Eggs contain 150 mg of omega-3.

Hallelujah Acres
704-481-1700
www.hacres.com
George Malkmus is founder of Hallelujah Acres and creator of the Hallelujah Diet.

Pilgrim's Pride Eggs Plus
1-800-824-1159
www.pilgrimspride.com/products/eggsplus
Hens are fed natural grain and flaxseed. Each egg contains 200 mg omega-3.

Diagnostic Laboratories

Great Plains Laboratories (GPL)
888-347-2781
www.greatplainslaboratory.com
gpl4u@aol.com

Great Smokies Diagnostic Laboratories
800-522-4762
www.gsdl.com

International Molecular Diagnostics, Inc.
714-596-6636
www.immed.org
Lab of Dr. Garth Nicolson. They do a wide variety of testing for mycoplasma, rickettsia, and other infectious organisms.

Medical Diagnostics Laboratories, LLC
877-269-0090
www.mdlab.com
This lab does extremely accurate testing for numerous viral, mycoplasmal, rickettsial, and bacterial diseases.

MetaMatrix Diagnostic Labs
800-734-1630
www.metamatrix.com

Other Information

American Nutraceutical Association
The ANA's goal is to provide professionals with current information concerning nutraceutical supplements as to their purity, standardization, medical use, and bio-availability. The quarterly *Journal of the American Nutraceutical Assocation (JANA)* contains excellent peer-reviewed articles on the latest research on nutraceutical supplements and review articles on current nutritional topics.

In addition, they publish a quarterly newsletter, *The Grapevine*, which contains interesting articles for the lay public as well as the medical professional. Membership and subscriptions for *JANA* and *The Grapevine* are reasonably priced.

Call 800-566-3622 for information (205-833-1750 outside the U.S.) or visit their web site at www.Ana-Jana.org.

Appendix II: Recommended Reading

The Antioxidant Miracle. Lester Packer and Carol Colman. John Wiley & Sons Publishing, 1999.

A Consumer's Dictionary of Food Additives. Ruth Winter. Crown Publishing, Inc., 1999.

The Crazy Makers: How the Food Industry is Destroying our Brains and Harming our Children. Carol Simontacchi. Tarcher Putnam Publishers, 2000. Highly recommended. It is well-researched and -written, and attacks some sacred cows.

Bioterrorism: How You Can Survive. Russell L. Blaylock, M.D. Self-published, 2001.

Excitotoxins: The Taste That Kills. Russell L. Blaylock, M.D. Health Press, 1994.

Fats that Heal. Fats that Kill. 11th printing. Udo Erasmus. Alive Books, 1993.

Feeding the Brain. How Foods Affect Children. C. Keith Conners. Plenum Press, 1989.

Fluoride. The Aging Factor. John Yiamouyiannis. Health Action Press, 1993. Currently out of print, but a wonderful read if you can find it.

Food Chemical Sensitivity. Robert Buist. Avery Publishing, 1988. Currently out of print.

Genetic Nutritioneering. Jeffrey S. Bland, PhD. Keats Publishing, Inc., 1999.

The Healing Power of Food. Michael T. Murray, M.D. Prima Press, Inc., 1993.

In Bad Taste: The MSG Symptom Complex. George R. Schwartz, M.D. Health Press, 1999.

The Iron Time Bomb. How Iron Adversely Affects Your Health. Bill Sardi, B. Sardi, 2003.

Moooove Over Milk: The Udder Side of Dairy. Dr. Vicky B. Griffin and Dane J. Griffin, Let's Eat!, 800-453-8732. An excellent book on the dangers of cows' milk.

Natural Medicines Comprehensive Database. April 2001. www.Natural Database.com. One of the most comprehensive encyclopedias of natural medicine. It is updated every year.

No More Heartburn. Stop the Pain in 30 Days—Naturally! Sherry A. Rogers, M.D. Kensington Publishing, 2000.

The Omega-3 Connection. Andrew L. Stoll, M.D. Simon & Schuster, 2001.

The Osteoporosis Solution. New Therapies for Prevention and Treatment. Carl Germano, RD, CNS, LDN & William Cabot, M.D., FAAOS, Kensington Press, Inc., 1999.

The Plutonium Files. America's Secret Medical Experiments in the Cold War. Ellen Welsome. The Dial Press, 1999.

Professional's Handbook of Complementary and Alternative Medicines. Charles W. Fetrow and Juan R. Avila. Springhouse Corporation, 1999.

Program for Reversing Heart Disease. Dean Ornish. Ballantine Books, 1992.

Smart Fats. Michael A. Schmidt. Frog, Ltd., 1997.

Total Wellness. Joseph Pizzorno. Prima Publishing, 1996.

Treating Epilepsy Naturally. Patricia A. Murphy. Keats Publishing, Inc., 2001.

Vaccinations: Deception and Tragedy. Michael Dye. Hallelujah Acres Publishing, 1999.

Vaccinations: Are They Really Safe and Effective? Neil Z. Miller. New Atlantean Press, 1992.

Why Zebras Don't Get Ulcers. Robert Sapolsky. W.H. Freeman & Co., 1998.

The Wonderful World Within You. Dr. Roger J. Williams. Biocommunications Press, 1998.

Your Miracle Brain. Jean Carper. HarperCollins, 2000. Excellent book on nutrition and brain health.

Index

A

C

E

M

T

U-V